ATLAS OF CARDIOTHORACIC SURGERY

ATLAS OF CARDIOTHORACIC SURGERY

David C. Sabiston, Jr., M.D.
James B. Duke Professor of Surgery
Chief of Staff
Duke University Medical Center
Durham, North Carolina

Illustrated by

Stanley M. Coffman
Robert G. Gordon

W.B. SAUNDERS COMPANY
A Division of Harcourt Brace & Company
Philadelphia London Toronto Montreal Sydney Tokyo

W.B. SAUNDERS COMPANY
A Division of
Harcourt Brace & Company

The Curtis Center
Independence Square West
Philadelphia, Pennsylvania 19106

Library of Congress Cataloging-in-Publication Data

Atlas of cardiothoracic surgery / [edited by] David C. Sabiston, Jr.—1st ed.

p. cm.

Includes bibliographical references and index.

ISBN 0–7216–3498–2

1. Heart—Surgery—Atlases. 2. Chest—Surgery—Atlases. I. Sabiston, David C.

[DNLM: 1. Thoracic Surgery—methods—atlases. 2. Heart Surgery—methods—atlases. WF 17 A861 1995]

RD598.A93 1995

617.4′12059′0222—dc20

DNLM/DLC 94–32213

Atlas of Cardiothoracic Surgery ISBN 0–7216–3498–2

Printed in the United States of America.

Last digit is the print number: 9 8 7 6 5 4 3 2 1

CONTRIBUTORS

JAMES L. COX, M.D. Evarts A. Graham Professor of Surgery, Division of Cardiothoracic Surgery, Washington University School of Medicine; Chief, Division of Cardiothoracic Surgery, Cardiothoracic Surgeon-in-Chief, Barnes Hospital, St. Louis, Missouri

JAMES M. DOUGLAS, JR., M.D. Assistant Professor of Surgery, Duke University School of Medicine, Durham, North Carolina; Senior Cardiac Surgeon, St. Joseph Hospital, Bellingham, Washington

DONALD D. GLOWER, M.D. Associate Professor of Surgery, Duke University Medical Center, Durham, North Carolina

IVO HANKE, M.D. Department of Surgery, Bohunice Hospital, Masaryk University, Brno, Czechoslovakia

CHUNG-PING HSU, M.D. Attending Surgeon, Division of Chest Surgery, Department of Surgery, Taichung Veterans General Hospital, Taichung, Taiwan

ROBERT H. JONES, M.D. Mary and Deryl Hart Professor of Surgery, Associate Professor of Radiology, Duke University Medical Center, Durham, North Carolina

PATRICK D. KENAN, M.D. Associate Professor of Otolaryngology, Duke University Medical Center, Durham, North Carolina

L. SCOTT LEVIN, M.D. Assistant Professor of Surgery, Divisions of Orthopaedic, Plastic and Reconstructive Surgery, Duke University Medical Center, Durham, North Carolina

JAMES E. LOWE, M.D. Professor of Surgery, Duke University Medical Center, Durham, North Carolina

SAMUEL M. MAHAFFEY, M.D. Assistant Professor of Pediatric Surgery, Duke University Medical Center, Durham, North Carolina

DAVID C. SABISTON, JR., M.D. James B. Duke Professor of Surgery and Chief of Staff, Duke University Medical Center, Durham, North Carolina

RICHARD L. SCHER, M.D. Assistant Professor of Otolaryngology, Duke University Medical Center, Durham, North Carolina

PETER K. SMITH, M.D. Professor of Surgery and Chief of Thoracic Surgery, Duke University Medical Center, Durham, North Carolina

ROSS M. UNGERLEIDER, M.D. Professor of Surgery, Chief of Pediatric Cardiac Surgery, Surgical Director of ECMO Program and PICU, Duke University Medical Center, Durham, North Carolina

PETER VAN TRIGT, III, M.D. Professor of Surgery, Surgical Director of Cardiopulmonary Transplantation, Duke University Medical Center, Durham, North Carolina

WALTER G. WOLFE, M.D. Professor of Surgery and Director of the Thoracic Surgery Training Program, Duke University Medical Center, Durham, North Carolina

W. GLENN YOUNG, JR., M.D. Professor of Surgery, Duke University Medical Center, Durham, North Carolina

PREFACE

The primary goal of the *Atlas of Cardiothoracic Surgery* is to provide the surgical profession with a complete collection of carefully drawn illustrations for the contemporary procedures used in cardiac and thoracic surgery. The drawings are arranged in a step-wise manner and are accompanied by a description beside each illustration. This permits the reader to gain a complete understanding of each part of the procedure without turning the page.

The *Atlas* is divided into 20 sections with 100 chapters and more than 700 illustrations. General thoracic procedures presented in the first part of the *Atlas* include endoscopy, thoracic incisions, tracheal procedures, operations for congenital deformities of the sternum, and correction of the thoracic outlet syndrome. The surgical aspects of the mediastinum and all types of pulmonary procedures are presented next. Seven chapters are devoted to operations on the esophagus, with special emphasis on the surgical management of hiatal hernia and the various forms of esophagectomy and options for reconstruction. Disorders of the diaphragm and the pericardium are individually described. Neoplasms of the chest wall are covered in detail, with emphasis on the role and technique of extensive resection and reconstruction of the chest wall for malignant neoplasms.

The subject of congenital heart disease is extensively covered with descriptions of 19 specific congenital abnormalities and their surgical correction. Acquired cardiac valvular disease is described and illustrated for 11 specific disorders. The surgical aspects of cardiac arrhythmias are depicted in three chapters, including pacemakers, surgical procedures for cardiac tachyarrhythmias, and the recently introduced surgical procedure for atrial fibrillation. This operation was devised by Dr. James L. Cox and is illustrated in 29 drawings. They show in great detail each step in this procedure in patients with refractory and life-threatening atrial fibrillation resistant to other means of therapy. These illustrations are published for the first time and introduce an exciting and technically exacting procedure that has yielded excellent results.

The surgical removal of cardiac neoplasms is emphasized. Cardiac, pulmonary, and cardiopulmonary transplantations are considered in detail, with illustrations depicting the preferred current techniques. The surgical management of ventricular aneurysms is reviewed with appropriate illustrations. Extracorporeal membrane oxygenation (ECMO) is described, with detailed illustrations of the technique employed for connecting the patient to this unit.

Of special significance is the attention given recently devised thoracoscopic procedures. This subject is depicted in a series of step-wise illustrations of a variety of thoracic disorders now amenable to this approach. The initial section is devoted to a consideration of the general principles of video-assisted thoracoscopic surgery. It is followed by individual illustrations and corresponding descriptions of thoracoscopic wedge resection for indeterminate pulmonary nodules, thoracoscopic pulmonary biopsy for diffuse lung disease, and thoracoscopic resection of blebs and pleurodesis. The thoracoscopic approach to aorticopulmonary window and the resection of mediastinal cysts and neoplasms are also shown. The thoracoscopic technique employed in creation of a pericardial window as well as the thoracoscopic approach to the anterior mediastinum is presented. Thoracoscopic esophagomyotomy (modified Heller procedure) for achalasia is depicted in several drawings. The thoracoscopic approach to the sympathetic and parasympathetic nervous systems is included, illustrating thoracoscopic sympathectomy, splanchnicectomy, and vagotomy. The final chapter of the text concerns thoracoscopic pulmonary lobectomy and the details of this type of pulmonary resection.

The illustrations in this *Atlas* have been meticulously drawn by two talented medical artists. Most of the drawings have been done by Mr. Stanley M. Coffman, who has given this *Atlas* his prime attention for the past two years. Mr. Robert G. Gordon, M.F.A., prepared the drawings for the thoracoscopic procedures. Both these medical artists are professionals who are thoroughly committed to their work and have discussed the illustrations in detail with the surgeons performing the procedures. Each drawing has been thoughtfully reviewed by the artist and the involved surgeon to ensure uniform accuracy and clarity. The editor is deeply grateful to these superb medical artists for their dedication and tireless efforts in making this *Atlas* a reality.

Much praise is due members of the faculty of the Division of Thoracic and Cardiovascular Surgery at Duke for the many hours spent in creation of this *Atlas*. All have been thoroughly committed to its excellence and have performed procedures that in their experience have proved to be successful.

David C. Sabiston, Jr., M.D.

ACKNOWLEDGMENTS

Much appreciation is due the faculty of the Division of Thoracic and Cardiovascular Surgery at Duke for their contributions to this *Atlas* and particularly for their promptness in completing the task on schedule. Our medical artists, Stanley M. Coffman and Robert G. Gordon, have been tireless in their efforts to maintain the schedule and simultaneously maintain both the quality and accuracy of the illustrations.

Thanks are due Ms. Lisette Bralow, Vice President and Editor-in-Chief, Medical Books, at W.B. Saunders, for her suggestions throughout the various phases of this *Atlas*. It would be difficult to overpraise the staff of the W.B. Saunders Company, because they consistently maintain the highest level of quality in medical publishing. Their promptness is especially appreciated, and my sincere thanks are due Ms. Carolyn Naylor, Assistant Director of Book Production, for her ever-present interest, advice, and thorough commitment to this *Atlas*. As in the past, her participation has been invaluable.

The editor has been indeed fortunate to have an extraordinary editorial assistant, Ms. Martha M. Dimes. Her distinguished background and editorial achievements have made this task much easier, with the confidence that everything relating to this *Atlas* has been carefully reviewed with attention to every detail. Her daily interest and conscientious approach in bringing this *Atlas* to fruition are deeply appreciated.

David C. Sabiston, Jr., M.D.

CONTENTS

SECTION I
Endoscopy

1 **Bronchoscopy** 3
JAMES M. DOUGLAS, JR., M.D., and RICHARD L. SCHER, M.D.

2 **Esophagoscopy** 14
RICHARD L. SCHER, M.D.

SECTION II
Thoracic Incisions

3 **Anterior Thoracotomy** 25
DONALD D. GLOWER, JR., M.D.

4 **Posterolateral Thoracotomy** 30
DONALD D. GLOWER, JR., M.D.

5 **Transaxillary Thoracotomy** 37
DONALD D. GLOWER, JR., M.D.

6 **Median Sternotomy** 40
JAMES M. DOUGLAS, JR., M.D.

7 **Cervicothoracic Incisions** 45
JAMES M. DOUGLAS, JR., M.D.

8 **Thoracoabdominal Incisions** 53
JAMES M. DOUGLAS, JR., M.D.

9 **Thoracostomy** 65
JAMES M. DOUGLAS, JR., M.D.

SECTION III
Tracheal Procedures

10 **Tracheostomy** 73
PATRICK D. KENAN, M.D.

11 **Correction of Tracheal Stenosis** 78
JAMES E. LOWE, M.D.

12 **Resection of Trachea for Neoplasms** 81
JAMES E. LOWE, M.D.

SECTION IV
Congenital Deformities of the Sternum

13 **Correction of Pectus Excavatum** 87
DAVID C. SABISTON, JR., M.D.

14 **Correction of Pectus Carinatum** 94
DAVID C. SABISTON, JR., M.D.

15 **Correction of Sternal Cleft** 97
DAVID C. SABISTON, JR., M.D.

SECTION V
Correction of Thoracic Outlet Syndrome

16 **Posterior Approach** 103
W. GLENN YOUNG, JR., M.D.

17 **Transaxillary Approach** 107
W. GLENN YOUNG, JR., M.D.

SECTION VI
The Mediastinum

18 Thymectomy 111
ROBERT H. JONES, M.D.

19 Excision of Mediastinal Tumor 115
DAVID C. SABISTON, JR., M.D.

20 Muscle and Omental Flaps for Mediastinitis 119
L. SCOTT LEVIN, M.D.

SECTION VII
Pulmonary Procedures

21 Pulmonary Wedge Excision 133
W. GLENN YOUNG, JR., M.D.

22 Excision of Large Pulmonary Bullae 135
W. GLENN YOUNG, JR., M.D.

23 Right Upper Lobectomy 136
WALTER G. WOLFE, M.D.

24 Right Middle Lobectomy 139
WALTER G. WOLFE, M.D.

25 Right Lower Lobectomy 142
WALTER G. WOLFE, M.D.

26 Left Upper Lobectomy 147
W. GLENN YOUNG, JR., M.D.

27 Left Lower Lobectomy 152
W. GLENN YOUNG, JR., M.D.

28 Right Pneumonectomy 158
WALTER G. WOLFE, M.D.

29 Left Pneumonectomy 162
W. GLENN YOUNG, JR., M.D.

30 Embolectomy for Acute Pulmonary Embolism 166
DAVID C. SABISTON, JR., M.D.

31 Embolectomy for Chronic Pulmonary Embolism 169
DAVID C. SABISTON, JR., M.D.

SECTION VIII
The Esophagus

A Benign Lesions

32 Esophageal Atresia with Distal Tracheoesophageal Fistula 177
SAMUEL M. MAHAFFEY, M.D.

33 Resection of Zenker's Diverticulum 182
WALTER G. WOLFE, M.D.

34 Correction of Hiatal Hernia: Belsey Procedure 185
WALTER G. WOLFE, M.D.

B Malignant Lesions

35 Left Transthoracic Approach for Esophagogastrectomy (Sweet Procedure) 191
WALTER G. WOLFE, M.D.

36 Ivor Lewis Esophagogastrectomy 199
WALTER G. WOLFE, M.D.

37 Transhiatal (Orringer) Esophagogastrectomy 207
WALTER G. WOLFE, M.D.

38 Correction of Achalasia 218
WALTER G. WOLFE, M.D.

SECTION IX
The Diaphragm

39 Congenital Diaphragmatic Hernia 223
SAMUEL M. MAHAFFEY, M.D.

40 Placement of Diaphragmatic Pacemaker 229
PETER VAN TRIGT, III, M.D.

SECTION X
Pericardium

41 Pericardial Window 235
DONALD D. GLOWER, JR., M.D.

42 Pericardiectomy for Effusion 238
DONALD D. GLOWER, JR., M.D.

43 Pericardiectomy for Chronic Constrictive Pericarditis 240
DONALD D. GLOWER, JR., M.D.

SECTION XI
Neoplasms of the Chest Wall

44 Resection of a Posterior Chest Wall Tumor 245
JAMES E. LOWE, M.D.

45 Resection and Reconstruction for a Large Anterior Chest Wall Tumor 249
JAMES E. LOWE, M.D.

SECTION XII
Congenital Heart Disease

46 Patent Ductus Arteriosus 255
ROSS M. UNGERLEIDER, M.D.

47 Aortopulmonary Window 260
ROSS M. UNGERLEIDER, M.D.

48 Coarctation of the Aorta 266
ROSS M. UNGERLEIDER, M.D.

49 Aneurysms of the Sinus of Valsalva 276
ROSS M. UNGERLEIDER, M.D.

50 Atrial Septal Defect, Secundum 279
ROSS M. UNGERLEIDER, M.D.

51 Atrial Septal Defect: Repair of Sinus Venosus 283
ROSS M. UNGERLEIDER, M.D.

52 Correction of Atrial Septal Defect, Primum (Partial Atrioventricular Septal Defect) 287
ROSS M. UNGERLEIDER, M.D.

53 Correction of Anomalous Pulmonary Venous Return 290
ROSS M. UNGERLEIDER, M.D.

54 Correction of Complete Atrioventricular Septal Defect (AV Canal) 297
ROSS M. UNGERLEIDER, M.D.

55 Ventricular Septal Defect 305
ROSS M. UNGERLEIDER, M.D.

56 Tetralogy of Fallot 311
ROSS M. UNGERLEIDER, M.D.

57 Truncus Arteriosus 320
ROSS M. UNGERLEIDER, M.D.

58 Congenital Aortic Stenosis 325
ROSS M. UNGERLEIDER, M.D.

59 Interruption of Aortic Arch 341
ROSS M. UNGERLEIDER, M.D.

60 Transposition of the Great Arteries 346
ROSS M. UNGERLEIDER, M.D.

61 Pulmonary Atresia with Intact Ventricular Septum 352
ROSS M. UNGERLEIDER, M.D.

62 Hypoplastic Left Heart Syndrome 356
ROSS M. UNGERLEIDER, M.D.

63 Tricuspid Atresia 362
ROSS M. UNGERLEIDER, M.D.

64 Ebstein's Anomaly 372
ROSS M. UNGERLEIDER, M.D.

SECTION XIII

Acquired Cardiac Valvular Disease

65 Closure of Wounds of the Heart 377
PETER VAN TRIGT, III, M.D.

66 Tricuspid Valve Replacement for Tricuspid Stenosis 381
PETER VAN TRIGT, III, M.D.

67 Tricuspid Valve Repair 384
JAMES M. DOUGLAS, JR., M.D.

68 Mitral Valve Replacement 389
JAMES M. DOUGLAS, JR., M.D.

69 Mitral Valve Repair 398
JAMES M. DOUGLAS, JR., M.D.

70 Aortic Valve Replacement for Aortic Stenosis 413
PETER VAN TRIGT, III, M.D.

71 Aortic Valve Replacement for Aortic Insufficiency 417
PETER VAN TRIGT, III, M.D.

72 Closure of Aortic Wounds 421
DONALD D. GLOWER, JR., M.D.

73 Aneurysms of the Ascending Aorta 426
WATLER G. WOLFE, M.D.

74 Aneurysms of the Transverse Aortic Arch 434
WALTER G. WOLFE, M.D.

75 Aneurysms of the Descending Aorta 438
WALTER G. WOLFE, M.D.

SECTION XIV
Cardiac Arrhythmias

76 Placement of Implantable Cardiac Defibrillator 445
JAMES E. LOWE, M.D.

77 Surgical Procedures for Cardiac Arrhythmias 448
JAMES E. LOWE, M.D.

78 The Maze III Procedure for Treatment of Atrial Fibrillation 460
JAMES L. COX, M.D.

SECTION XV
Myocardial Revascularization

79 Coronary Artery Bypass Grafts 479
ROBERT H. JONES, M.D.

80 Reoperation for Coronary Artery Bypass Grafting 489
PETER K. SMITH, M.D.

81 Correction of Anomalous Left Coronary Artery Arising from the Pulmonary Artery 493
DAVID C. SABISTON, JR., M.D.

SECTION XVI
Cardiac Neoplasms

82 Excision of Left Atrial Myxoma 503
DAVID C. SABISTON, JR., M.D.

SECTION XVII
Transplantation

83 Cardiac Transplantation 509
PETER VAN TRIGT, III, M.D.

84 Right Lung Transplantation 514
PETER VAN TRIGT, III, M.D.

85 Cardiopulmonary Transplantation 521
PETER VAN TRIGT, III, M.D.

SECTION XVIII
Ventricular Aneurysms

86 Resection and Repair of Left Ventricular Aneurysm 529
JAMES E. LOWE, M.D.

SECTION XIX
Extracorporeal Membrane Oxygenation

87 Cannulation 537
ROSS M. UNGERLEIDER, M.D.

SECTION XX
Thoracoscopic Procedures

88 General Approach to Video-Assisted Thoracoscopic Surgery 541
IVO HANKE, M.D., and JAMES M. DOUGLAS, JR., M.D.

89 Thoracoscopic Wedge Resection for Indeterminate Pulmonary Nodule 546
CHUNG-PING HSU, M.D., and JAMES M. DOUGLAS, JR., M.D.

90 Thoracoscopic Pulmonary Biopsy for Diffuse Lung Disease 551
CHUNG-PING HSU, M.D., and JAMES M. DOUGLAS, JR., M.D.

91 Thoracoscopic Resection of Blebs and Pleurodesis 553
IVO HANKE, M.D., and JAMES M. DOUGLAS, JR., M.D.

92 Thoracoscopic Approach to the Aorticopulmonary Window 556
CHUNG-PING HSU, M.D., and JAMES M. DOUGLAS, JR., M.D.

93 Video-Assisted Thoracoscopic Surgery for Posterior Mediastinal Tumors 558
CHUNG-PING HSU, M.D., and JAMES M. DOUGLAS, JR., M.D.

94 Pericardial Window 561
IVO HANKE, M.D., and JAMES M. DOUGLAS, JR., M.D.

95 Video-Assisted Thoracoscopic Surgical Approach to the Anterior Mediastinum 563
IVO HANKE, M.D., and JAMES M. DOUGLAS, JR., M.D.

96 Modified Heller Esophagomyotomy for Achalasia 565
JAMES M. DOUGLAS, JR., M.D.

97 Thoracoscopic Sympathectomy 573
CHUNG-PING HSU, M.D., and JAMES M. DOUGLAS, JR., M.D.

98 Thoracoscopic Splanchnicectomy 576
JAMES M. DOUGLAS, JR., M.D.

99 Thoracoscopic Truncal Vagotomy 580
JAMES M. DOUGLAS, JR., M.D.

100 Thoracoscopic Lobectomy for Lung Cancer 584
CHUNG-PING HSU, M.D., and JAMES M. DOUGLAS, JR., M.D.

Index 589

SECTION I

Endoscopy

JAMES M. DOUGLAS, JR., M.D.
RICHARD L. SCHER, M.D.

1 Bronchoscopy

RIGID BRONCHOSCOPY

Rigid bronchoscopy can be used for both diagnostic and therapeutic purposes. Diagnostic procedures include biopsy of endobronchial and extraluminal lesions, cytologic brushings and washings, and bronchography. The therapeutic uses of rigid bronchoscopy include the extraction of foreign bodies, control of hemorrhage, tracheobronchial toilet, and emergent control of the airway.

Rigid bronchoscopy is performed with the patient in the supine position on an operative or endoscopy table that allows full extension and flexion of the head. Positioning that allows full lateral head movement is also necessary to provide adequate visualization during the bronchoscopy. The procedure is performed under general anesthesia with full muscle relaxation. The eyes, teeth, and lips should be protected to prevent inadvertent injury from the endoscope or the endoscopist's hands. The rigid bronchoscope has a ventilating port that allows maintenance of ventilation by the anesthesiologist during the procedure. If bronchoscopy is performed in a region distal to one of the main stem bronchi for a prolonged period, the bronchoscope should be withdrawn intermittently to allow adequate ventilation of both lungs. The rigid bronchoscope also has an attachment for an illuminated telescope, which should be used to provide adequate magnification and visualization of the tracheobronchial lumen.

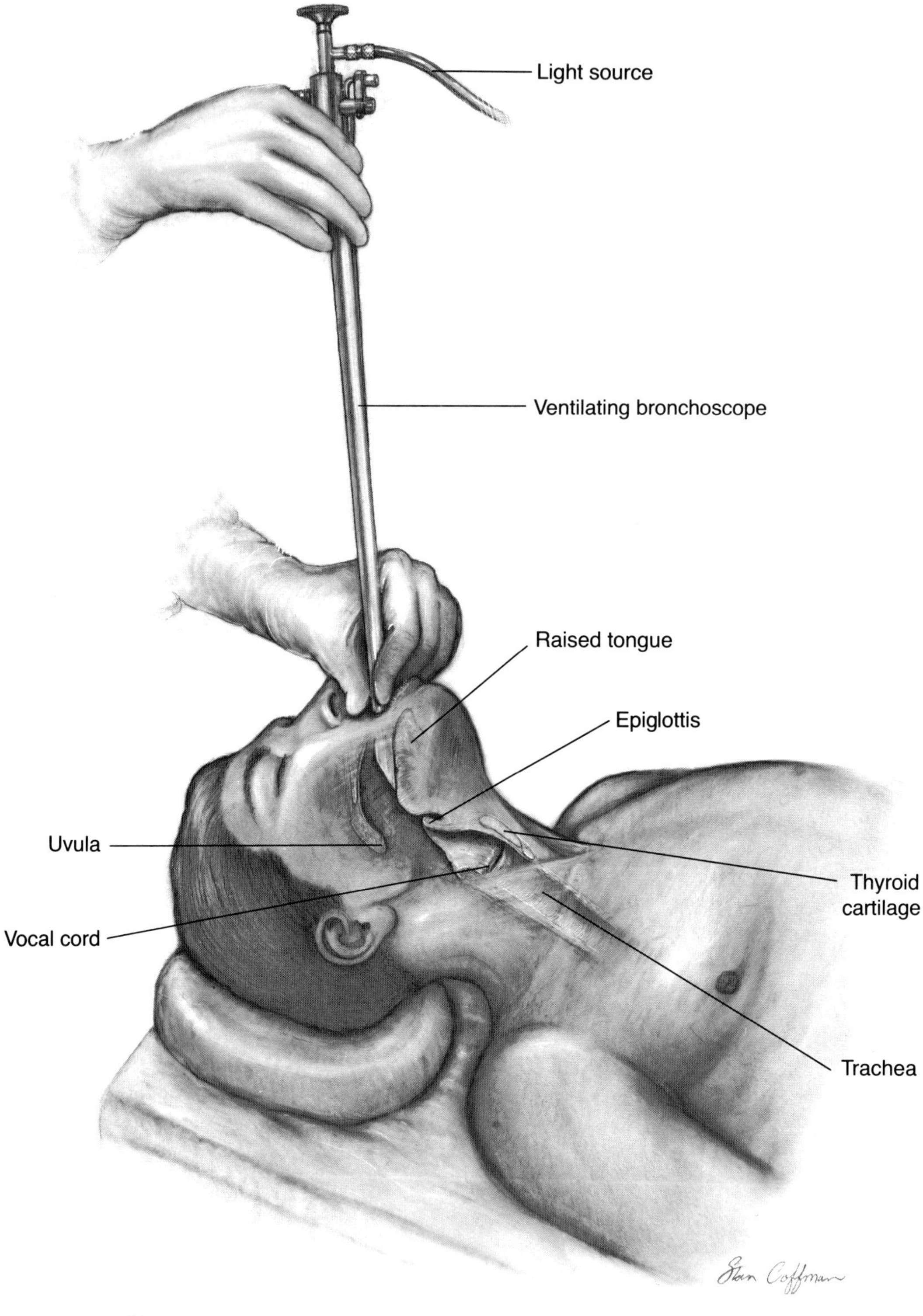

FIGURE 1–1. The rigid bronchoscope is inserted into the patient's oral cavity, with the surgeon's left hand used to support the bronchoscope and protect the patient's upper teeth and lips. The surgeon's left thumb acts as a rest for the bronchoscope and serves as a guide for the insertion of the instrument. The bronchoscope should be inserted in the midline along the dorsum of the tongue, or to the right of the tongue along the right lingual sulcus. If an endotracheal tube is in place, it can be followed as a guide to the larynx.

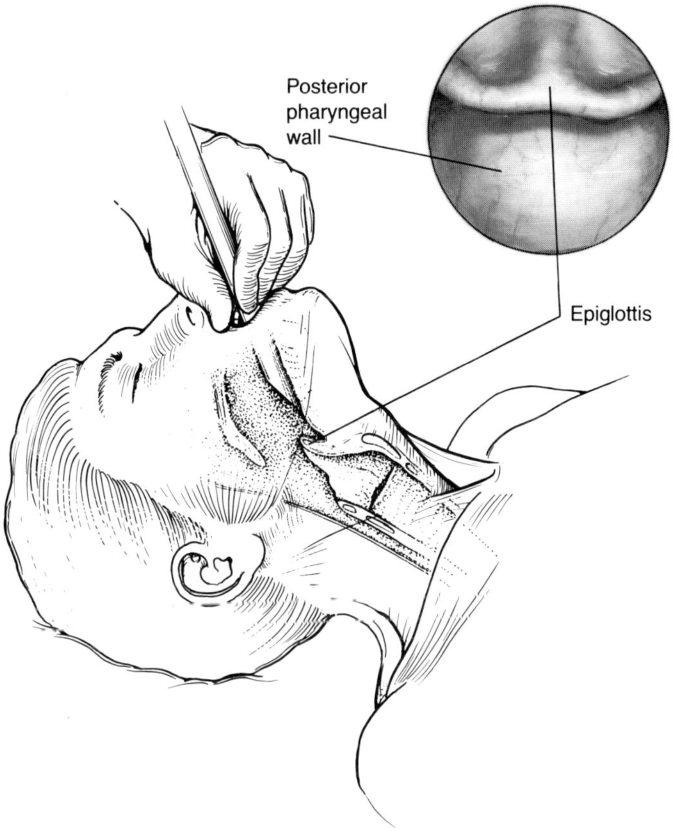

FIGURE 1–2. As the bronchoscope is passed through the oral pharynx, the vallecula and epiglottis are visualized in the midline. As these structures are identified, the bronchoscope is slowly lowered toward the horizontal plane, with the left hand and thumb continuing to control the bronchoscope and provide protection to the patient's teeth and lips.

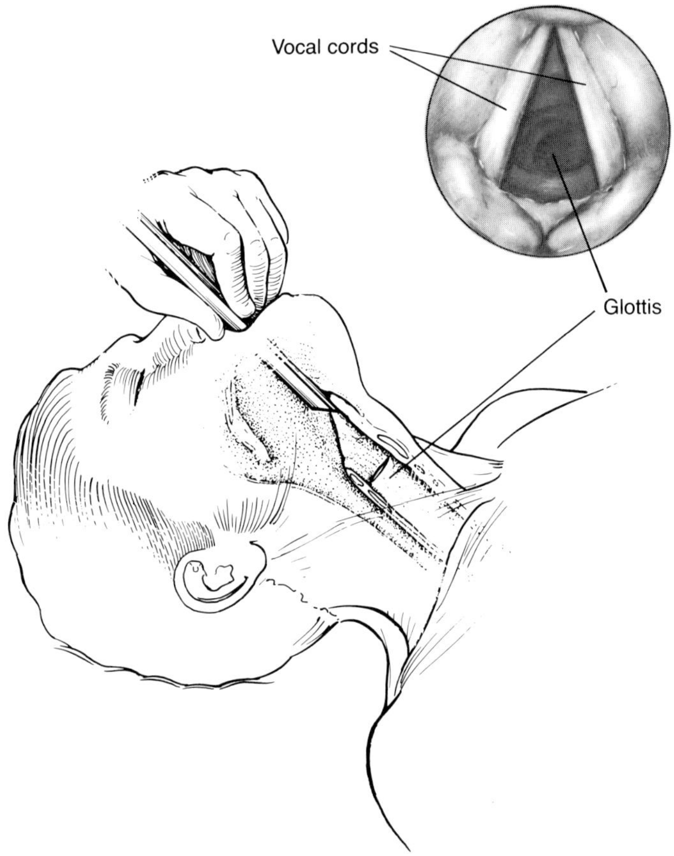

FIGURE 1–3. Once the epiglottis is visualized, the tip of the bronchoscope is used to lift the epiglottis, exposing the vocal cords and posterior laryngeal cartilages. With direct visualization, the bronchoscope is slowly advanced toward the true vocal cords. If an endotracheal tube is in place, the bronchoscope should be advanced along its superior surface into the glottic airway. The smallest size endotracheal tube that allows adequate ventilation should be used. If difficulty is encountered exposing the vocal cords with the bronchoscope, a laryngoscope can be used to lift the epiglottis. The bronchoscope can then be passed into the larynx under direct visualization. Failure to adequately expose the larynx may lead to pharyngeal trauma. A common mistake involves placement of the bronchoscope laterally into the pyriform sinuses.

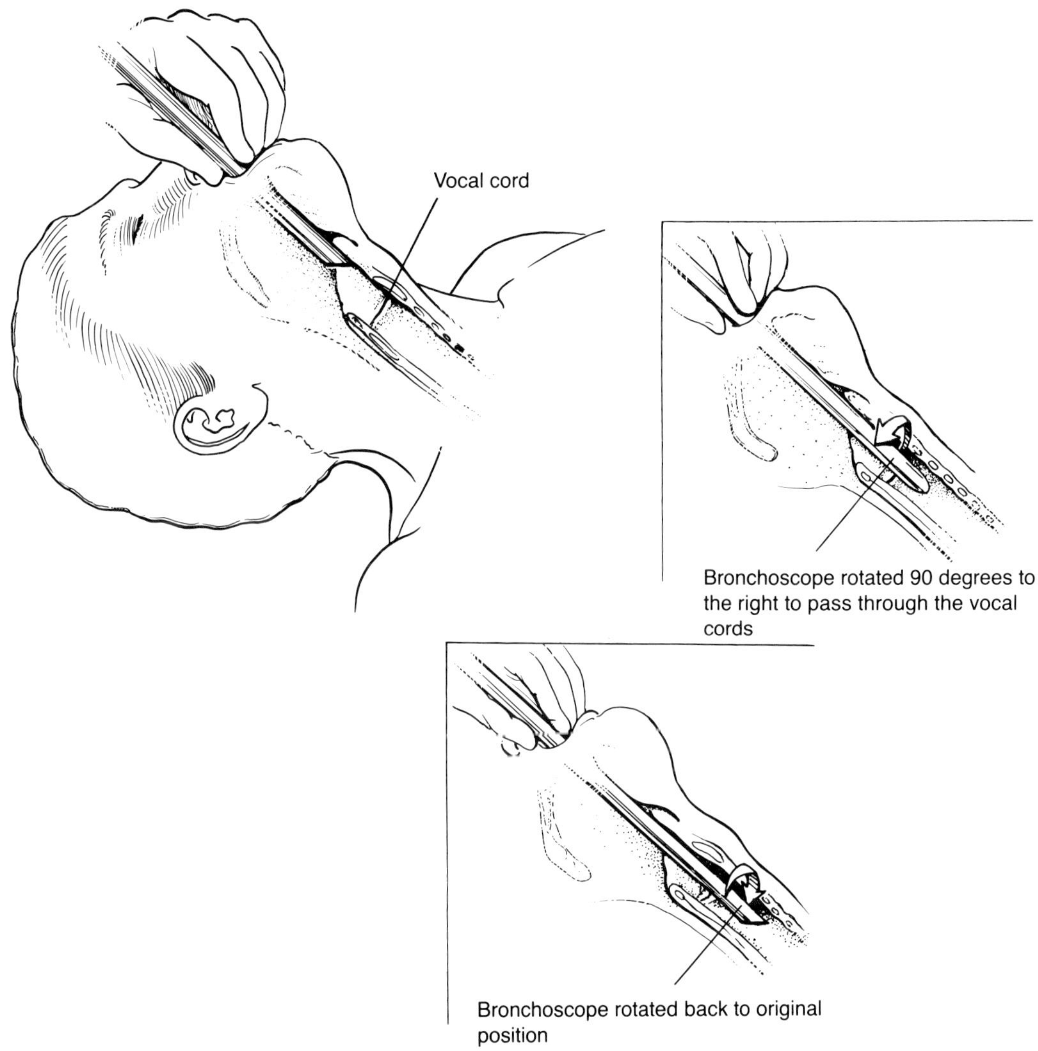

FIGURE 1–4. The bronchoscope is rotated 90 degrees to the right to allow the beveled tip to fit between the true vocal cords. Once the bronchoscope is passed into the subglottic region, it is rotated 90 degrees back to the midline to provide vertical orientation of the tracheal lumen. If an endotracheal tube is present, its cuff is deflated, allowing passage of the bronchoscope distal to the endotracheal tube.

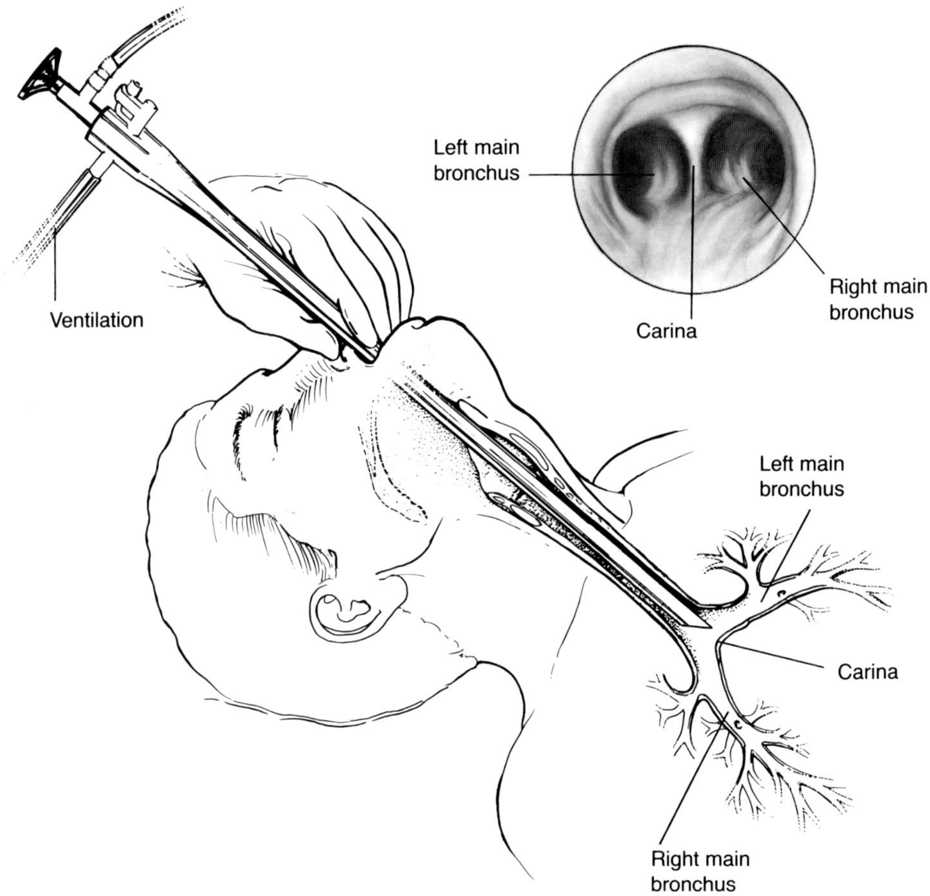

FIGURE 1–5. At this point, the bronchoscope should be in direct alignment with the tracheal lumen, with the scope supported at the mouth by the surgeon's left hand. The bronchoscope can be advanced distally to visualize the carina and prepare for examination of the right and left main stem bronchi. Ventilation is accomplished either via the endotracheal tube or directly through the bronchoscope.

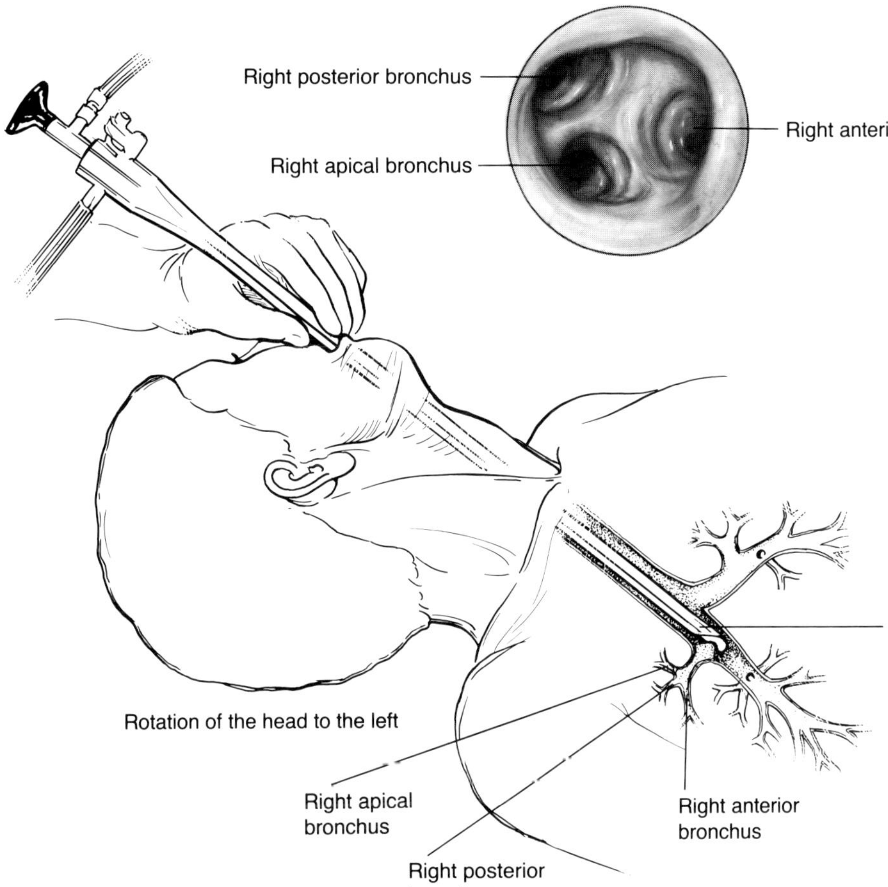

FIGURE 1–6. Proper positioning of the patient's head is necessary for adequate examination of the right and left main stem bronchi and segmental bronchi. Rotation of the head to the left allows direction of the bronchoscope into the right main stem bronchus. Examination of the right main stem bronchus is easier than examination of the left because the right has less acute angulation from the trachea. Complete evaluation of the right endobronchial tree is possible. Angled-view telescopes passed through the rigid bronchoscope allow adequate visualization of the right upper and middle lobes. A 90-degree telescope is used to visualize the right upper lobe bronchus and its segmental bronchi. A 60-degree or 70-degree telescope can be used to examine the right middle lobe bronchus. Direct viewing with a 0-degree telescope is adequate for examination of the lower lobe. During examination of each individual bronchus, care must be taken not to exert undue pressure along the lateral bronchial wall, which can tear or perforate the lumen.

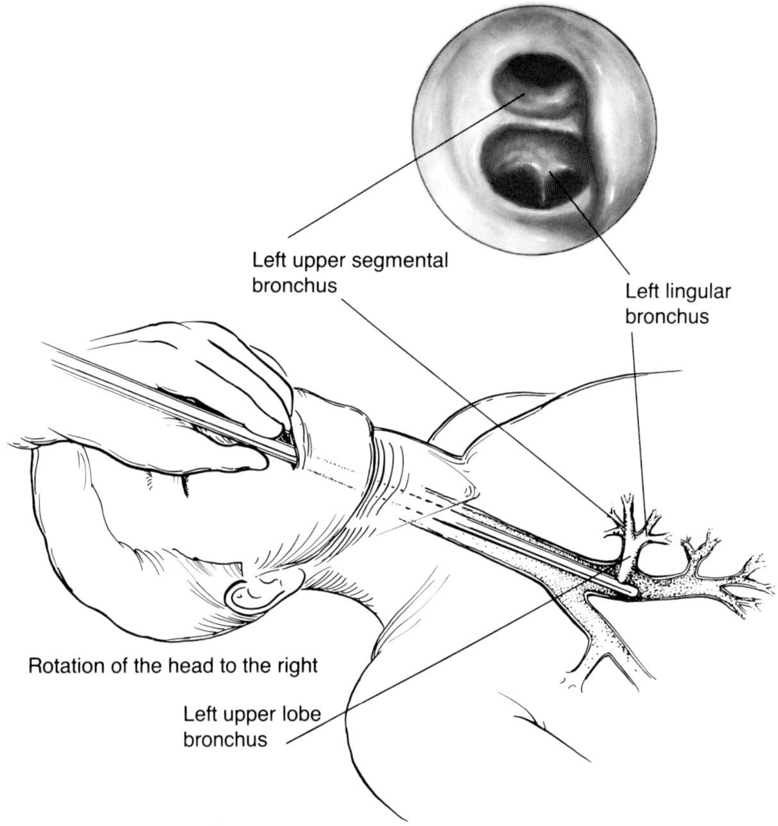

FIGURE 1–7. Examination of the left main stem bronchus is more difficult because of its increased angulation from the trachea. The patient's head must be rotated to the right as far as possible to allow advancement of the rigid bronchoscope into the left main stem bronchus. Examination of the left upper lobe bronchus is facilitated by the use of an angled telescope. The lower lobe bronchus is usually easily examined with a 0-degree telescope.

Withdrawal of the bronchoscope should be done with the same care used with insertion. If an endotracheal tube is in place, its position should be carefully maintained and observed during removal of the bronchoscope, and the surgeon's left hand should be used to continuously support the bronchoscope. Direct visualization of the endobronchial lumen should be performed until the bronchoscope is at the level of the vallecula, preventing any inadvertent damage to the tracheobronchial lumen or the larynx.

FLEXIBLE BRONCHOSCOPY

The patient should be maintained with nothing by mouth for a minimum of four hours prior to the procedure. The details of the procedure are discussed carefully with the patient to minimize anxiety. Pharmacologic preparation may include a combination of a sedative, a narcotic, and an anticholinergic; alternatively, a benzodiazepine alone may be given. For a 70-kg adult patient, a typical regimen would be the administration of Demerol 50 mg IM (intramuscularly) and Phenergan 25 mg IM, with atropine 0.04 mg IM on call to the procedure. Diazepam 10 mg by mouth one-half hour prior to the procedure has also been used as a solo agent. The choice of agents must be modified according to the patient's associated diseases, age, and body size.

The flexible fiberoptic bronchoscope, suction attachment, bronchoscopy forceps, sputum trap, and bronchoscopic brush should be available for each procedure. Additional instruments are necessary for more technically advanced procedures. For the safety of the patient, oxygen should be available, and a standard hospital resuscitation cart for unexpected cardiac arrest should be in the room.

Most flexible bronchoscopies can be performed with the patient under topical anesthesia. When general anesthesia is required, the bronchoscopy may be performed through a T-piece attachment placed on the endotracheal tube.

The topical anesthetics are usually administered with the patient in the sitting position, but this is not a requirement. The actual bronchoscopic procedure is most frequently done with the patient in the supine position with a 45-degree elevation of the upper body. Because of the versatility of the flexible bronchoscope, patient position is a minor consideration and should minimally affect the ability to perform this procedure. Typically, the patient is approached from behind. A towel covering the eyes prevents substances from falling into them and relieves some of the anxiety experienced by some patients. The scope is passed through the nares or the mouth under direct visualization, and this should be done slowly and carefully. Excessive pressure on the turbinates causes pain even in the presence of topical anesthetic. Additionally, the operator should avoid inducing coughing spells by too hurried an approach. The areas that appear to be poorly anesthetized should be retreated to ensure a comfortable, effective examination.

As the bronchoscope is passed, all anatomic structures should be noted, including the nasopharynx and hypopharynx, prior to passing behind the epiglottis. Following passage behind the epiglottis, the vocal cords are visualized. The patient is asked to say "E," and the mobility of the cords is noted. If a transtracheal anesthetic has not been administered, 2 ml of tetracaine (1% or 2%) may be administered by way of the bronchoscope through the cords. The subglottic area is visualized carefully while the scope is passed through the cords. The course of the trachea is examined, as is its mucosa. Both external compression and intrinsic lesions may be visualized. The carina should appear sharp and mobile in the normal patient. In the adequately anesthetized, relaxed patient, the suspected normal portion of the tracheobronchial tree should be examined first. If it appears that the patient is not tolerating the examination well, the pathologic area must be managed quickly prior to removal of the scope. However, this occurs rarely if the patient has been properly prepared. Following visual inspection of the entire accessible tracheobronchial anatomy, bronchial washings, brushings, and biopsies may be performed as indicated.

FIGURE 1–8. Typically, flexible bronchoscopy is performed via a transnasal route. However, the procedure may be performed transorally when technical factors limit the ability to perform the procedure through the nose. The nasopharynx and pharyngeal mucosa are anesthetized with topical anesthetic spray. We have typically used a combination anesthetic, Cetacaine. The patient is allowed to swallow a small portion of the solution sprayed into the pharynx. Two or three sprays through the nose and through the mouth are usually adequate. At this point, the tracheobronchial tree may also be anesthetized directly with a transtracheal injection of 6 ml of tetracaine. If this method is chosen, a small skin wheal of anesthetic is raised over the hyoid membrane using a 27- or 25-gauge needle. A 21-gauge needle is then passed percutaneously through the hyoid membrane into the trachea while aspiration confirms the presence of air. The patient is asked to take a deep breath while the tetracaine is quickly flushed into the trachea, which invariably induces coughing; however, the anesthetic is frequently distributed quite well throughout the tracheobronchial tree with this method. Alternatively, the tracheobronchial tree may be anesthetized by way of injections passed through the flexible bronchoscope as it enters the trachea.

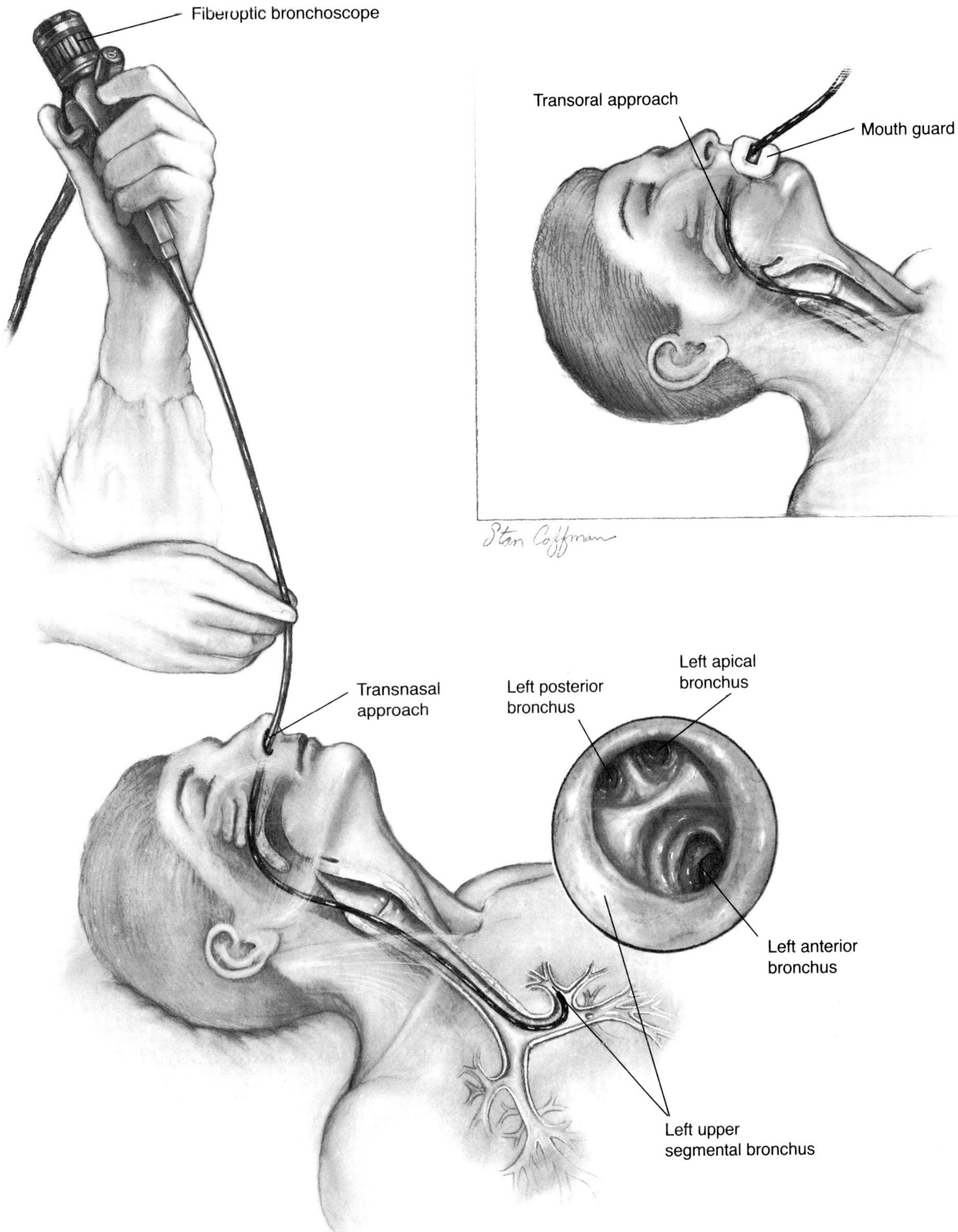

FIGURE 1–8 *See legend on opposite page*

RICHARD L. SCHER, M.D.

2
Esophagoscopy

Esophagoscopy can be performed with either a rigid or a flexible esophagoscope for both diagnostic and therapeutic purposes. Diagnostic uses include the assessment of malignant or benign tumors, functional esophageal disease, stenoses, and caustic or corrosive injuries, and suspicion of esophageal foreign bodies; therapeutic uses include removal of foreign bodies from the esophagus, dilatation of stenoses by bougienage, and treatment of esophageal varices. Rigid esophagoscopy is contraindicated when the patient's medical condition precludes the performance of a procedure under general or relaxant anesthesia or when severe deformities of the cervical or thoracic spine make head positioning difficult. In these patients, flexible esophagoscopy may be performed for the same diagnostic purposes as rigid esophagoscopy and can be used therapeutically for balloon dilatation of stenoses and injection of esophageal varices.

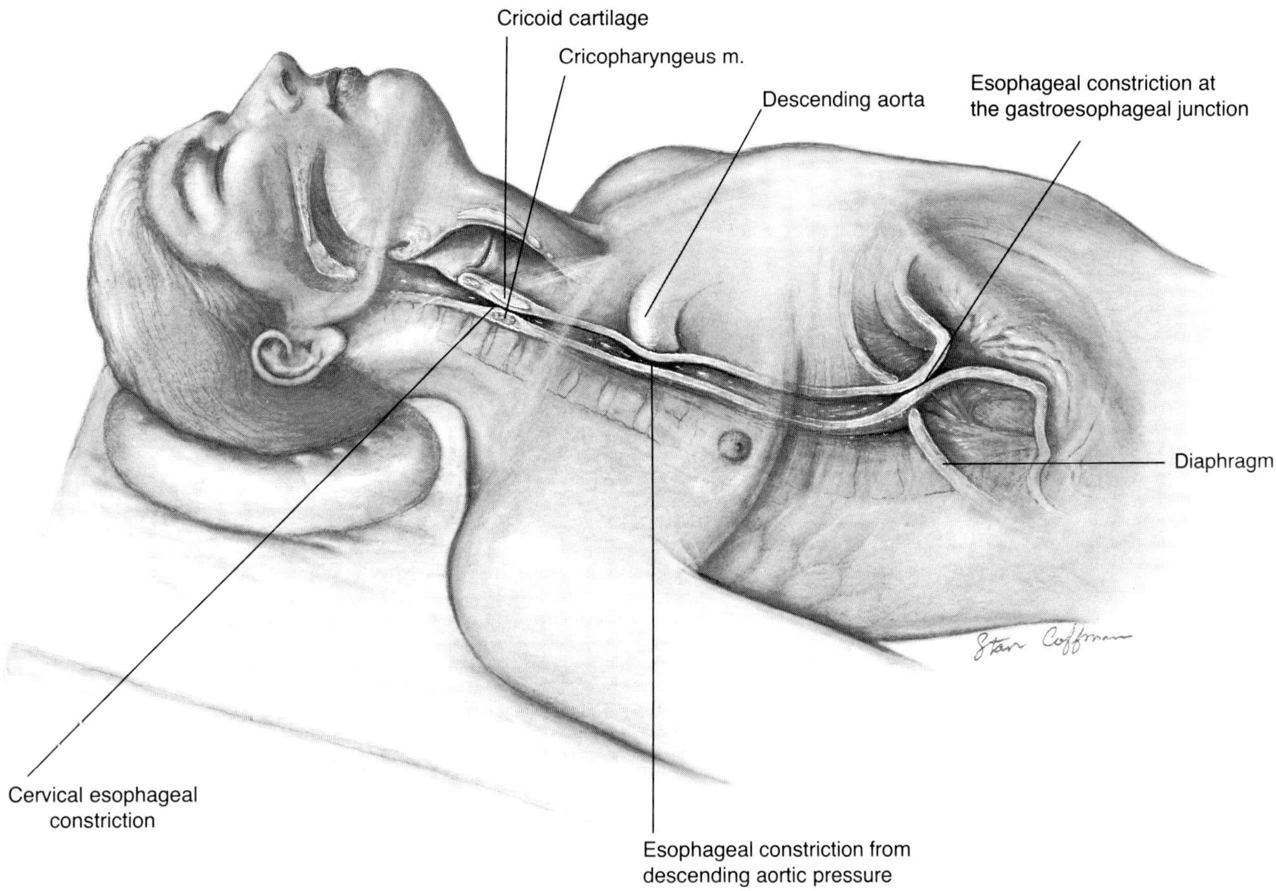

FIGURE 2–1. Knowledge of pharyngoesophageal anatomy is essential for the safe performance of esophagoscopy, and the three natural anatomic constrictions of the esophagus must always be considered during the performance of this procedure. The first narrowing occurs in the proximal esophagus at the cricopharyngeus muscle distal to the cricoid cartilage. The second narrowing occurs at the midthoracic level, where the descending aorta produces an indentation on the left posterolateral surface of the esophagus; and the third narrowing occurs at the gastroesophageal junction (GEJ). Extra care must be taken when passing the esophagoscope at these points to prevent injury to the esophageal lumen.

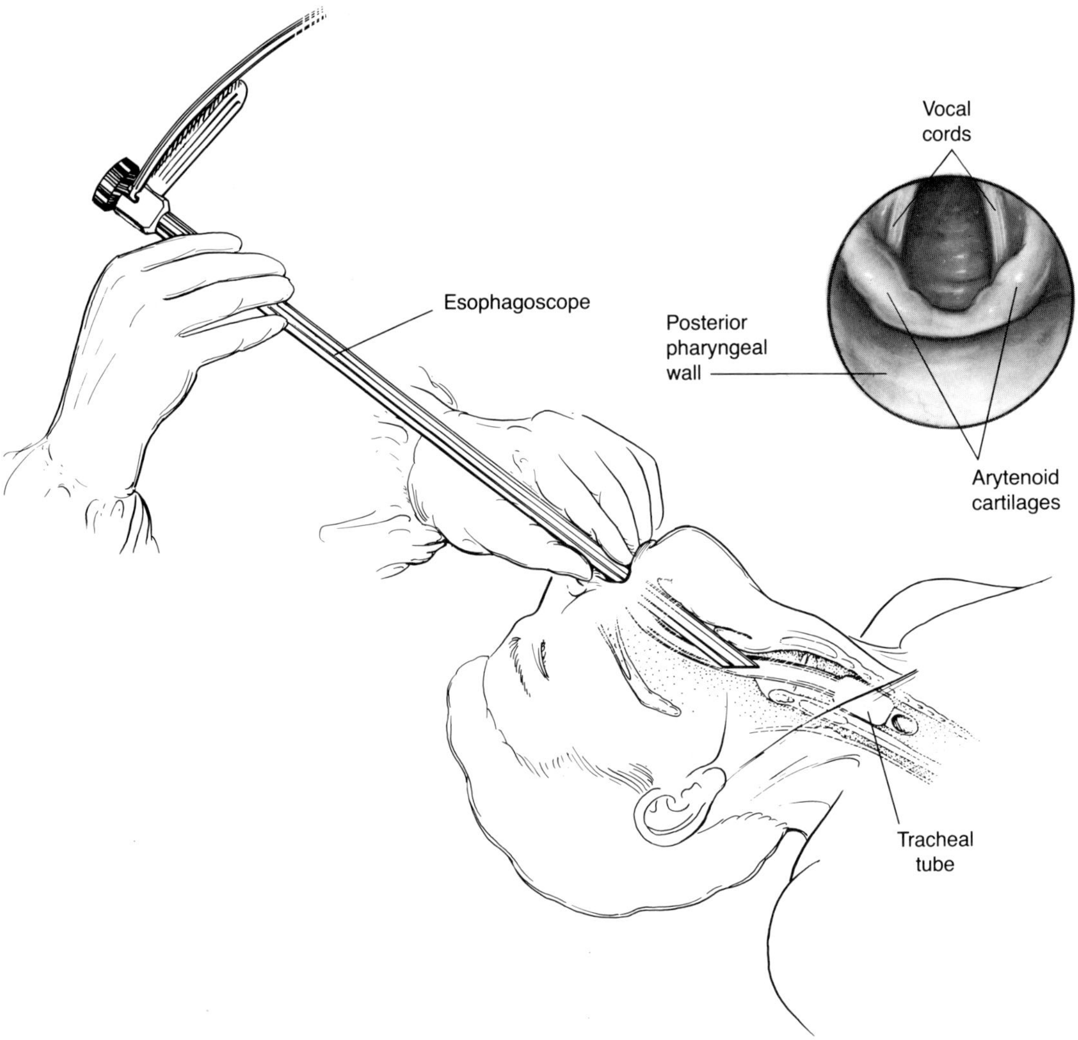

FIGURE 2–2. The patient is placed in the supine position on an operative table that allows for multiple levels of head extension and flexion, and the procedure is performed with the patient under general anesthesia with muscle relaxation. A rigid esophagoscope with an attachment for an illuminated telescope allows precise examination of the esophageal mucosa. With the patient's head in slight extension and the teeth, lips, and eyes protected, the rigid esophagoscope is inserted into the oral cavity. The esophagoscope is supported by the surgeon's left hand and advanced with gentle pressure into the right side of the oral cavity, displacing the tongue anteriorly and toward the midline. It is advanced along the posterior pharyngeal wall to the level of the larynx. Identification of the arytenoid cartilages posteriorly provides orientation for the endoscopist. The endotracheal tube can also be used as a guide to locate the larynx.

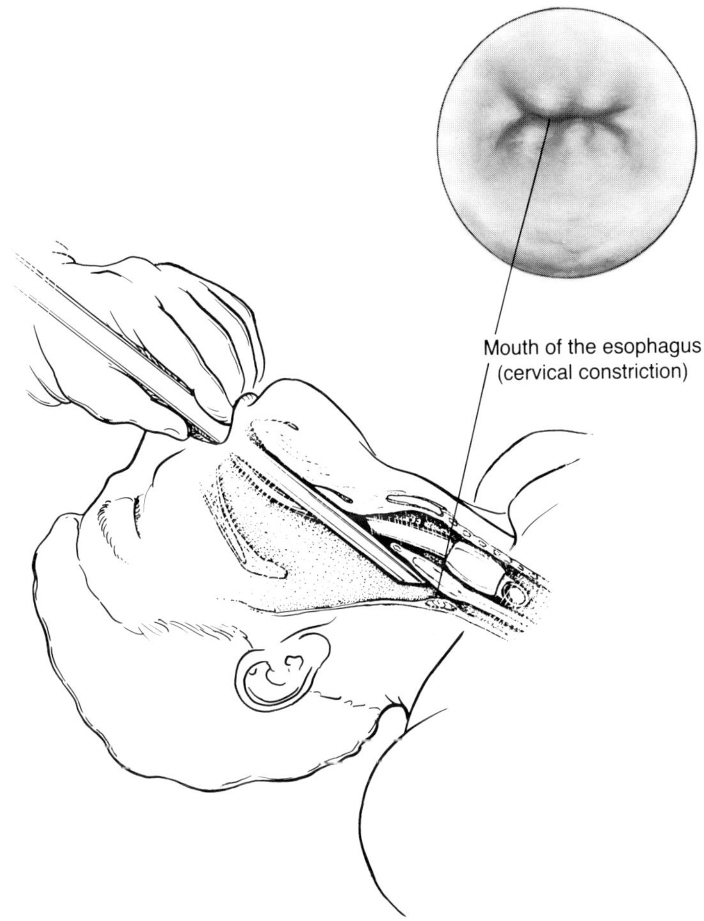

FIGURE 2–3. The proximal opening of the esophagus is identified by elevating the postcricoid mucosa and cricoid cartilage with the tip of the esophagoscope, exposing the cricopharyngeus muscle. This sphincter-like opening appears as a transversely oriented structure delineating the proximal extent of the esophagus. Care must be taken at this point to prevent placement of the esophagoscope laterally into the pyriform sinuses, because the risk of perforation of the pharynx increases during this maneuver. The esophageal lumen may be difficult to identify because of obstruction from tumor, fibrotic stenosis, or anatomic abnormalities such as cervical vertebral osteophytes, and identification can be assisted by passing a nasogastric tube or long suture preoperatively to serve as a guide during the endoscopy. Under no circumstance should the rigid esophagoscope be passed blindly without visualization of the esophageal lumen.

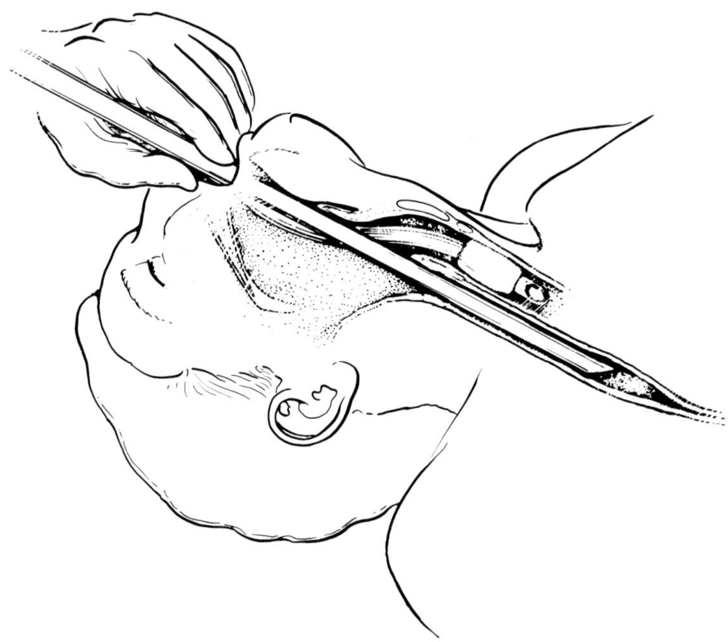

FIGURE 2–4. Once the cricopharyngeus muscle is recognized, gentle pressure is exerted on the esophagoscope to allow passage into the proximal esophagus. As the esophagoscope is passed beyond the cricopharyngeus, slightly greater extension of the head is necessary to allow passage of the scope through the thoracic esophagus. Passage of the esophagoscope should be controlled by gentle pressure exerted by the fingers of the operator's left hand. The scope should not be advanced if the esophageal lumen is not visualized, and care must be taken to prevent posterior advancement of the scope to avoid injury to the esophageal wall. During advancement of the scope, the overall quality and appearance of the mucosa should be noted; it should appear pink, moist, and smooth. Identification of diverticula, tumors, varices, or stenoses should be noted, and their location measured in reference to the maxillary incisor teeth. Gentle pressure exerted at the tip of the scope against the esophageal wall can provide some idea of possible extraluminal compression or esophageal wall thickening.

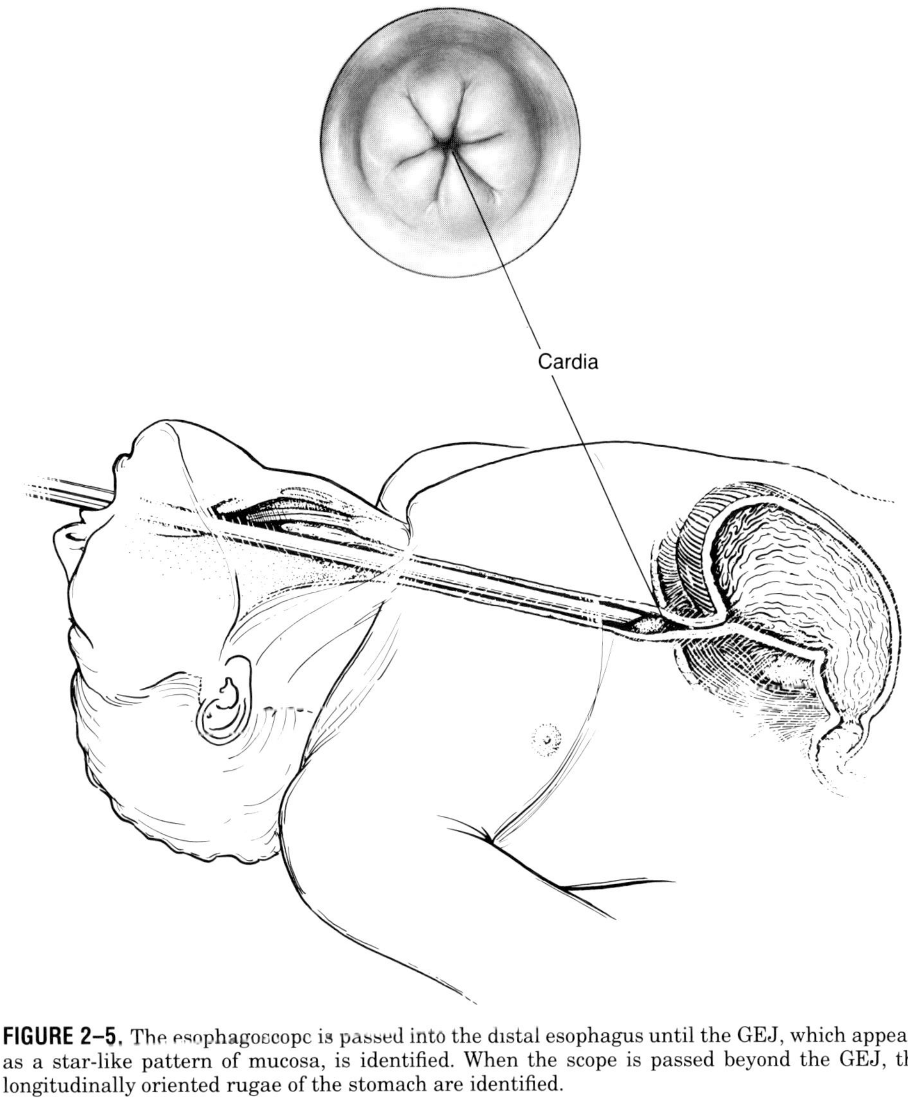

FIGURE 2–5. The esophagoscope is passed into the distal esophagus until the GEJ, which appears as a star-like pattern of mucosa, is identified. When the scope is passed beyond the GEJ, the longitudinally oriented rugae of the stomach are identified.

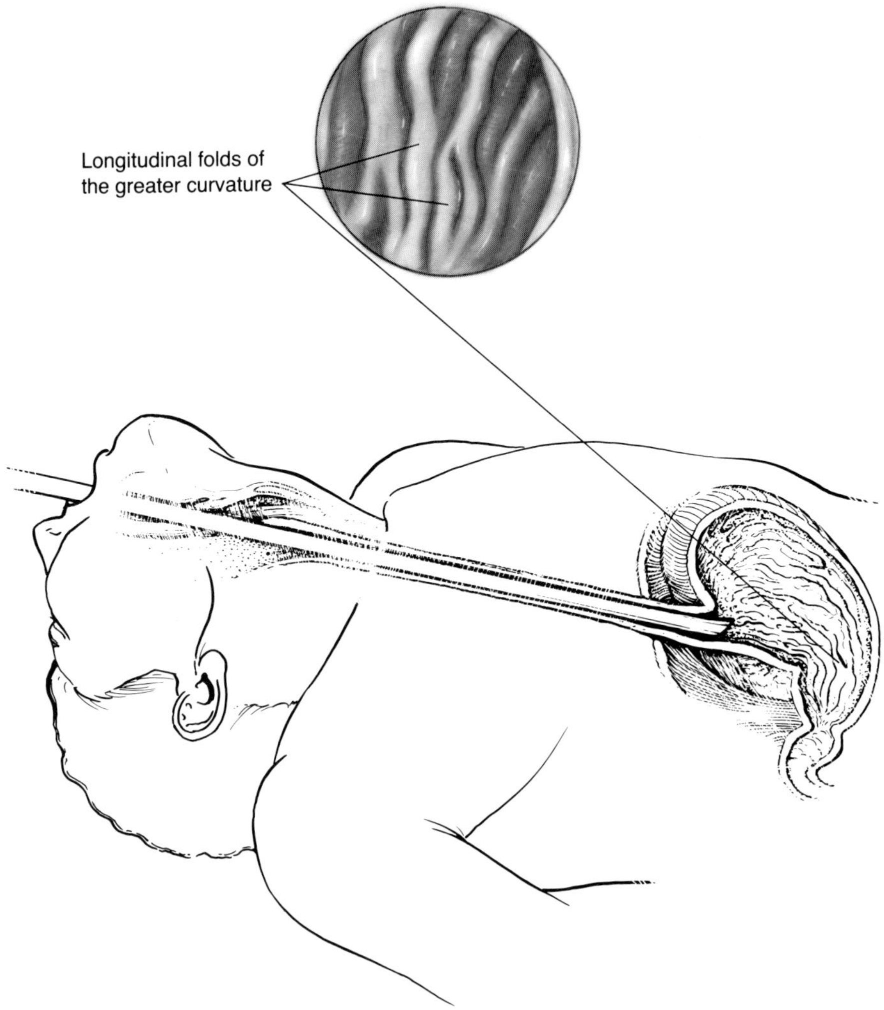

FIGURE 2–6. The mucosa of the stomach is reddened and has a rough-appearing quality in comparison with the esophageal mucosa. When the esophagoscope is in the distal esophagus and stomach, the patient's head must be maximally extended to provide adequate exposure of the esophageal lumen. After the esophagoscope is advanced into the stomach, it can be gently withdrawn from the esophagus. During withdrawal, the mucosa should be observed again in great detail for the assessment of any abnormalities, and care must be taken not to exert undue pressure on the esophageal wall, which may cause laceration or perforation. In addition, the position of the endotracheal tube must be maintained to prevent displacement from the airway.

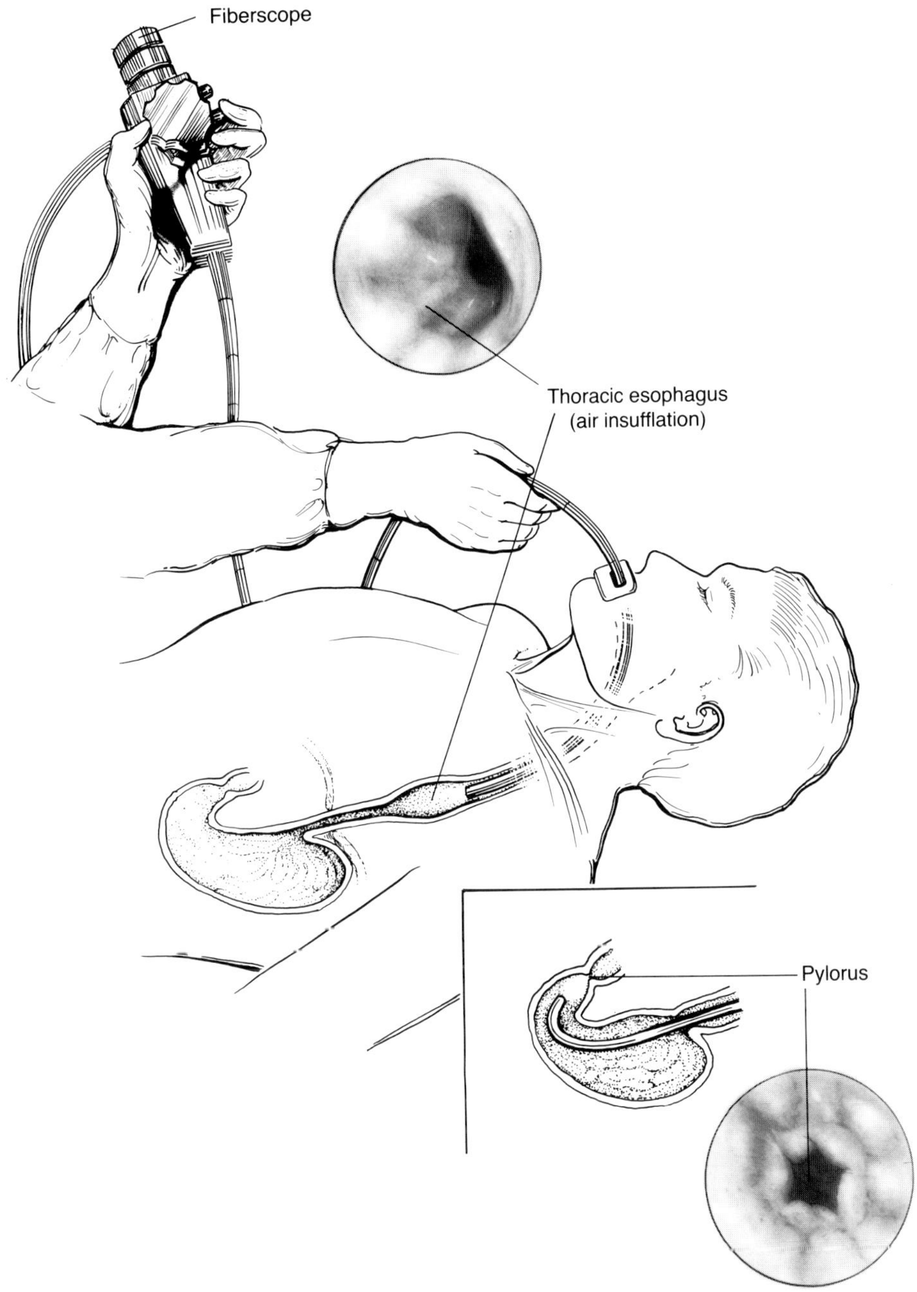

FIGURE 2–7. Flexible esophagoscopy may be performed under either general anesthesia or topical anesthesia with intravenous sedation. When used in conjunction with other upper aerodigestive tract endoscopy, such as direct laryngoscopy or bronchoscopy, it is performed under general anesthesia, and the patient is placed supine on the operative table. With topical anesthesia, the procedure is usually accomplished with the patient in the left lateral decubitus position. A mouth guard is used between the teeth to prevent bite injury to the endoscopist as well as to allow passage of the endoscope in the midline. The flexible esophagoscope is passed through the oral cavity with direct visualization of the pharynx. The body of the endoscope is held in the left hand to allow fingertip control of the vertical and lateral tip rotating wheels. The left hand also controls the air insufflation and suction valves. The right hand is used to gently pull, advance, and torque the esophagoscope to allow adequate visualization during the examination.

Under direct visualization, the midline raphe of the tongue is identified in the superior field of view. The endoscope is advanced to the level of the larynx, where the arytenoid cartilages and aryepiglottic folds are visualized (see Fig. 2–2). If an endotracheal tube is in place, it can be used as a guide to the larynx. With identification of the arytenoid cartilages, the endoscope is allowed to drop posteriorly into the hypopharynx. At this point, the cricopharyngeus is identified (see Fig. 2–3). With gentle pressure by the scope against the cricopharyngeus and gentle air insufflation, relaxation of the cricopharyngeus muscle allows passage of the scope into the proximal esophagus. Once the scope has passed the cricopharyngeus muscle, gentle insufflation of air allows continued identification of the esophageal lumen, and the endoscope can be passed into the distal esophagus and stomach. It should be noted that perforation of the esophageal lumen and pharynx is possible with the flexible esophagoscope. Any resistance to passage of the scope requires gentle withdrawal of the scope and, under direct visualization, reassessment for the presence of the esophageal lumen prior to any additional attempt at passage.

The esophagoscope can be used exclusively for examination of the esophagus, or it can be used to examine the stomach and the proximal duodenum. If the scope is extended into the stomach, care must be taken to prevent overinsufflation of air, which causes gastric distention and discomfort to the patient when performed under topical anesthesia, and may cause reflux of gastric contents and aspiration in a patient under general anesthesia. The esophagoscope is withdrawn with direct visualization and examination of the esophageal mucosa.

SECTION II

Thoracic Incisions

DONALD D. GLOWER, JR., M.D.

3

Anterior Thoracotomy

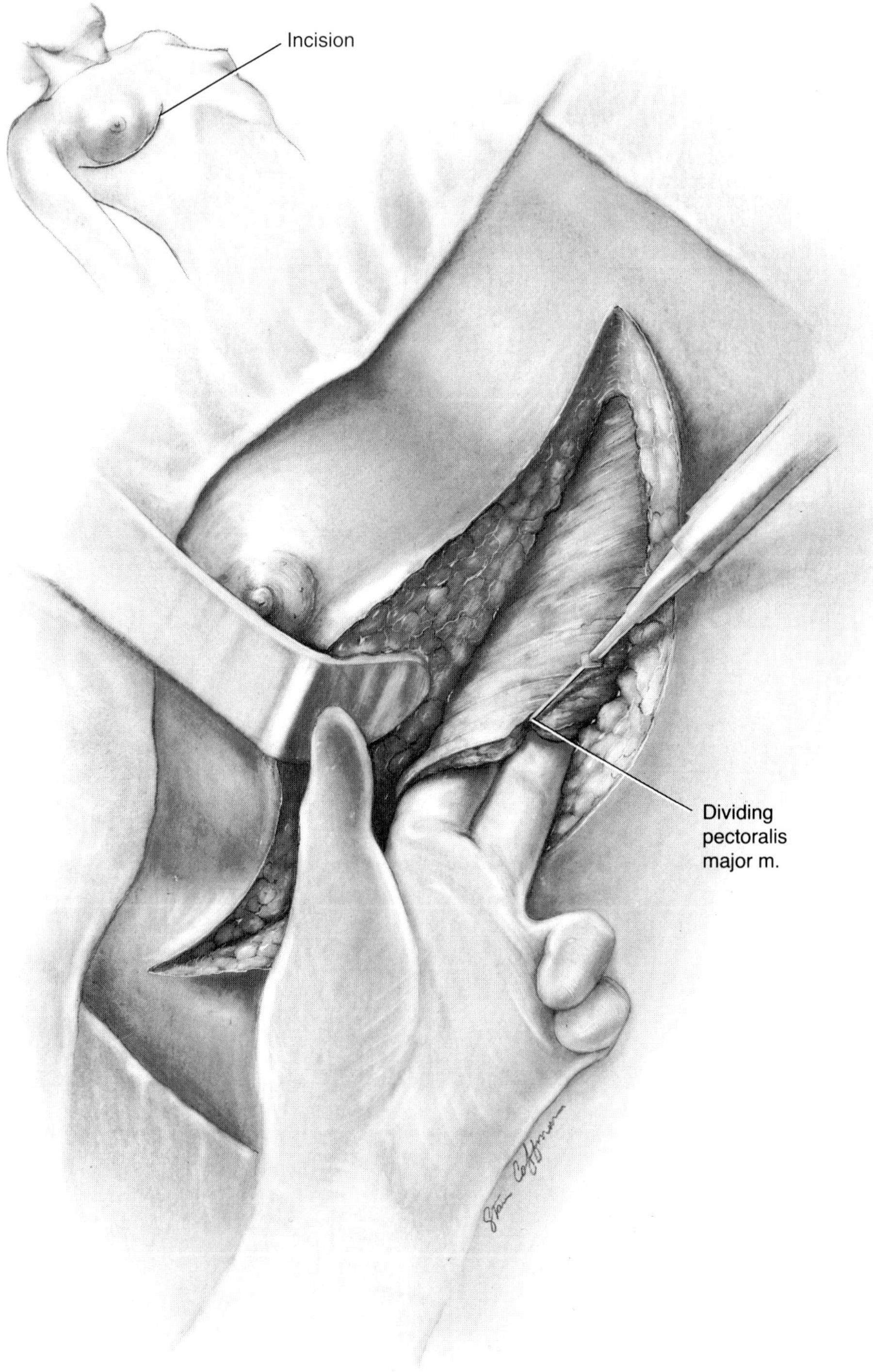

FIGURE 3–1. The ipsilateral chest is rolled anteriorly 45 degrees, with the ipsilateral arm at the side. An inframammary incision is made, and the pectoralis major muscle is incised.

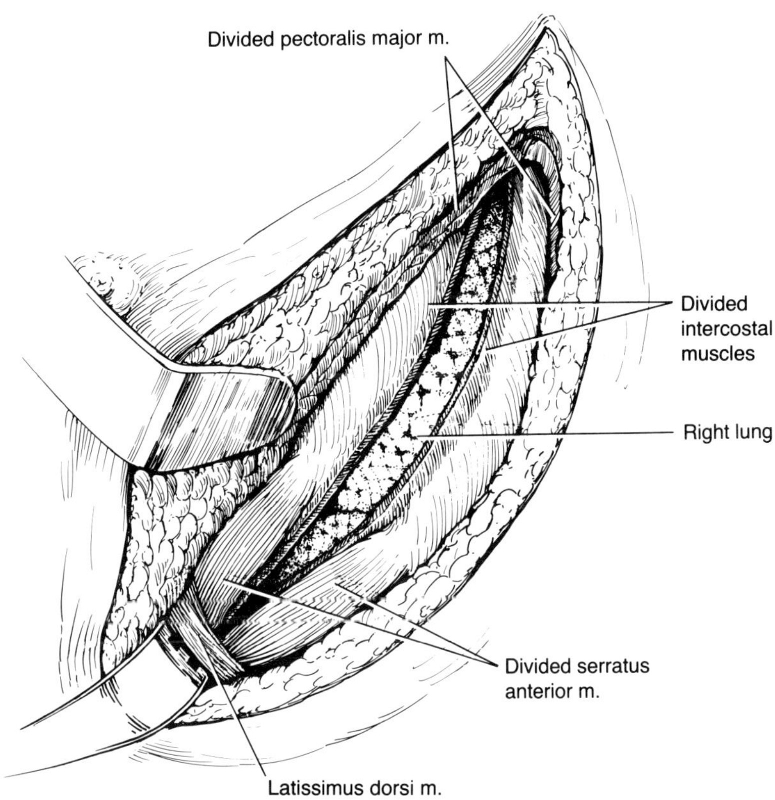

FIGURE 3–2. The fourth or fifth intercostal space is entered, and the incision may be extended medially to the internal mammary artery or to the sternum, as needed, and laterally to the latissimus dorsi muscle.

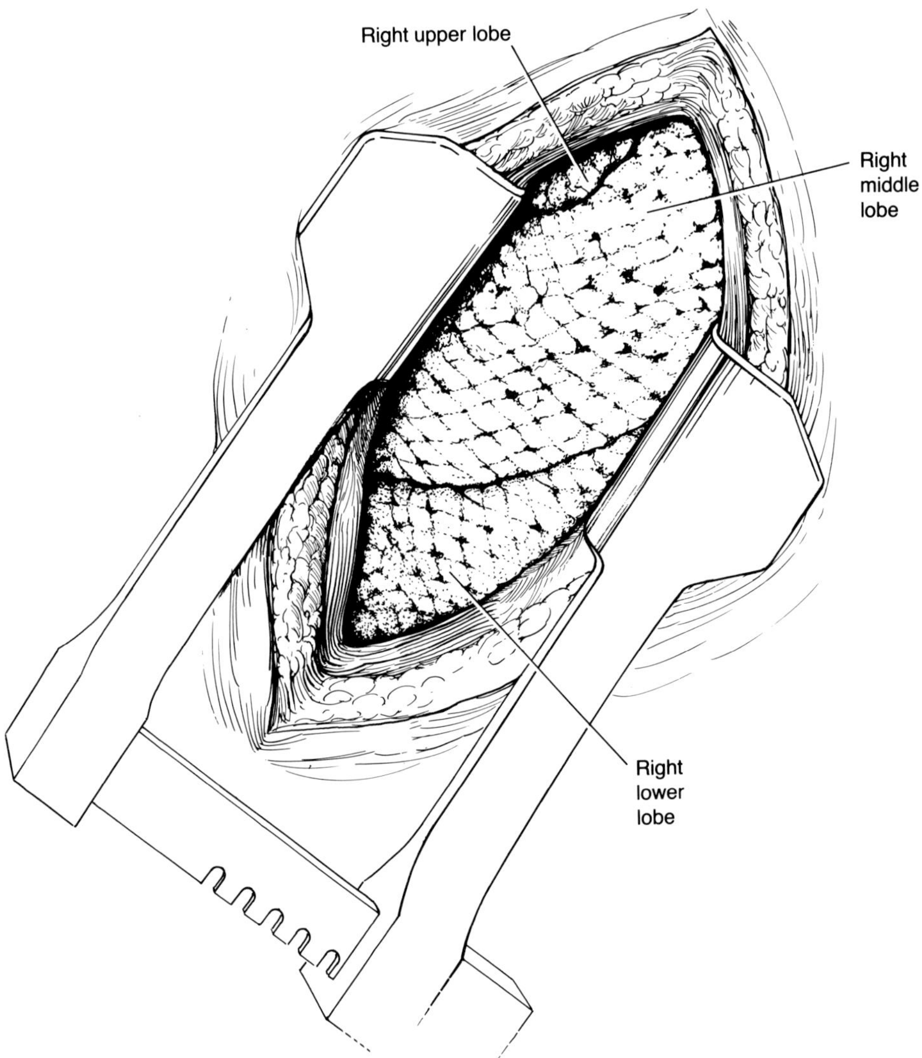

FIGURE 3–3. The anterior thoracotomy provides exposure to the mediastinum, pericardium, hilum, lower lobe, and middle lobe or lingula.

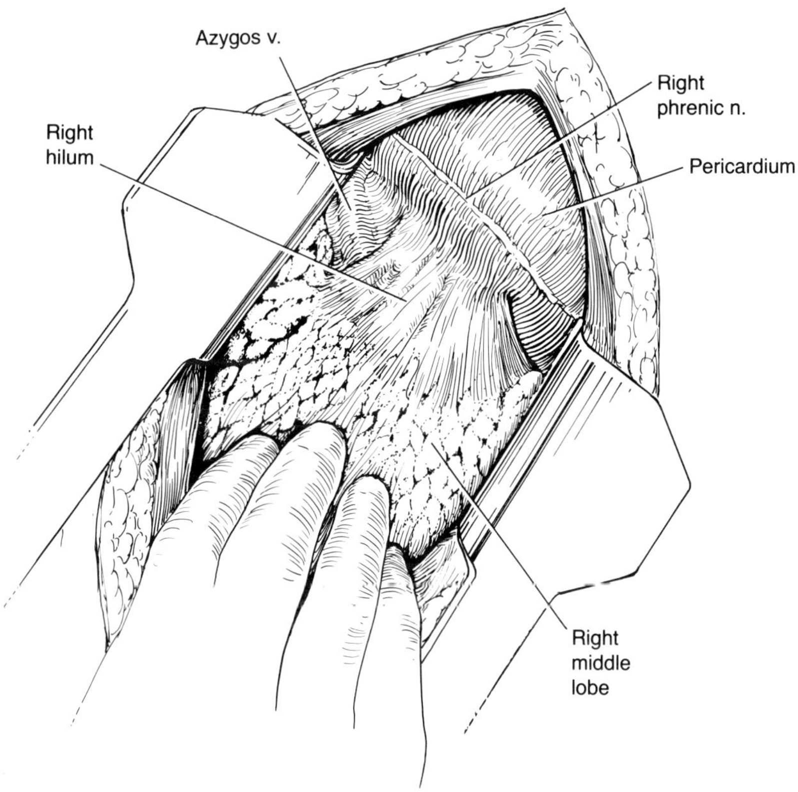

FIGURE 3–4. With retraction of the lung, the mediastinum, pericardium, and hilum are exposed. The incision is closed in the standard manner.

DONALD D. GLOWER, JR., M.D.

4
Posterolateral Thoracotomy

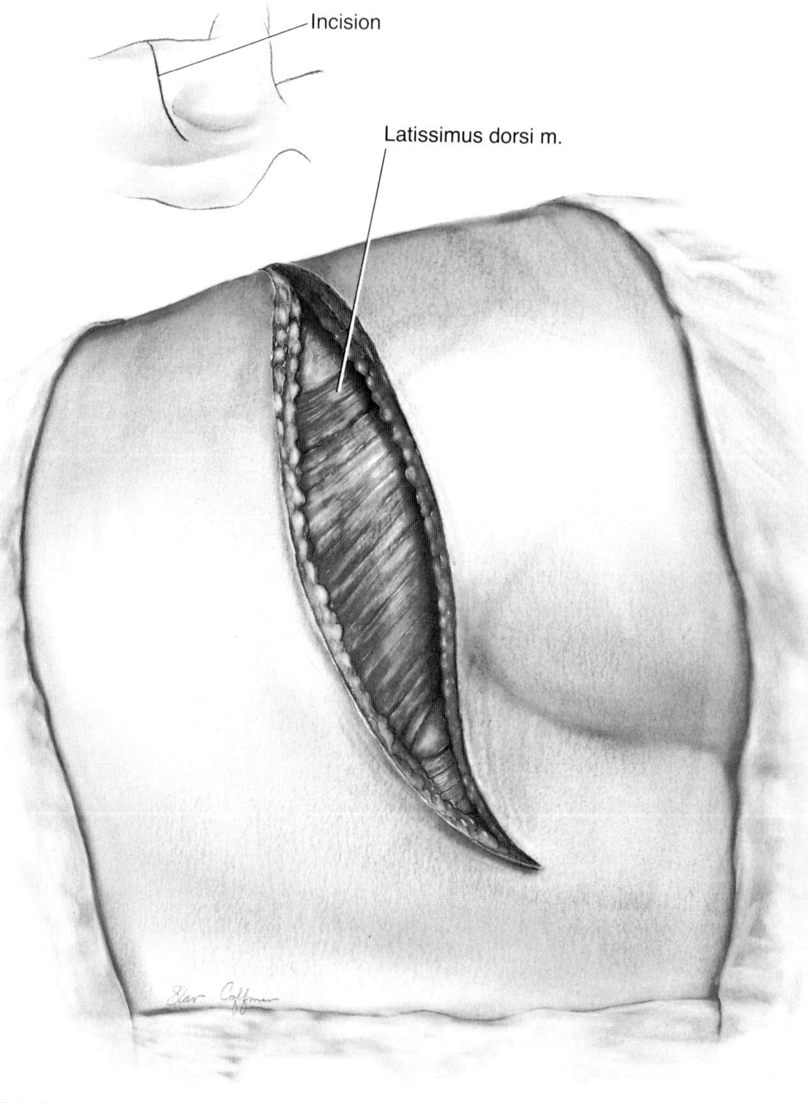

FIGURE 4–1. The chest is in the straight lateral position, with a roll placed under the dependent axilla and the upper arm extended anteriorly. The skin is incised along the inframammary line anteriorly to 1 cm below the tip of the scapula and midway between the scapula and the spine posteriorly.

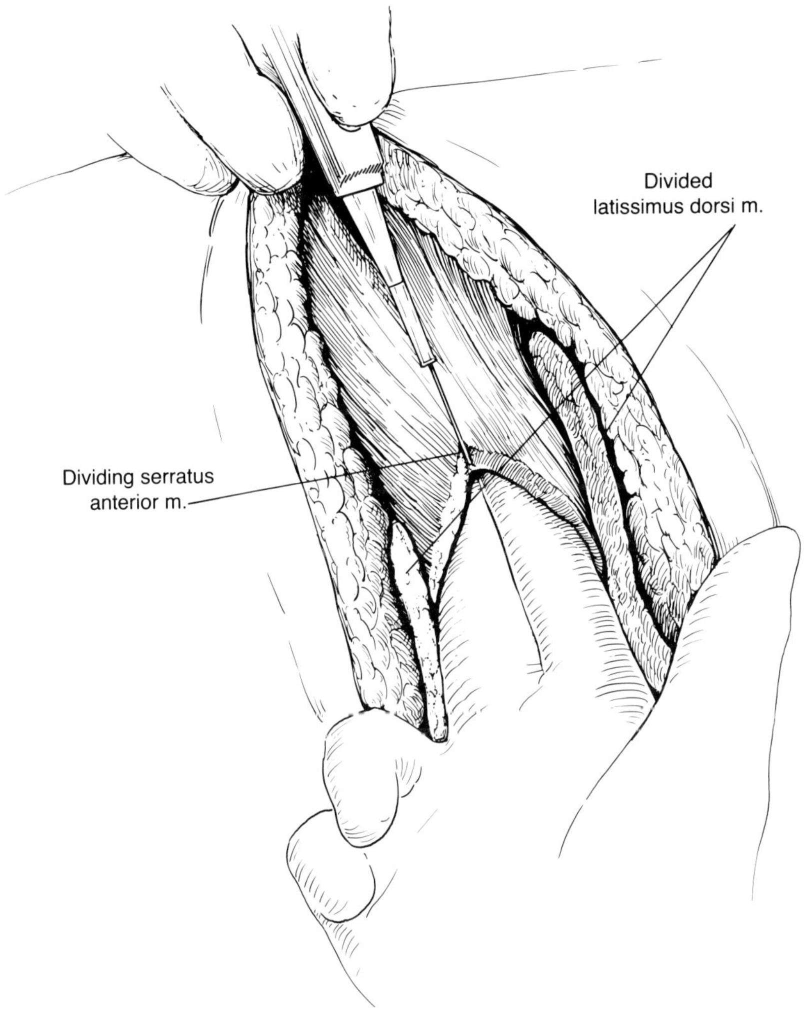

FIGURE 4–2. The serratus anterior and the latissimus dorsi muscles are divided. Alternatively, they may be spared by retracting them anteriorly and posteriorly under superior and inferior skin flaps (not shown).

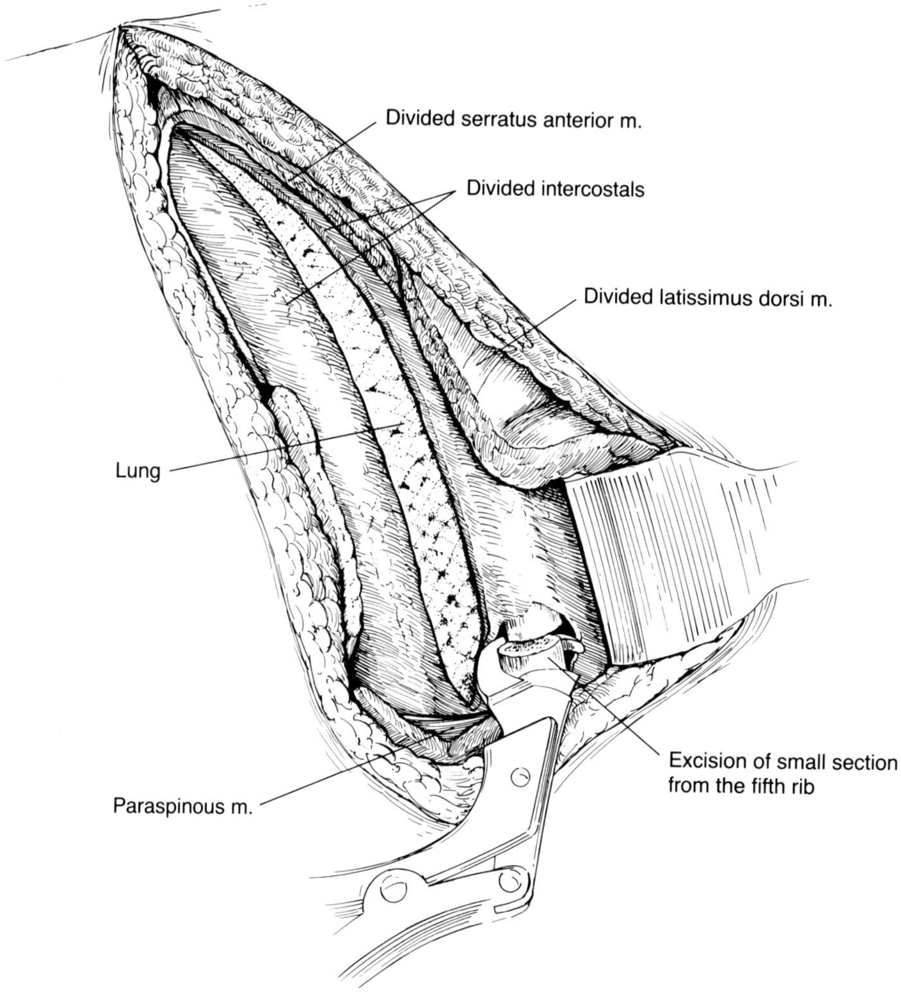

FIGURE 4–3. The fifth (or fourth or sixth) intercostal space is entered, or the fifth rib may be removed and the pleural space entered through the bed of the fifth rib. Additional exposure may be obtained by resecting a 1-cm section of rib above or below, preserving the intercostal neurovascular bundle. The trapezius and rhomboid muscles may be incised posteriorly as necessary up to the paraspinous muscle, which is spared.

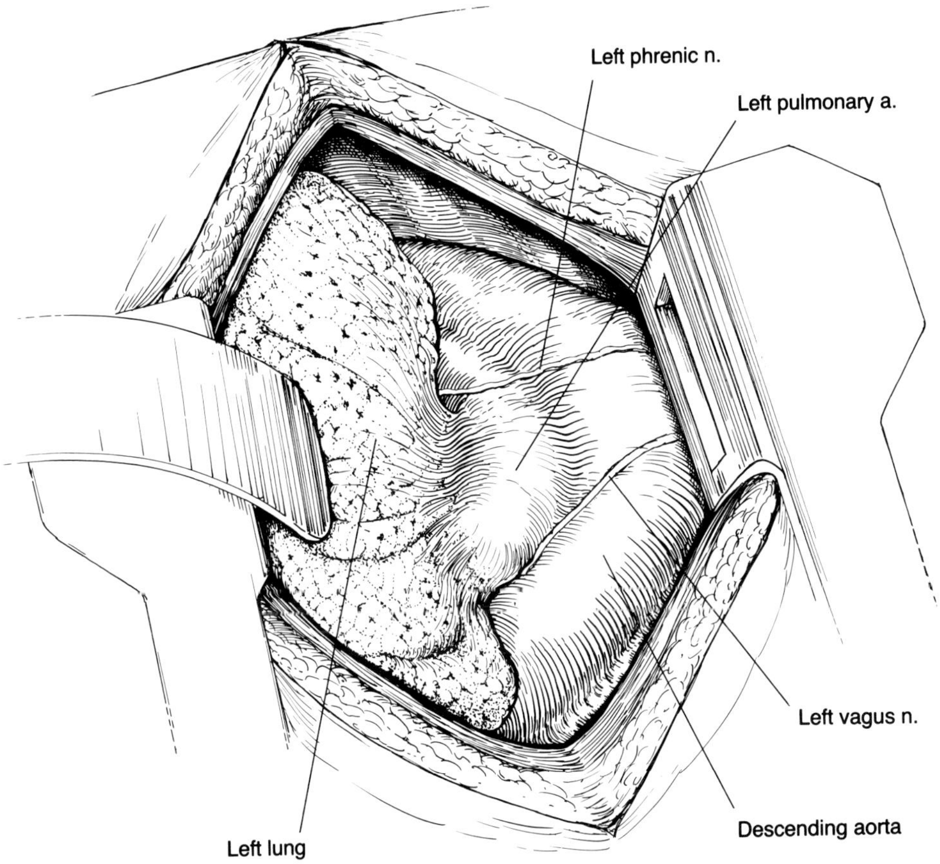

FIGURE 4–4. Exposure is gained to the entire pleural space and the lateral mediastinum.

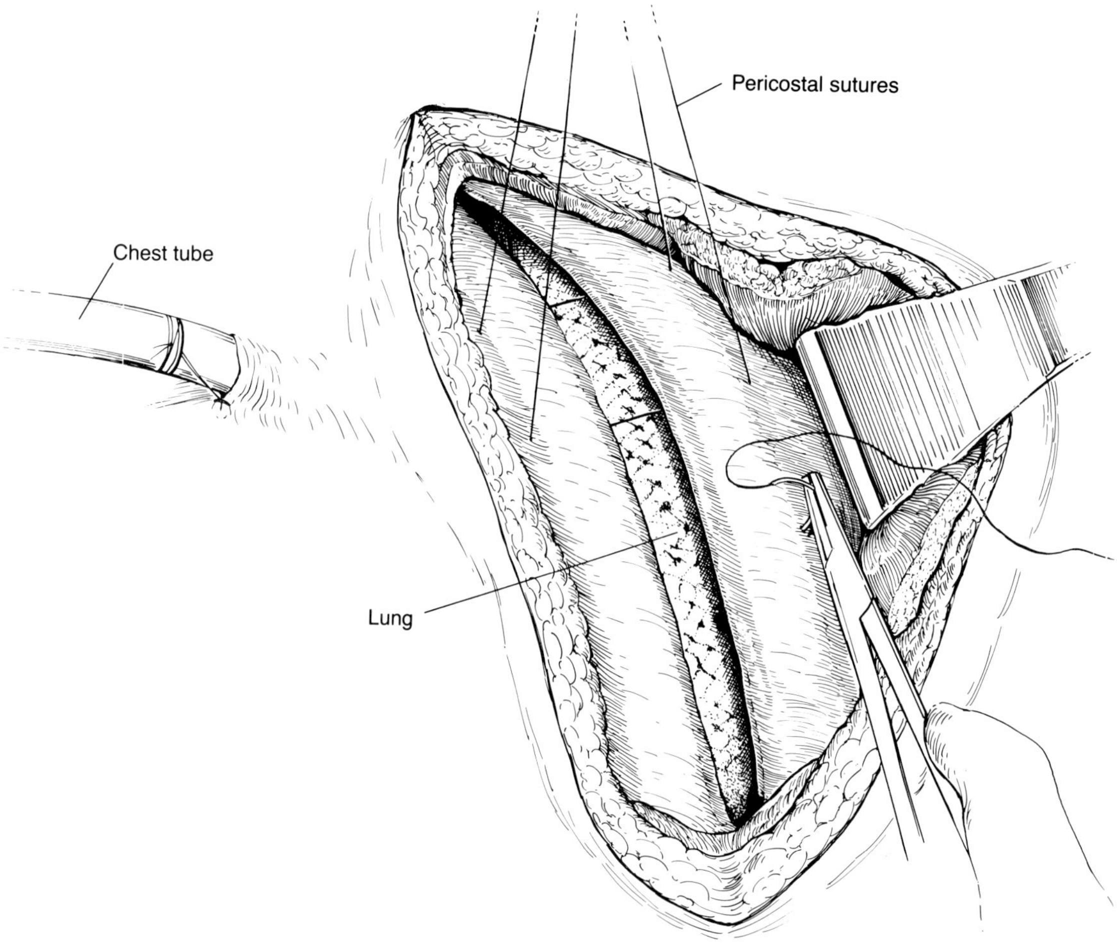

FIGURE 4–5. One or two chest tubes are placed in the pleural space one to two interspaces below the incision. The ribs are reapproximated with heavy pericostal sutures.

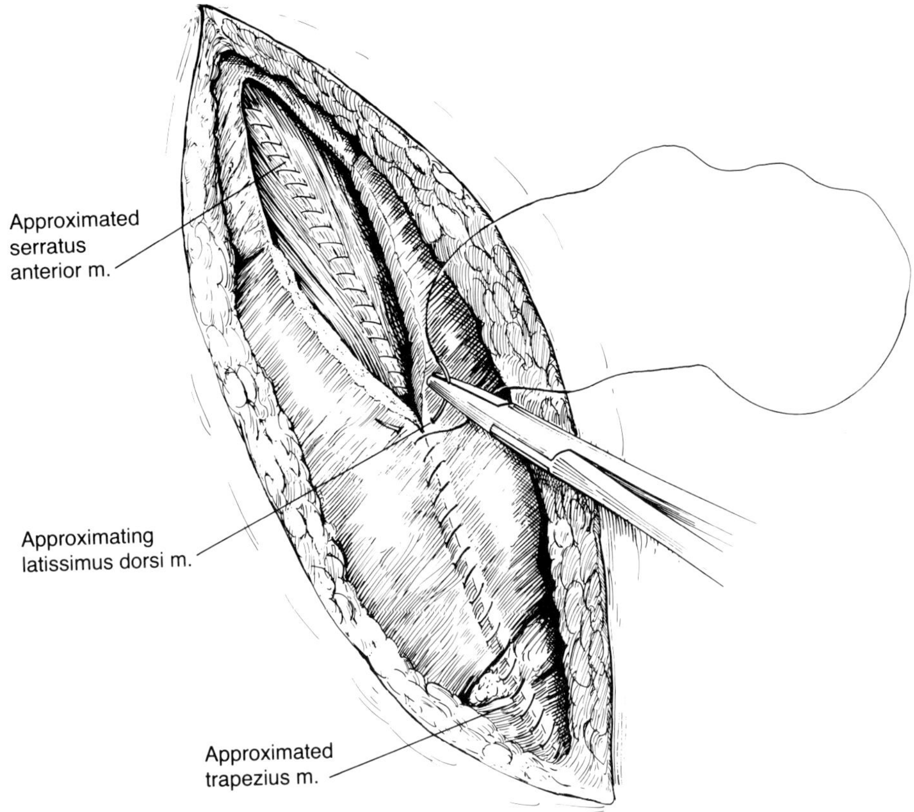

FIGURE 4–6. The serratus anterior and latissimus dorsi muscles with associated fascia are closed with continuous 1–0 Vicryl suture.

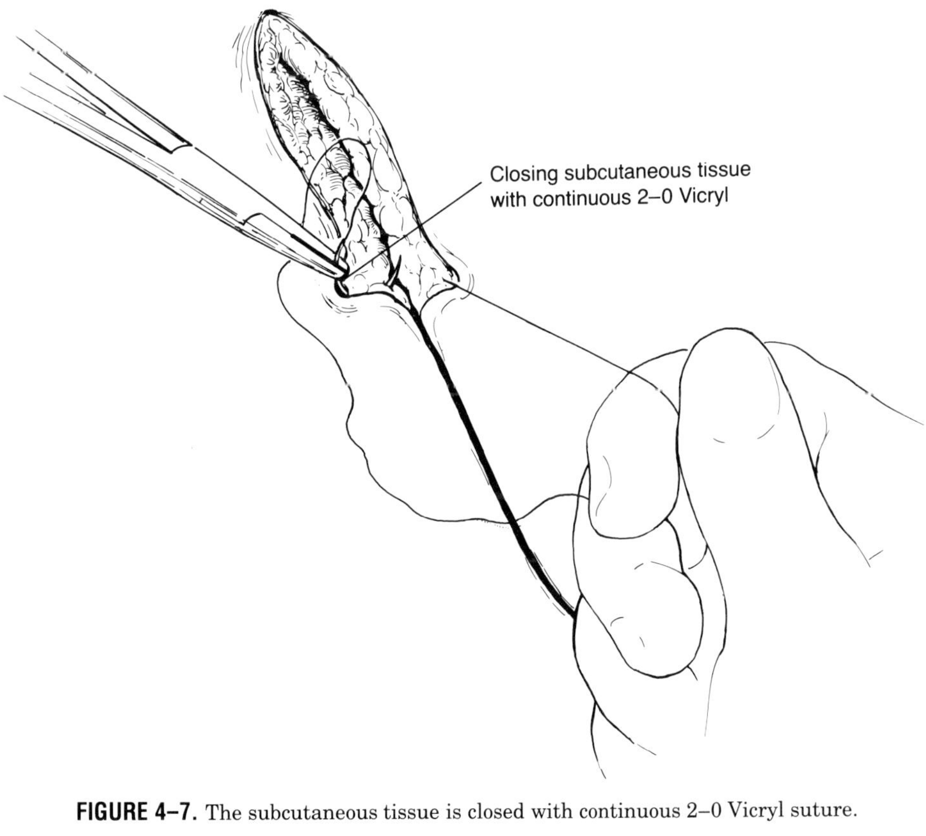

FIGURE 4–7. The subcutaneous tissue is closed with continuous 2–0 Vicryl suture.

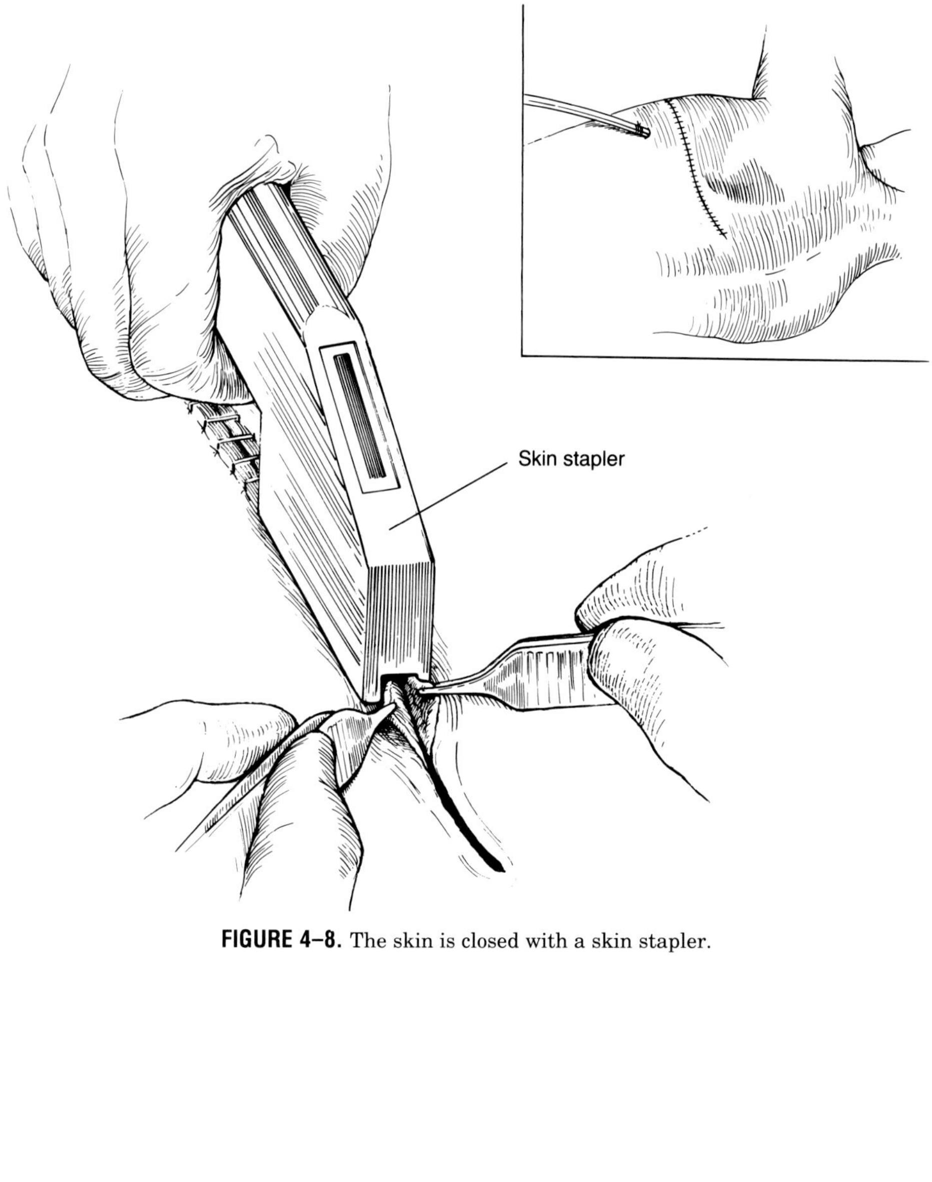

FIGURE 4–8. The skin is closed with a skin stapler.

DONALD D. GLOWER, JR., M.D.

5
Transaxillary Thoracotomy

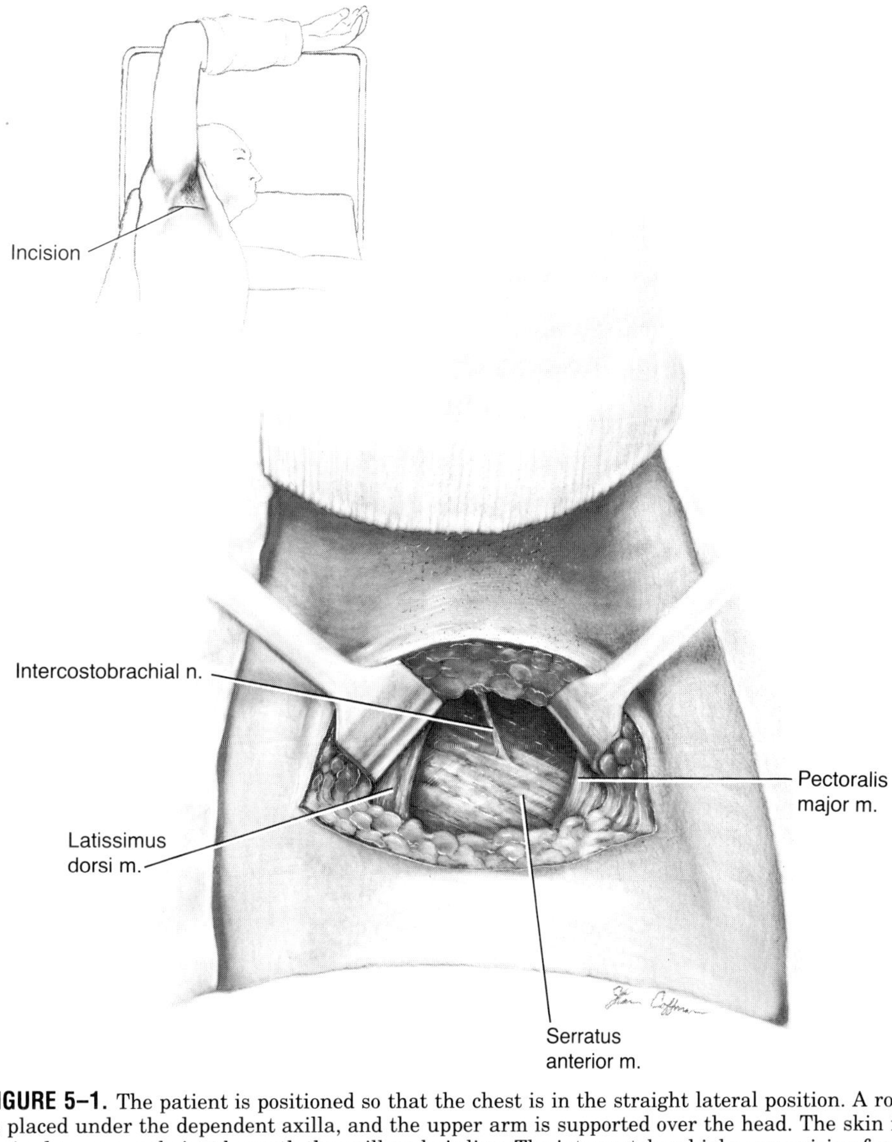

FIGURE 5–1. The patient is positioned so that the chest is in the straight lateral position. A roll is placed under the dependent axilla, and the upper arm is supported over the head. The skin is incised transversely just beneath the axillary hair line. The intercostobrachial nerve arising from the second intercostal space should be avoided.

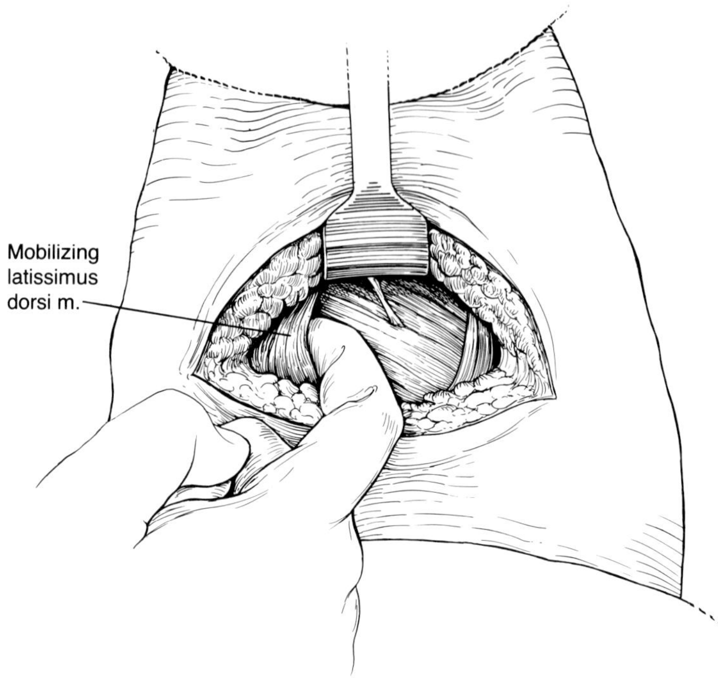

FIGURE 5–2. The pectoralis major and latissimus dorsi muscles are mobilized as needed.

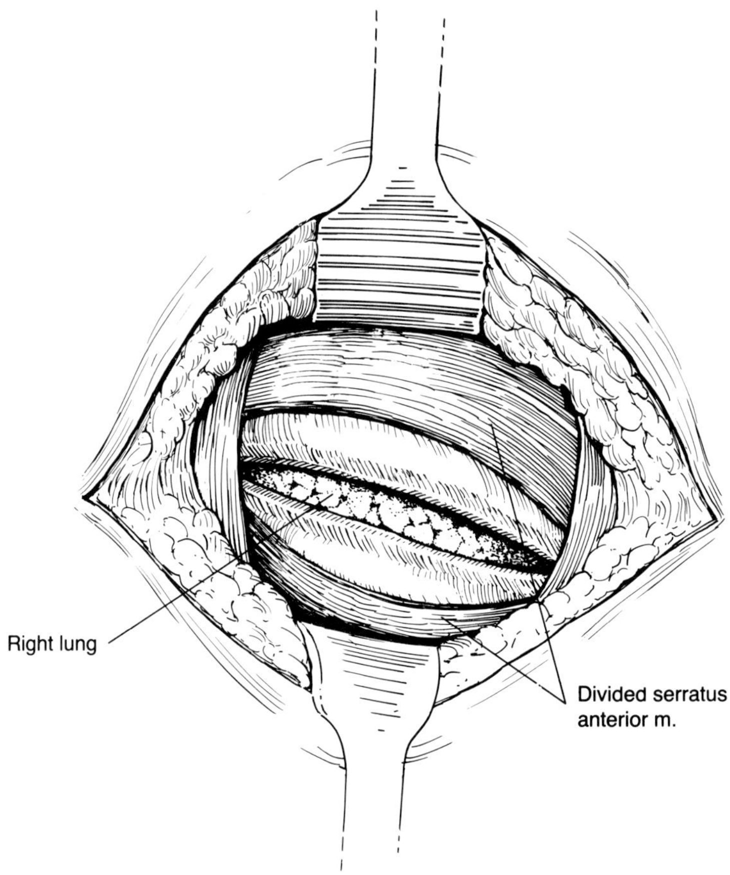

FIGURE 5–3. The third intercostal space is entered after dividing the serratus anterior muscle in the direction of its fibers.

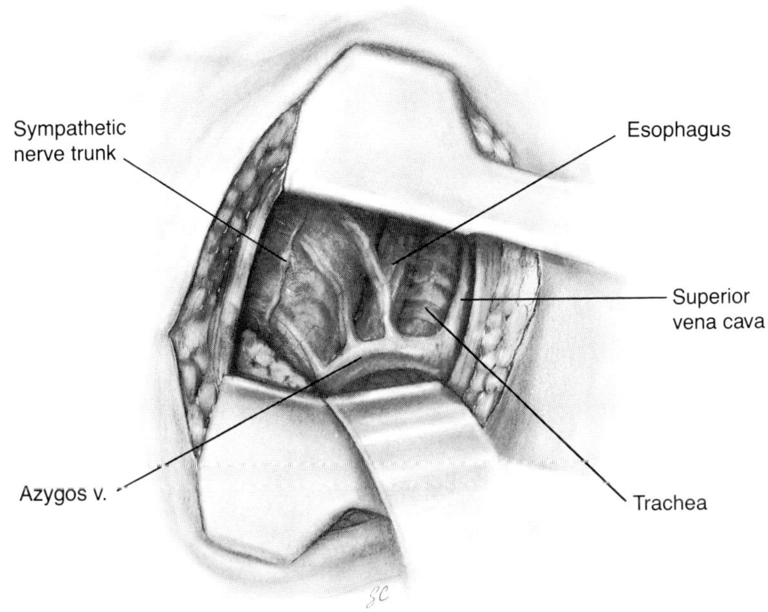

FIGURE 5–4. Exposure is gained to the superior posterior mediastinum, including the sympathetic nerve trunk. The incision is closed in the standard manner.

JAMES M. DOUGLAS, JR., M.D.

6

Median Sternotomy

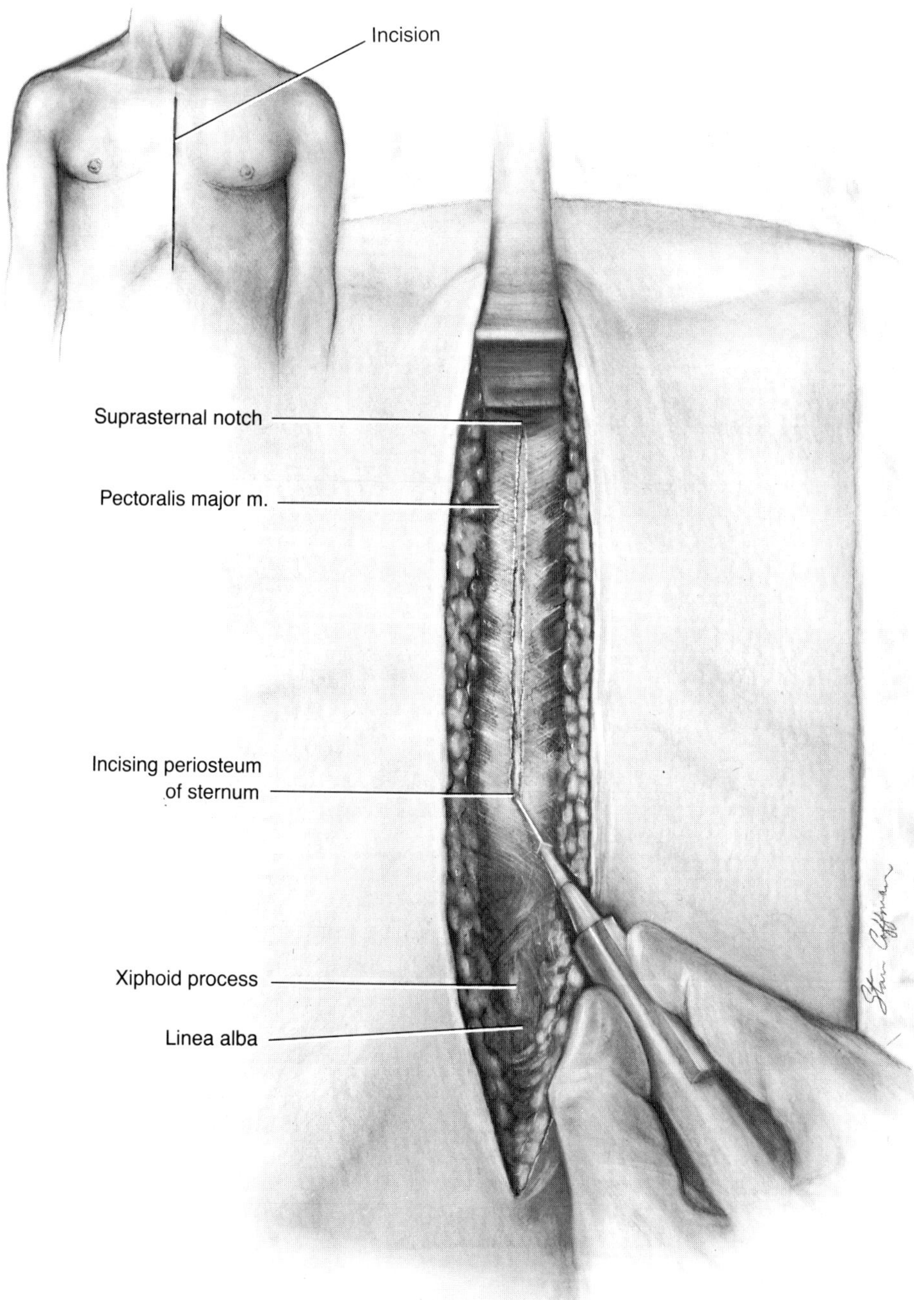

FIGURE 6–1 *See legend on opposite page*

FIGURE 6–1. The intended line of incision may be identified with ink or by pinpoint skin depressions defining the starting point, midpoint, and completion point of the incision. Every effort should be made to ensure that the incision is straight and exactly in the midline over the sternum. The sternal notch and tip of the xiphoid process are identified by palpation. The incision is begun approximately 2 cm below the sternal notch and extended approximately 2 cm beyond the distal tip of the xiphoid process and is usually extended with the electrocautery down to the sternal periosteum. A midline approach can be ensured by careful attention to the insertion points of the pectoralis major muscles onto the sternum; the incision should lie directly midway between these insertion points. This method is preferable to estimation of the midline by palpation of the intercostal notches.

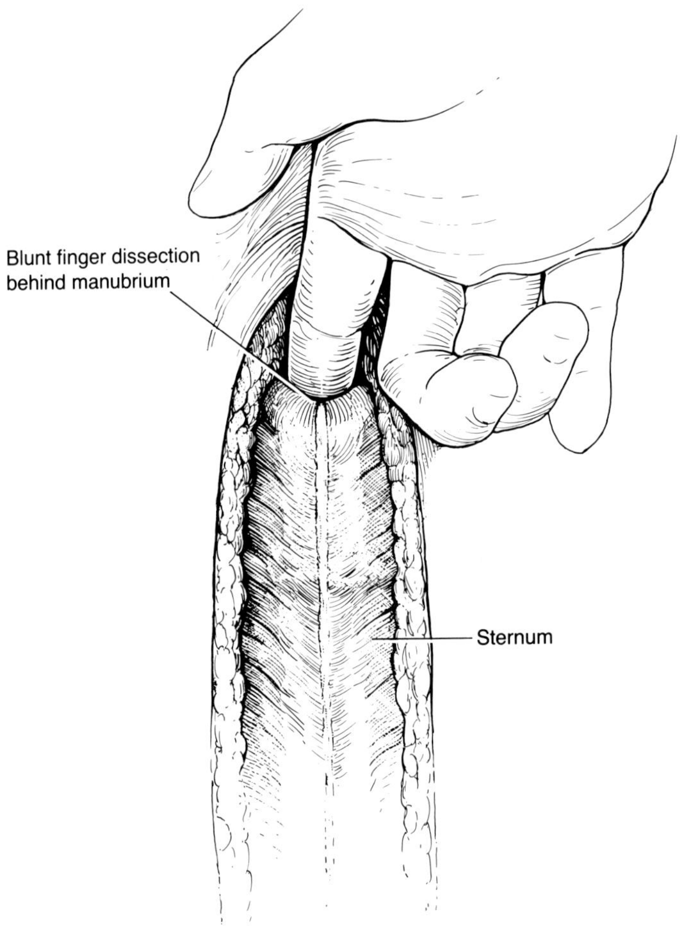

FIGURE 6–2. Following complete delineation of the midportion of the sternum by a line of electrocautery, preparation is made for sternal splitting. Using blunt finger dissection, a pathway is created above the suprasternal ligament and continued beneath the manubrium. No attempt at direct division of the suprasternal ligament by scissors, electrocautery, or other means is necessary. These techniques are to be avoided because of the risk of injury to the innominate artery as it passes upward to the neck. Division of the suprasternal ligament with the sternal saw is quite simple and much safer.

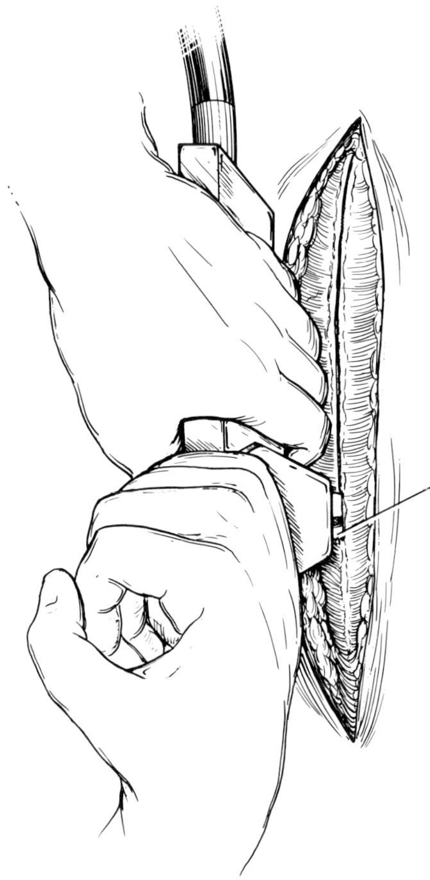

FIGURE 6–3

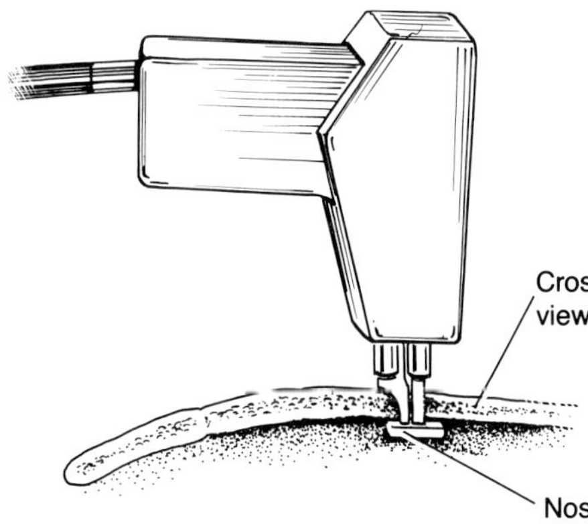

FIGURE 6–4

FIGURES 6–3 and 6–4. In most cases, the sternum is divided in a cephalad to caudad direction. The nose plate of the sternal saw is hooked underneath the suprasternal ligament, and the saw is grasped with both hands for stability. As the sternum is split, upward lifting on the sternal saw allows safe passage and helps avoid injury to the underlying pleura and mediastinal structures. It may be helpful to retreat slightly within the midportion of the sternotomy to allow release of any gathered pleura before completing the sternotomy .

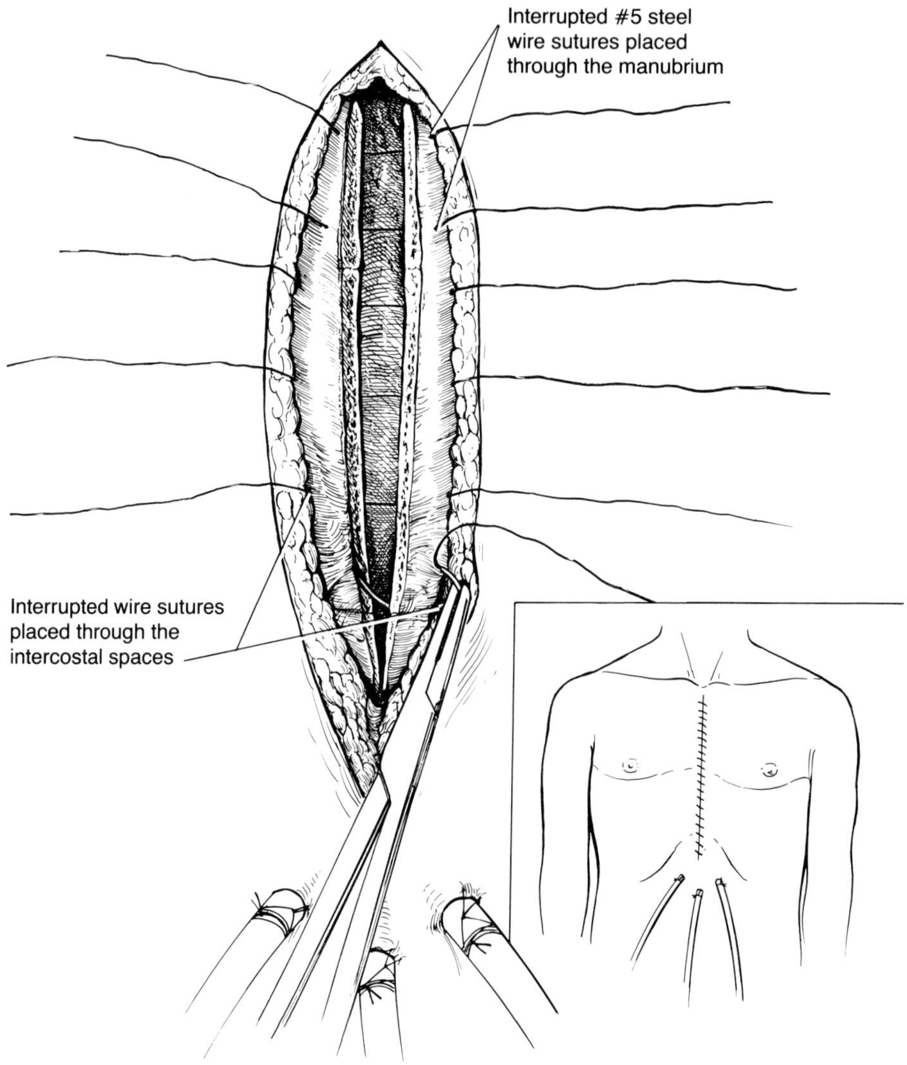

FIGURE 6–5. Following complete hemostasis and placement of mediastinal drains, preparation is made for closure. The sternum is approximated with #5 stainless steel wire sutures. Two sutures are typically passed through the manubrium. The remaining sutures are passed through the intercostal spaces close to the notch and the superior portion of the rib to avoid the internal mammary arteries and the intercostal neurovascular bundle. Following placement of wires, each sternal edge is lifted and the underside examined for possible bleeding. The wires are crossed and the sternum is elevated while the wires are twisted closed. This elevation is important to avoid inadvertent entrapment of the underlying mediastinal tubes. The wires are twisted for firm closure, but overzealous twisting may cause primary or delayed sternal wire breakage. The uppermost portion of the linea alba is closed either with interrupted fascial sutures or as part of a continuous heavy monofilament suture. Typically, the pectoralis fascia is closed with a continuous monofilament suture. The subcutaneous tissue is closed with absorbable suture, and the skin is closed with staples or sutures of the surgeon's preference.

JAMES M. DOUGLAS, JR., M.D.

7

Cervicothoracic Incisions

Trauma to the base of the neck or upper chest may cause major vascular injury requiring well-planned incisions that allow surgical treatment under optimal visualization and control. This chapter details the operative approaches to a variety of important structures in this area and focuses primarily on access to vascular structures. The exposure afforded to portions of the trachea and cervical esophagus and other surrounding soft tissues and bones is also discussed.

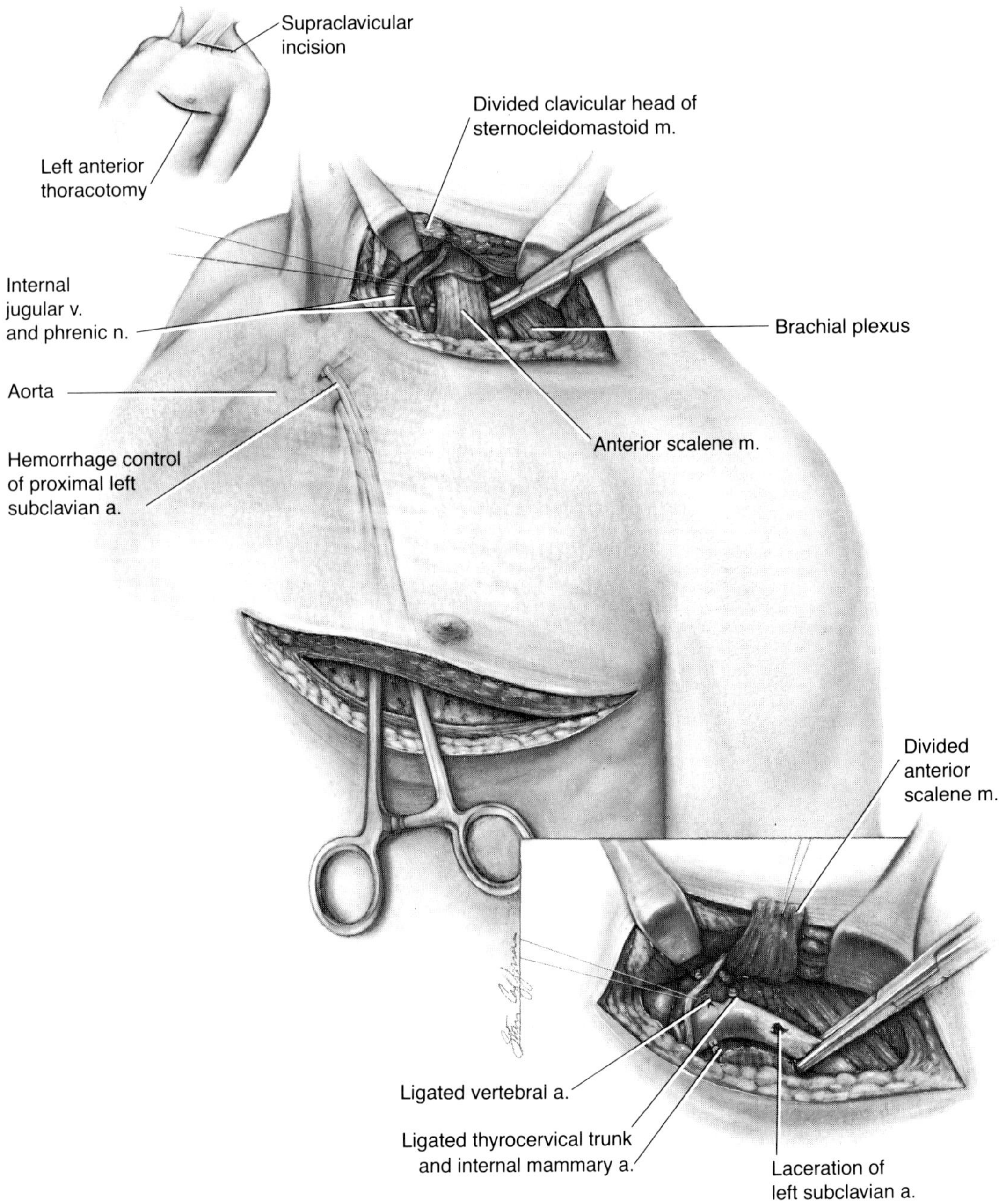

FIGURE 7–1. Injuries to the left subclavian artery must be approached with the understanding that the vessel originates to the left and posteriorly from the aortic arch. In elective operations on the subclavian vessel, a standard posterolateral thoracotomy through the fourth or fifth intercostal space exposes the base of this vessel. However, under emergency circumstances, control of this vessel can be rapidly gained through a left anterior thoracotomy through the fourth intercostal space. This incision also allows good access to the heart for compression or repair.

Lower inset, Once proximal control is achieved, the distal subclavian artery is exposed through a left supraclavicular incision. The platysma is divided, as is the clavicular attachment of the sternocleidomastoid muscle, exposing the fascia overlying the internal jugular vein just lateral to the left common carotid artery. Care must be taken to identify the phrenic nerve just lateral to the internal jugular vein as it courses over the medial border of the anterior scalene muscle. The nerve is retracted medially as the anterior scalene muscle is divided. The subclavian artery lies immediately behind this muscle and may be dissected from surrounding tissues, with a clamp placed on the distal vessel. Control of the vertebral artery and thyrocervical trunk in addition to the internal mammary artery is necessary to minimize continued bleeding through the subclavian artery.

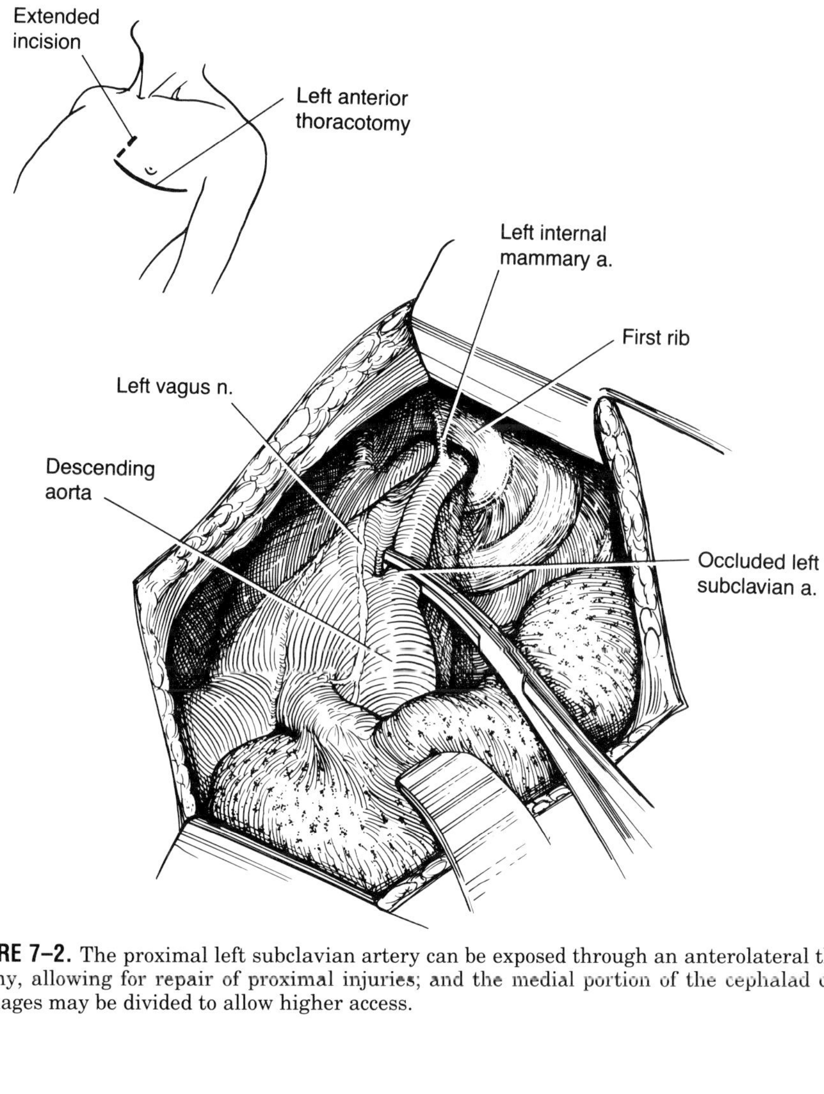

FIGURE 7–2. The proximal left subclavian artery can be exposed through an anterolateral thoracotomy, allowing for repair of proximal injuries; and the medial portion of the cephalad costal cartilages may be divided to allow higher access.

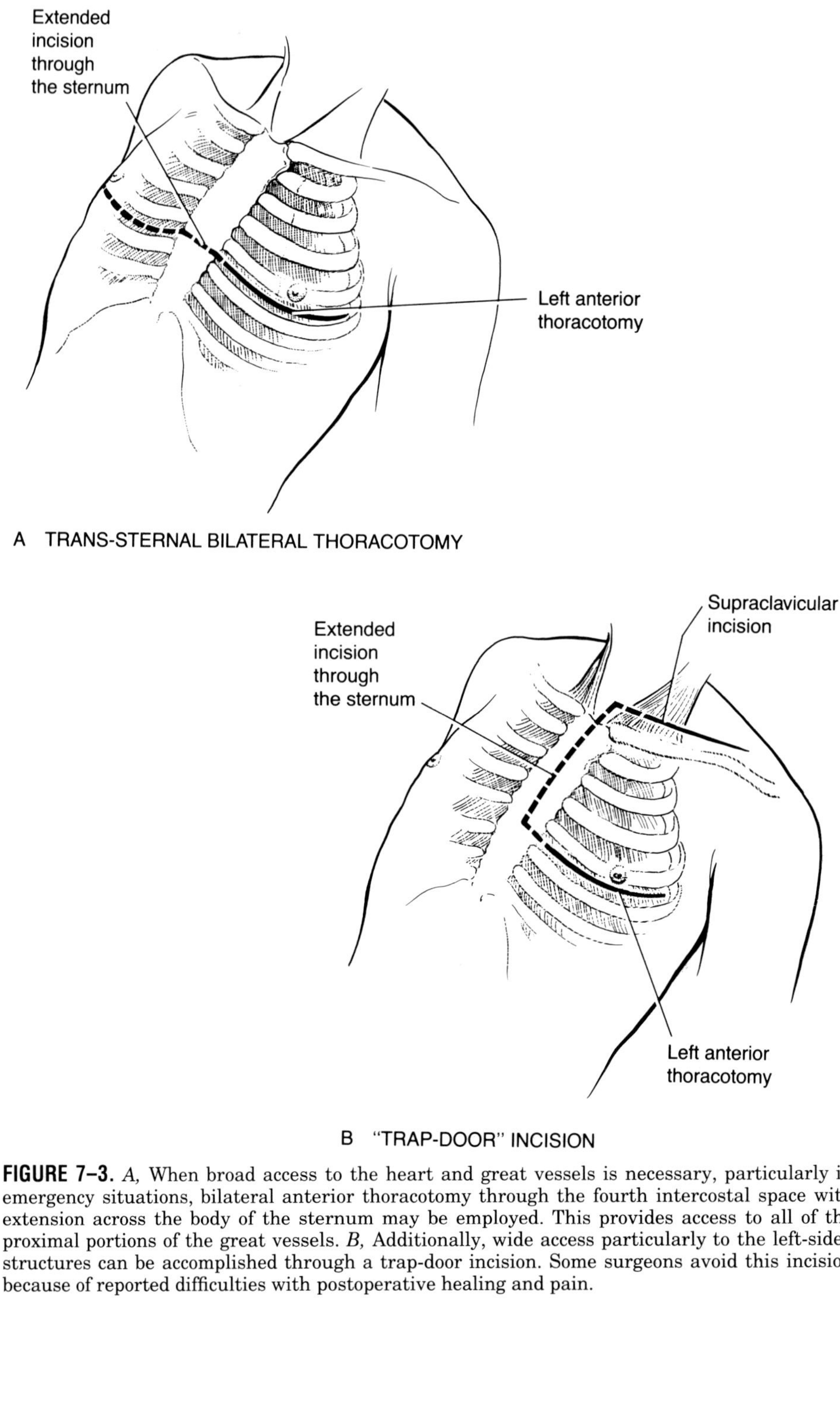

FIGURE 7–3. *A,* When broad access to the heart and great vessels is necessary, particularly in emergency situations, bilateral anterior thoracotomy through the fourth intercostal space with extension across the body of the sternum may be employed. This provides access to all of the proximal portions of the great vessels. *B,* Additionally, wide access particularly to the left-sided structures can be accomplished through a trap-door incision. Some surgeons avoid this incision because of reported difficulties with postoperative healing and pain.

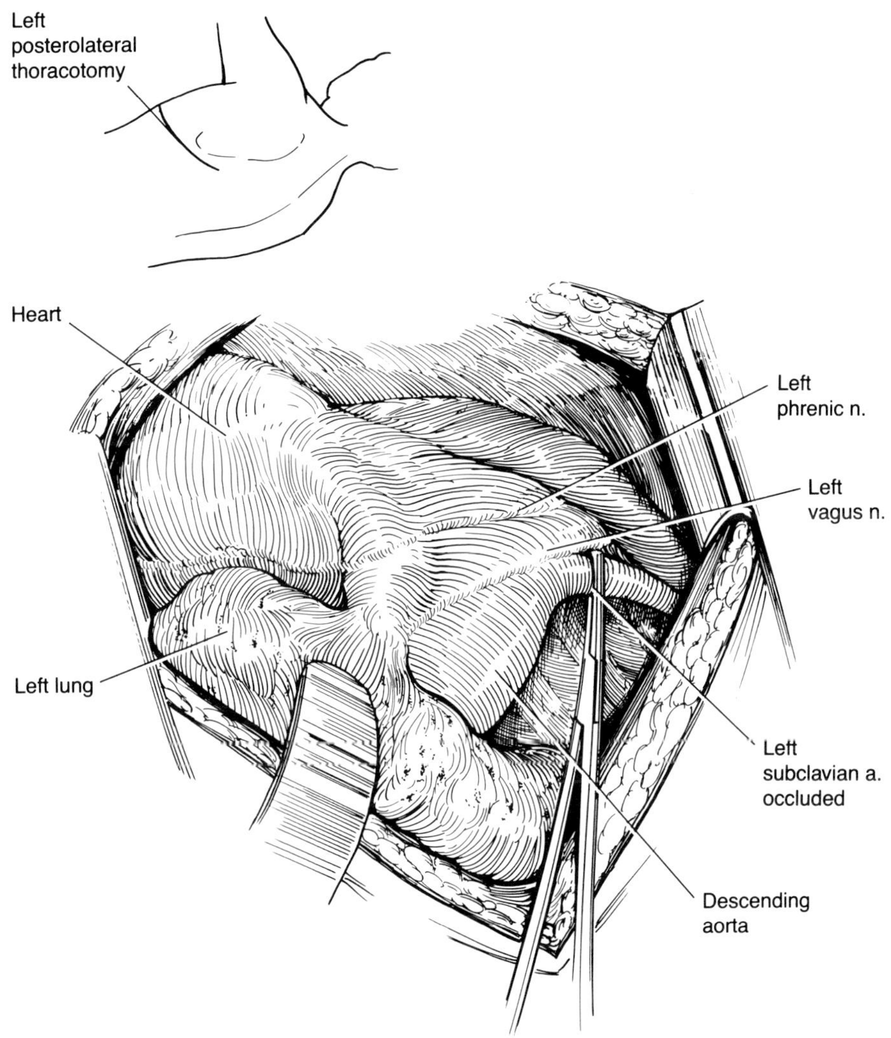

FIGURE 7–4. Shown is the exposure afforded by a standard *left posterolateral thoracotomy* through the fourth or fifth intercostal space, an incision that provides optimal access to the proximal left subclavian artery and good visualization of the distal aortic arch and proximal descending aorta. This incision may be particularly useful in the setting of associated lung injury.

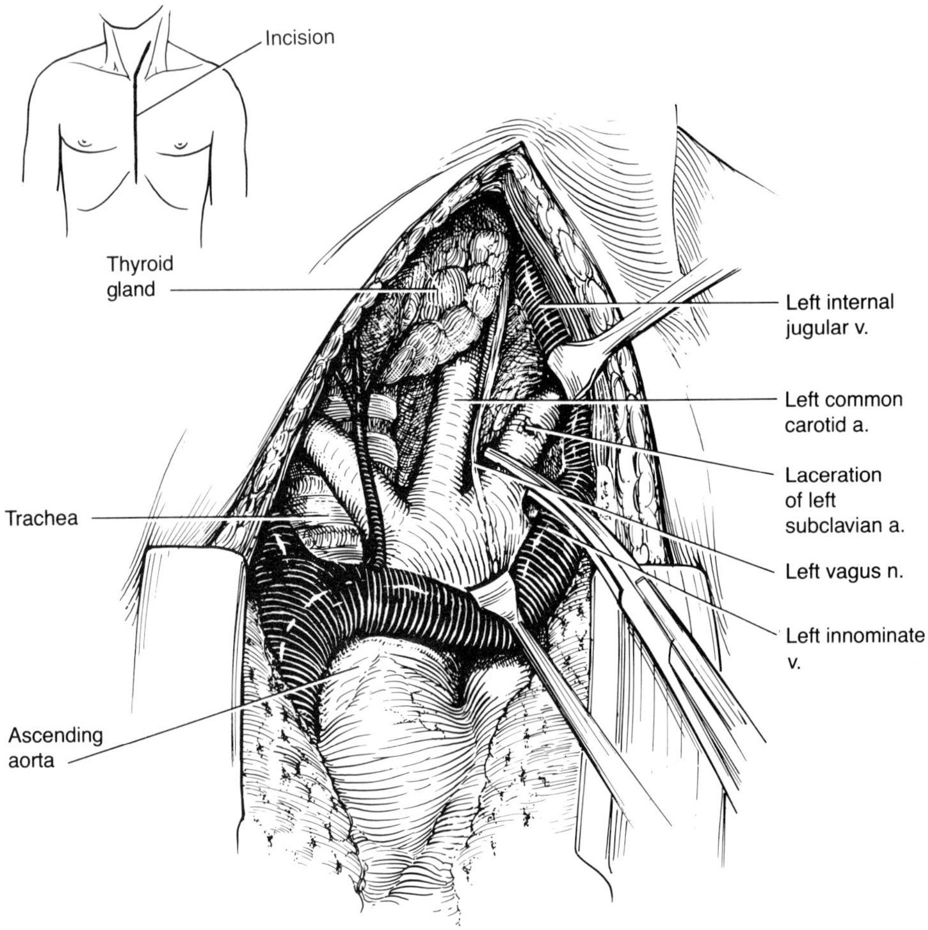

FIGURE 7–5. A *left cervicothoracic incision* involves a standard median sternotomy with extension of the incision cephalad anterior to the left sternocleidomastoid muscle. It provides access to the aortic arch, left common carotid artery, proximal innominate artery, proximal left subclavian artery, left vertebral artery, left internal jugular vein, innominate vein, proximal left subclavian vein, midtrachea, cervical esophagus, and lower anterior cervical spine.

A standard median sternotomy is performed as described in the previous chapter, the skin incision is carried anterior to the left sternocleidomastoid muscle, and the platysma is divided. Dissection is carried along the border of the sternocleidomastoid muscle down to the desired anatomic region. The strap muscles are retracted or divided near their attachments to the sternum and clavicle as necessary to provide optimal exposure. The left common carotid artery is easily identified just lateral to the trachea. The accompanying left vagus nerve and left internal jugular vein are also easily seen. Care must be exercised when mobilizing the trachea toward the right to avoid damage to the recurrent laryngeal nerve, which traverses posteriorly in the tracheoesophageal groove. The phrenic nerve courses anteriorly across the anterior scalene muscle and courses medially just posterior to the subclavian vein near its junction with the internal jugular vein. It then continues caudally just lateral to the internal mammary artery at its junction with the proximal subclavian artery before coursing more medially along the upper mediastinum and pericardium.

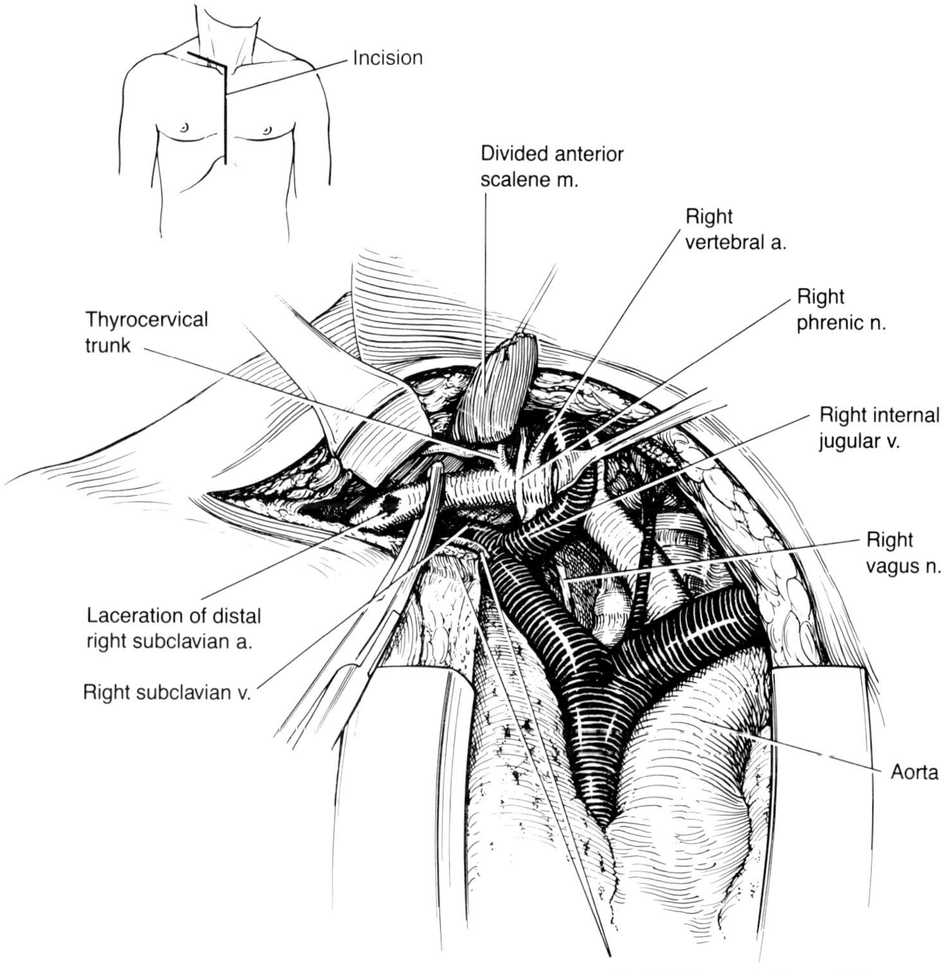

FIGURE 7–6. The *right thoracosupraclavicular incision* provides access to the ascending aorta, the innominate artery and vein, proximal right carotid artery, right subclavian artery and vein, origin of the right internal jugular vein, and the superior vena cava. Following a standard median sternotomy, the incision is extended over the border of the right clavicle. The platysma and sternocleidomastoid muscles are divided. The right subclavian artery is exposed following division of the anterior scalene muscle, and care is taken to avoid the right phrenic nerve.

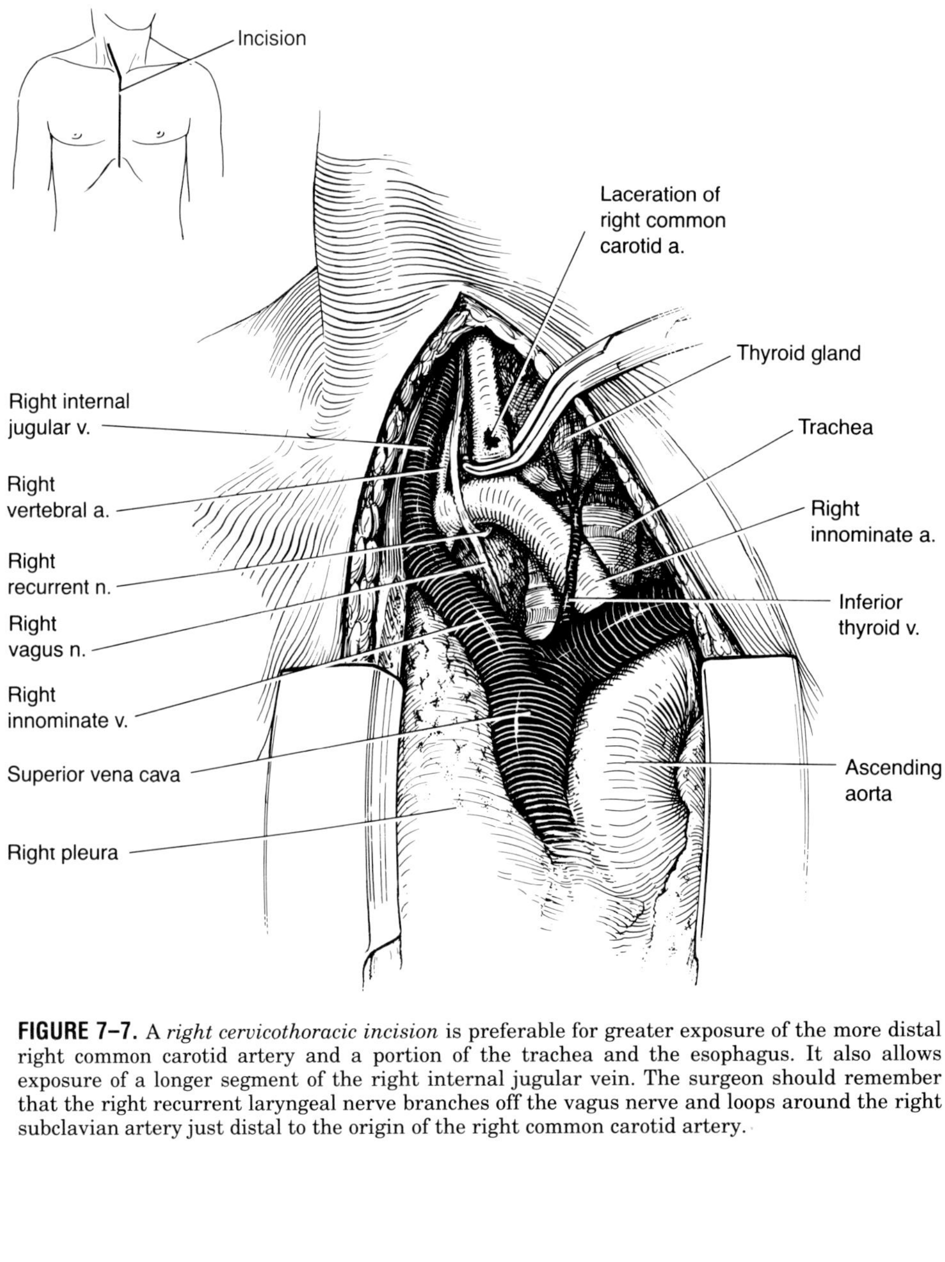

FIGURE 7–7. A *right cervicothoracic incision* is preferable for greater exposure of the more distal right common carotid artery and a portion of the trachea and the esophagus. It also allows exposure of a longer segment of the right internal jugular vein. The surgeon should remember that the right recurrent laryngeal nerve branches off the vagus nerve and loops around the right subclavian artery just distal to the origin of the right common carotid artery.

JAMES M. DOUGLAS, JR., M.D.

8

Thoracoabdominal Incisions

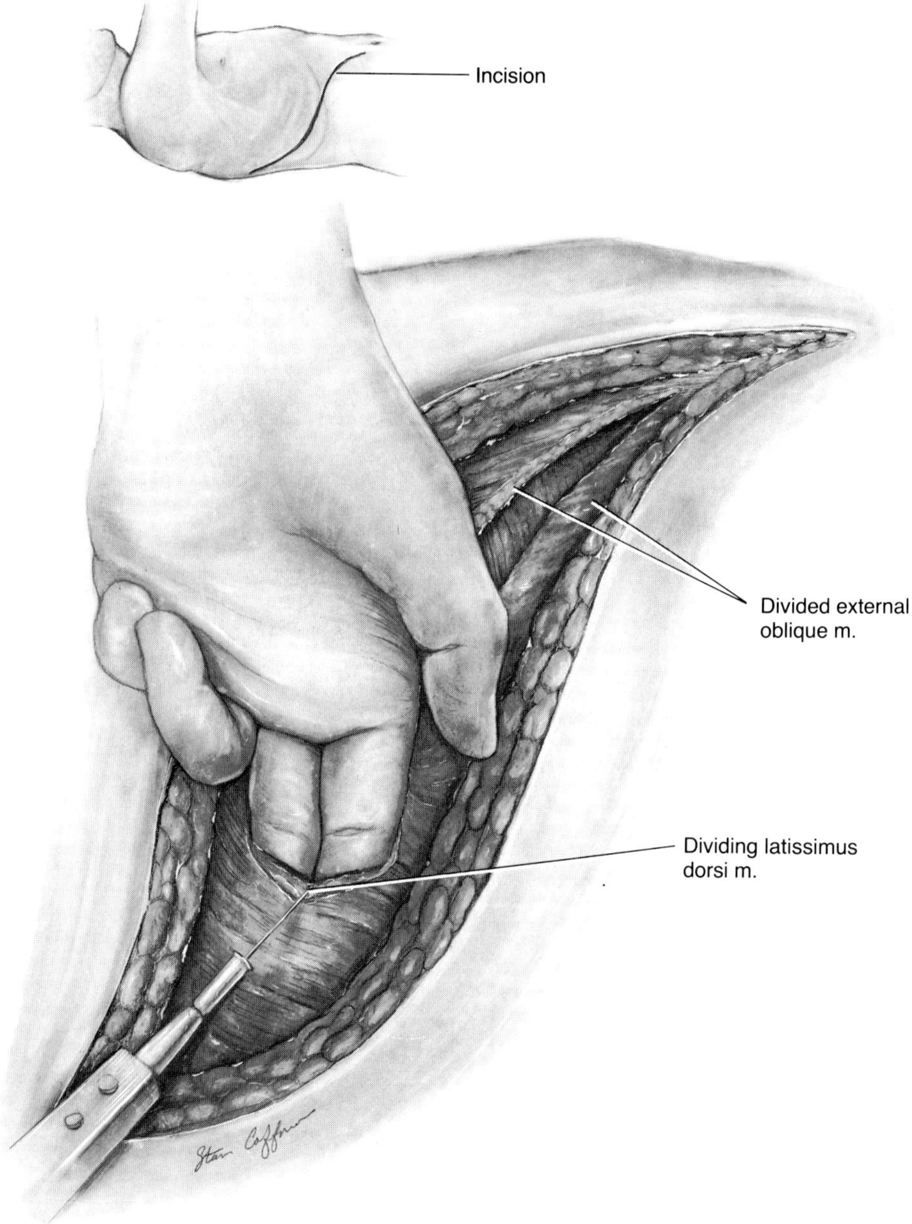

FIGURE 8–1. The exact placement of the thoracoabdominal incision is determined by the specific operation being performed, and the various incisions may be used for approach to the thoracic and abdominal aorta, stomach and esophagus, vena cava and liver, or thoracolumbar spine. The patient is usually placed in the left or right lateral decubitus position with some outward rotation of the pelvis to better expose the ventral surface of the abdomen. It is helpful to outline the proposed incision following identification of the desired landmarks. The typical incision is made beginning at a point midway between the spine and a line extending from the tip of the scapula parallel to the spine, following a curve overlying the ninth or tenth rib, and extending a variable distance onto the abdominal wall toward the rectus musculature.

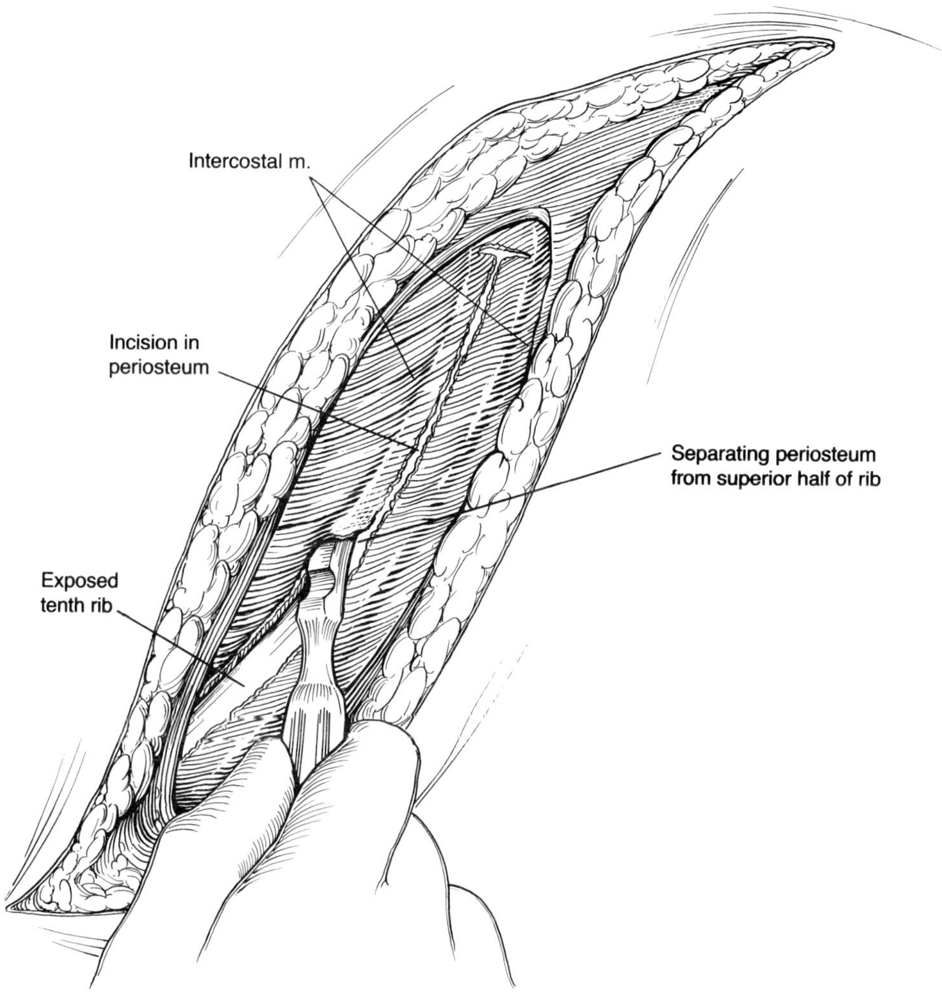

FIGURE 8–2. If rib excision is to be performed, the periosteum over the rib is divided in the midportion of the rib with the electrocautery. A periosteal elevator is employed to strip the periosteum superiorly and inferiorly, which is performed from anterior to posterior on the inferior surface of the rib and from posterior to anterior on the superior portion of the rib.

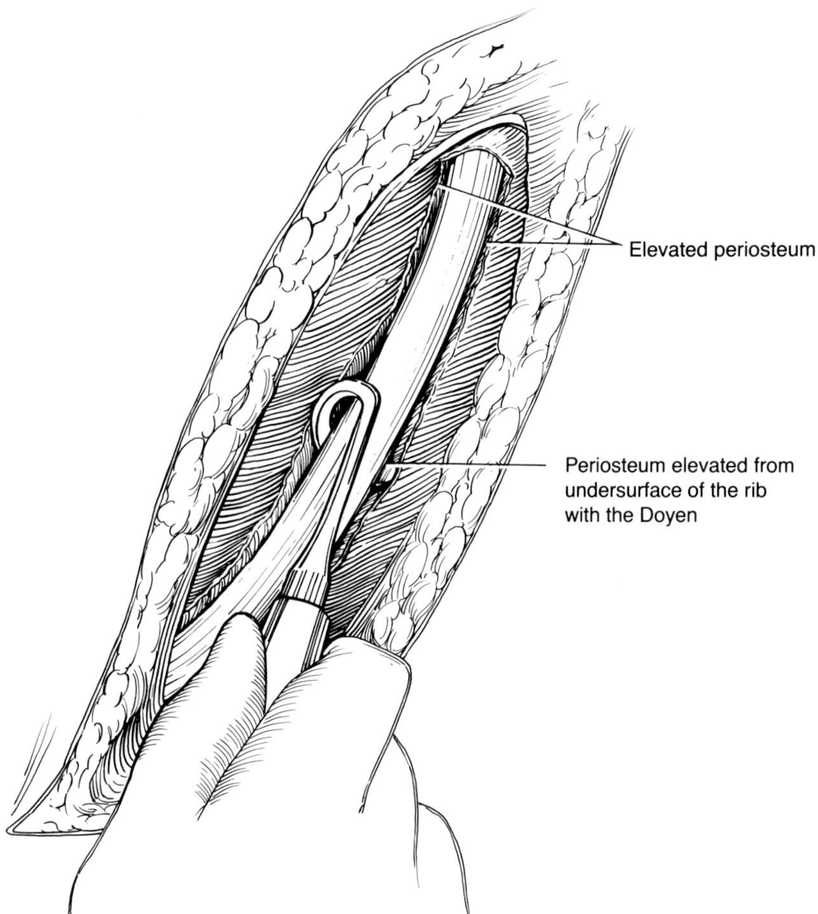

FIGURE 8–3. A Doyen periosteal elevator is employed to separate the medial surface of the periosteum, and the rib is divided with a rib cutter.

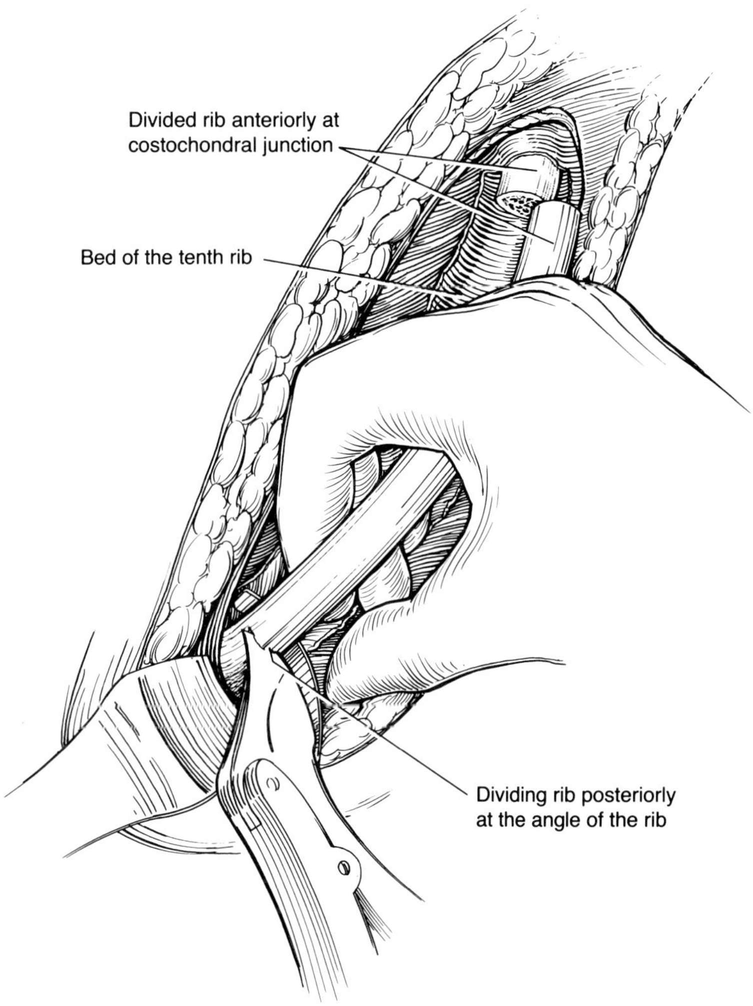

FIGURE 8–4. Anteriorly, the junction between the rib and cartilage is identified, and the cartilage is divided in the direction of the skin incision. This typically leaves a very small fragment inferiorly with the remainder of the costal cartilage proceeding toward the attachment to the sternum anteriorly.

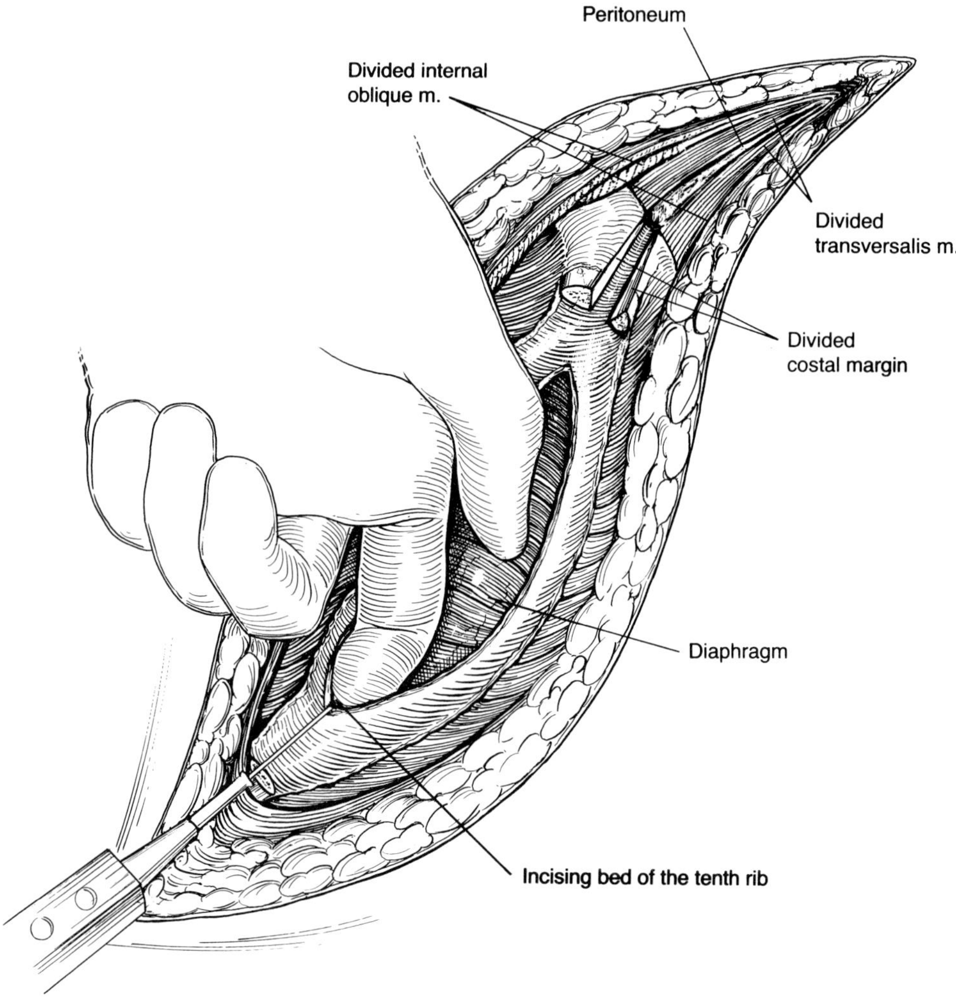

FIGURE 8–5. Division to this level allows easy identification of the muscular layers of the anterior abdominal wall. The internal and external oblique muscles along with the transversalis muscle may be divided in a stepwise manner. The parietal pleura is opened, and the chest entered. The ribs are spread; the lung is retracted; and exposure of the stomach, abdominal aorta, or liver requires division of the diaphragm.

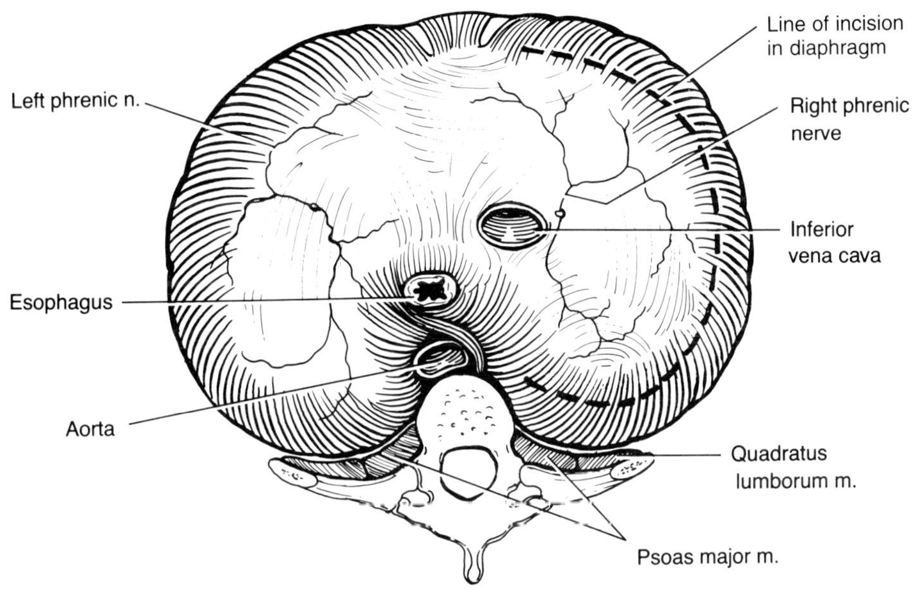

FIGURE 8–6. Division of the diaphragm should be performed in a circumferential manner to minimize damage to the phrenic nerves. The line of incision is parallel to the chest cavity, approximately 2 cm from the insertion of the diaphragm to the chest wall. Posteriorly, the incision extends to the spine, aortic hiatus, esophageal hiatus, or foramen of the inferior vena cava, depending on the structures being exposed. Anteriorly, the line of incision extends to the point of division of the costal cartilage. It is helpful to outline the proposed incision on the diaphragm by scoring its surface with the flat side of the electrocautery blade.

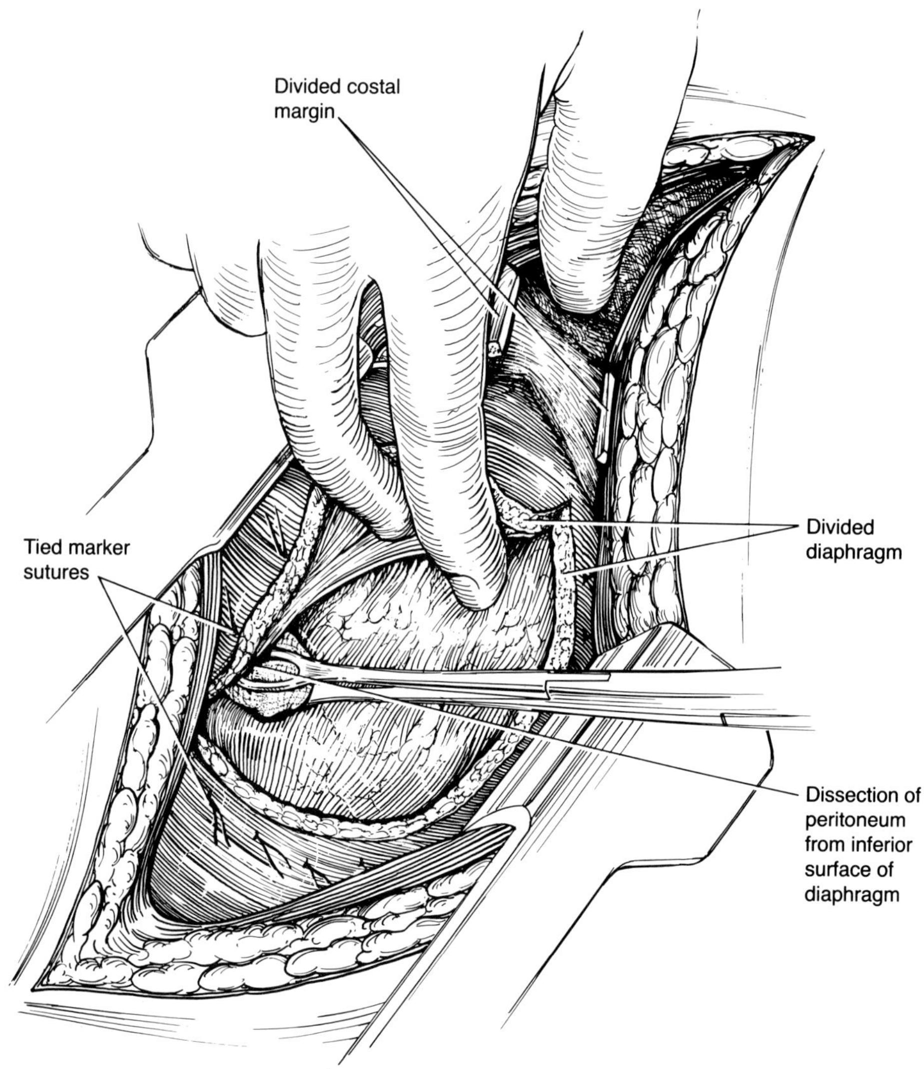

FIGURE 8–7. The diaphragm is divided from the anterior portion of the incision to the most posterior portion. If a retroperitoneal approach is desired, care is taken to avoid entry into the peritoneal cavity during the dissection. Blunt mobilization of the peritoneum away from the inferior diaphragmatic surface can usually be accomplished by combination of sponge stick and finger dissection. In making the incision, it is also helpful to periodically mark corresponding sides of the diaphragm with tied sutures to assist in the later accurate closure of this muscle.

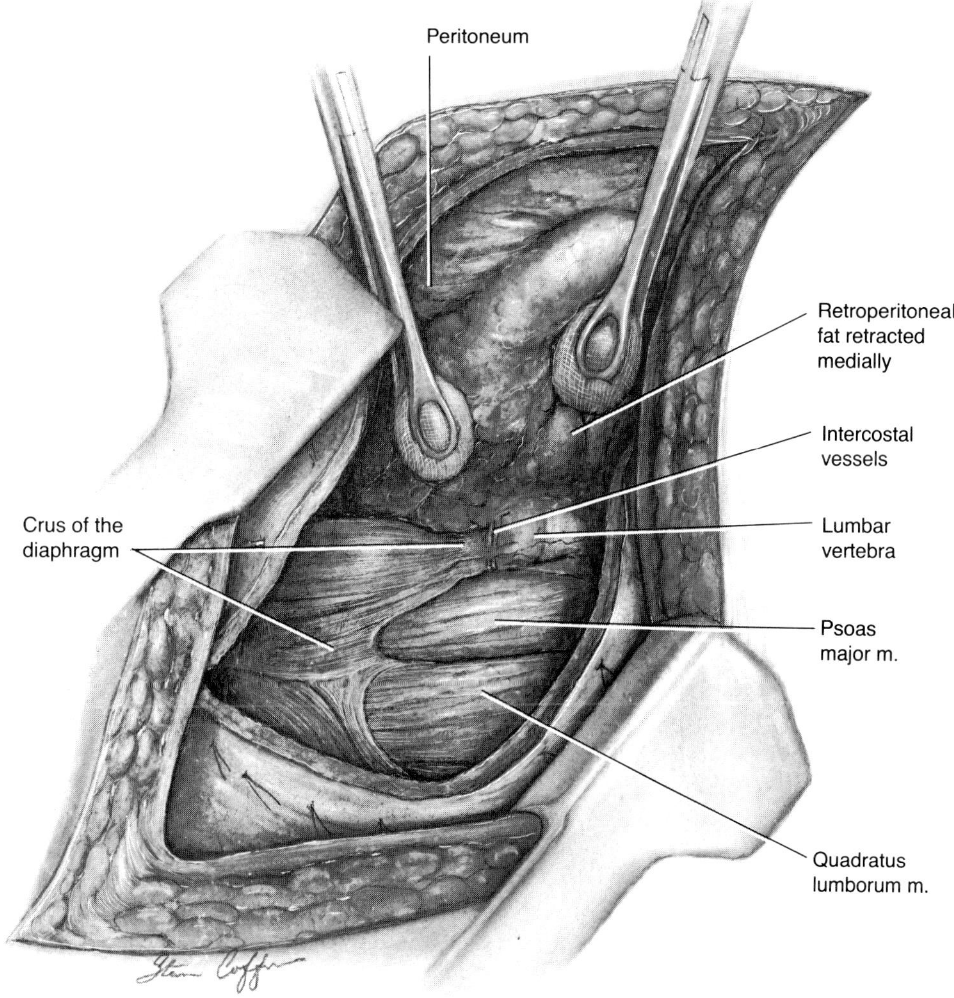

FIGURE 8–8. Retroperitoneal dissection can usually be performed with minimal bleeding when the proper plane has been established. Occasional crossing vessels should be cauterized as necessary.

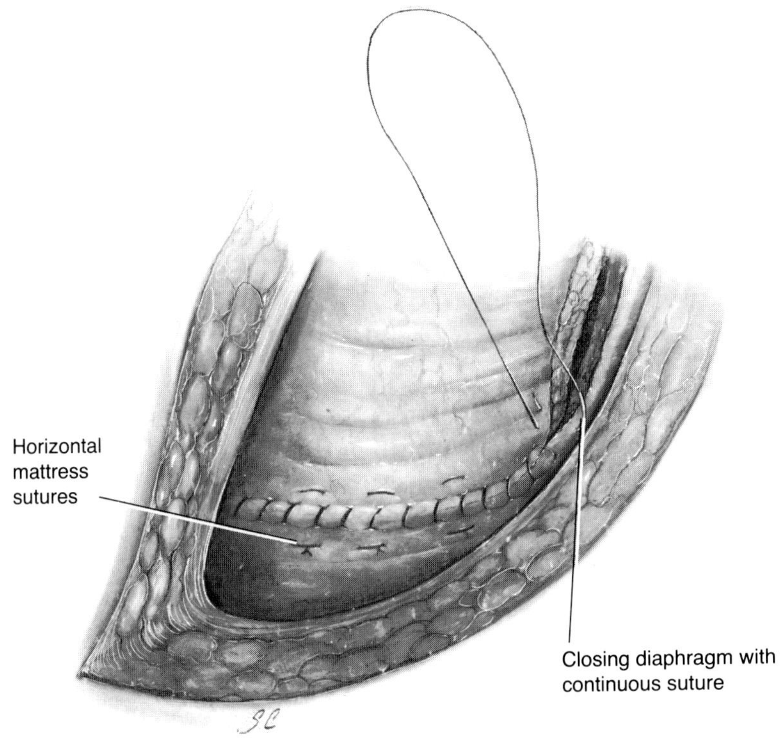

FIGURE 8–9. Following completion of the operative procedure, closure is begun with attention to the diaphragm. Although many different approaches are suitable, it is preferred to place multiple, widely spaced interrupted horizontal mattress sutures of nonabsorbable 2–0 braided material followed by a continuous suture of 3–0 monofilament. The previously placed marking stitches ensure accurate reapproximation. Retroperitoneal drainage is rarely needed. One or two chest tubes are placed two intercostal spaces below the chest incision if the seventh or higher interspace has been chosen for the incision. Otherwise, the chest tube exit site may be placed above the incision. In this instance, a right-angle tube is frequently used to ensure dependent drainage. The exit sites of the chest tubes are designed to be anterior to the midaxillary line for increased patient comfort.

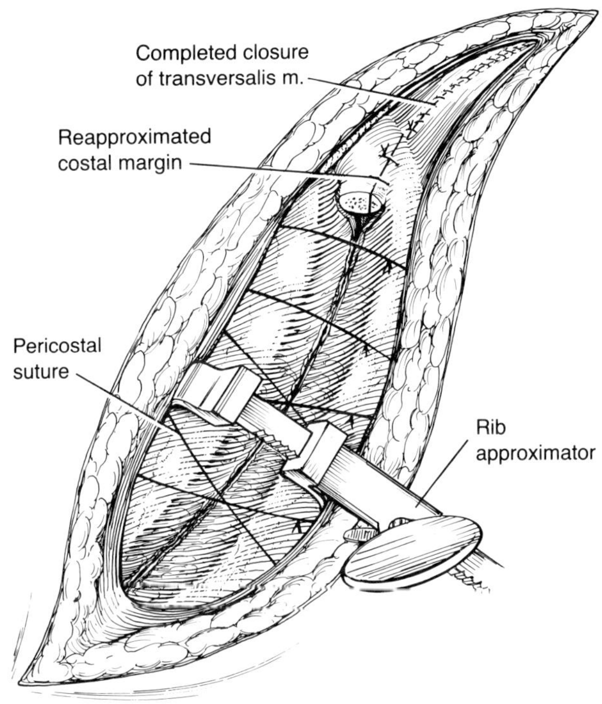

FIGURE 8–10

FIGURES 8–10 through 8–12. The chest tubes are fixed securely to the skin level with 2–0 or 1–0 sutures, and the ribs are reapproximated with #l chromic catgut suture. Care is taken to be certain that the sutures are placed to avoid the neurovascular bundles. If a rib has been excised, the periosteum is closed with a continuous suture. The fascial layers of the abdomen and chest are closed in an anatomic pattern. The previously divided costal margin is specifically reapproximated. Subcutaneous layers and skin are closed in the routine manner.

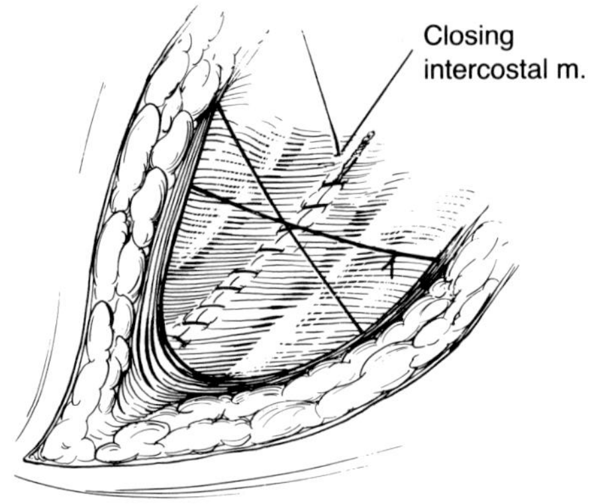

FIGURE 8–11

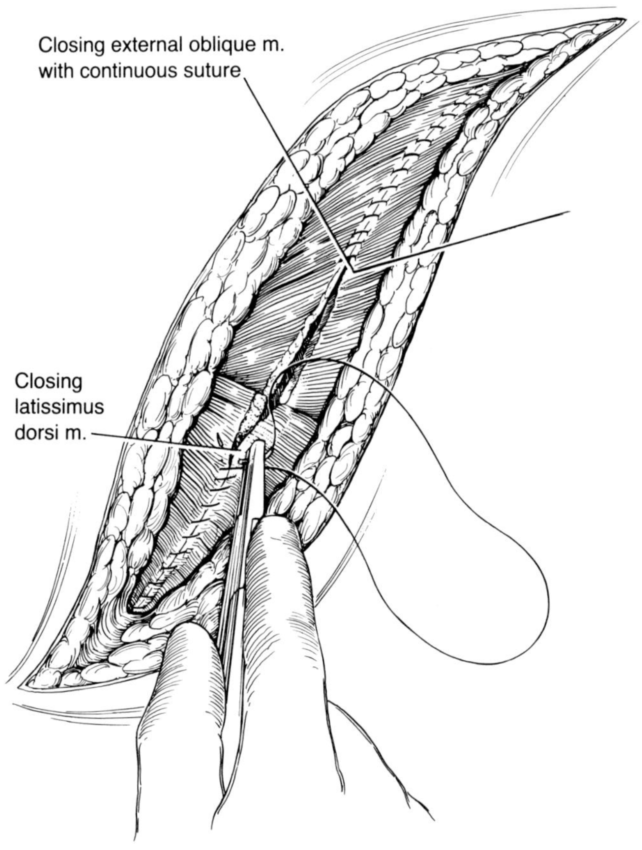

FIGURE 8–12

JAMES M. DOUGLAS, JR., M.D.

9

Thoracostomy

The presence of a pneumothorax may be considered an indication for chest tube placement and underwater drainage. However, there are certain situations in which chest tube placement is mandatory and others in which observation is an acceptable course. Clearly, patients showing signs and symptoms of a tension pneumothorax with respiratory and hemodynamic compromise require immediate placement of a chest tube. Likewise, simple pneumothorax in a patient with signs of respiratory distress should be treated with placement of a chest tube; and it is advisable in asymptomatic patients who have baseline respiratory compromise, signs of increasing pneumothorax, or a requirement for mechanical ventilatory support. Simple needle aspiration of a pneumothorax may be attempted in stable patients who are unlikely to have a source for continued air leakage into the pleural space. It should be remembered that when in doubt, one should err on the side of insertion of a chest tube in the presence of a documented pneumothorax. The procedure is easily performed using local anesthesia and, with proper attention to detail, can be accomplished with minimal patient discomfort.

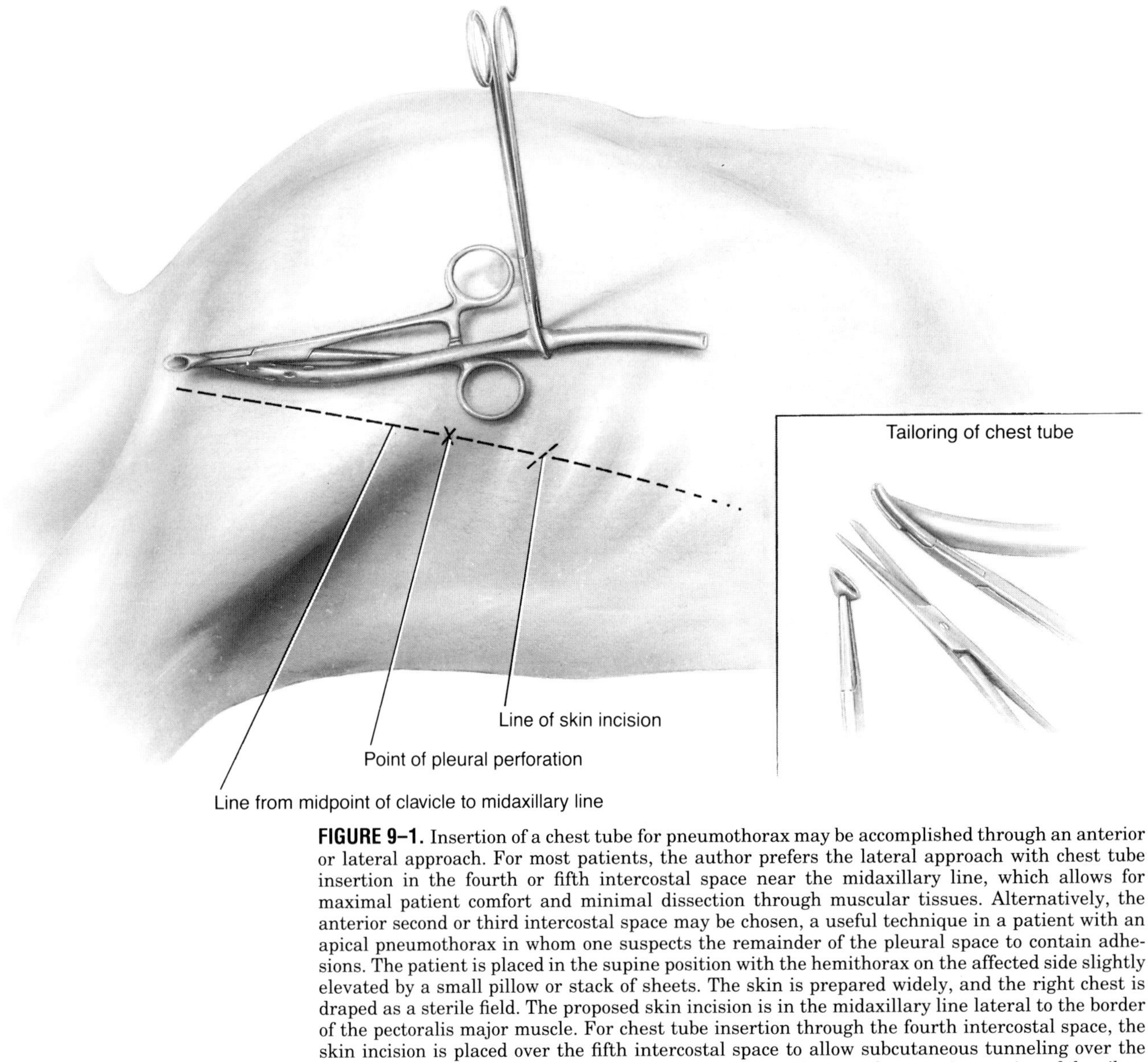

FIGURE 9–1. Insertion of a chest tube for pneumothorax may be accomplished through an anterior or lateral approach. For most patients, the author prefers the lateral approach with chest tube insertion in the fourth or fifth intercostal space near the midaxillary line, which allows for maximal patient comfort and minimal dissection through muscular tissues. Alternatively, the anterior second or third intercostal space may be chosen, a useful technique in a patient with an apical pneumothorax in whom one suspects the remainder of the pleural space to contain adhesions. The patient is placed in the supine position with the hemithorax on the affected side slightly elevated by a small pillow or stack of sheets. The skin is prepared widely, and the right chest is draped as a sterile field. The proposed skin incision is in the midaxillary line lateral to the border of the pectoralis major muscle. For chest tube insertion through the fourth intercostal space, the skin incision is placed over the fifth intercostal space to allow subcutaneous tunneling over the span of one rib, with subsequent insertion of the chest tube over the superior portion of the rib.

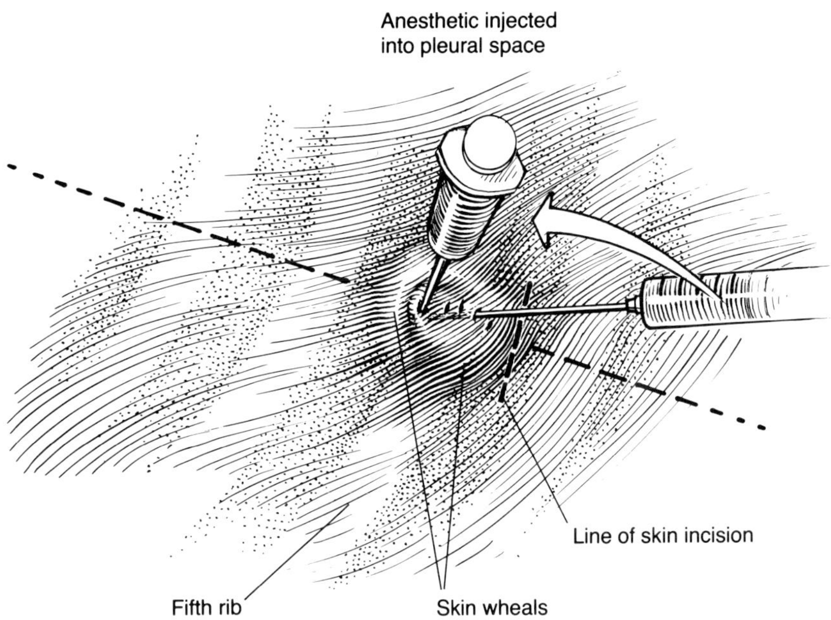

FIGURE 9–2. The proposed angle of insertion is outlined. It should be emphasized that the subsequent course of the chest tube is dictated by the angle between the skin incision and the chest entry site. If the angle is too medial, the chest tube passes across the mediastinum. If it is too posterior, the tube passes posterior to the lung. A skin wheal is raised at the proposed site of skin incision, with 1% lidocaine (without epinephrine) being sufficient. The subcutaneous tissue is infiltrated along the proposed tract overlying the fifth rib. A tiny skin wheal is raised over the fourth intercostal space. The longer 21-gauge needle is passed perpendicular to the skin, and lidocaine is infiltrated as the needle is passed over the superior border of the fifth rib into the intercostal space. As soon as aspiration of air confirms entry into the pleural space, the needle is withdrawn slightly and the bulk of the anesthetic agent is infused at the pleural surface and around the periosteum of the rib. It is important that an adequate volume of anesthetic be infused to allow diffusion throughout the sensitive pleural and periosteal regions. Usually, 15 to 20 ml of anesthetic agent is used.

While the anesthetic agent is diffusing through the tissues, attention is turned to selection of the chest tube and its preparation. A #24 or #28 French tube is typically selected, although smaller tubes may suffice. To assess the proper length of the tube to be inserted following accurate tube placement, the distal tip of the tube is placed at the level of the clavicle, and the proximal end is clamped at the level of the proposed skin incision.

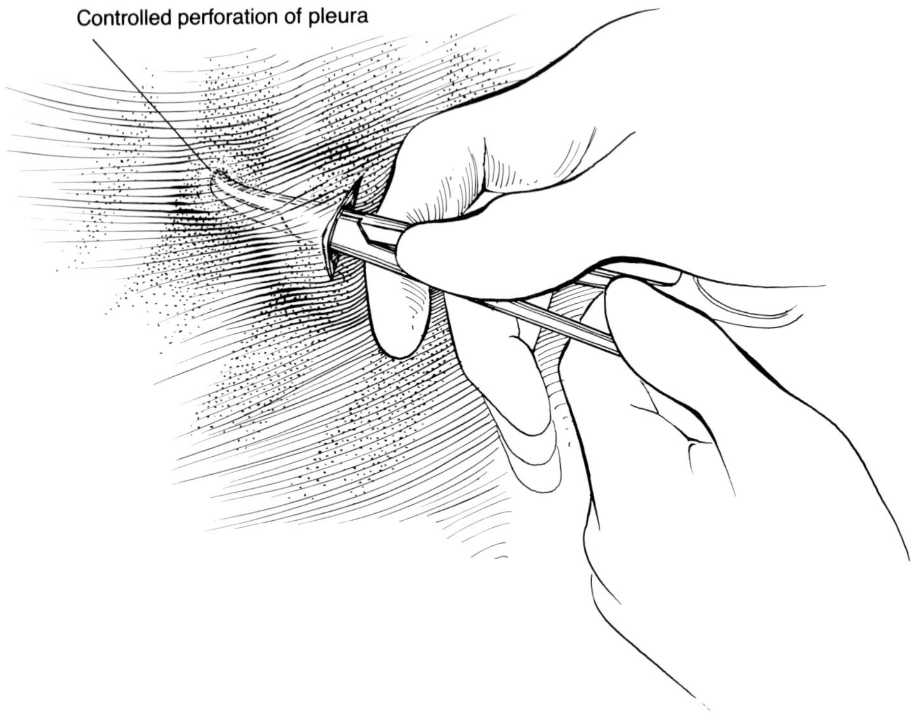

FIGURE 9–3. A Kelly clamp is placed on the tip of the chest tube, and the distal tip is tailored with the scissors to allow smooth passage through the patient's tissues. A skin incision approximately 1.5 cm in length is made, and the subcutaneous tissue is bluntly dissected using a second Kelly clamp. The tip of the clamp is passed over the top of the fifth rib, and downward pressure is applied to the underlying periosteum. The patient is questioned regarding possible pain generated by this pressure. If the anesthetic has been adequately administered, the patient should feel no pain. While the surgeon applies firm pressure with the dominant hand and countercontrol with the other hand, the Kelly clamp is passed forcefully over the top of the rib and through the intercostal space into the pleural cavity. Care should be taken to limit the degree of penetration to *just inside* the pleura. The underlying lung tissue may be damaged if the clamp is inserted too vigorously or placed improperly at the site of pleural adhesion.

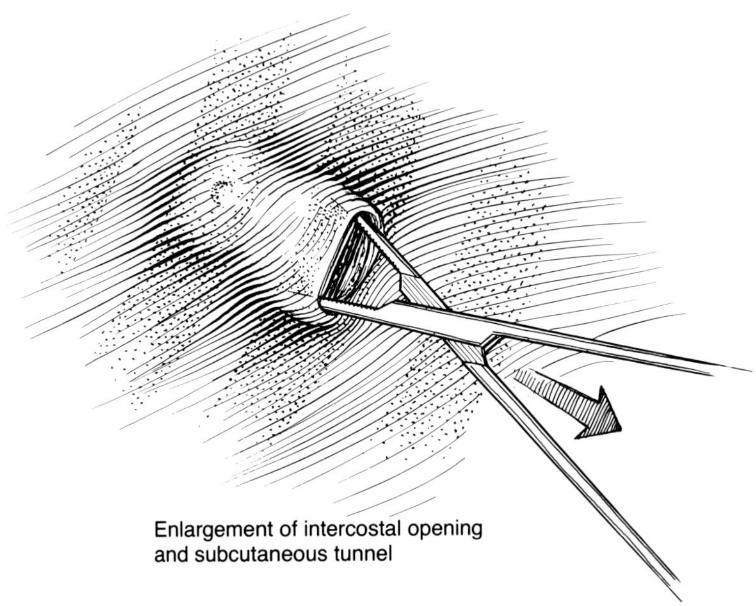

FIGURE 9–4. Once the pleural space has been entered, the Kelly clamp is spread open and a hiss of air exiting the pleural space is frequently heard. The Kelly clamp should be spread vigorously while it is being removed to produce a widely patent tract. If underlying adhesions are suspected, the gloved finger is inserted through the tract to palpate the pleural surfaces.

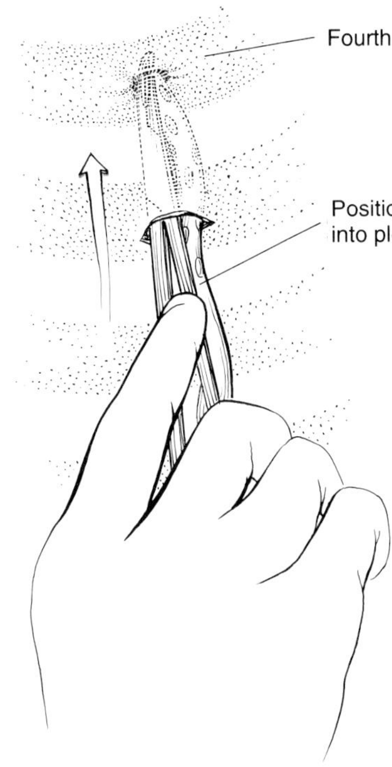

FIGURE 9–5

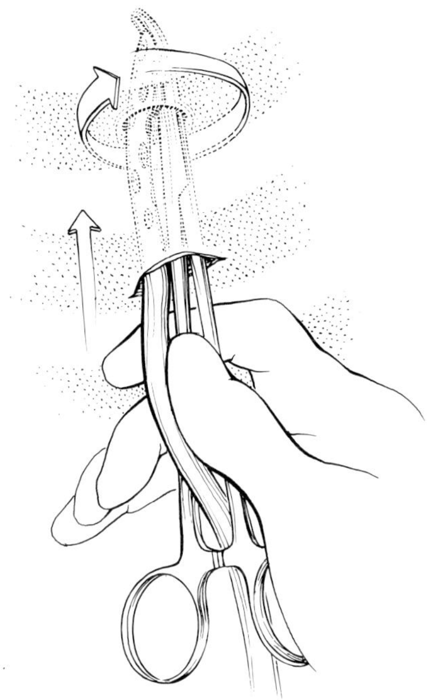

FIGURE 9–6

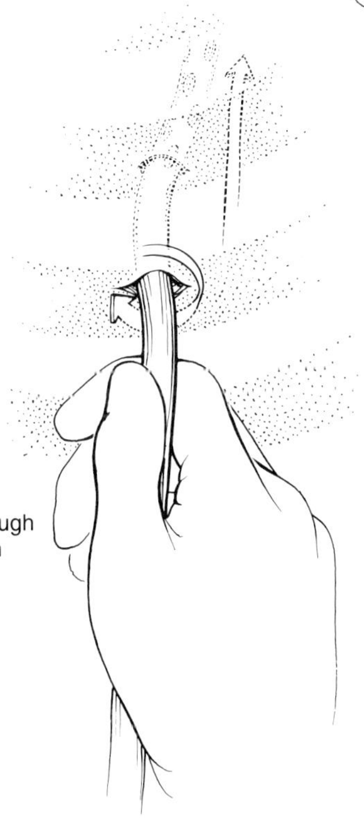

FIGURE 9–7

FIGURE 9–5. With the aid of the attached Kelly clamp, the chest tube is passed through the tract and into the pleural space.

FIGURE 9–6. The curve of the clamp should face downward as the tube is passed into the interspace and then turned upward toward the apex of the chest upon entry into the pleural space. This causes the tube to be directed toward the apex of the chest in a lateral or anterior position for optimal evacuation of air. Once the chest tube is confirmed within the pleural space, the Kelly clamp is withdrawn, with care taken to avoid dislodging the chest tube.

FIGURE 9–7. The tube is passed to the apex of the chest. As the tube is passed, it should be rotated gently to confirm that kinking of the tube has not occurred. It must be emphasized that passage of the tube should be smooth and facile; otherwise, improper placement must be suspected.

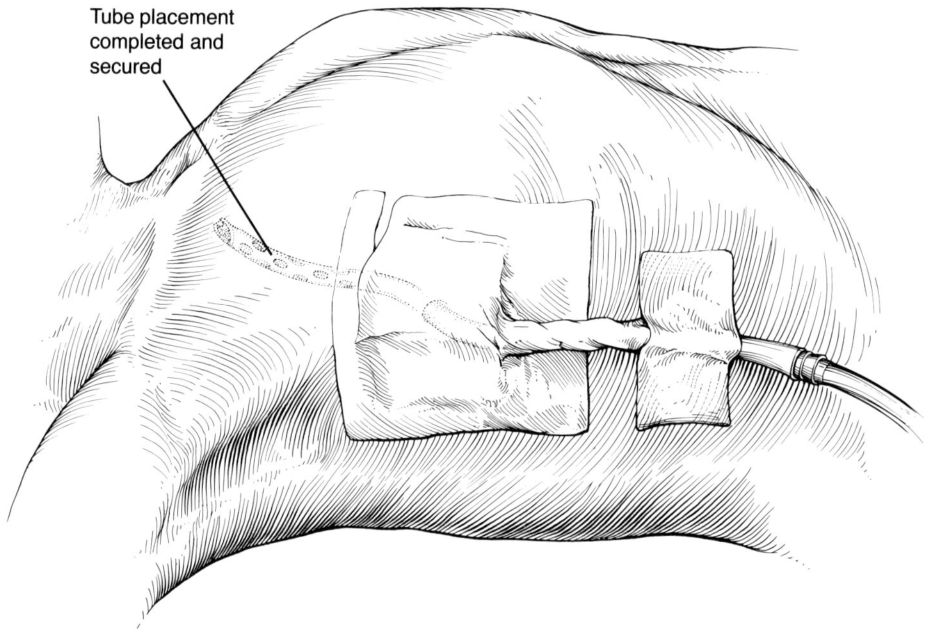

FIGURE 9–8. The chest tube is connected to underwater drainage and fixed at the skin level with two heavy sutures. The site is dressed sterilely, and the tube fixation reinforced with tape applied to the skin. An immediate chest film is obtained to confirm the proper position of the tube and evacuation of the pneumothorax cavity.

SECTION III

Tracheal Procedures

PATRICK D. KENAN, M.D.

10

Tracheostomy

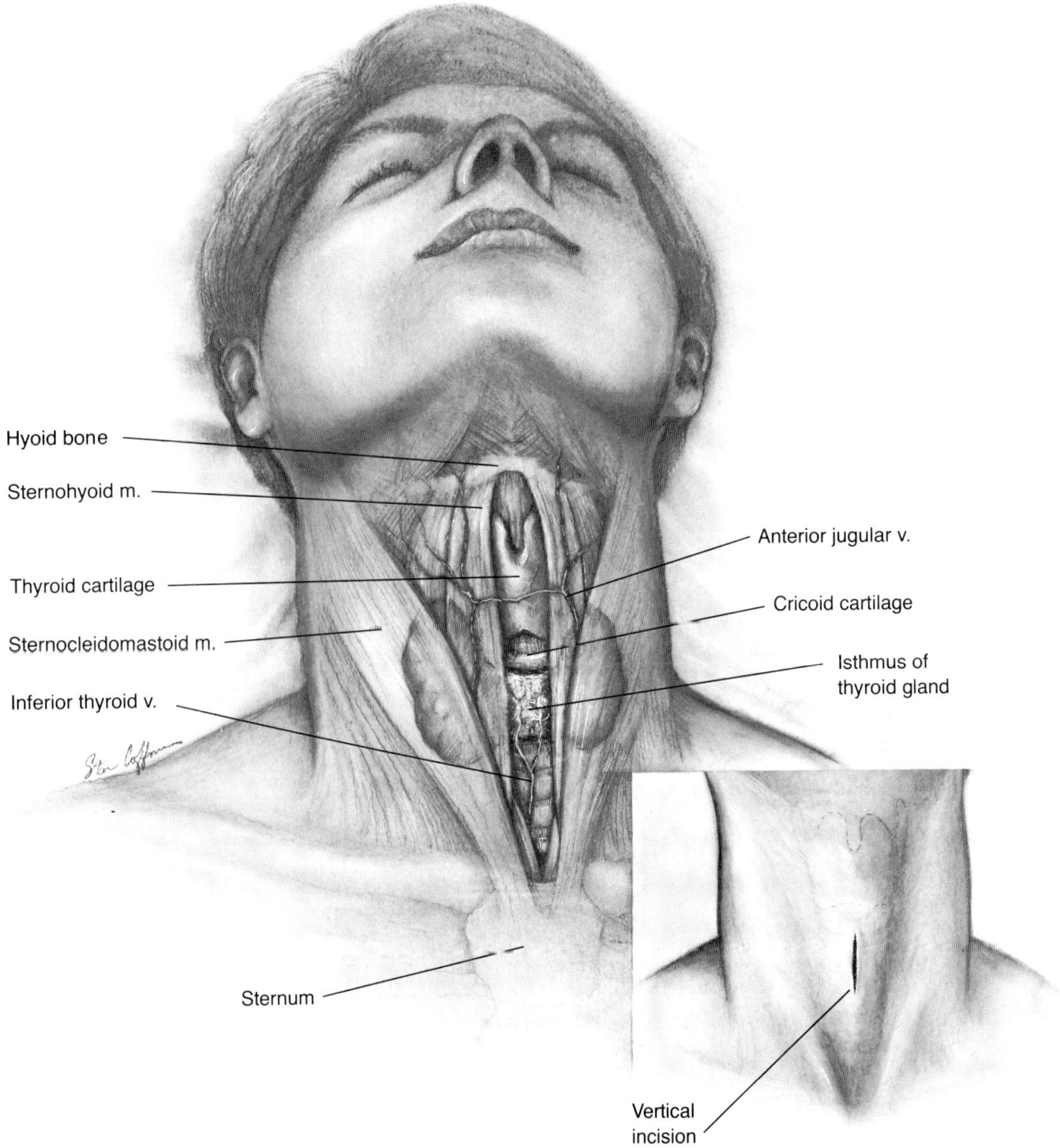

FIGURE 10–1. The anatomy of the anterior neck varies widely, creating problems of tracheal access in the short "bull neck" patient. Careful palpation of the surface anatomy should clearly identify the cricoid cartilage and, therefore, the trachea that is to be exposed immediately below the cricoid. Except in extraordinary circumstances, a tracheostomy should be done in the operating room, because adequate headlight illumination and operating room support systems and monitors, including anesthesia, pulse oximetry, suction, cautery, cardioscope, and so forth, are required. When chest tubes, intravascular catheters, and monitors make transfer to an operating table difficult, tracheostomy may be performed with the patient in a hospital bed, but the procedure is preferably performed in the operating room.

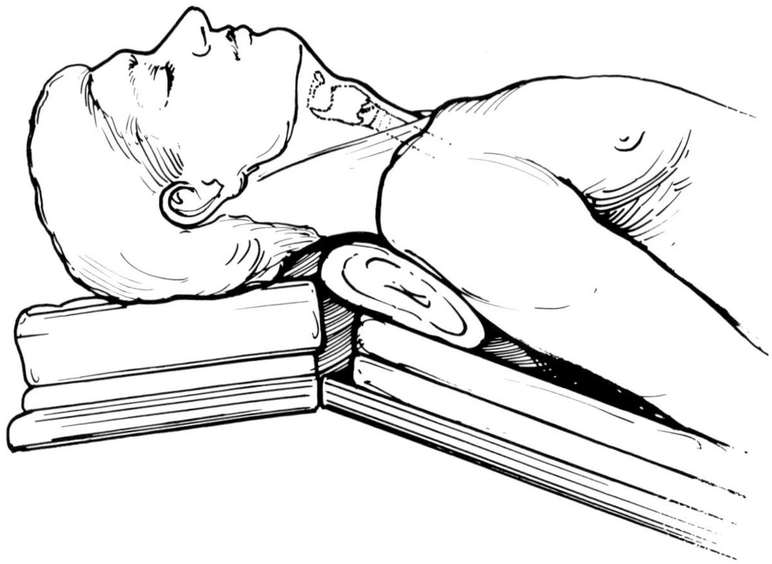

FIGURE 10–2. The patient's position is that of reverse Trendelenburg or the semi-Fowler position, with the trunk elevated, thus reducing venous pressure in the neck and abdominal visceral pressure against the diaphragm. The shoulders are further elevated with a folded sheet to produce slight hyperextension of the neck, and the area is prepped from above the hyoid bone to below the clavicles.

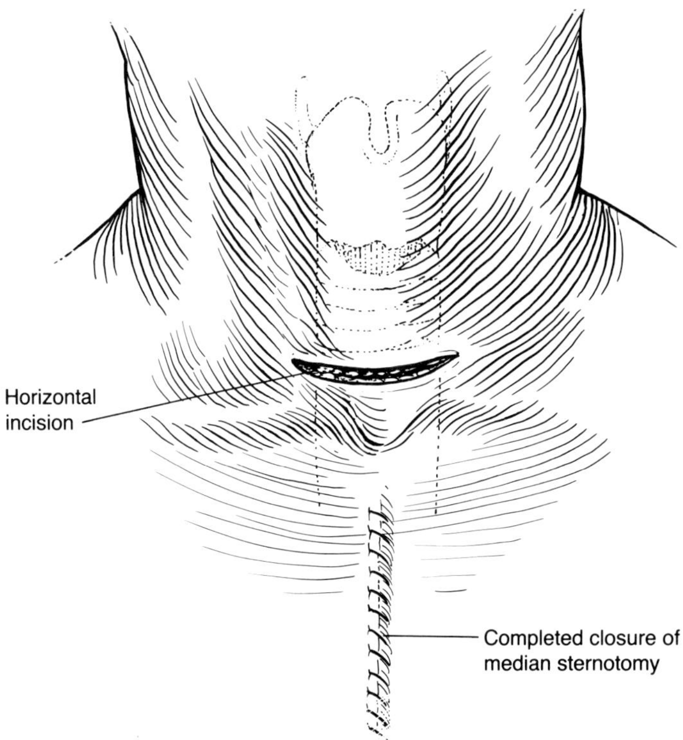

FIGURE 10–3. Except for temporary, emergency tube placement, cricothyrotomy is discouraged because of increased risk of subglottic stenosis. A vertical skin incision is usually desirable and minimizes the pressure erosion of the flange of the tracheotomy tube. However, a transverse incision is preferred if a fresh sternotomy incision is present, to avoid communication between the tracheostomy wound and the mediastinum. Bleeding sites are carefully cauterized for hemostasis.

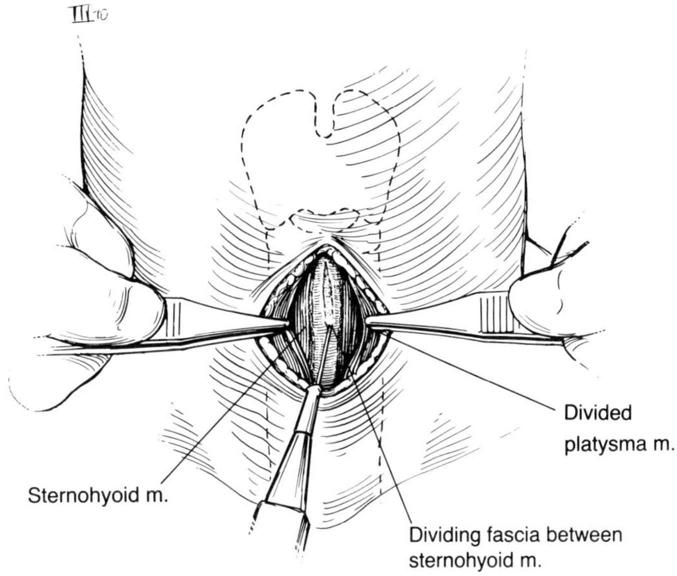

FIGURE 10–4. The incision is continued through the platysma muscle. Retraction is by forceps or right-angle retractors, applied in equal and opposite directions at the same tissue depth. Dissection continues in the midline, either by scissors or Bovie cautery, separating the two layers of strap muscles. Hemostasis is maintained throughout, with smaller vessels cauterized and the larger veins and arteries ligated. The thyroid isthmus is usually visible after the strap muscles are separated and retracted.

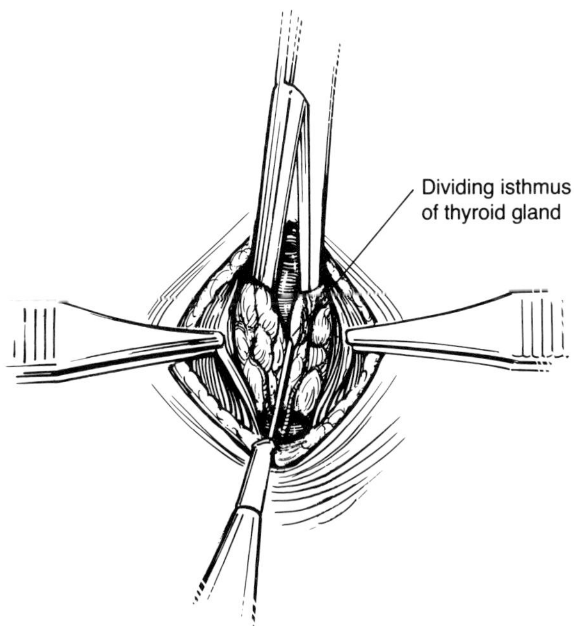

FIGURE 10–5. Because of the vascularity of the thyroid, the isthmus can be divided either by clamping, cutting, and ligating the cut edges, or, in some cases, by slow cautery dissection, usually over an opened clamp beneath the isthmus.

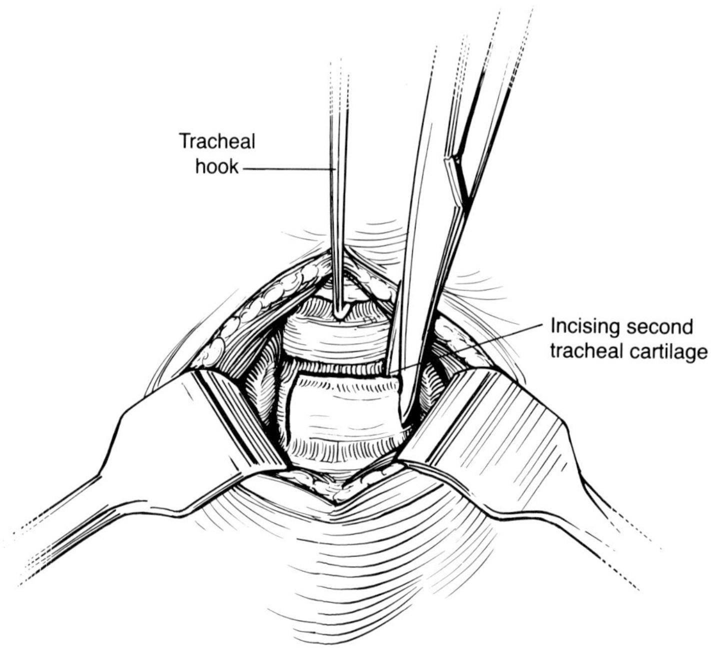

FIGURE 10–6. The upper trachea is exposed by triangulated retraction using a tracheal hook at the cricoid and angled retractors laterally and inferiorly. The pretracheal fascia is separated to expose the cartilage rings, and the cuff of the endotracheal tube is deflated to allow an incision to be made into the trachea without the risk of rupturing the cuff. Several different types of tracheal incisions may be made, including cruciate and T incision, or excised buttons of anterior tracheal wall. The author prefers an inferiorly based flap of anterior tracheal wall, made by incising horizontally between the first and second, or second and third, tracheal rings and making vertical lateral incisions through the ring below the incision. Later, following extubation, this type of flap allows healing with the least stricturing effect. Although the incised tracheal mucosa may bleed briskly, it is not appropriate to use cauterization for hemostasis if oxygen is being delivered, because of risk of airway fire. The tracheotomy tube itself is usually sufficient tamponade to control bleeding of the mucosa. Once the tracheal incision is made, use of the Trousseau dilator is not recommended, because it tears rather than dilates the incision.

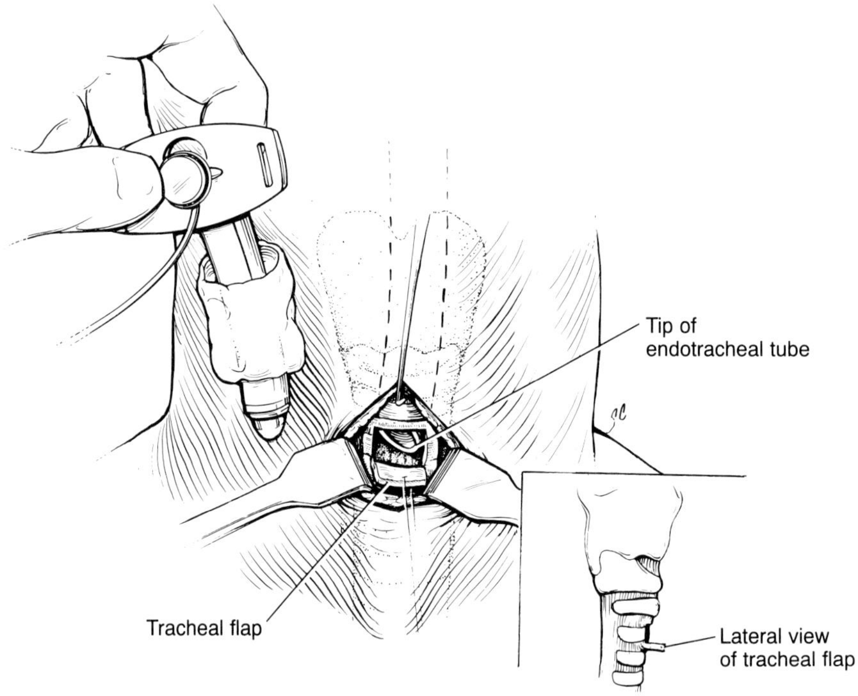

FIGURE 10–7. The tracheal flap may be retracted anteriorly or anchored to the skin with stay sutures to permit easier change of tracheotomy tubes if desired. The endotracheal tube is retracted under visual control until the tip of the tube clears the tracheal stoma sufficient to introduce the tracheotomy tube.

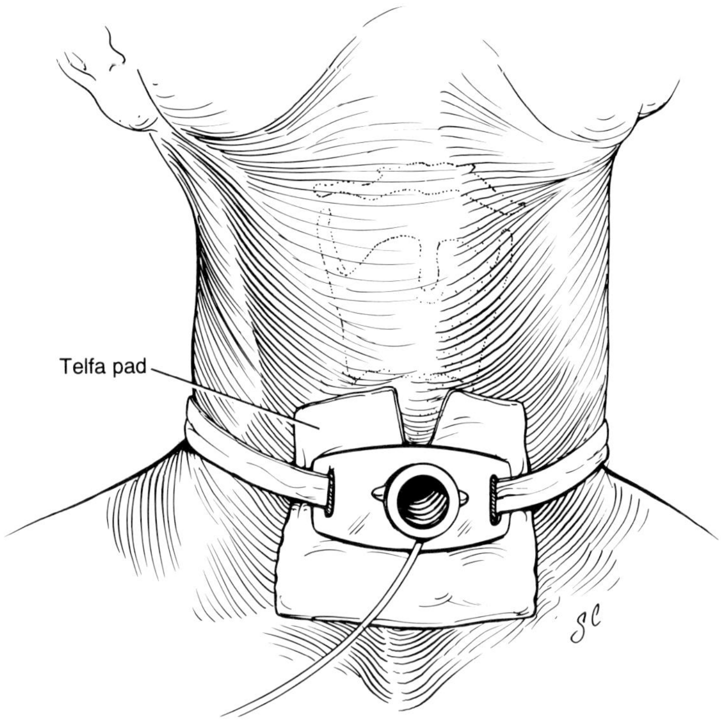

FIGURE 10–8. With the tracheotomy tube fully introduced into the trachea, the cuff is inflated and ventilatory support is transferred to the tracheostomy. The tube is secured by tying the neck straps. The endotracheal tube is removed only when it is evident that satisfactory ventilation is present via tracheostomy. The wound may be loosely closed with one or more skin sutures. A pad is placed under the tracheotomy tube. Meticulous suction using a sterile catheter is appropriate to clear the tracheobronchial tree after the tracheotomy tube is placed and secured, and again before the patient is returned from the operating room.

EXTUBATION NOTES

(1) Change to smaller and uncuffed metal (or plastic) tracheotomy tube when the patient no longer has a compromised airway or requires ventilatory support. (2) Consider 24 hours of full cork application, because there is rarely a need for partial corks. (3) If the patient is breathing well around a fully corked tracheotomy tube, extubation can be done with full expectation of an adequate airway. (4) Usually a dry dressing is applied over the stoma and is all that is necessary during healing by secondary intention. The patient should be instructed to use hand or finger pressure to reinforce the dressing when talking or coughing until the stoma is sealed. (5) Silver nitrate cauterization may be necessary to eliminate stomal granulation. (6) Fiberoptic monitoring of endotracheal healing can be done if one suspects endotracheal granulations, which, if present, may warrant laser or other endoscopic removal.

JAMES E. LOWE, M.D.

11

Correction of Tracheal Stenosis

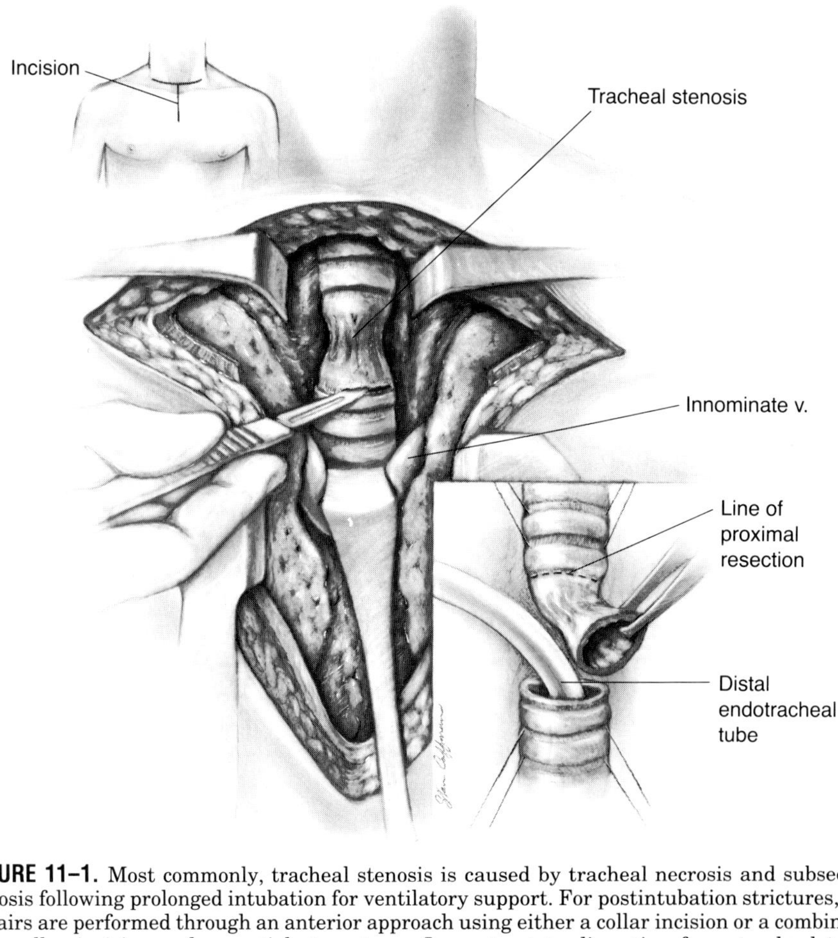

FIGURE 11–1. Most commonly, tracheal stenosis is caused by tracheal necrosis and subsequent fibrosis following prolonged intubation for ventilatory support. For postintubation strictures, most repairs are performed through an anterior approach using either a collar incision or a combination of a collar incision and a partial sternotomy. In contrast to dissection for a tracheal tumor, dissection for this problem is kept very close to the trachea to avoid injury to the recurrent laryngeal nerves. As recommended by Grillo, stenoses are dilated prior to anesthesia if they are smaller than 6 mm in diameter to provide adequate intraoperative ventilation. The trachea is divided just below the stenotic lesion, and the distal trachea is then intubated directly.

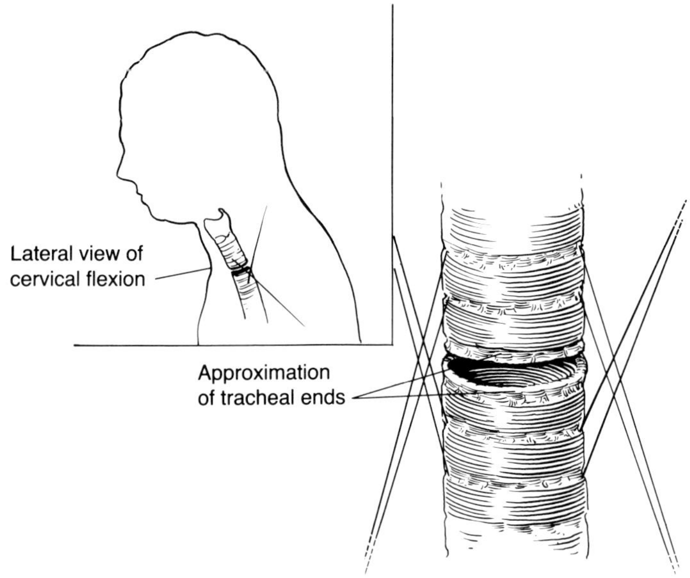

FIGURE 11–2. The dissection proceeds superiorly, allowing for separation of the area of stricture, which may be densely adherent to the esophagus posteriorly. Following complete resection of the stenosis, traction sutures can be temporarily placed for approximation of the tracheal ends.

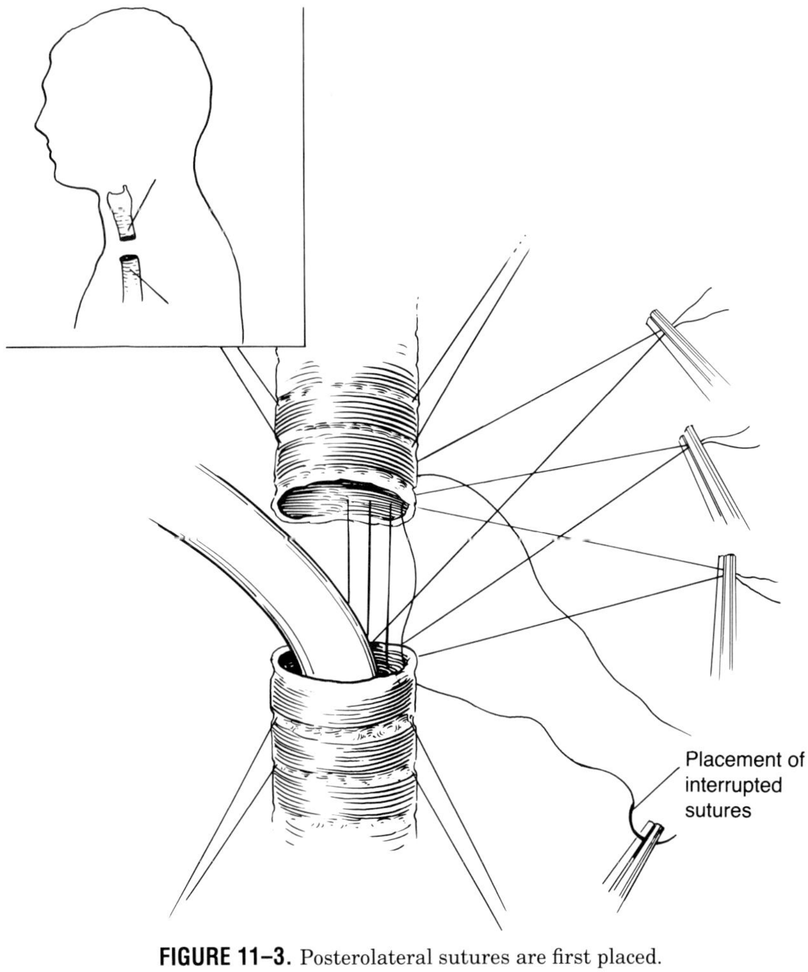

FIGURE 11–3. Posterolateral sutures are first placed.

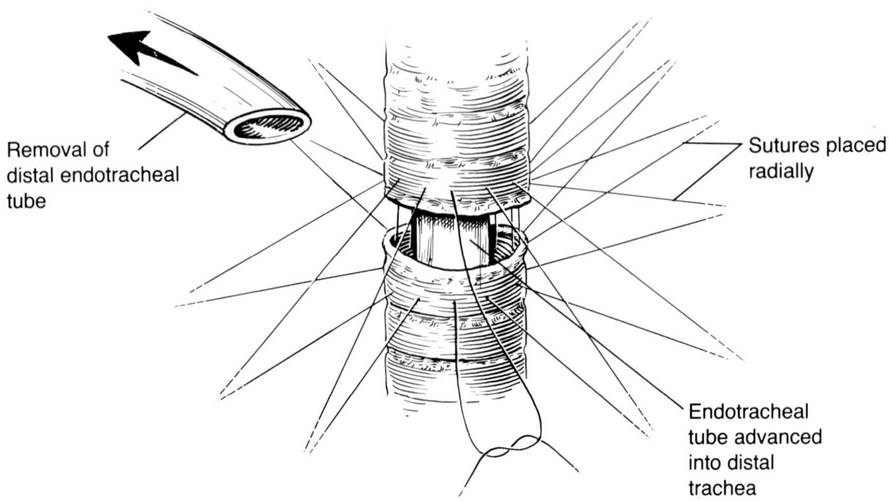

FIGURE 11–4. The endotracheal tube in the distal trachea is removed and advanced back into the trachea from above.

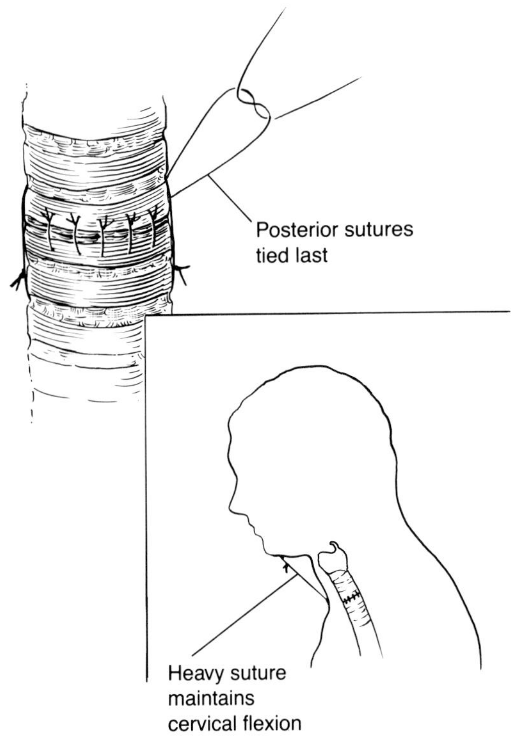

FIGURE 11–5. Sutures are tied from front to back, and all knots are placed on the outside of the trachea. Absorbable sutures of 4–0 Vicryl are used for the anastomosis. The posterior sutures are tied last, and cervical fixation is maintained using a heavy suture from the chin to the fascia over the sternum to prevent tension on the tracheal anastomosis.

JAMES E. LOWE, M.D.

12

Resection of Trachea for Neoplasms

For many years, surgical resection of tracheal tumors was limited because it was thought that only 2 cm of the trachea (approximately four rings) could be removed with the ends safely reanastomosed. However, various techniques pioneered by Grillo have permitted resection of as much as half of the trachea with primary reconstruction. In all dissections involving the trachea, it is of critical importance that the lateral segmental blood supply be preserved. Tumors involving the upper trachea are generally approached through a collar incision, combined if necessary with a partial sternotomy, as described earlier for the treatment of tracheal stenoses. Tumors of the lower trachea are best approached through a right posterolateral thoracotomy in the fourth intercostal space. However, the cervical region is prepared into the operative field in the event that laryngeal release or another lengthening maneuver is required.

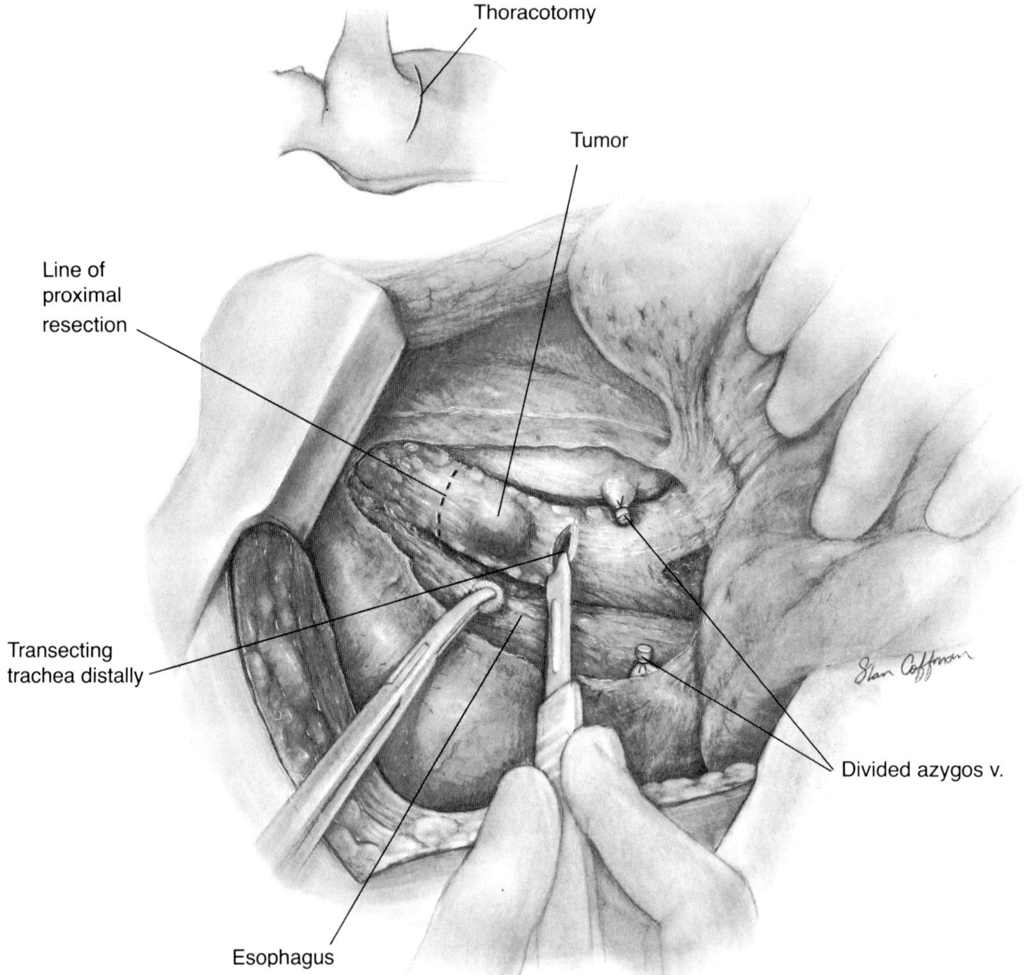

FIGURE 12–1. Through a right posterolateral thoracotomy in the fourth intercostal space, the distal trachea containing the tumor mass is gently mobilized. If necessary, the inferior pulmonary ligament may be divided and the hilar region dissected to provide mobilization of the distal trachea.

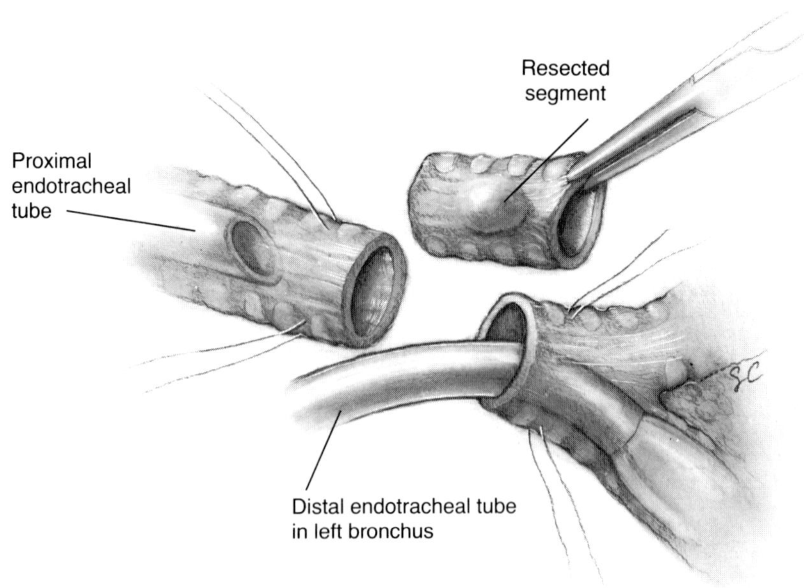

FIGURE 12–2. The distal trachea containing the tumor is resected with adequate margins based on intraoperative frozen sections, and the left lung is intubated across the operative field.

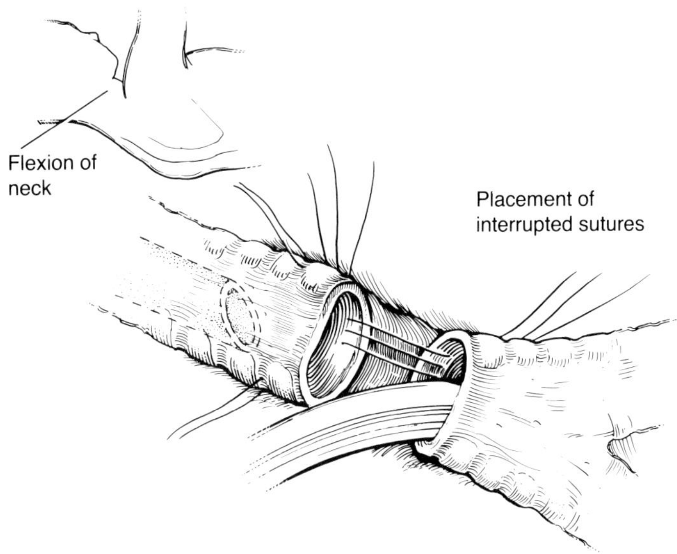

FIGURE 12–3

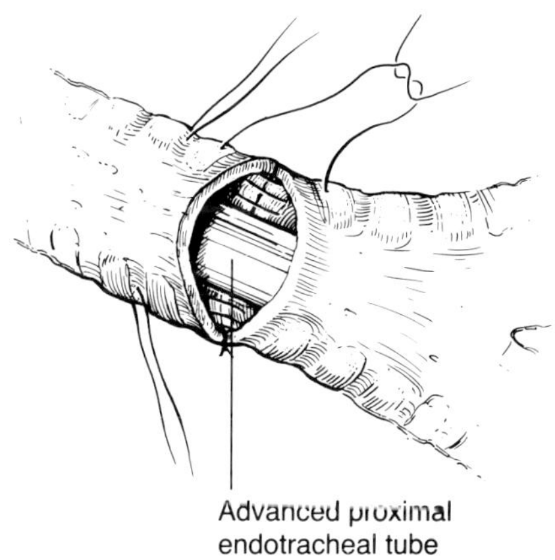

FIGURE 12–4

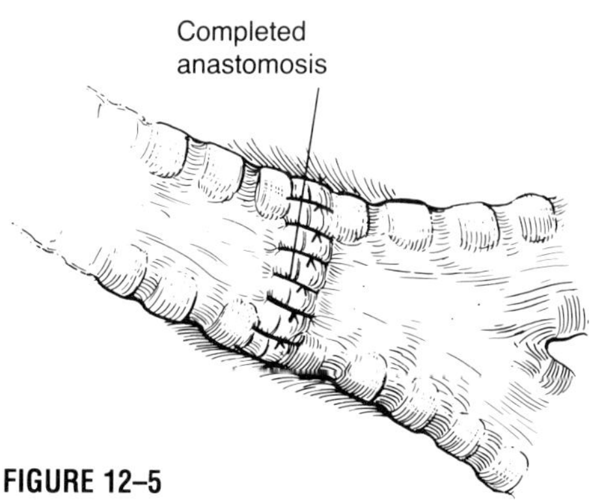

FIGURE 12–5

FIGURE 12–3. The right pulmonary artery may be temporarily clamped if there is significant shunting and hypoxemia. Left lateral and anterior tracheal sutures are placed.

FIGURE 12–4. The endotracheal tube is removed from the left main bronchus and replaced with a long endotracheal tube from above.

FIGURE 12–5. The primary anastomosis is completed using simple interrupted sutures of 4–0 Vicryl.

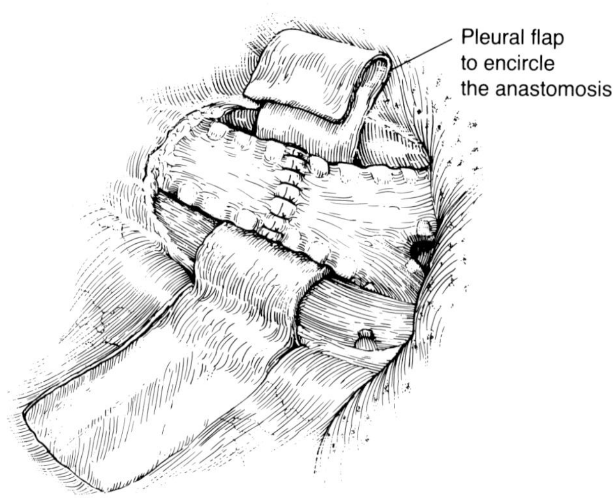

FIGURE 12–6. The suture line is protected using a pleural flap placed around the anastomosis.

SECTION IV

Congenital Deformities of the Sternum

DAVID C. SABISTON, JR., M.D.

13

Correction of Pectus Excavatum

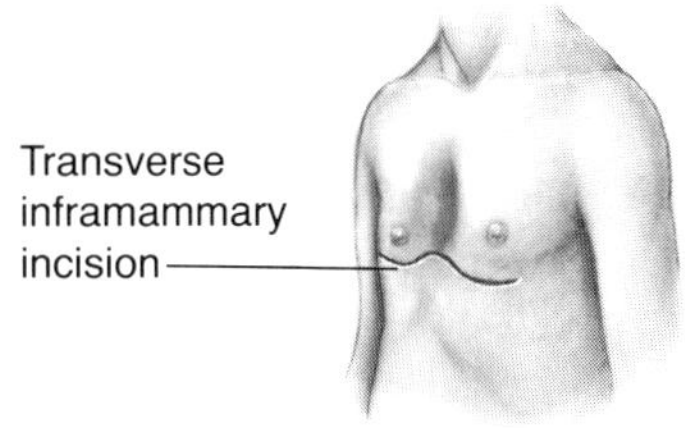

FIGURE 13–2

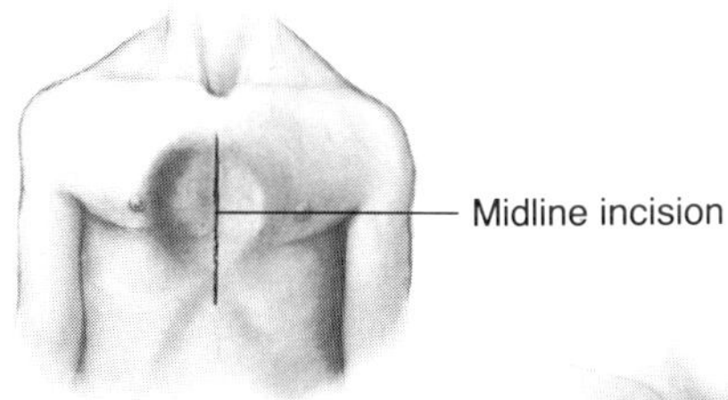

FIGURE 13–1

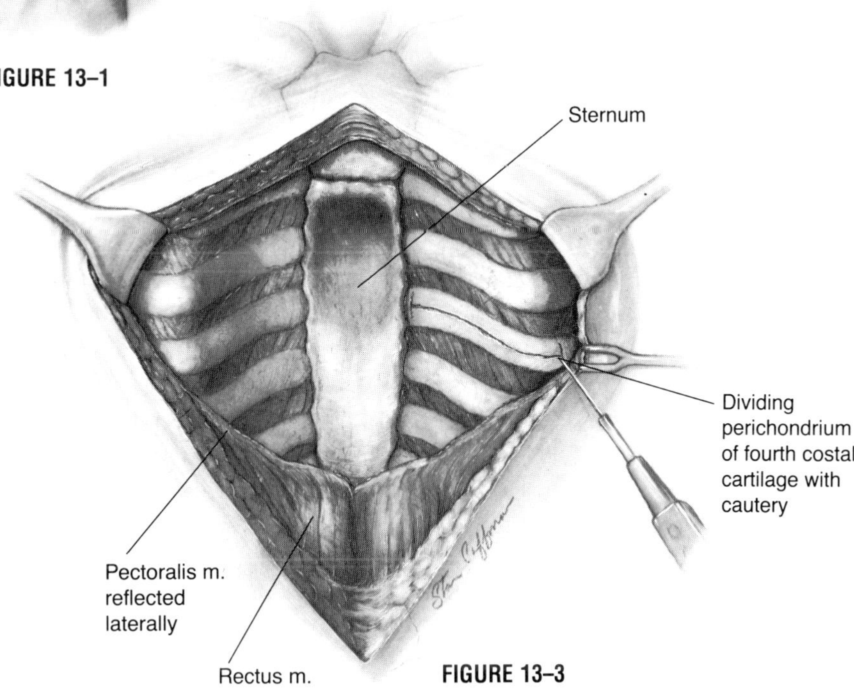

FIGURE 13–3

FIGURE 13–1. In most adult males and in children, the incision is generally vertical in the midline from approximately the sternomanubrial junction to the epigastrium.

FIGURE 13–2. In females, the incision is often transverse (submammary) in the fold of the breast to improve the cosmetic appearance of the scar.

FIGURE 13–3. The costal cartilages are exposed by elevation of the pectoral muscles. The plane of dissection is in the fascial layer beneath the pectoralis major muscles, which exposes the sternum and the costal cartilages. The dissection is preferably performed with a fine-needle cautery. It is especially important to dissect the lower costal cartilages. All of the involved cartilages are exposed.

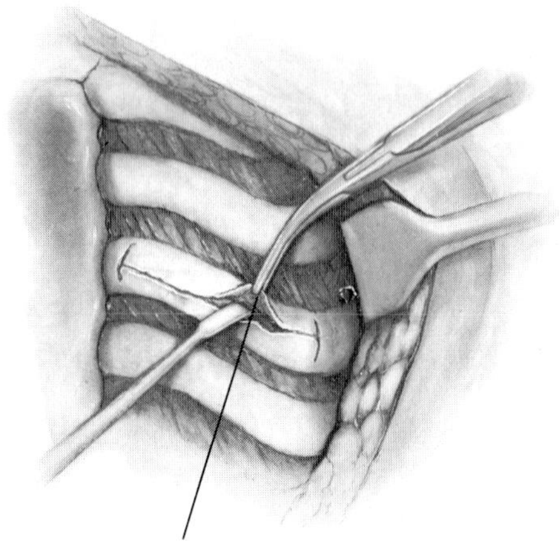

FIGURE 13–4

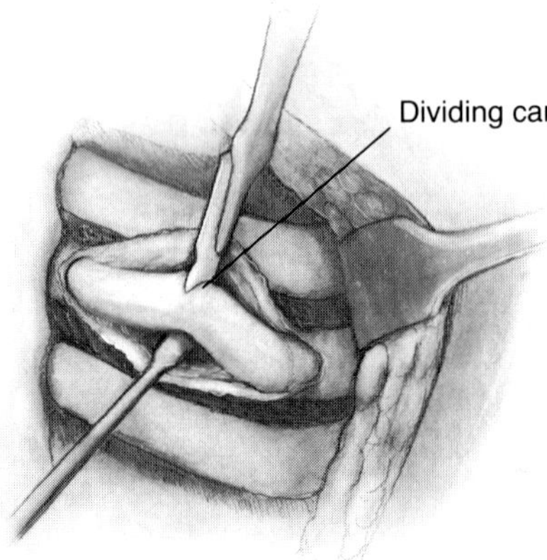

FIGURE 13–5

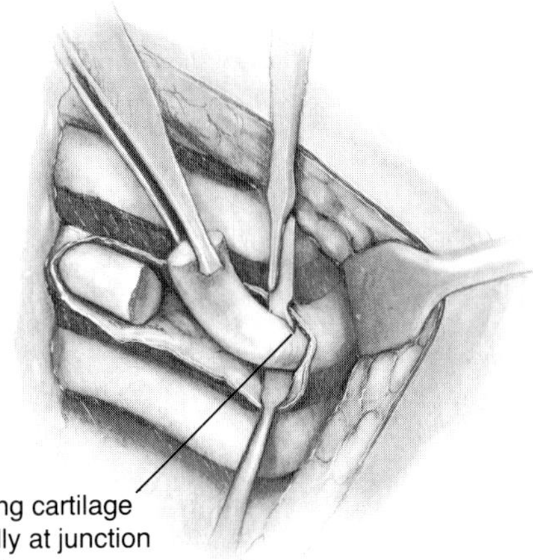

FIGURE 13–6

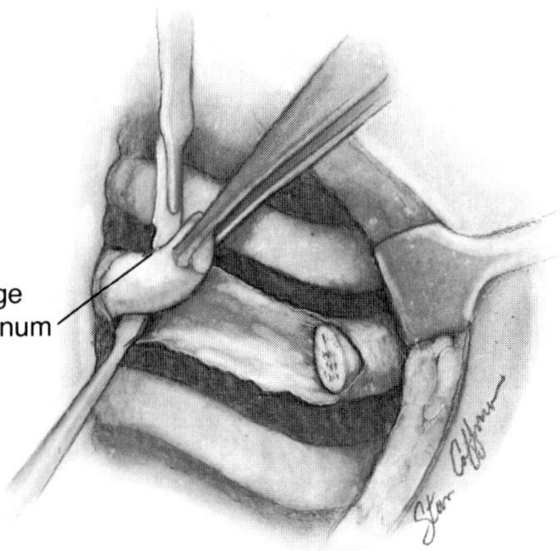

FIGURE 13–7

FIGURE 13–4. The perichondrium is dissected from the cartilage by first incising the perichondrium with the electrocautery and elevating it with a Joseph or similar elevator.

FIGURE 13–5. A tunnel is made using the periosteal elevator beneath the costal cartilage in its midposition, with the perichondrium being completely freed in this tunnel. A scalpel is introduced to divide the cartilages, with the cutting edge of the blade directed superiorly to prevent damage to important posterior structures should the blade slip while the cartilage is being divided.

FIGURE 13–6. With anterior traction on the costal segments, the anterior and posterior perichondrium can easily be stripped from the cartilage.

FIGURE 13–7. The dissection is taken laterally to the costochondral junctions and medially to the sternum. The deformed cartilages are then excised. From the perichondrial bed that remains, new costal cartilages will develop in the correct position. The cartilages are dissected from the second cartilage to those inferiorly.

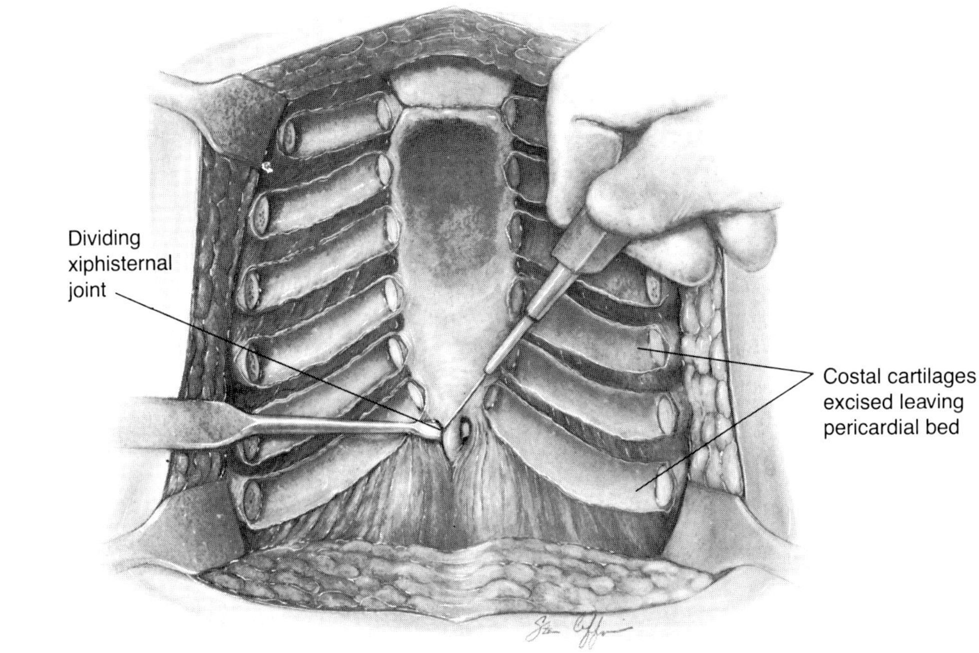

FIGURE 13–8. The deformed costal cartilages have been removed subperichondrially for the complete extent of the defect, and the xiphoid process is dissected prior to division from the sternum. The dissection is performed with a combination of the needle cautery and an elevator.

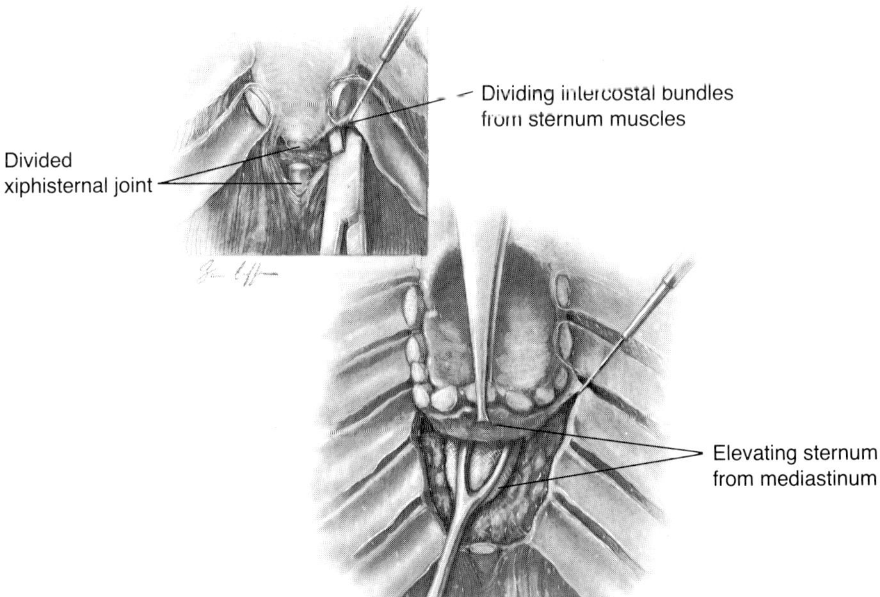

FIGURE 13–9. The lowest attachment of the perichondrium to the sternum is divided bilaterally. The sternum is elevated anteriorly by an assistant as the index finger is inserted beneath the xiphoid and the sternum to free the attached tissue between the posterior sternum and the pleura bilaterally. The perichondrial attachments are divided, and the retrosternal dissection extends proximally to the sternomanubrial junction. All intercostal bundles are completely divided from the sternum with the cautery, with the line of division being *medial* to the internal mammary arteries.

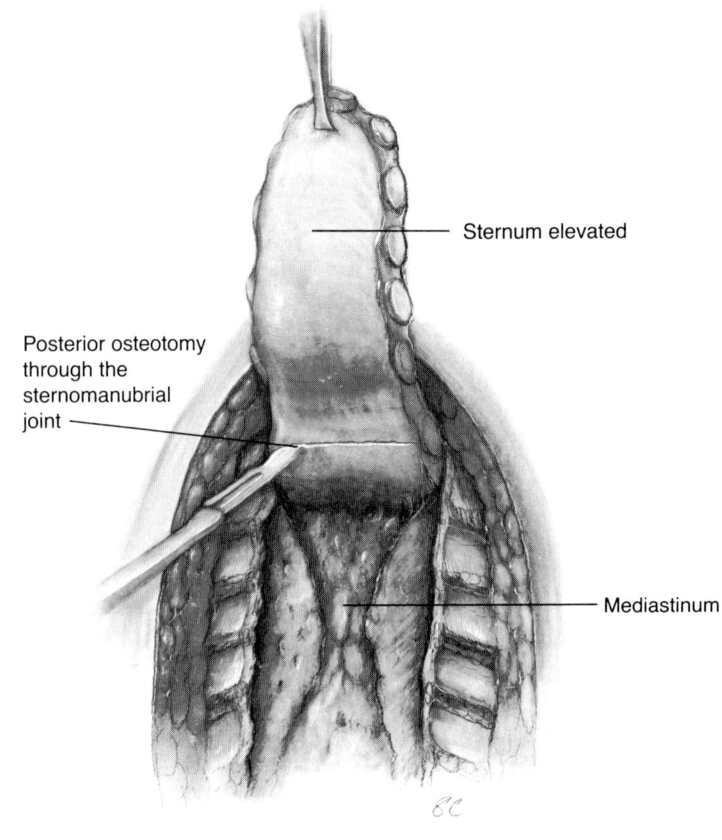

FIGURE 13–10. The posterior sternum is completely freed of attachments to the mediastinum, and a posterior osteotomy is made in the sternomanubrial junction.

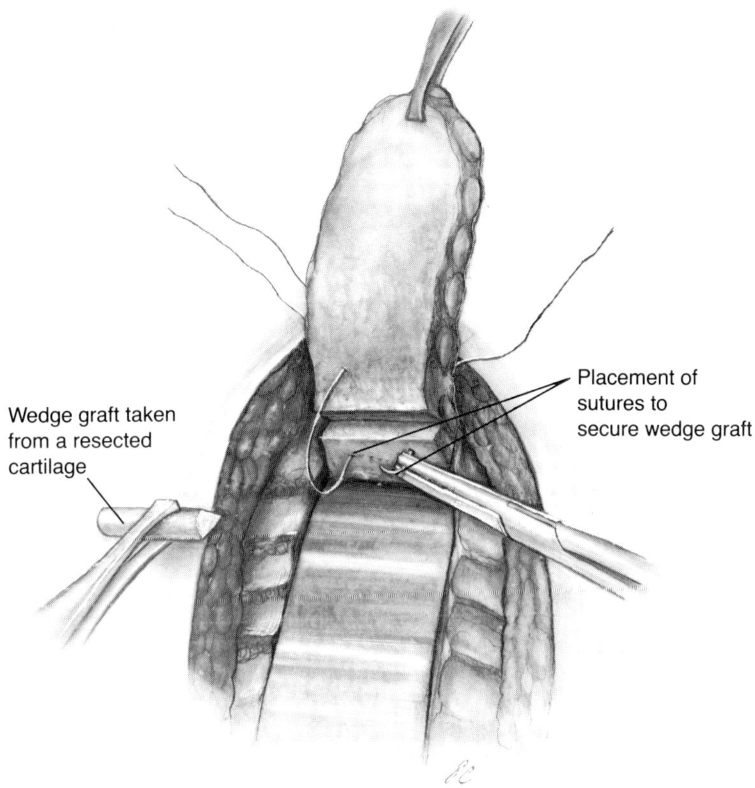

FIGURE 13–11. Two sutures are placed as shown using a cutting needle and a 2–0 monofilament suture above and below the osteotomy. A wedge of rib or of cartilage is inserted posteriorly and encircled by the sutures, which are tied in place. This permits an anterior "overcorrection" of the defect to achieve the best cosmetic result.

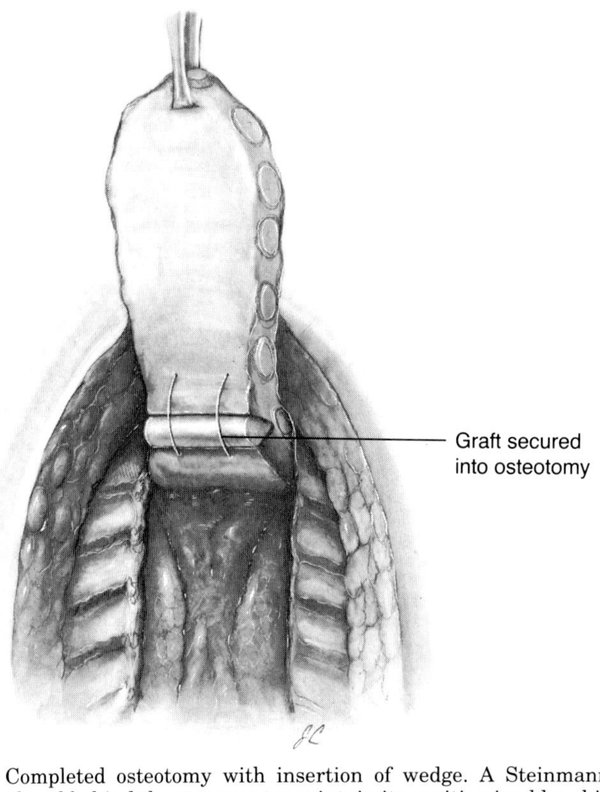

FIGURE 13–12. Completed osteotomy with insertion of wedge. A Steinmann pin (or similar support) is often placed behind the sternum to maintain its position in older children and adults.

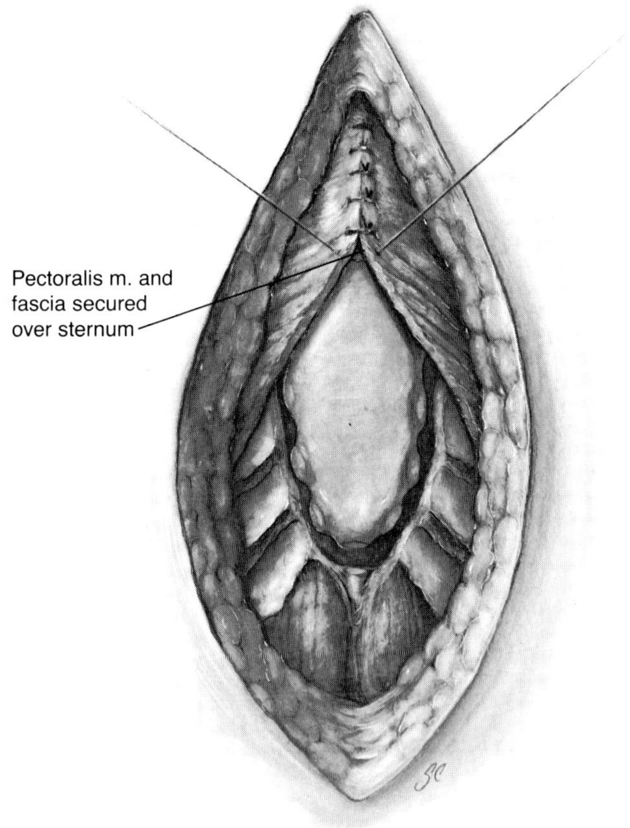

FIGURE 13–13. The pectoralis fascia is sutured in the midline, followed by closure of the subcutaneous tissue and the skin. A suction drain (Jackson-Pratt) is placed in the mediastinum and led out laterally through a separate stab wound for drainage.

DAVID C. SABISTON, JR., M.D.

14

Correction of Pectus Carinatum

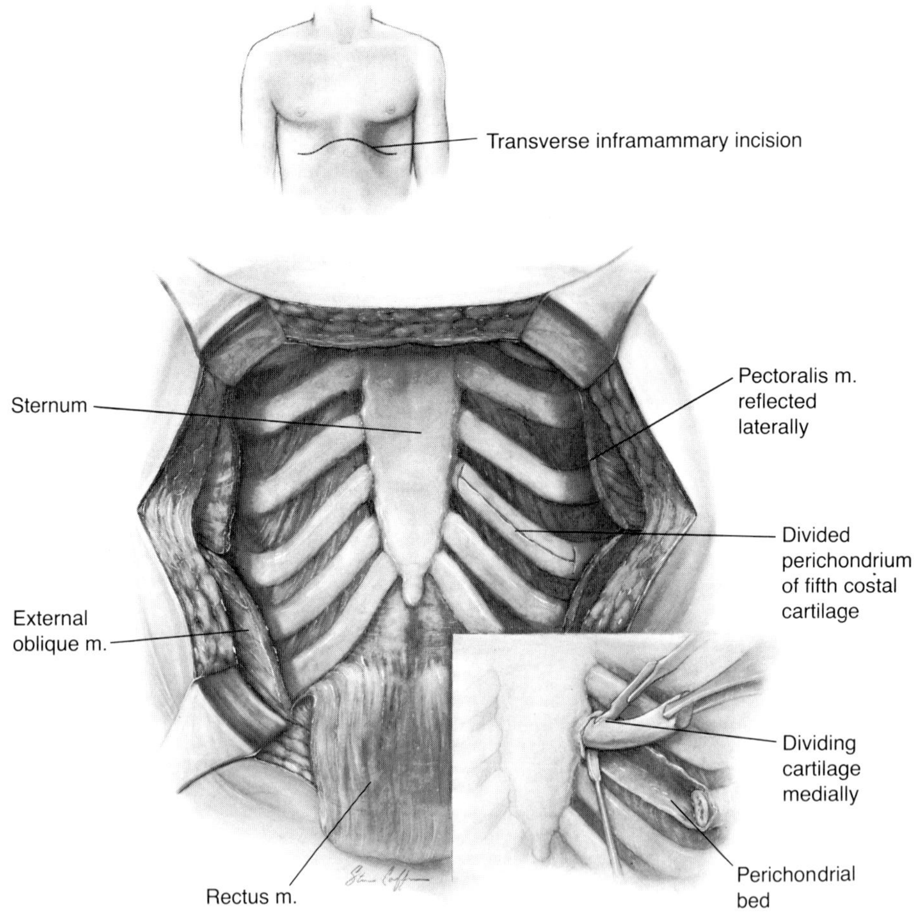

FIGURE 14–1. A transverse (or vertical) incision is made. The subcutaneous tissues are divided, exposing the pectoral muscles. With retraction of the skin flaps, a longitudinal incision is made overlying the sternum in the pectoral fascia. The dissection is directed toward the right and left with elevation of the pectoral muscles bilaterally, thus widely exposing the costal cartilages bilaterally on both sides. The rectus muscles are freed inferiorly and retracted. *Lower inset,* The perichondrium of each costal cartilage is then dissected as in the procedure for correction of pectus excavatum. The costal cartilages are removed, leaving the perichondrium.

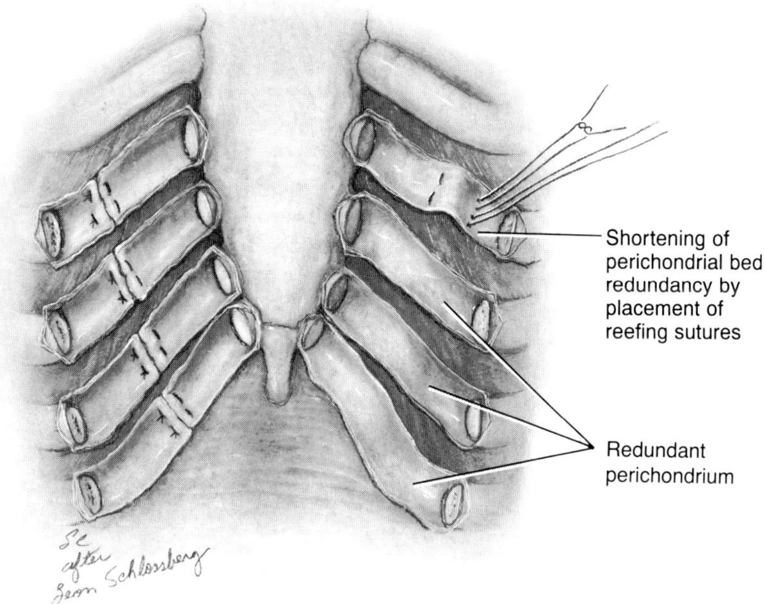

FIGURE 14–2. If the perichondrial bed is redundant, reefing sutures may be taken in the midportion of the perichondrium to tighten this layer. (Redrawn from Ravitch MM: *In* Shields TW [ed]: General Thoracic Surgery. Philadelphia, Lea & Febiger, 1972.)

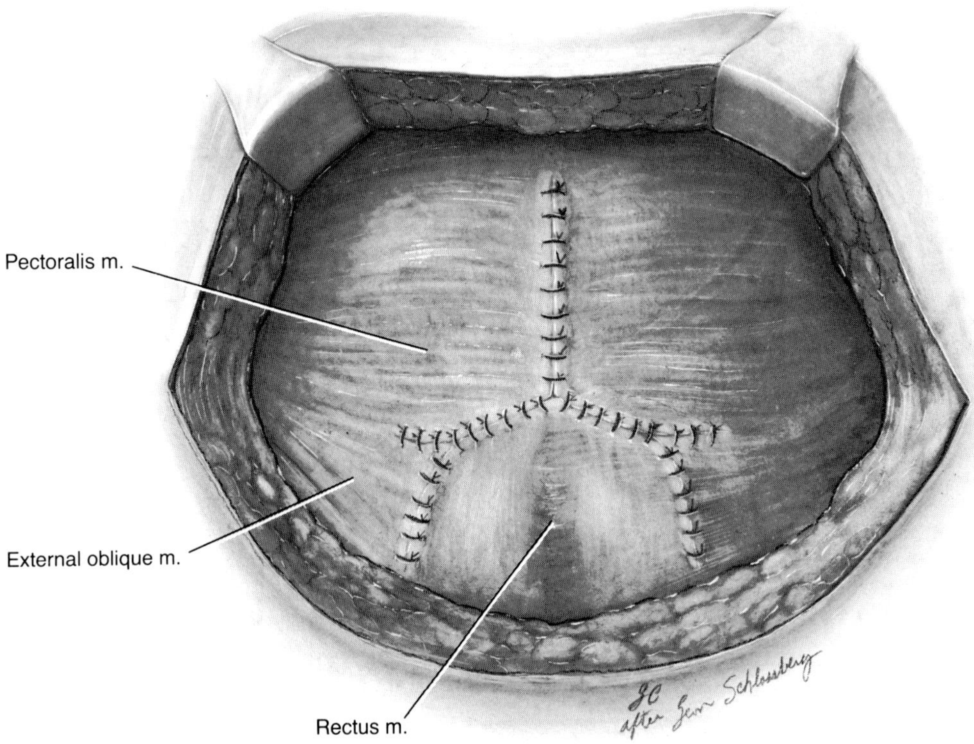

FIGURE 14–3. The pectoral fascia is sutured in the midline with interrupted sutures, and the rectus muscle is reattached. The subcutaneous tissues are closed with interrupted sutures, followed by closure of the skin. A suction drain (Jackson-Pratt) is placed in the mediastinum and led out laterally through a separate stab wound for drainage. (Redrawn from Ravitch MM: *In* Shields TW [ed]: General Thoracic Surgery. Philadelphia, Lea & Febiger, 1972.)

DAVID C. SABISTON, JR., M.D.

15

Correction of Sternal Cleft

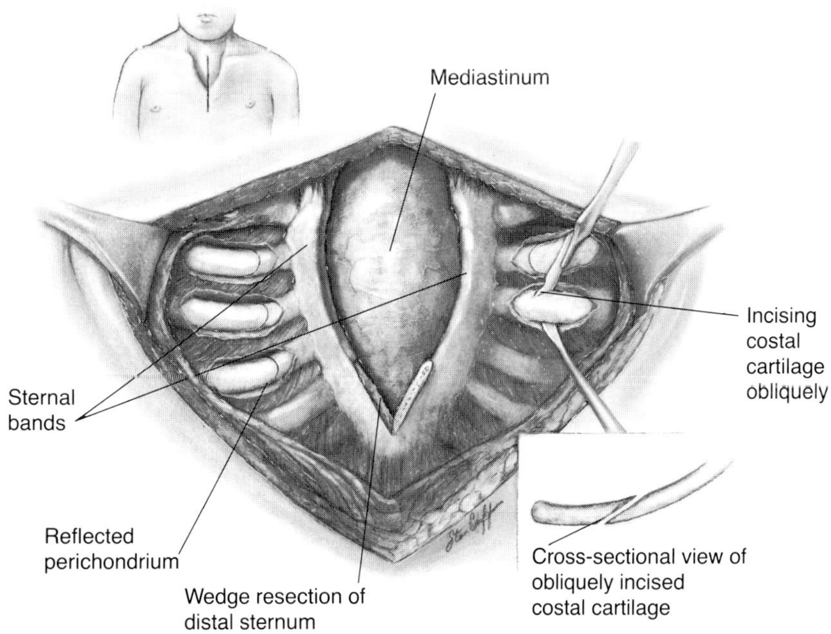

FIGURE 15–1. A vertical incision is made overlying the cleft. The pectoral fascia is divided as it inserts on the anterior surface of the sternal bands, and the skin flaps are retracted laterally, completely exposing the sternal cleft and costal cartilages that join the two sternal bands. The perichondrium is incised anteriorly in the midline of each costal cartilage and elevated. *Lower inset,* The costal cartilages are divided obliquely so they can spread easily.

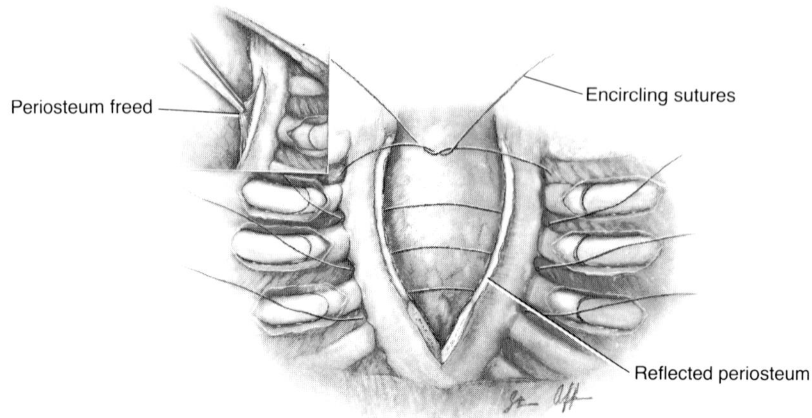

FIGURE 15–2. The perichondrium is freed from both sternal bands, allowing better healing to occur when they are approximated. A small wedge is excised from the confluence of the bands at the lower end of the sternum where they are joined.

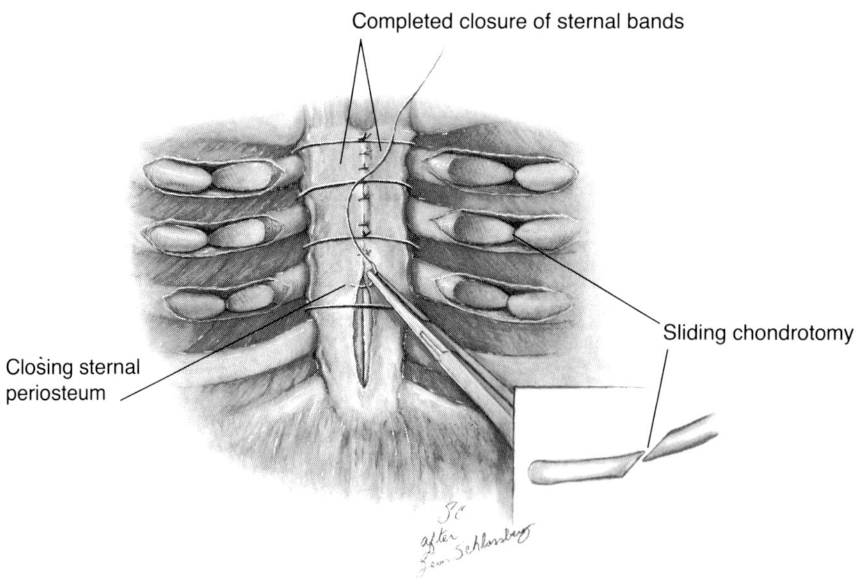

FIGURE 15–3. The sternal bands are approximated with encircling sutures. (Redrawn from Ravitch MM: Congenital Deformities of the Chest Wall and Their Operative Correction. Philadelphia, WB Saunders, 1977, p. 29.)

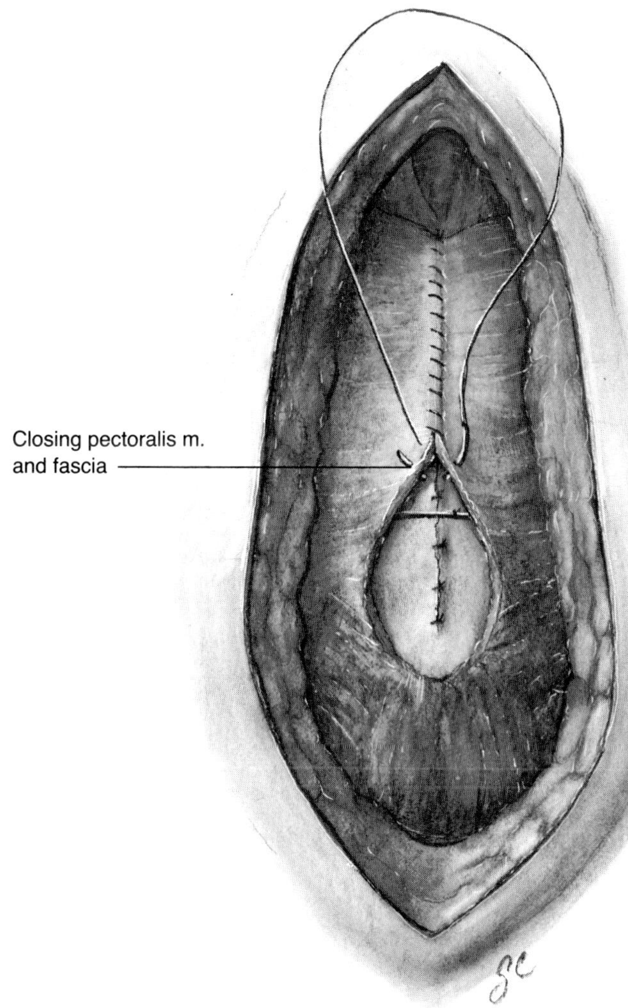

FIGURE 15–4. The pectoral muscles are reapproximated by closure of the pectoral fascia in the midline. A Jackson-Pratt closed drain is inserted and led out through a separate stab wound incision inferiorly.

SECTION V

Correction of Thoracic Outlet Syndrome

W. GLENN YOUNG, JR., M.D.

16

Posterior Approach

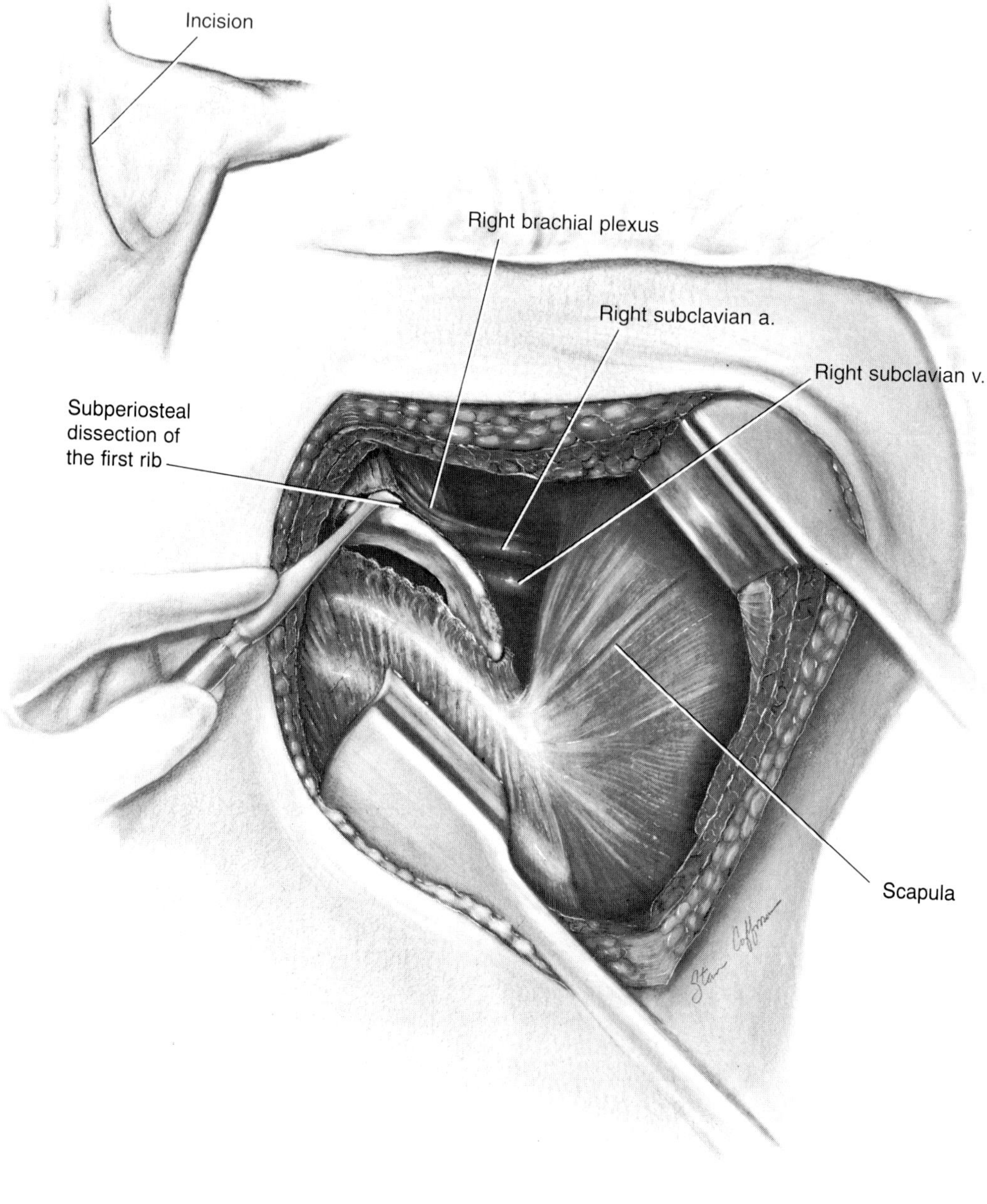

FIGURE 16–1. The first rib and, if present, a cervical rib are removed to decompress the thoracic outlet. This procedure can be accomplished via several approaches, and we usually employ the posterior, or Clagett, operation. The incision is a somewhat shortened version of that used for the old first-stage thoracoplasty, extending from the second thoracic spinous process to the auscultatory triangle midway between the scapula and spine. The trapezius and rhomboid muscles are divided, and the scapula is mobilized. The incision is not carried too far superiorly to protect the spinal accessory nerve. A Tuffier retractor is helpful in exposing the first rib, and subperiosteal dissection around it is begun on its outer and inferior borders to prevent damage to the brachial plexus and subclavian artery and vein, which lie close to the superior and medial aspects of this rib.

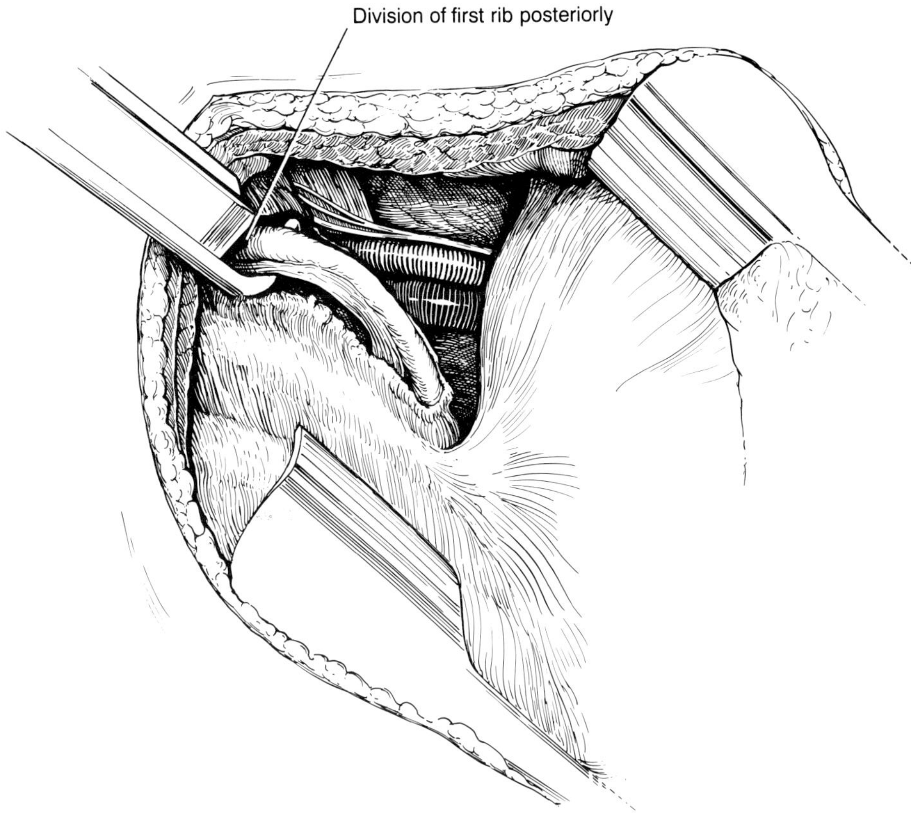

FIGURE 16–2. After the first rib has been encircled posteriorly, it can be divided.

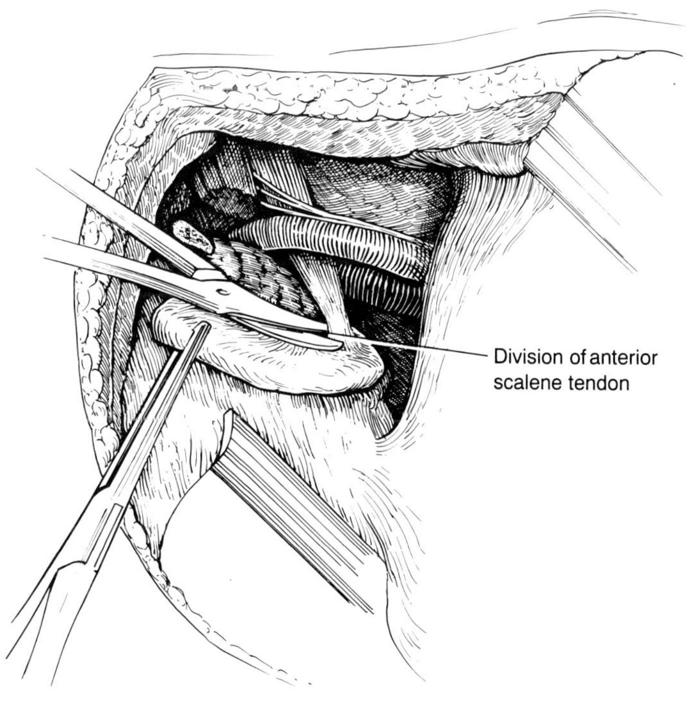

FIGURE 16–3. Grasping the rib posteriorly and drawing it downward with a Kocher clamp allows further dissection of the superior aspect of the rib and division of the anterior scalene tendon under direct vision.

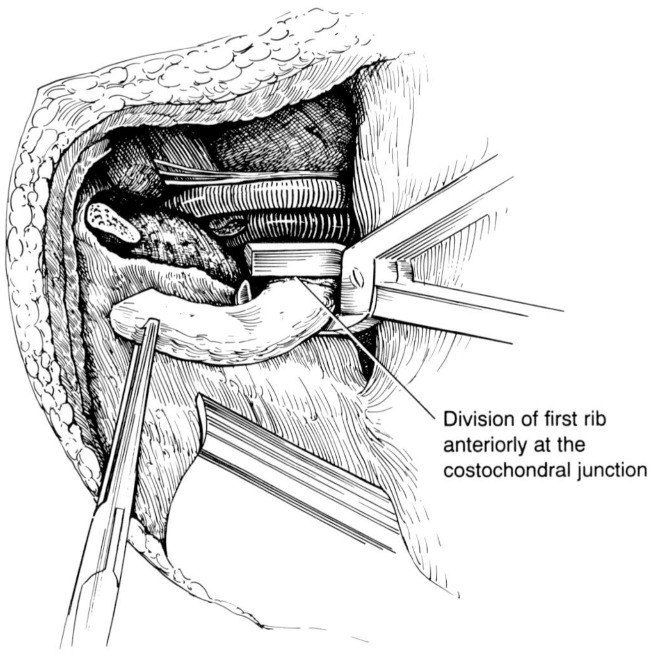

FIGURE 16–4. Dissection of the rib can be continued anteriorly quite safely, and the rib is divided at the costochondral junction. Any fibrous bands or thickened periosteal remnants are removed, ensuring that the neurovascular bundles are completely freed. The pleura is usually not entered, but if this occurs, a chest tube is inserted prior to closure of the wound, which is accomplished without drainage.

W. GLENN YOUNG, JR., M.D.

17
Transaxillary Approach

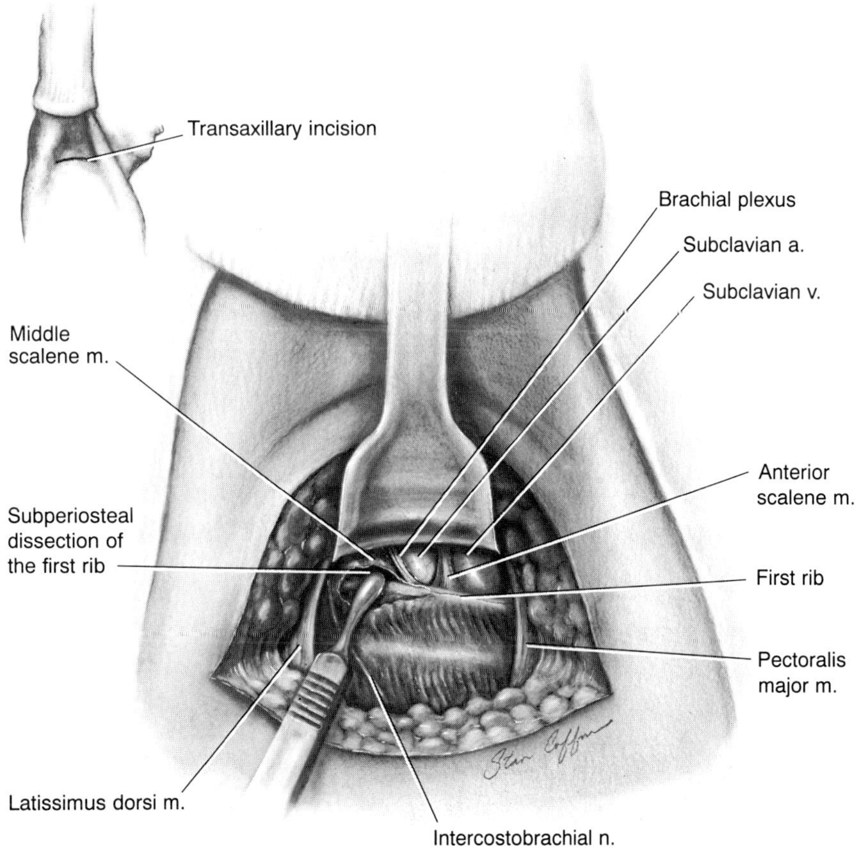

FIGURE 17–1. The transaxillary approach for resection of the first rib is favored by many surgeons and has the advantage of being a more cosmetic incision without the necessity to divide the large muscles. It is performed with the patient in the lateral position and the arm draped in the field with a stockinette so that it can be elevated from time to time by an assistant to lift the neurovascular structures away from the rib. The incision lies below the hairline and extends from the edge of the pectoralis major muscle anteriorly to the edge of the latissimus dorsi muscle posteriorly.

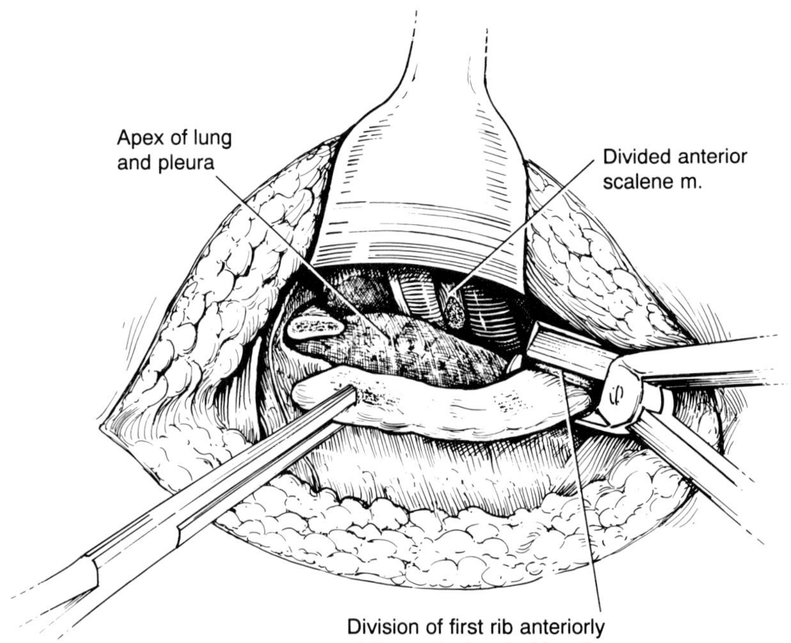

FIGURE 17–2. The subperiosteal resection of the first rib proceeds as described for the posterior approach. After the rib is divided posteriorly, it can be retracted away from the vital structures, facilitating the further dissection anteriorly.

SECTION VI

The Mediastinum

ROBERT H. JONES, M.D.

18

Thymectomy

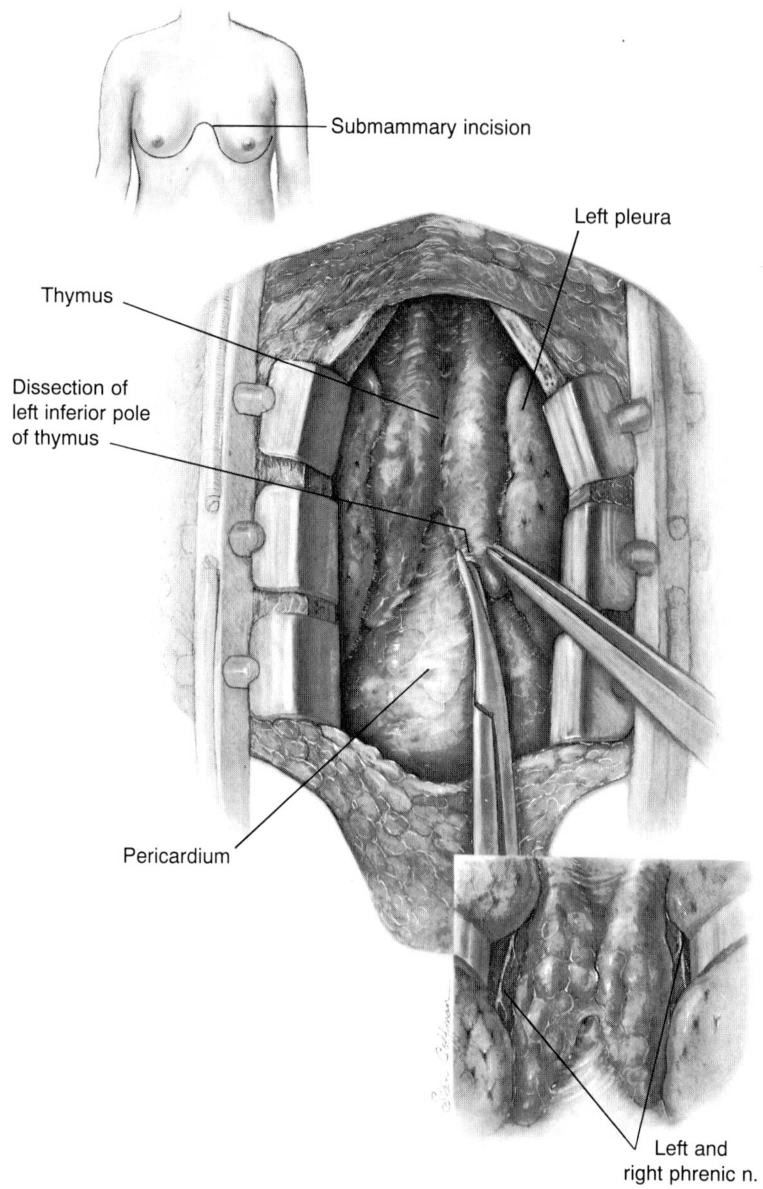

FIGURE 18–1. A vertical midline incision beginning 3 cm inferior to the sternal notch and extended to the xiphoid is most commonly used with a median sternotomy for thymectomy. A bilateral submammary incision provides a more pleasing cosmetic result in females and can be accomplished when desired by the patient without compromise of the operation. The submammary incision is made in the inferior breast crease bilaterally and connected in the midline with a gentle arc. Skin flaps are elevated anterior to the pectoralis fascia to the level of the sternal notch and as far laterally as required to relieve tension as the sternum is opened. Inferiorly, they are elevated and extended to the rectus fascia to the level of the xiphoid. The median sternotomy is completed, and the operation is continued in a manner identical to that using a vertical incision.

The thymus typically is an H-shaped gland, with the lower poles larger and fanning out onto the pericardium, and the upper poles extending into the neck. The poles are often asymmetrical and are connected with an isthmus of irregular shape. Considerable anatomic variation occurs, and the border of the thymus is often difficult to delineate from mediastinal and pleural fat. Therefore, the operative plan should be *en bloc* removal of all tissue suggestive of thymus that is anterior to the pericardium bordered by each phrenic nerve and extending to the neck. Dissection begins along the inferior border of this tissue mass with the pericardium, beginning in the midline and continuing laterally on both sides. Laterally this tissue extends between the pleura and pericardium and must be separated from pleural fat.

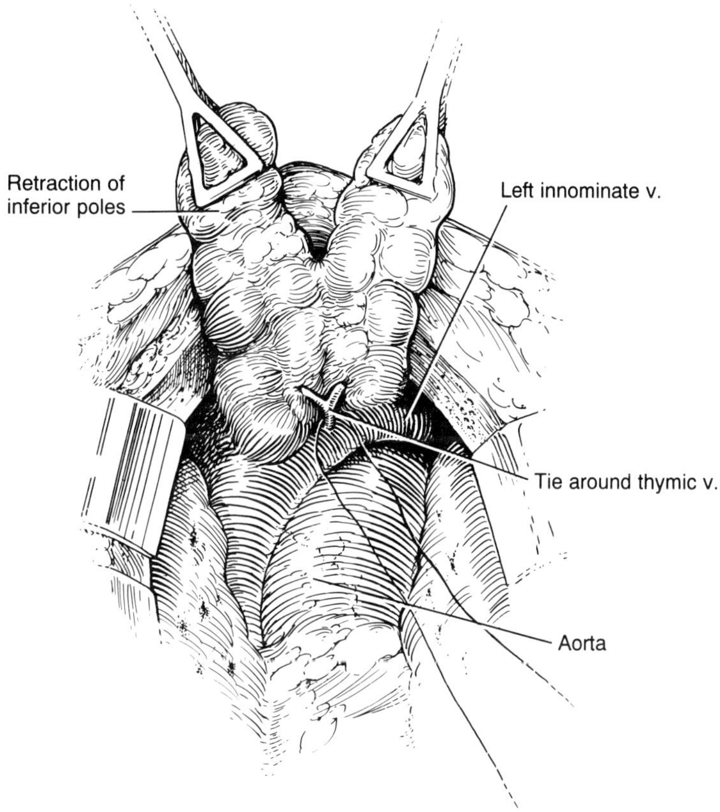

FIGURE 18–2. After delineation of the lower end of both inferior poles, dissection continues cephalad, avoiding injury to the phrenic nerve by traction or electrocautery. As dissection is extended near the upper extent of the sternum, lateral attachments often contain vessels that require ligation.

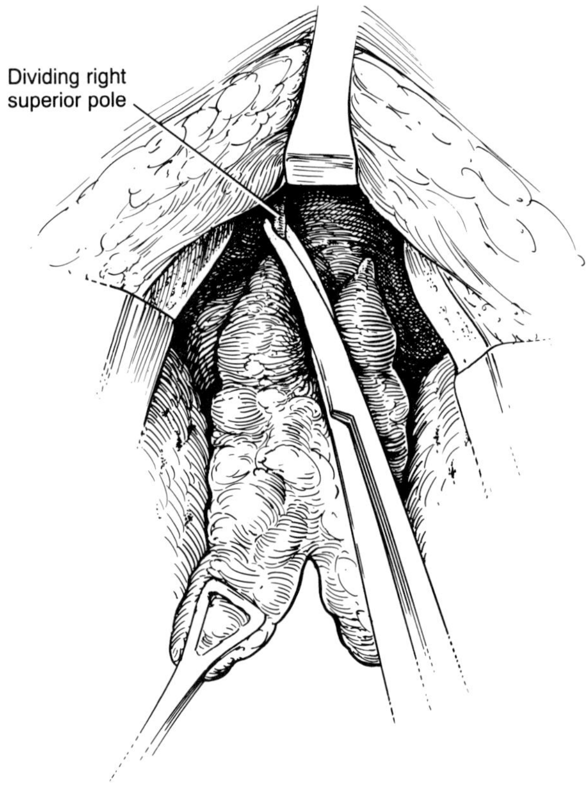

FIGURE 18–3. The two upper poles of the thymus usually pass anterior to the innominate vein and course inferior to the strap muscles. Absence of fat permits the border of these lobes to be well identified and sharply dissected from the surrounding neck structures. Commonly, small vessels that require ligation are encountered near the upper extent of both superior poles. During dissection of the thymus from the innominate vein, a large tributary is commonly encountered and should be carefully ligated to avoid tearing the innominate vein.

Thymectomy is commonly performed for myasthenia gravis. In this condition, the thymus is usually normal with some hyperplasia or cystic change. In patients with malignant thymoma, the gland may be enlarged, firm, and densely adherent to surrounding structures. The conduct of an extended thymectomy must be planned by balancing the risk of excision with the possible benefit. Entry into the pericardium often aids assessment of the extent of involvement. In most patients with thymectomy for malignancy, it is wise to attempt to preserve the phrenic nerve.

DAVID C. SABISTON, JR., M.D.

19

Excision of Mediastinal Tumor

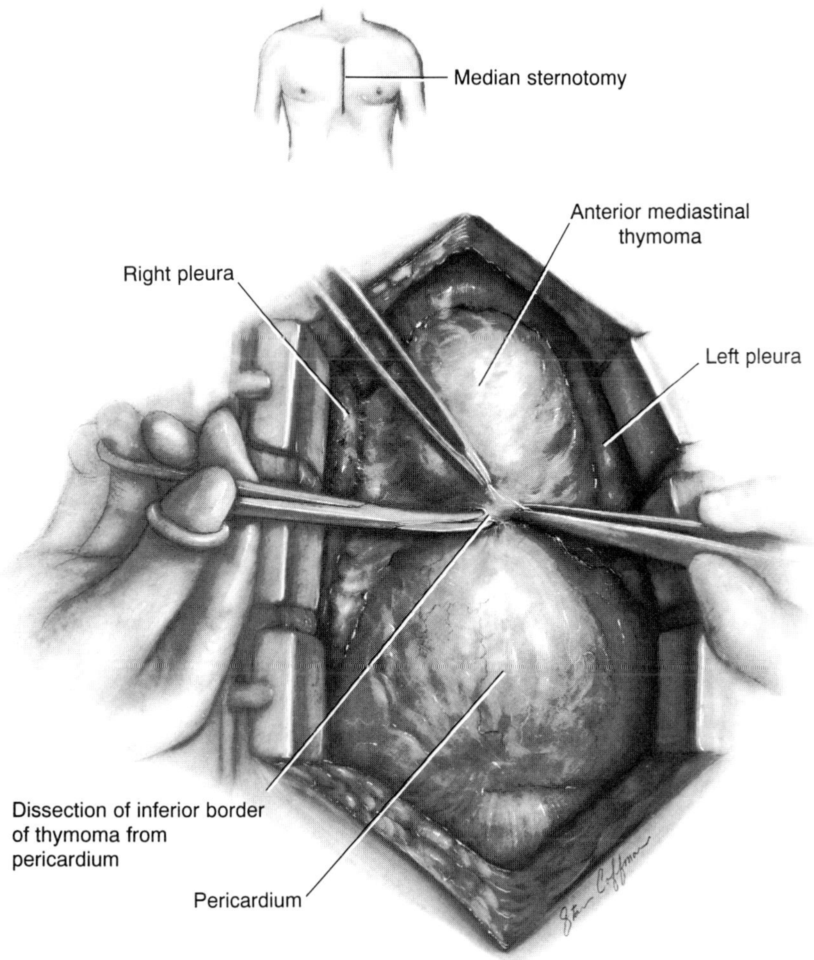

FIGURE 19–1. A median sternotomy is used to approach a thymoma in the anterior mediastinum. A sternal spreader is inserted, and dissection is initiated with separation of the tumor from the surrounding structures.

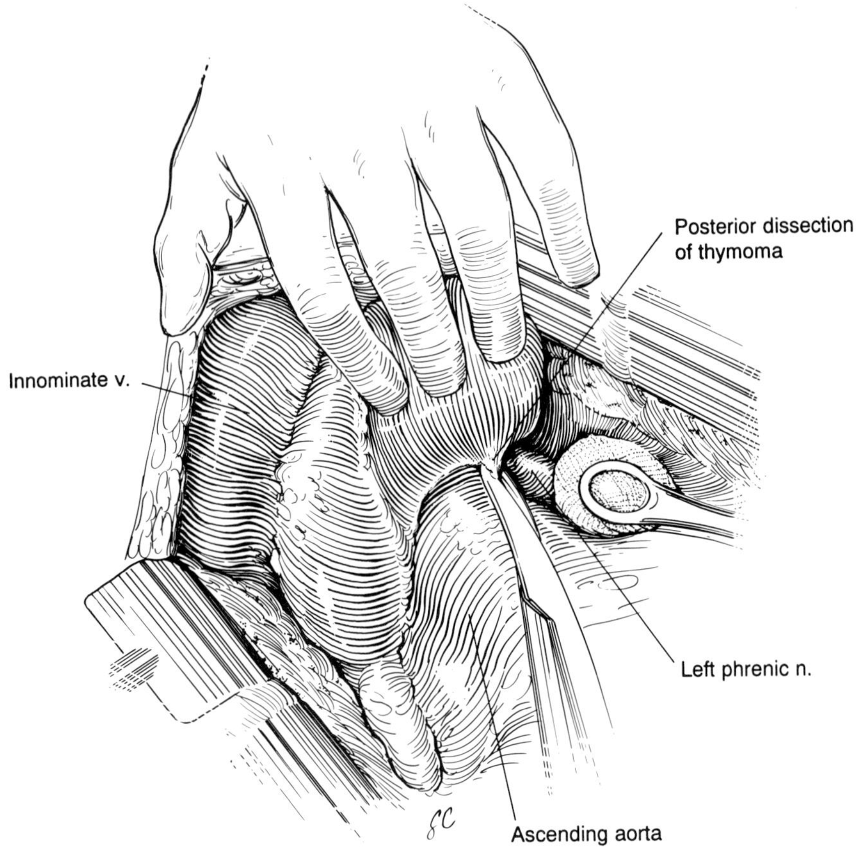

FIGURE 19–2. Care should be taken to protect the phrenic nerve. The posterior portion of the tumor is retracted anteriorly as its capsule is separated from the main pulmonary artery.

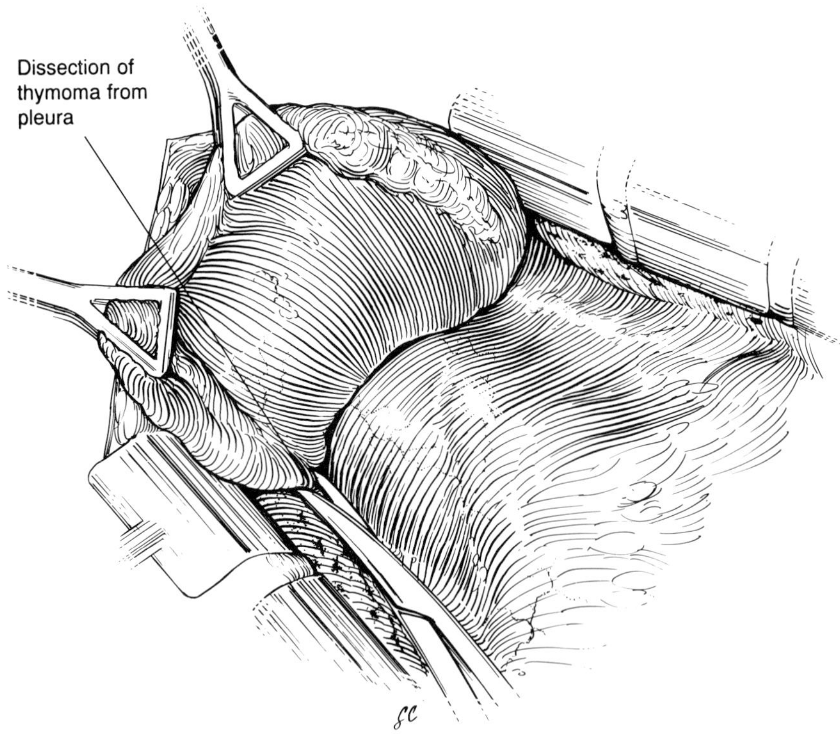

FIGURE 19–3. With retraction directed superiorly, the pleura is separated from the posterior border of the tumor.

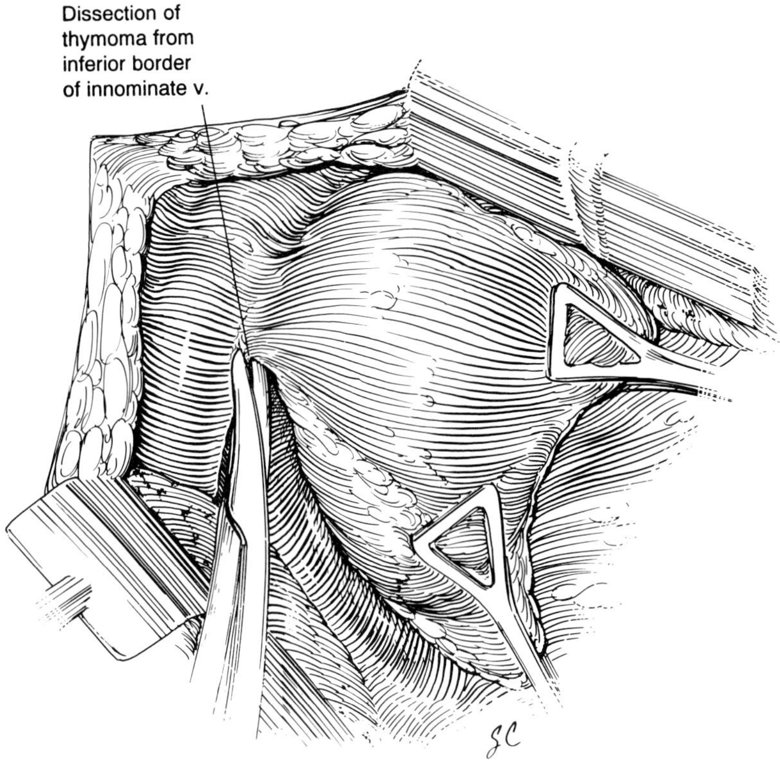

FIGURE 19–4. The inferior border of the innominate vein is dissected free of the thymoma.

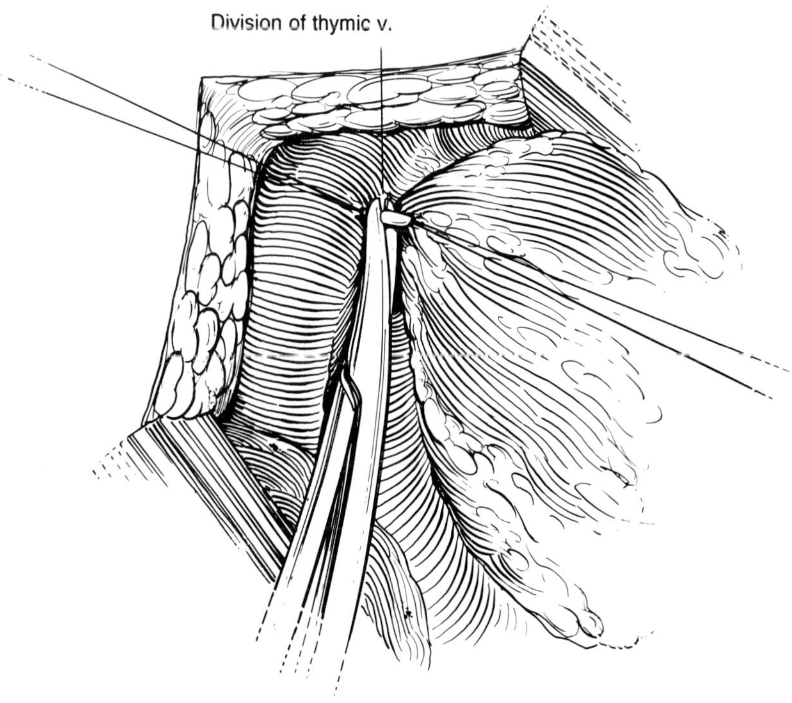

FIGURE 19–5. The thymic veins are divided between clamps, and the vessels are securely ligated.

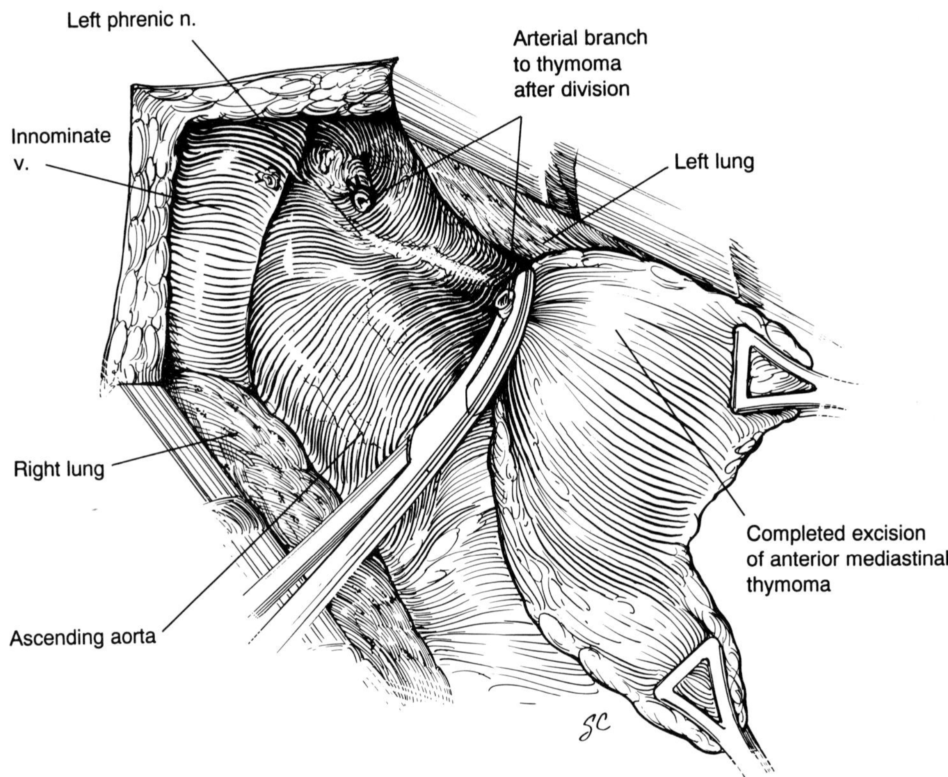

FIGURE 19–6. The arterial supply to the thymoma is clamped and doubly ligated at the completion of the dissection. The neoplasm is then removed from the mediastinum, and the median sternotomy is closed in the standard manner.

L. SCOTT LEVIN, M.D.

20
Muscle and Omental Flaps for Mediastinitis

Postoperative wound infections after open heart surgery can cause mediastinitis and acute or chronic osteomyelitis that involves the sternum and chondritis of adjacent ribs. This condition is usually refractory to open drainage alone and must be treated with aggressive debridement and filling of the dead space with muscle flaps or omentum, which can restore vascular supply and deliver nutrients and antibiotics to the compromised tissues. The method of management of mediastinitis depends on the patient presentation and clinical signs. The presence of fever, elevated leukocyte count, and local erythema and spontaneous drainage often indicates deep infection. If it presents acutely, mediastinitis is treated in one stage, and if it is chronic, it is treated in two stages with debridement and dressing changes followed by subsequent soft tissue reconstruction.

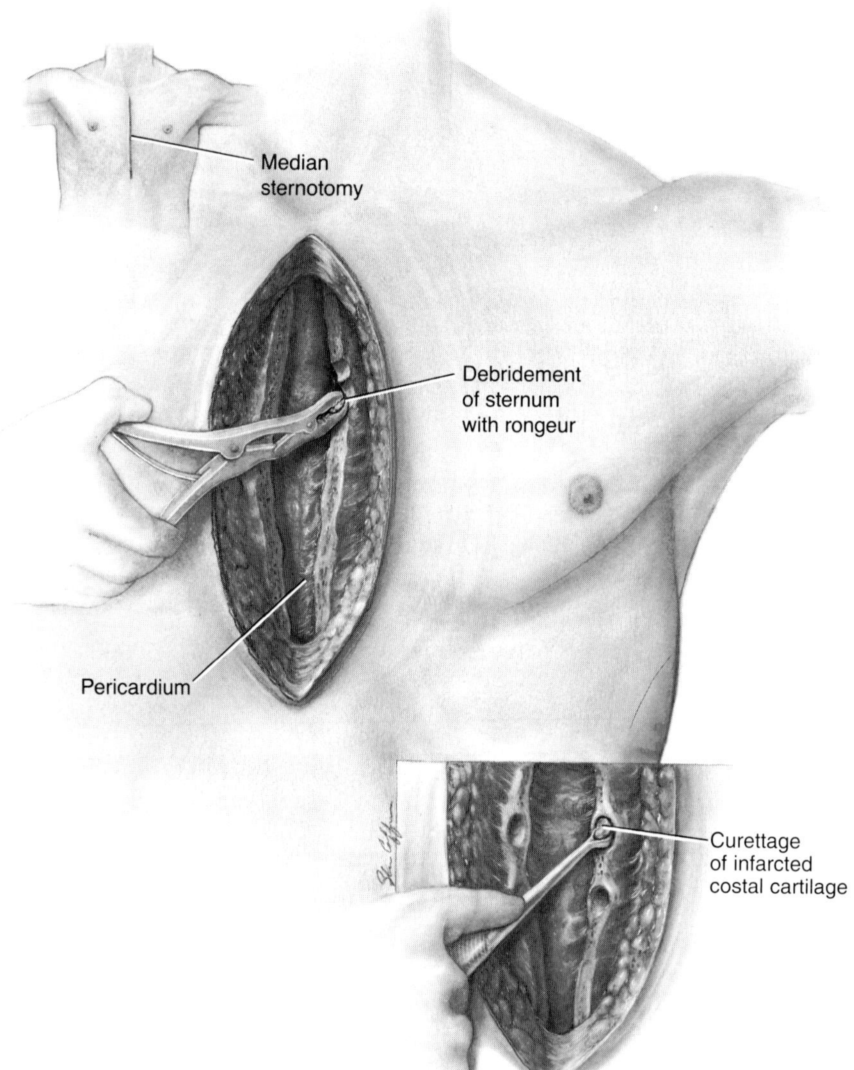

FIGURE 20–1. The original median sternotomy incision is opened. The wound edges are not debrided, but subcutaneous and nonviable deep tissue is sharply debrided. The sternal wires should be removed along the length of the incision unless the sternum is stable. In acute cases, the sternum has not had time to heal sufficiently, and, therefore, all wires should be removed. Debridement of the osseous and soft tissue structures is done with a large rongeur. A large curette is used to remove infarcted cartilage. Leaving any nonviable osteomyelitic bone or desiccated cartilage in the wound often causes a recurrence of the infection within weeks to months after coverage by the muscle flap. The pericardium can be scraped with a pericardial rasp, and care is taken not to dislodge vascular bypass grafts that may be exposed.

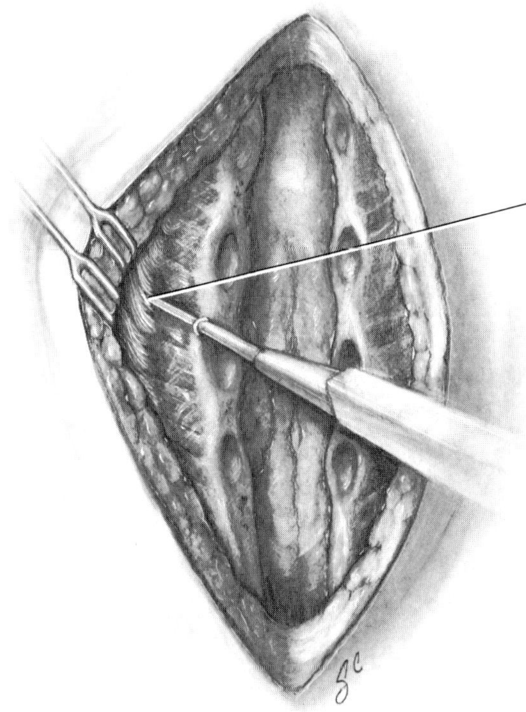

FIGURE 20–2. After completion of mediastinal debridement and resection of all nonviable bone and cartilage, the pectoralis muscle flaps are raised. The internal mammary artery, which is harvested from the left side of the chest, is often used for bypass. The dual blood supply of the pectoralis major muscle necessitates that the thoracoacromial trunk be the sustaining artery of the pectoralis on the left side if the internal mammary is used. On the right side of the chest, the internal mammary is preserved, and subsequently the intercostal perforators are available to nourish the muscle as secondary blood supply. Epimysium is preserved over the pectoralis, and the subcutaneous tissue is raised to the level of the tendinous insertion of the pectoralis major muscle on the humerus. Sharp skin hooks are used to hold the skin flaps when starting this procedure. Caution should be taken not to enter the epimysium but to stay just above this layer to preserve the architecture of the pectoralis muscle.

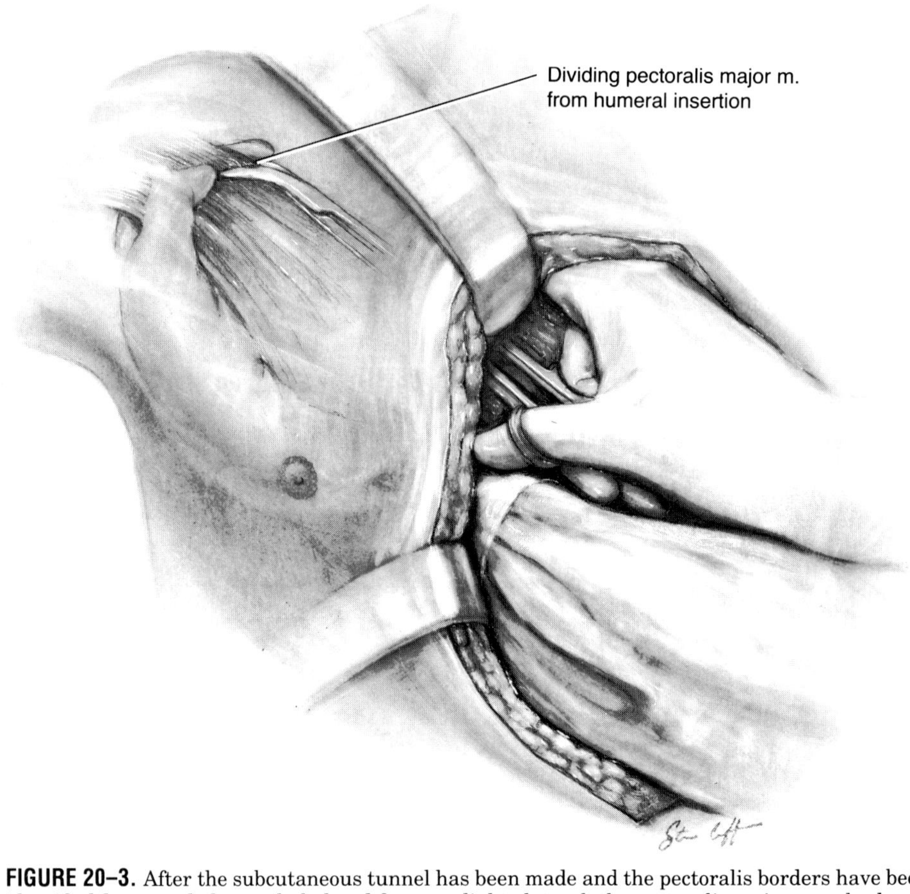

FIGURE 20–3. After the subcutaneous tunnel has been made and the pectoralis borders have been identified from caudad to cephalad and from medial to lateral, the pectoralis major muscle should be grasped at its insertion into the humerus, with care taken *not* to include the tail of the pectoralis minor. A special curved cutting scissors can be used to transect the muscle toward the insertion of the pectoralis major; and with adequate visualization, the cautery can be used. An incision may be made over the humeral insertion for better visualization if necessary.

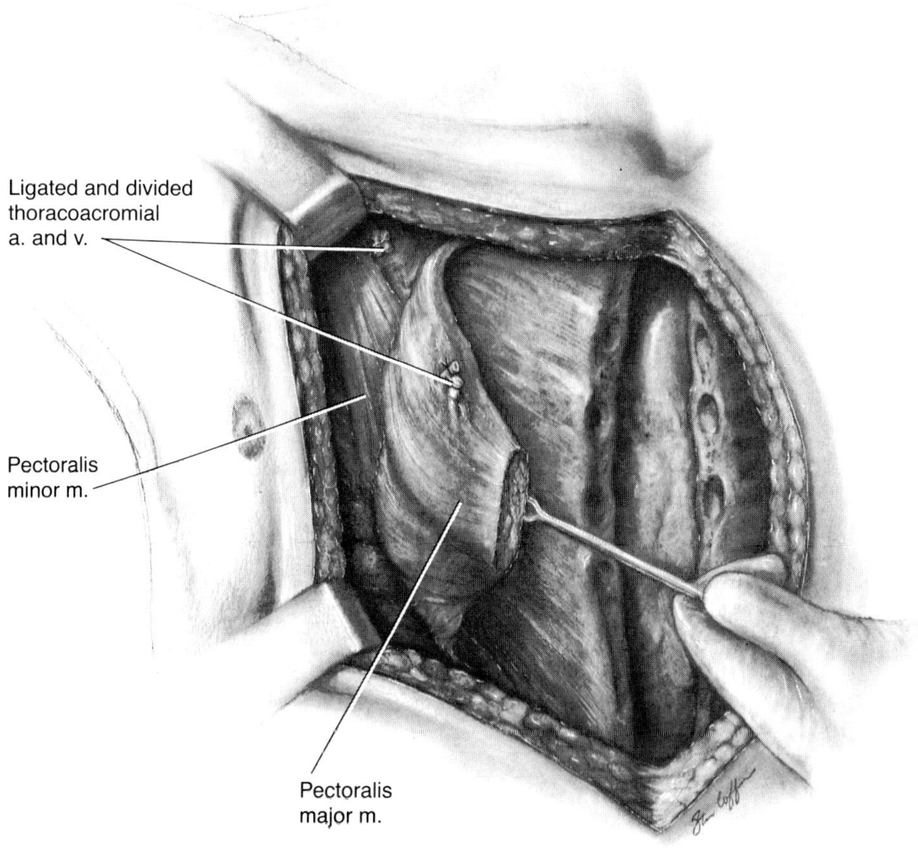

FIGURE 20–4. After the muscle insertion is transected, the pectoralis major is dissected from lateral to medial, taking care to leave the pectoralis minor on the chest wall. The thoracoacromial artery and vein are identified at approximately the midpoint of the clavicle, and artery and vein, respectively, are separated and suture ligated. The dissection is continued, mobilizing the pectoralis to the level of the intercostal perforators, allowing it to be delivered into the mediastinal defect.

If indicated, the pectoralis can be split transversely in the line of its fibers, with half of the right pectoralis filling the defect cephalad and the other half filling the defect caudad. However, in most cases, the volume of dead space is so great that both the left and right pectoralis muscles are utilized. Care is taken not to disrupt the intercostal perforators that are just lateral to the sternal debridement site, because they supply blood to this muscle.

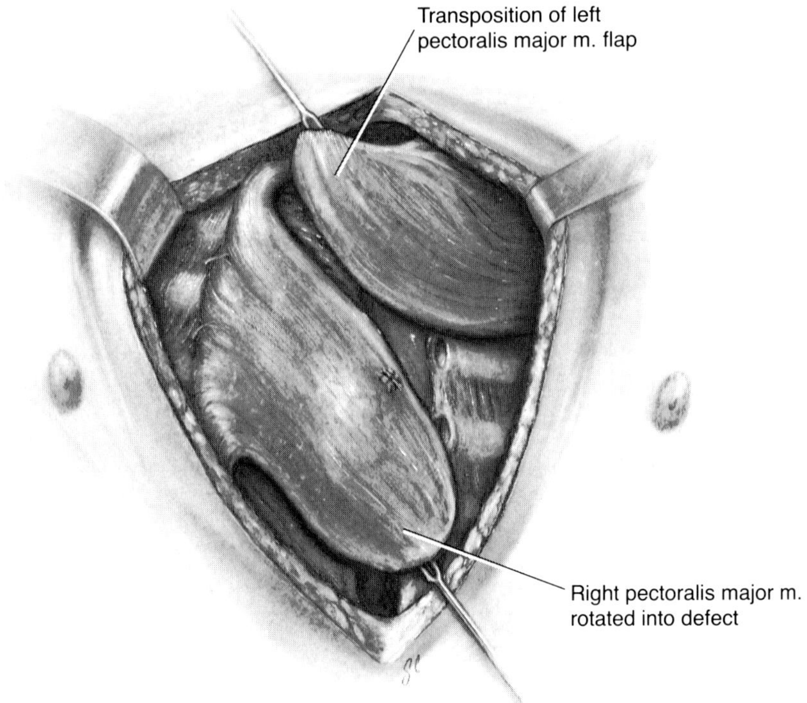

FIGURE 20–5. The left pectoralis muscle is similarly divided after the skin envelope is raised. The origin of the left pectoralis is mobilized off the chest wall, preserving the thoracoacromial trunk. The left pectoralis is transposed usually to the cephalad portion of the mediastinal defect to obliterate dead space. On the left side, the intercostal perforators are identified and clipped or ligated, allowing the inferior and medial aspect of the pectoralis to be mobilized off of the chest wall.

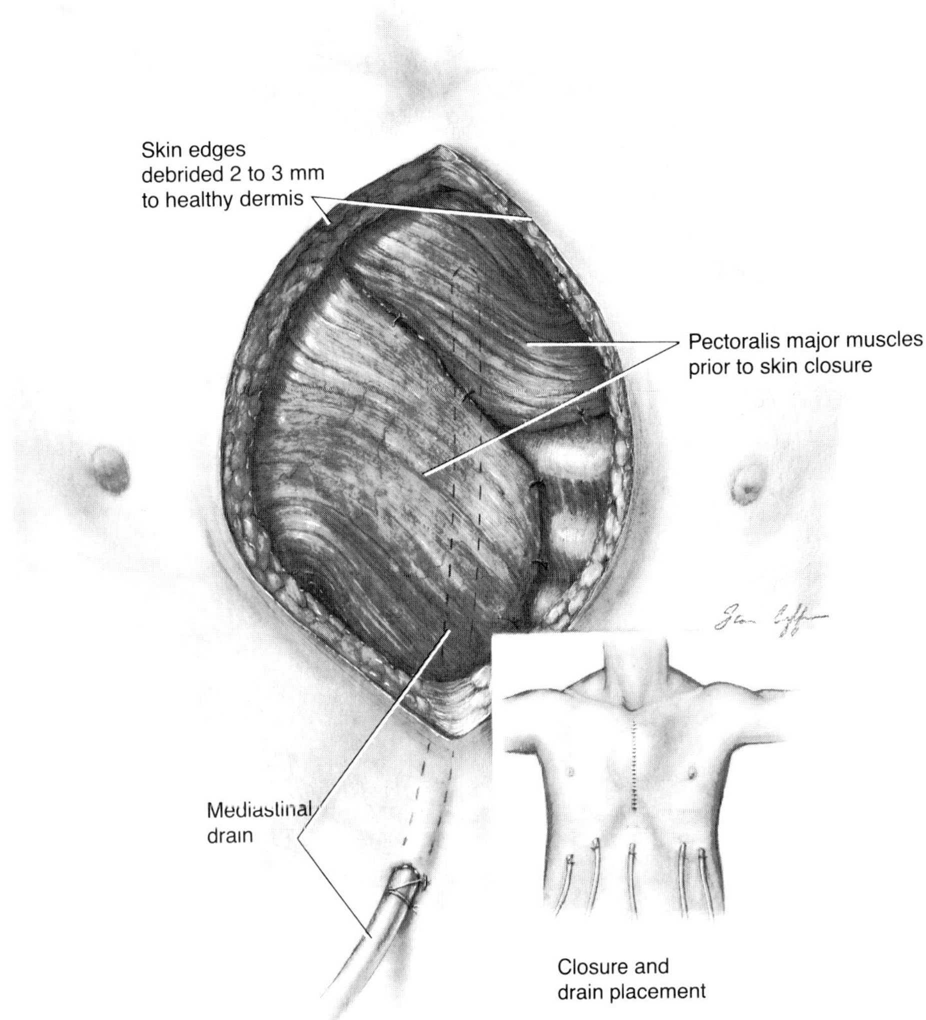

FIGURE 20–6. After both muscles are identified, they are transposed into the defect. The epimysium of the left and right pectoralis can be sutured in the midline, and the perichondrium can serve as an anchor site for the edge of the pectoralis. A large mediastinal drain is placed under the muscle at the midline, and subsequently, at least two large drains are placed in the axilla and anterior chest on both the left and right sides. Prior to insetting muscles and closure, both cavities are explored for residual bleeding, particularly at the insertion of the origin of the pectoralis major muscle.

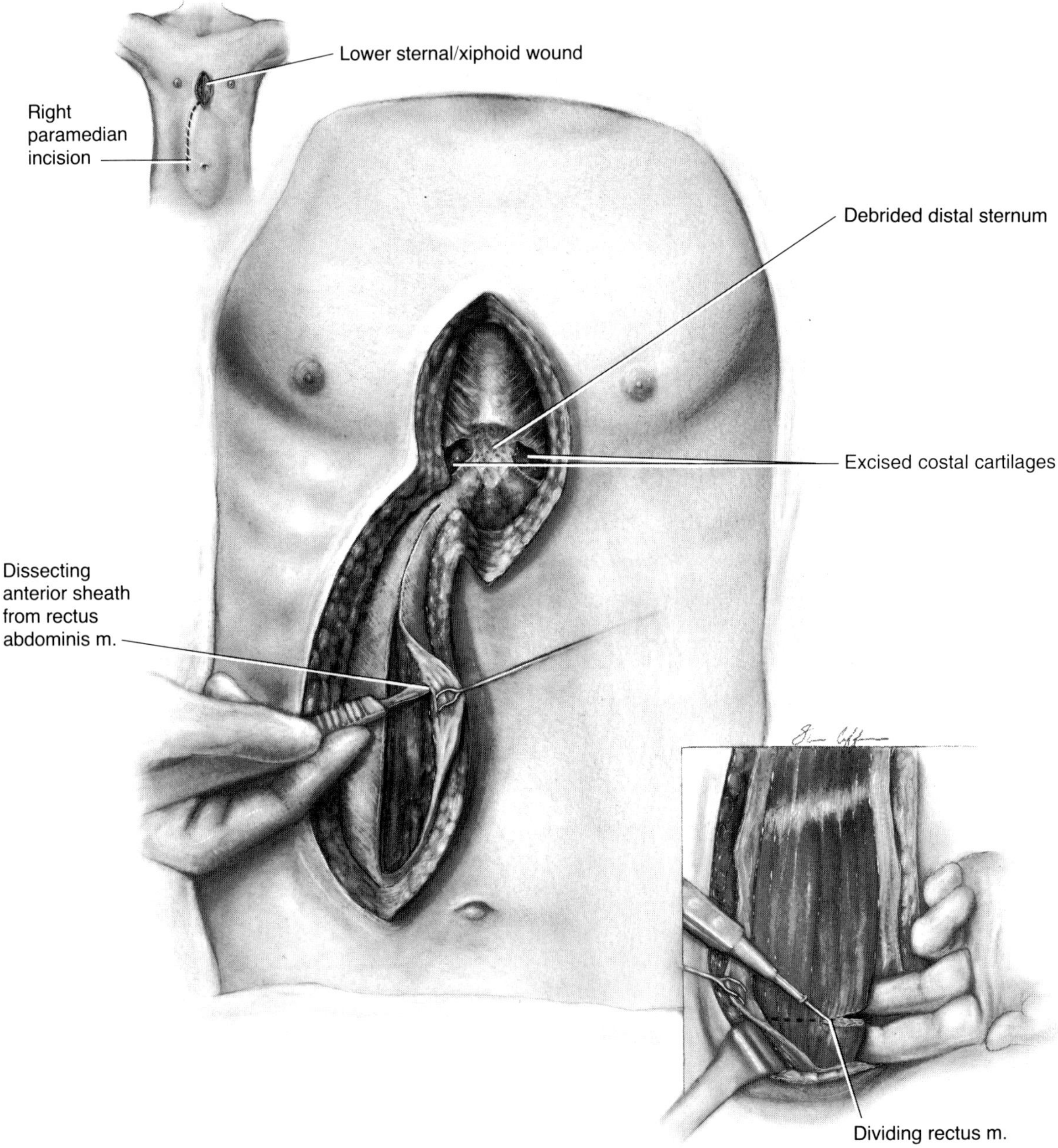

FIGURE 20–7. When there is a lower paraxiphoid defect for chronic osteomyelitis involving the xiphoid, the rectus abdominis muscle can be used. If the left internal mammary artery has been used for bypass grafting, the right superior epigastric artery supplies the rectus. A right paramedian incision is made that is angled toward the xiphoid. Necrotic costal cartilage is excised, and the xiphoid is debrided in a similar manner to the mediastinum, with care being taken to remove all nonviable tissue. The anterior rectus sheath is then opened, and the muscle is dissected inferiorly to the line of Douglas. The muscle is transected and folded on itself, transposing it into the defect of the xiphoid region. The skin is subsequently closed. The skin edges should always be debrided last to ensure fresh dermal bleeding at the time of skin closure.

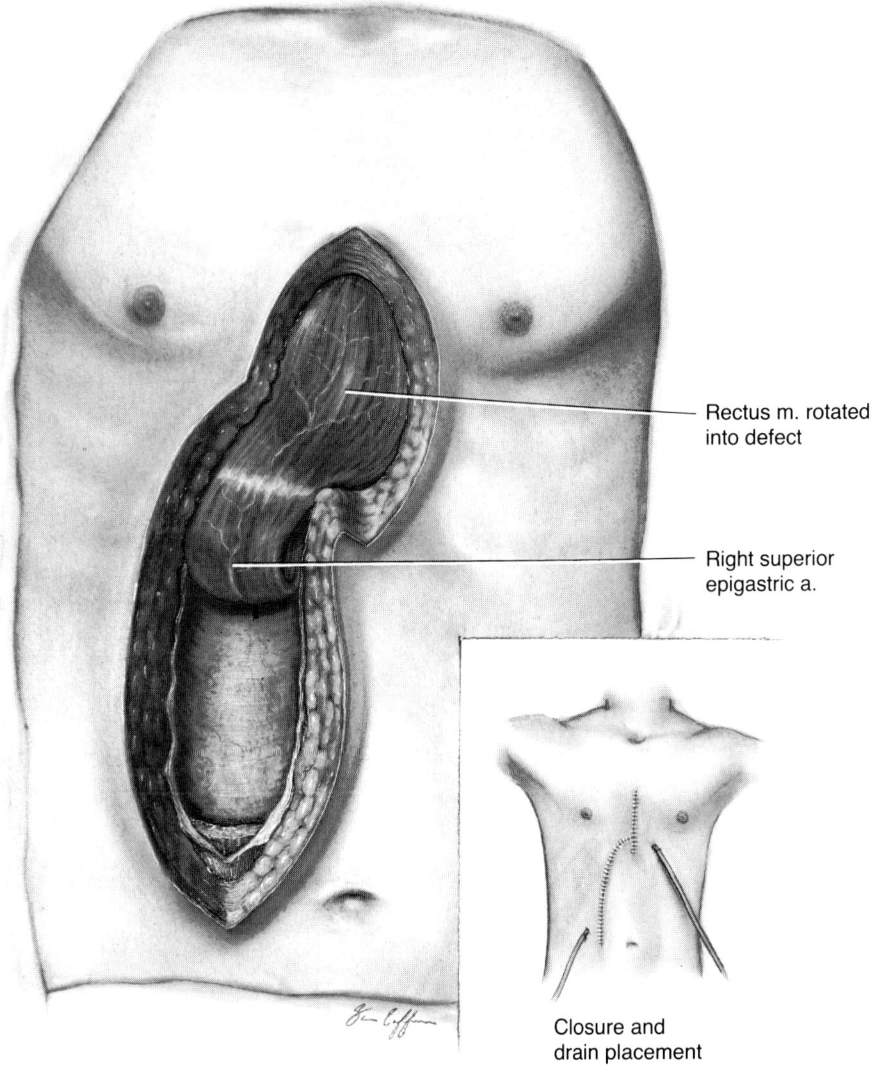

FIGURE 20–8. A drain is placed at the level of the rectus sheath.

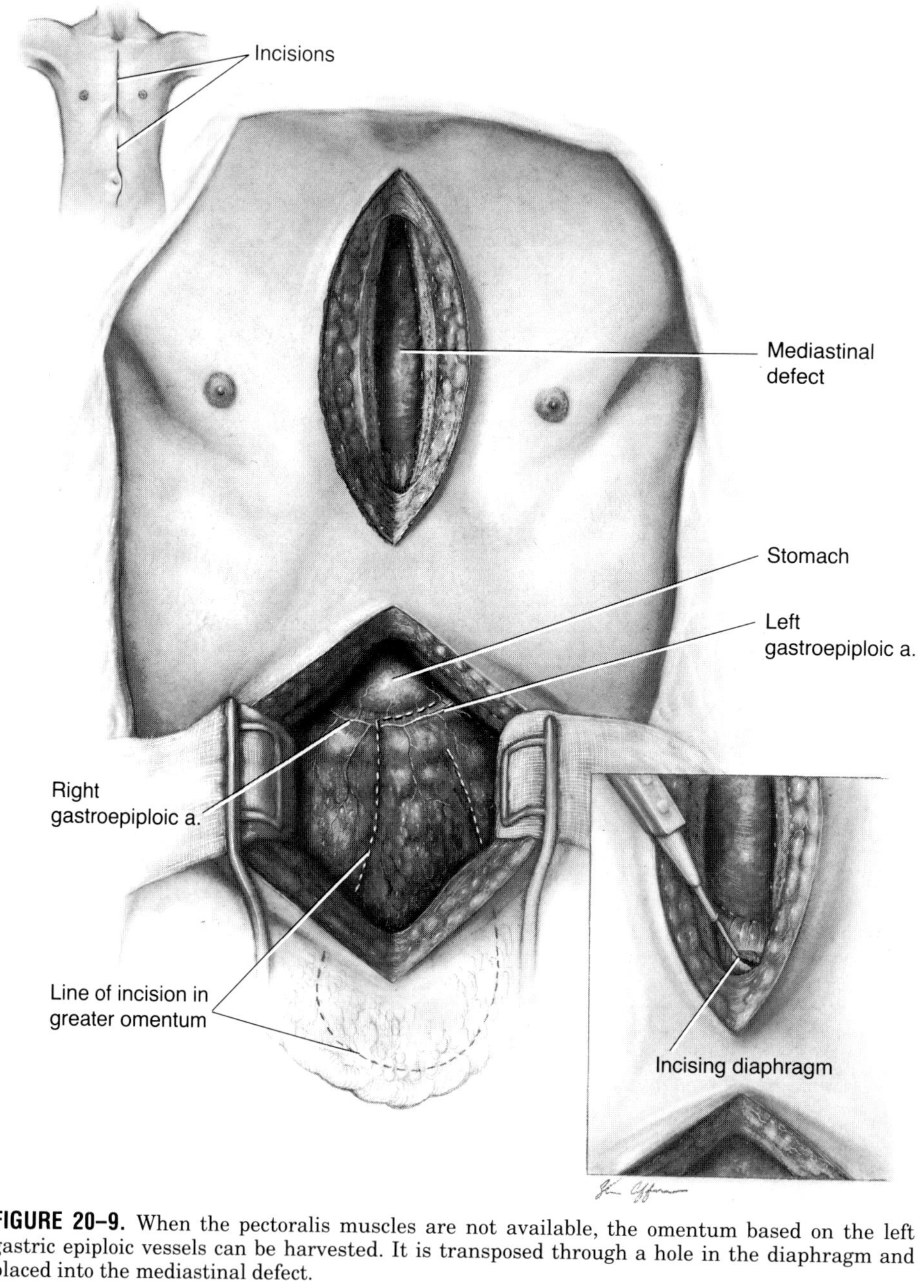

FIGURE 20–9. When the pectoralis muscles are not available, the omentum based on the left gastric epiploic vessels can be harvested. It is transposed through a hole in the diaphragm and placed into the mediastinal defect.

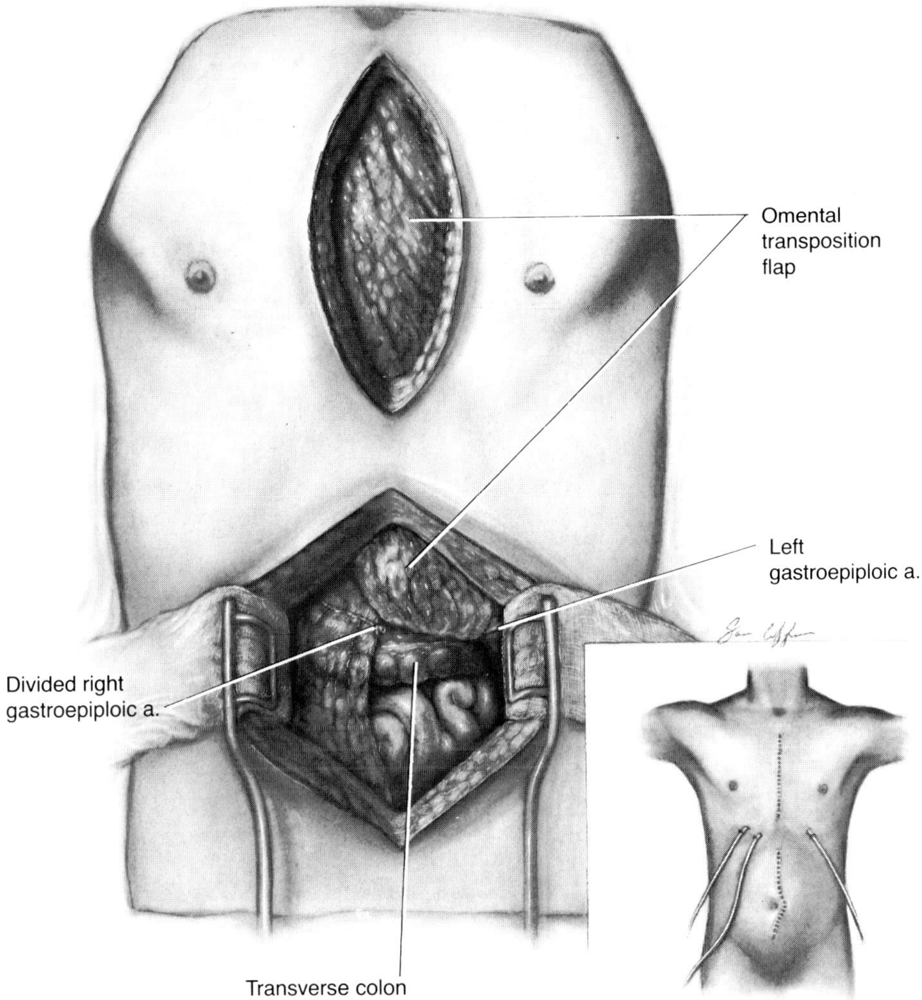

FIGURE 20–10. The left gastric epiploic artery is the vascular pedicle for the omental transposition flap.

SECTION VII

Pulmonary Procedures

W. GLENN YOUNG, JR., M.D.

21

Pulmonary Wedge Excision

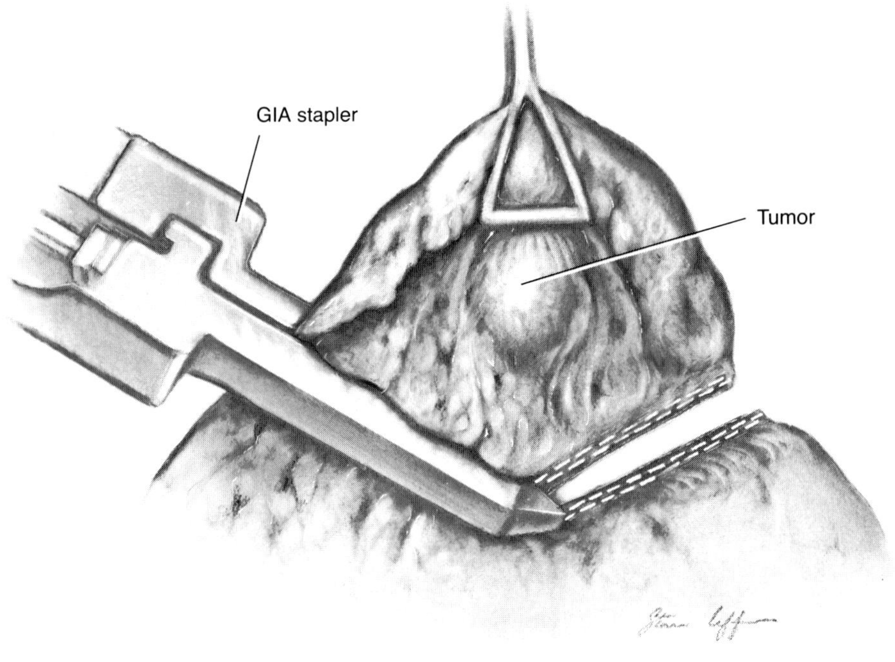

FIGURE 21–1

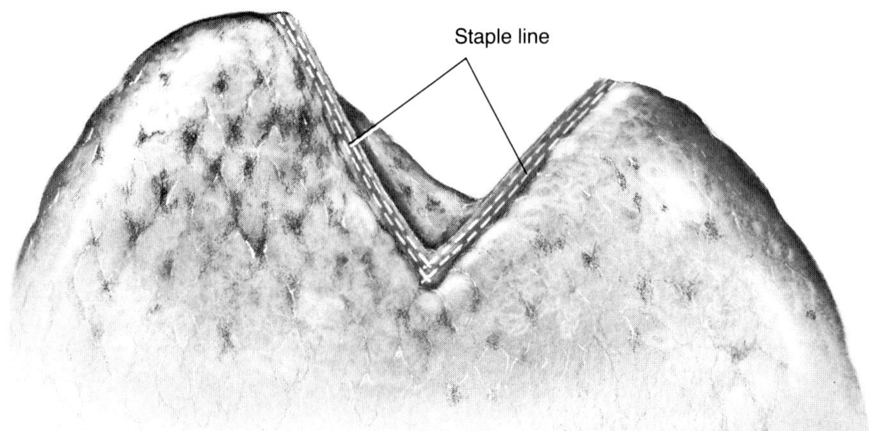

FIGURE 21–2

FIGURES 21–1 and 21–2. Wedge resection has been greatly simplified by the use of the GIA stapler. Application of the stapling device is facilitated by allowing the lung to collapse. An adequate margin should be ensured if the lesion is suspected to be malignant.

W. GLENN YOUNG, JR., M.D.

22

Excision of Large Pulmonary Bullae

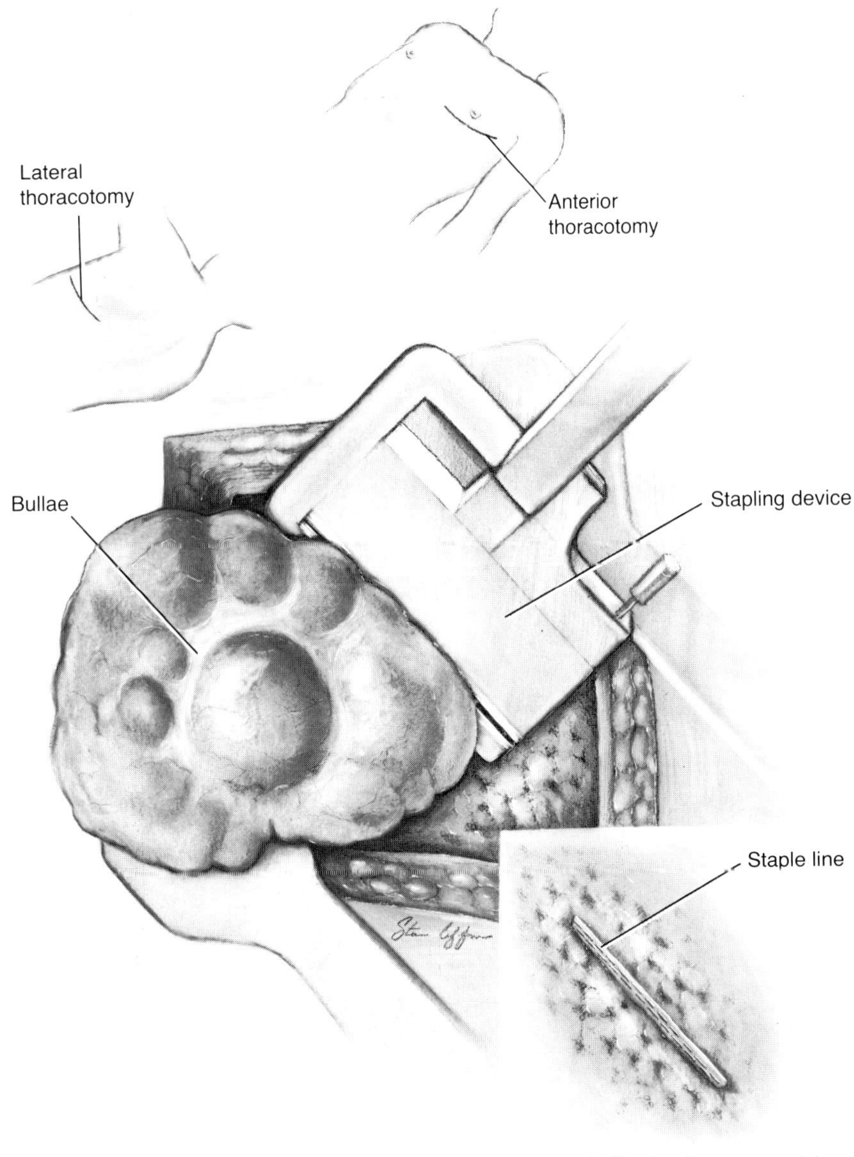

FIGURE 22–1. If resection is planned of a large emphysematous bulla that is compromising more normal surrounding lung, it is important not to perform a lobectomy or other major resection. Either a short lateral or anterior thoracotomy may be employed. Use of the large stapling device allows excision of the bulla with conservation of as much lung tissue as possible.

WALTER G. WOLFE, M.D.

23

Right Upper Lobectomy

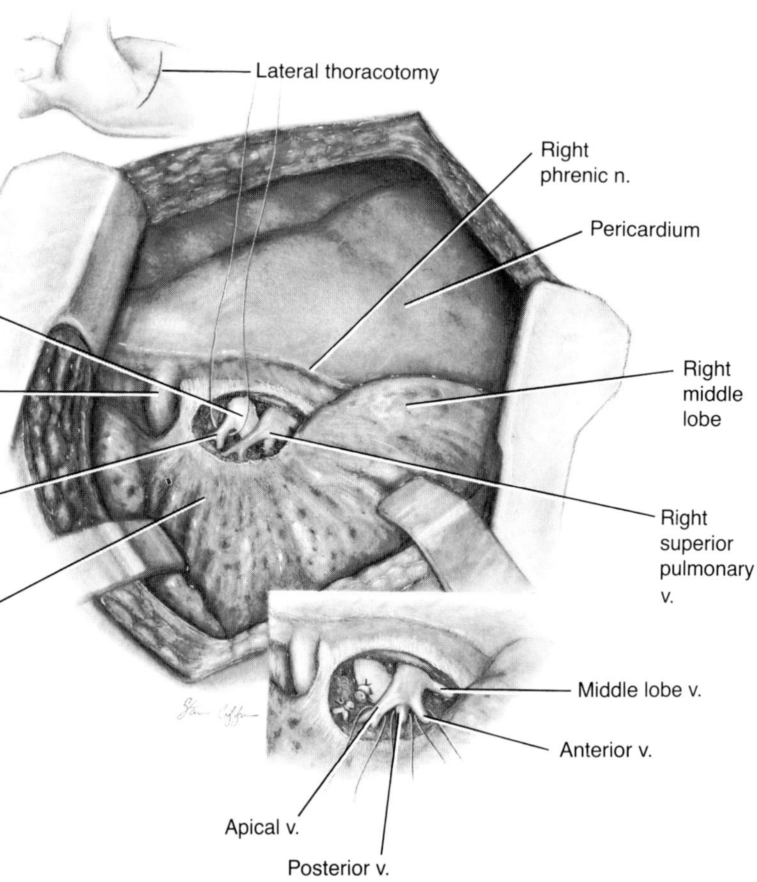

FIGURE 23–1. The patient is positioned, and a right posterolateral thoracotomy is made. The chest is entered through the fifth interspace. The hilum and lung are mobilized, and suspicious or abnormal lymph nodes in the area of the azygos vein, hilum, and mediastinum are sent for frozen section.

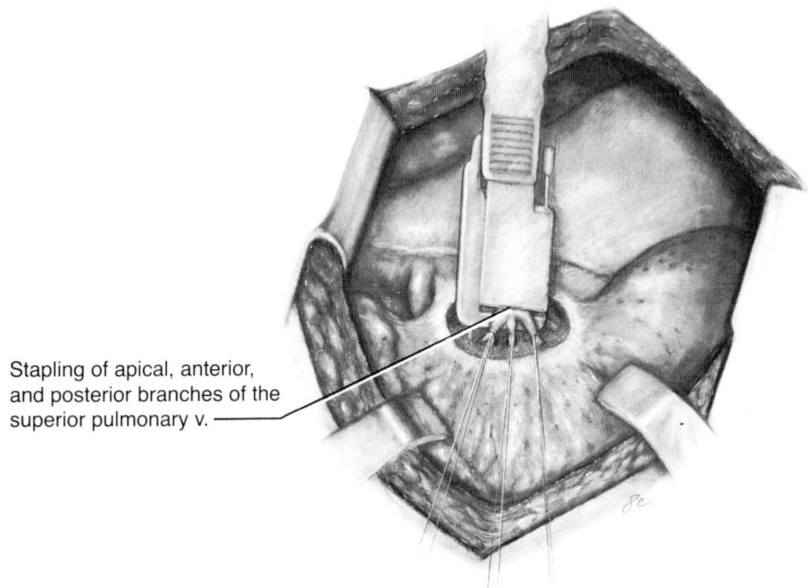

FIGURE 23–2. The pulmonary artery to the upper lobe is dissected free, with the branches usually being suture ligated and divided. The middle lobe vein is identified from the superior pulmonary vein, and the branches of the superior vein to the upper lobe are ligated and divided with silk transfixion sutures.

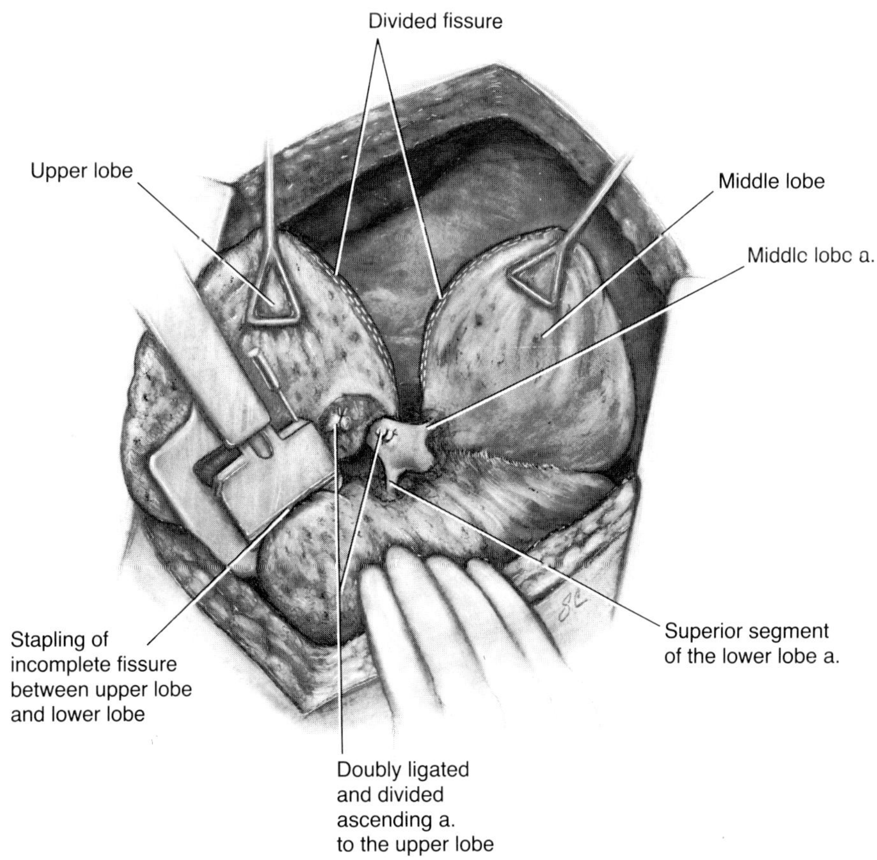

FIGURE 23–3. In general, the fissure lines, either between the middle lobe and upper lobe or the superior segment and the upper lobe, are not complete and must be divided, usually using stapling devices.

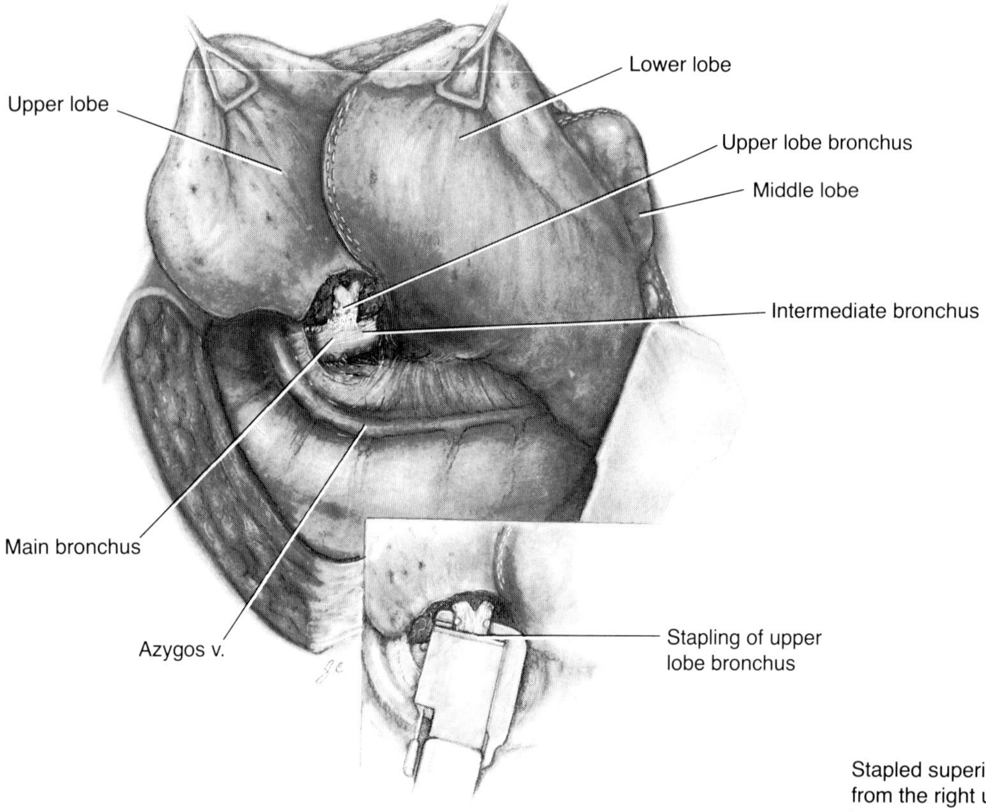

FIGURE 23–4

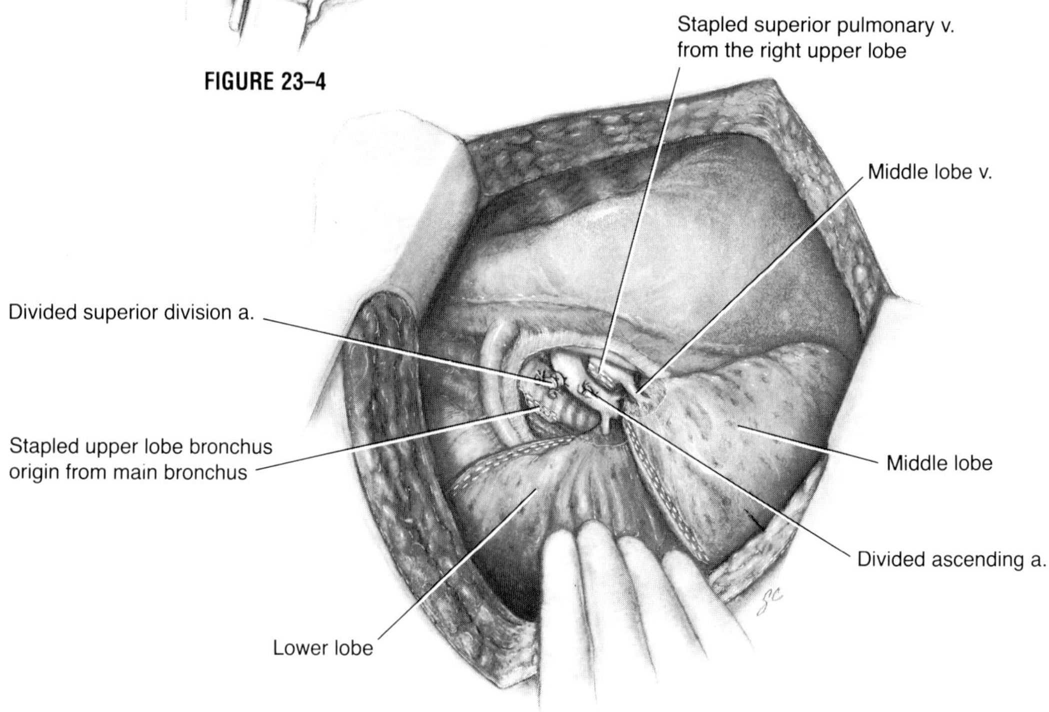

FIGURE 23–5

FIGURES 23–4 and 23–5. The posterior segmental artery is identified, ligated, and divided, after which the bronchus is cleaned and stapled and the upper lobe is removed. Two chest tubes are placed within the pleural space, one anteriorly and one laterally. The chest is closed in layers in the usual manner.

WALTER G. WOLFE, M.D.

24
Right Middle Lobectomy

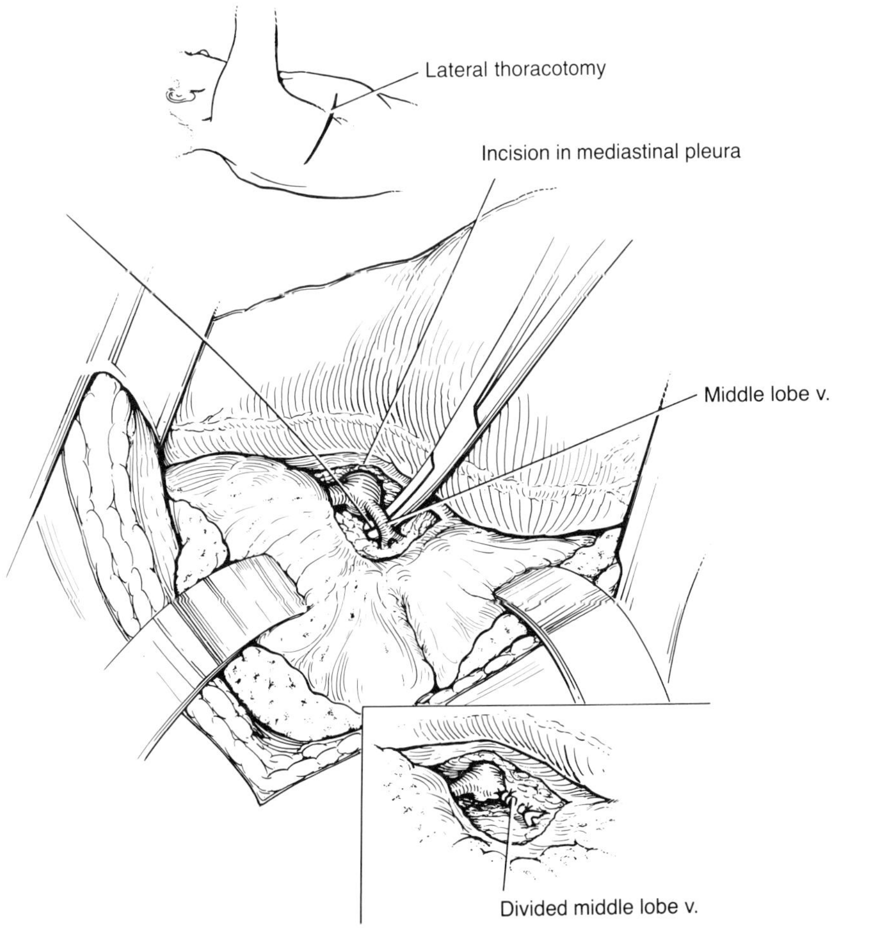

FIGURE 24–1. The patient is approached through a lateral incision usually in the fifth interspace with the cutting of the fifth rib posteriorly.

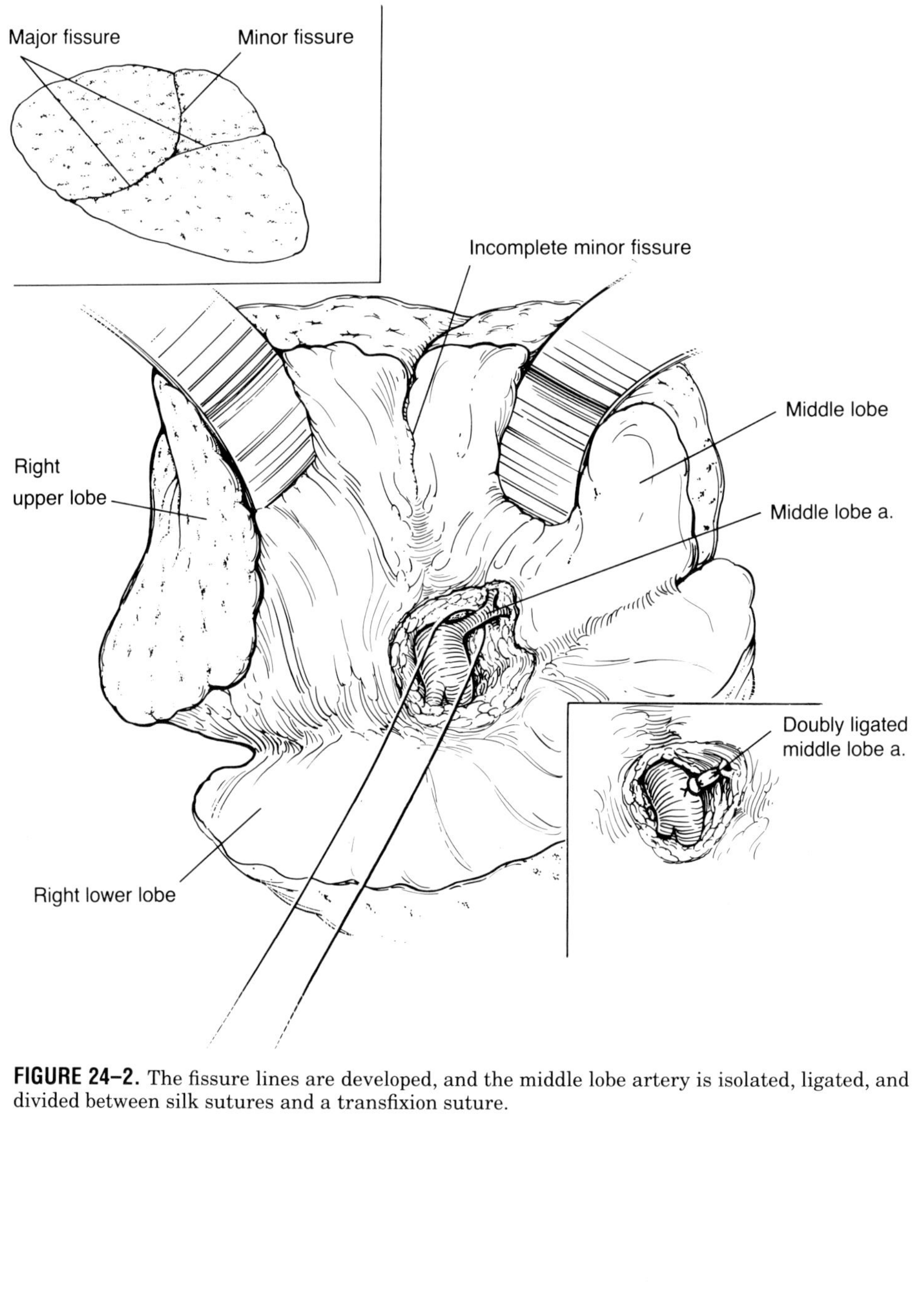

FIGURE 24–2. The fissure lines are developed, and the middle lobe artery is isolated, ligated, and divided between silk sutures and a transfixion suture.

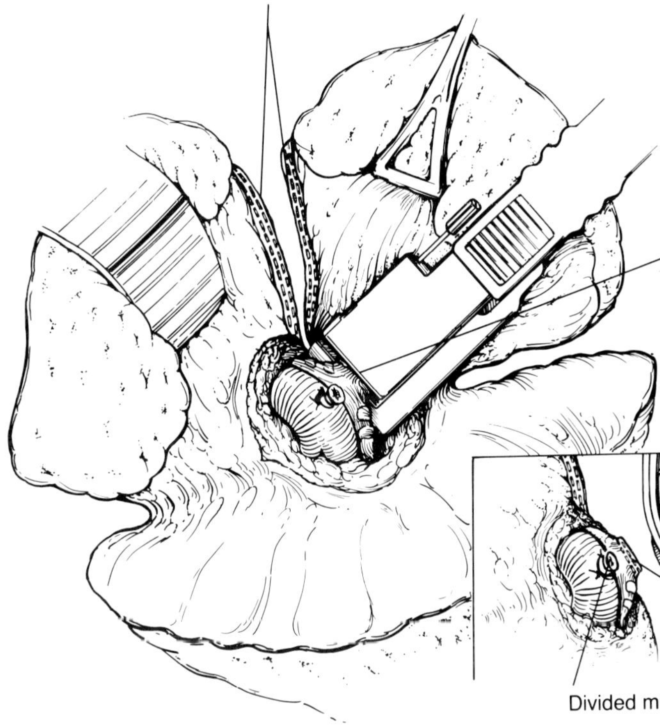

FIGURE 24–3. The vein is identified, ligated, and divided. The remaining fissures are completed, usually with the stapler, and the bronchus is divided and closed with interrupted sutures or with a stapling device. Once the stapler is placed and closed, the upper and lower lobes are inflated, having been previously collapsed with the use of a divided tube, to ensure that the lower lobe bronchus or the bronchus intermedius has not been compromised. Chest tubes are placed, and the chest is closed in the usual manner.

WALTER G. WOLFE, M.D.

25
Right Lower Lobectomy

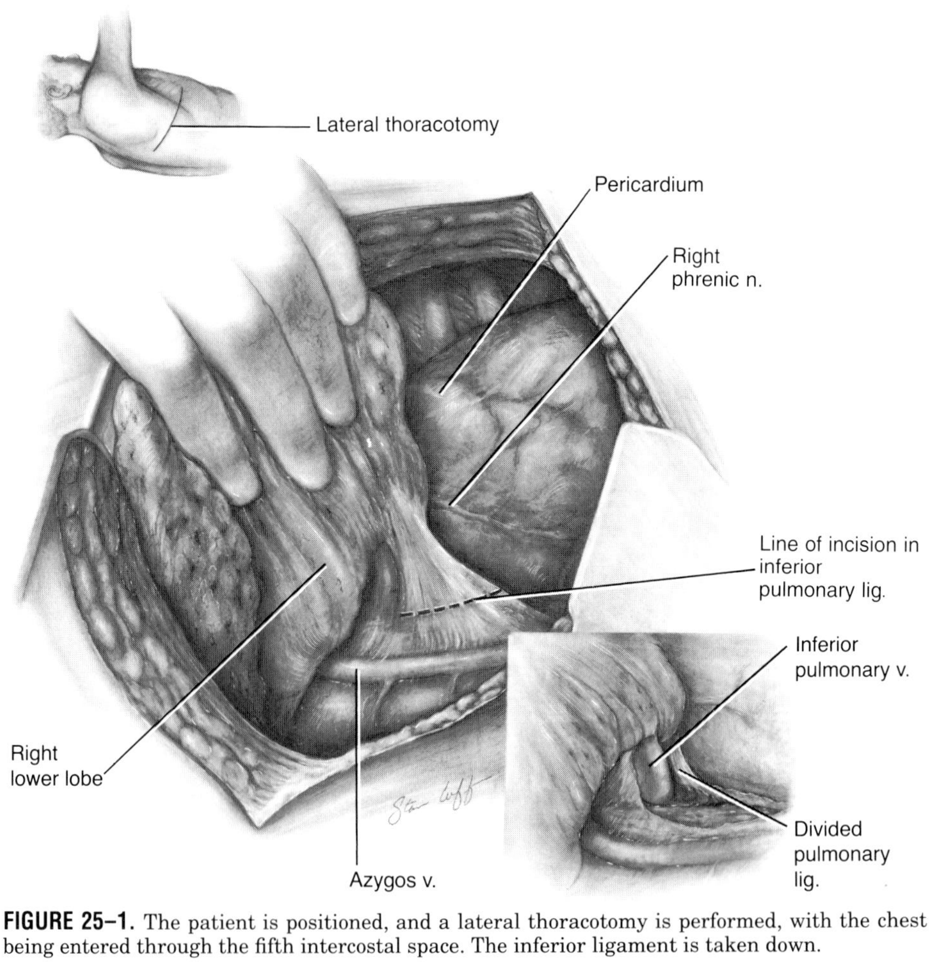

FIGURE 25–1. The patient is positioned, and a lateral thoracotomy is performed, with the chest being entered through the fifth intercostal space. The inferior ligament is taken down.

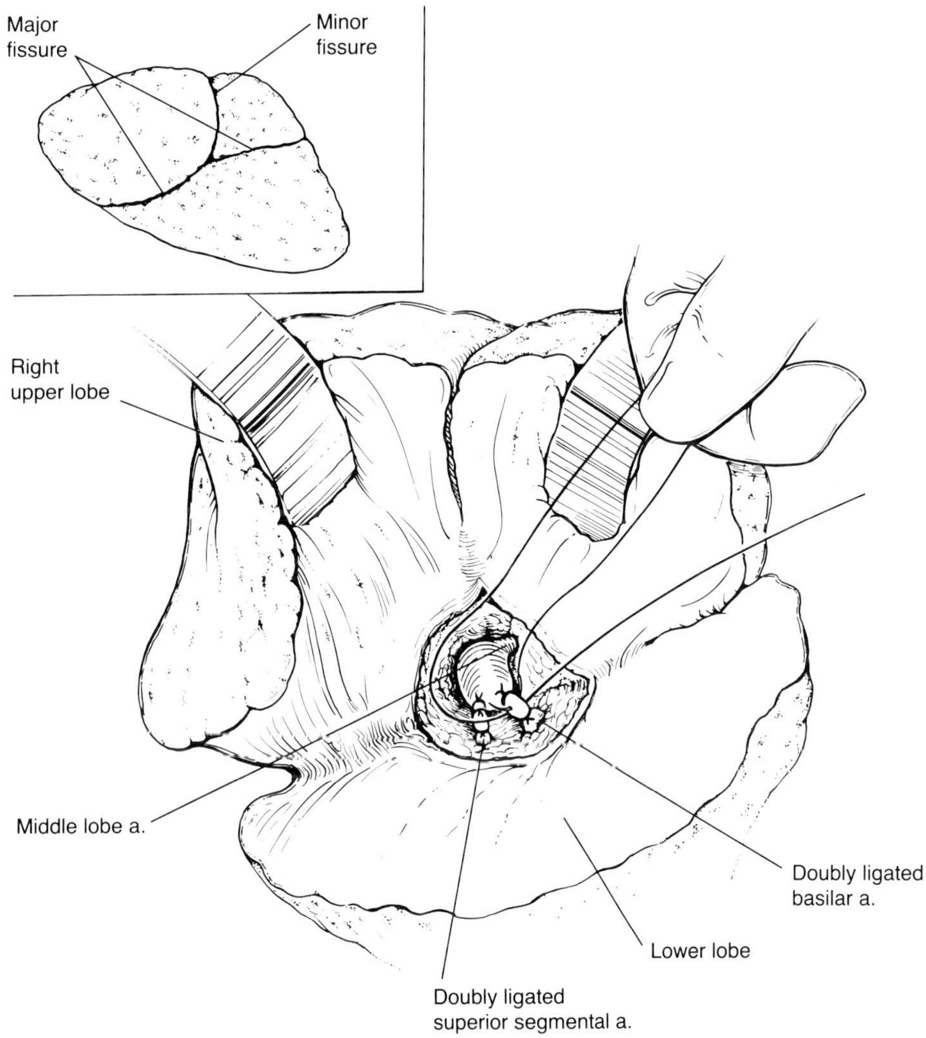

FIGURE 25–2. After the hilum and mediastinum have been explored, the vein is usually isolated. The fissure is opened and the superior segmental artery is identified, ligated, and divided between transfixion sutures.

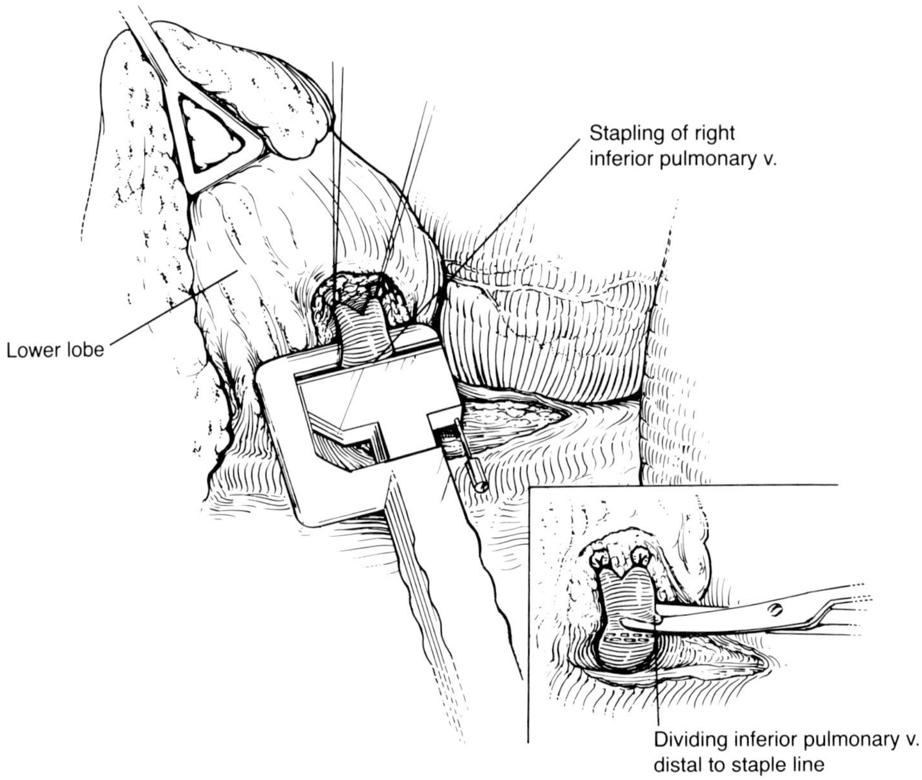

FIGURE 25–3. The remaining artery to the lower lobe is ligated and divided, and the vein is stapled and divided.

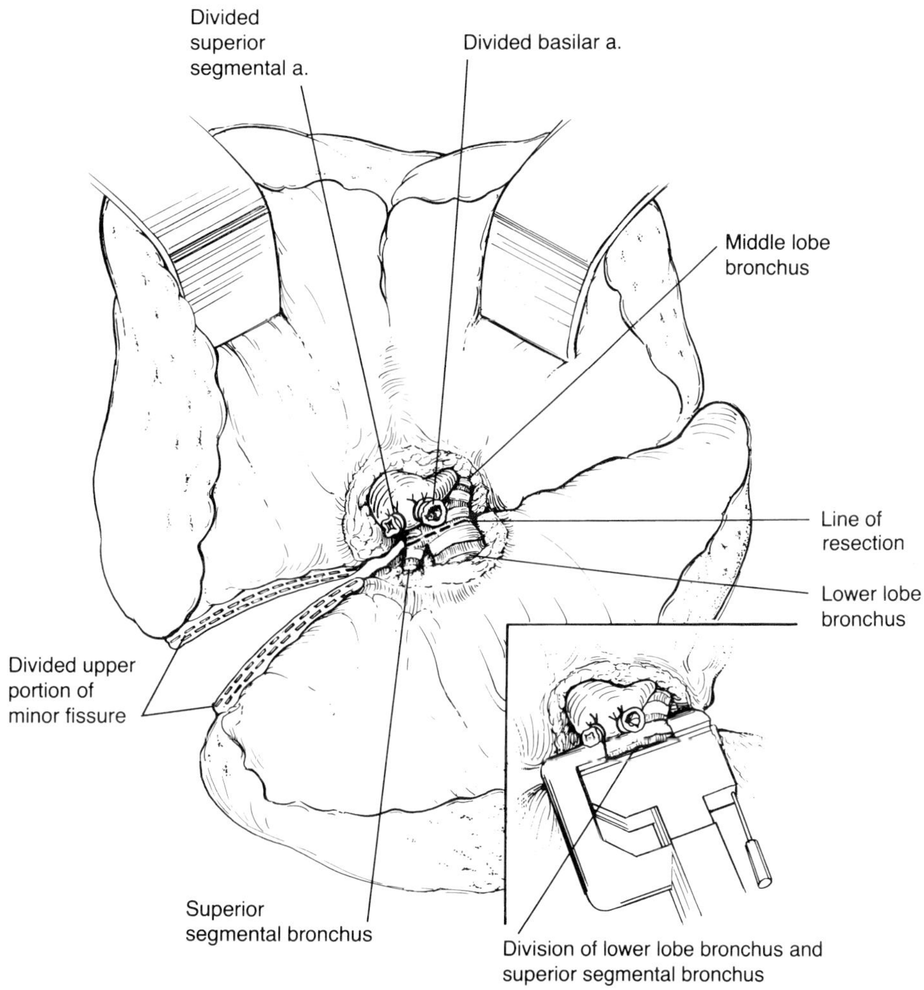

FIGURE 25–4. The bronchus is dissected of surrounding tissue, the stapler is positioned and closed, and the upper and middle lobes are ventilated again to ensure no compromise to the middle lobe bronchus.

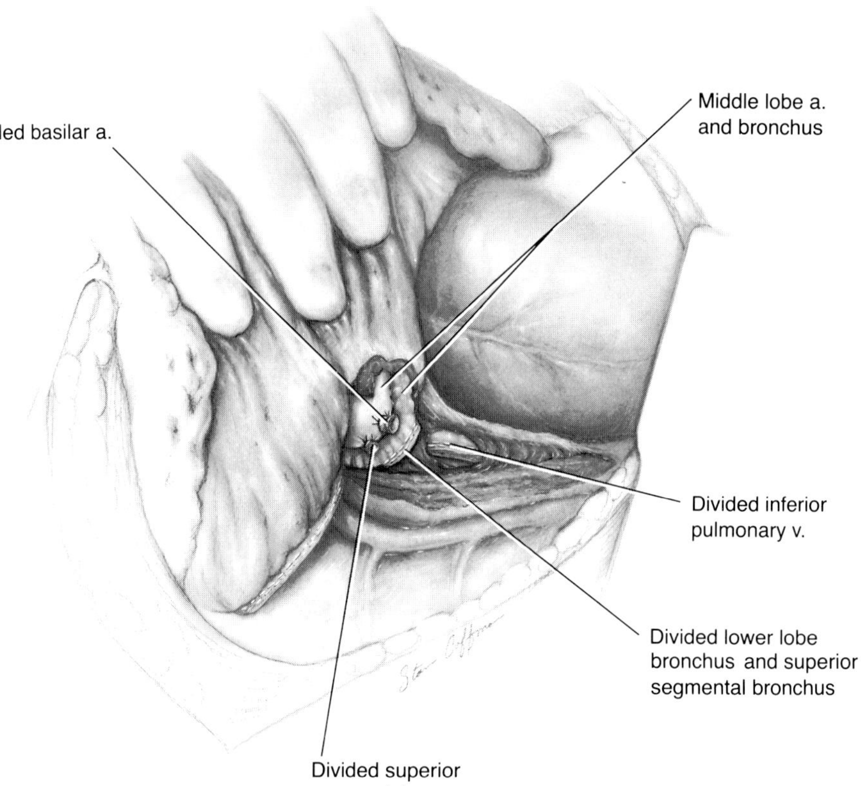

FIGURE 25–5. The stapler is fired, and the lower lobe is removed. Two chest tubes are placed anterior and posterolateral, and the chest is closed in the usual manner.

W. GLENN YOUNG, JR., M.D.

26

Left Upper Lobectomy

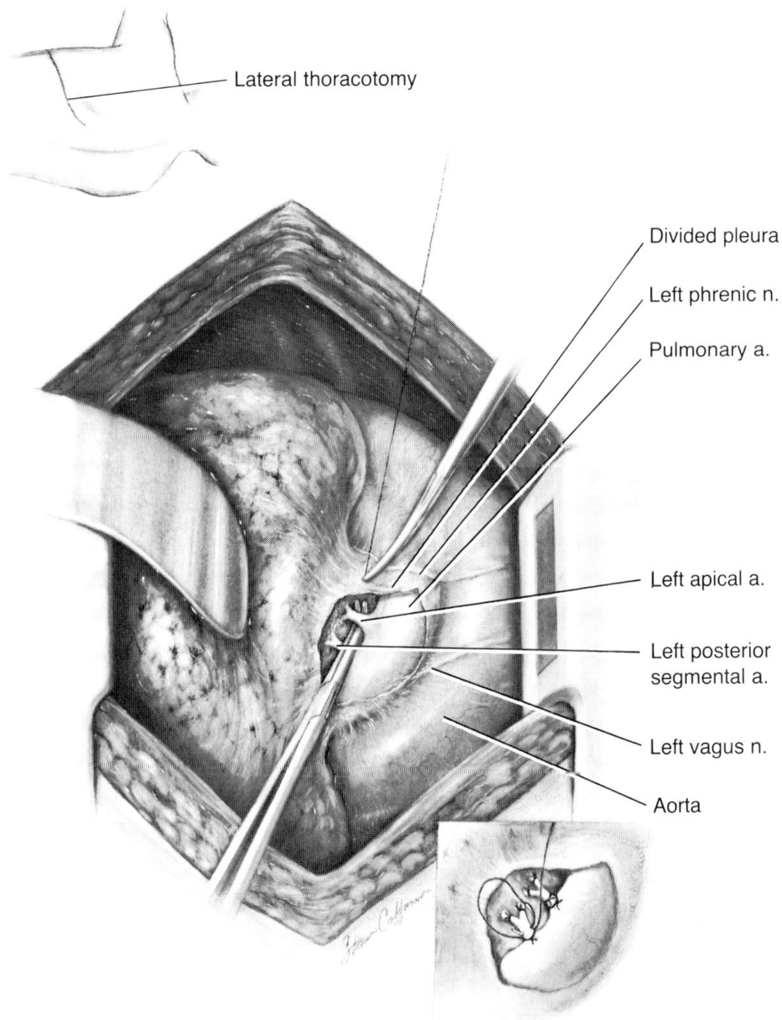

FIGURE 26–1. This resection is usually performed through a standard lateral thoracotomy, often with mobilization of the latissimus and serratus muscles to avoid their division. A double-lumen endotracheal tube is used to collapse the involved lung. With the upper lobe retracted downward, the pleura overlying the main left pulmonary artery posterior to the phrenic nerve is divided.

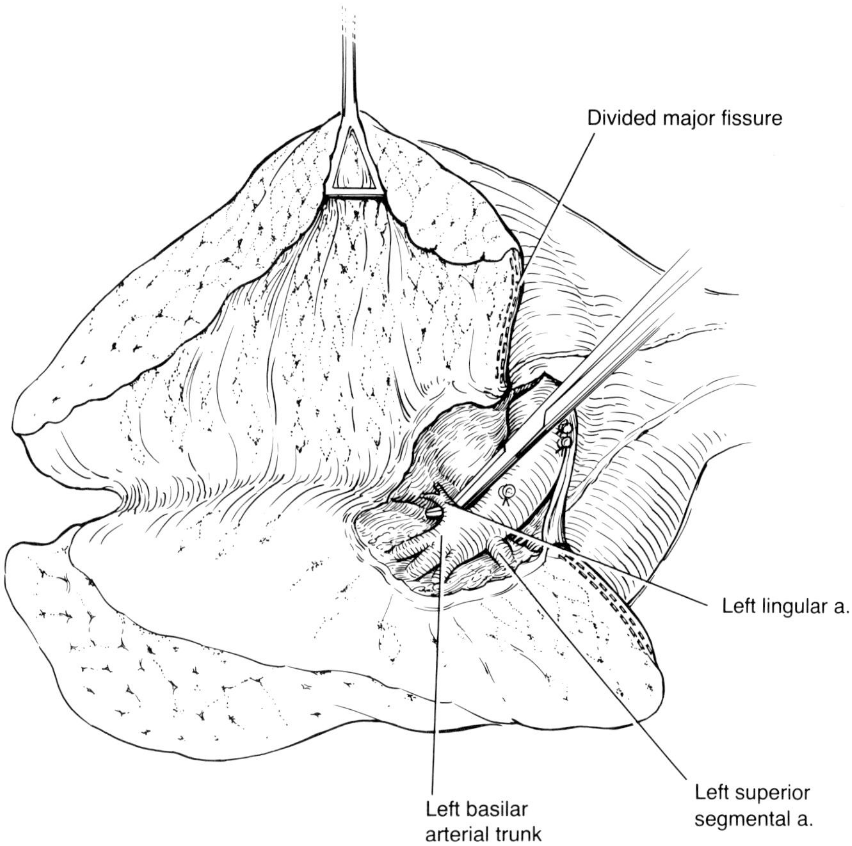

FIGURE 26–2. On the left side, the upper lobe has four or five or more individual branches originating from the main trunk, each of which is carefully dissected and doubly ligated, transfixed, and divided. Incomplete portions of the major fissure are divided using the GIA stapler.

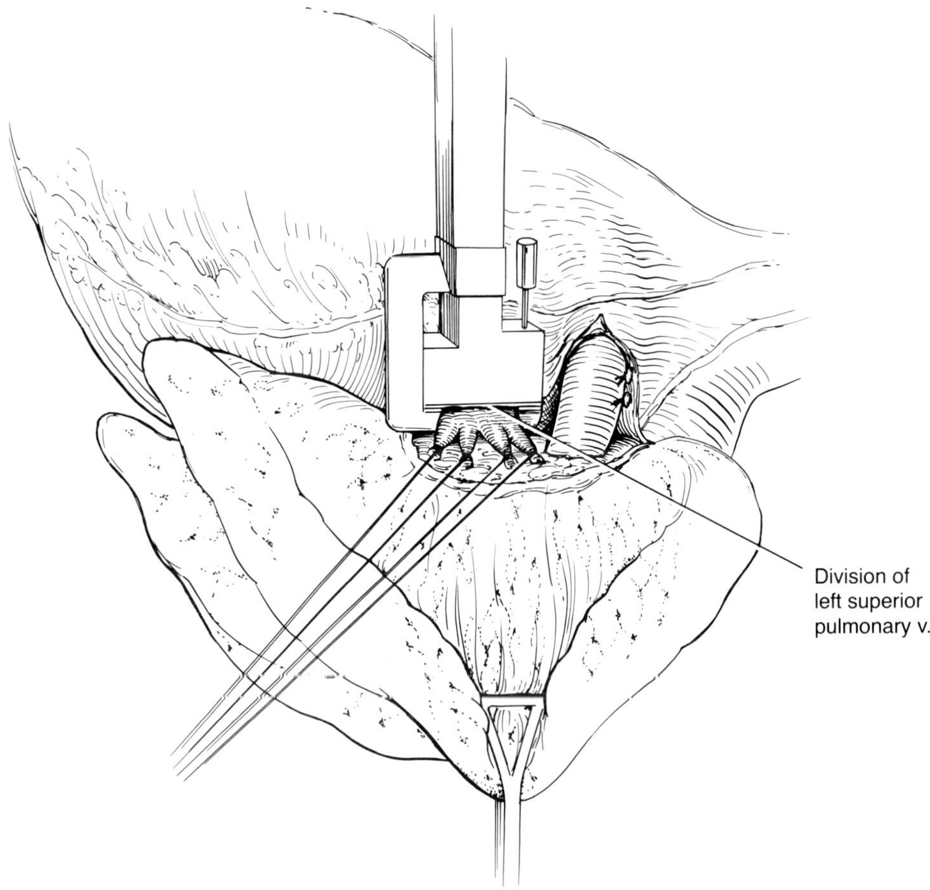

FIGURE 26–3. With the upper lobe retracted posteriorly, the superior pulmonary vein is isolated as it enters the pericardium anteriorly. The distal venous branches are ligated, and the proximal vein is occluded using the vascular TA-30 stapler. The stapler is released prior to division of the vein to ensure that the staples fired correctly.

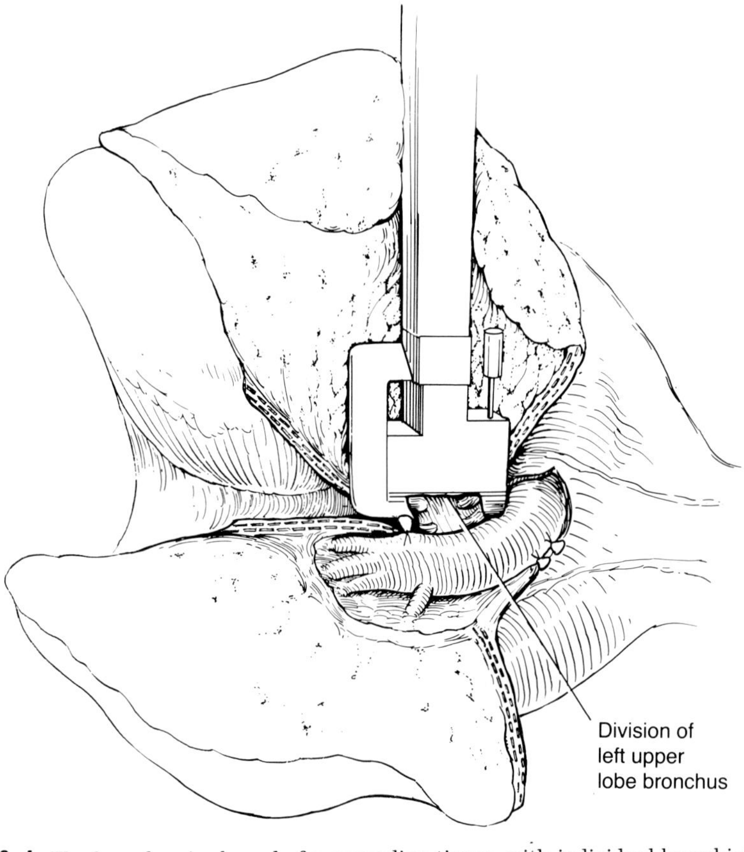

FIGURE 26–4. The bronchus is cleared of surrounding tissue, with individual bronchial arteries being ligated as encountered. The bronchus is closed with the TA-30 stapler close to its junction with the lower lobe bronchus. After the bronchus has been divided and the specimen removed, the inferior pulmonary ligament may be divided to allow the upper lobe to better fill the remaining pleural cavity.

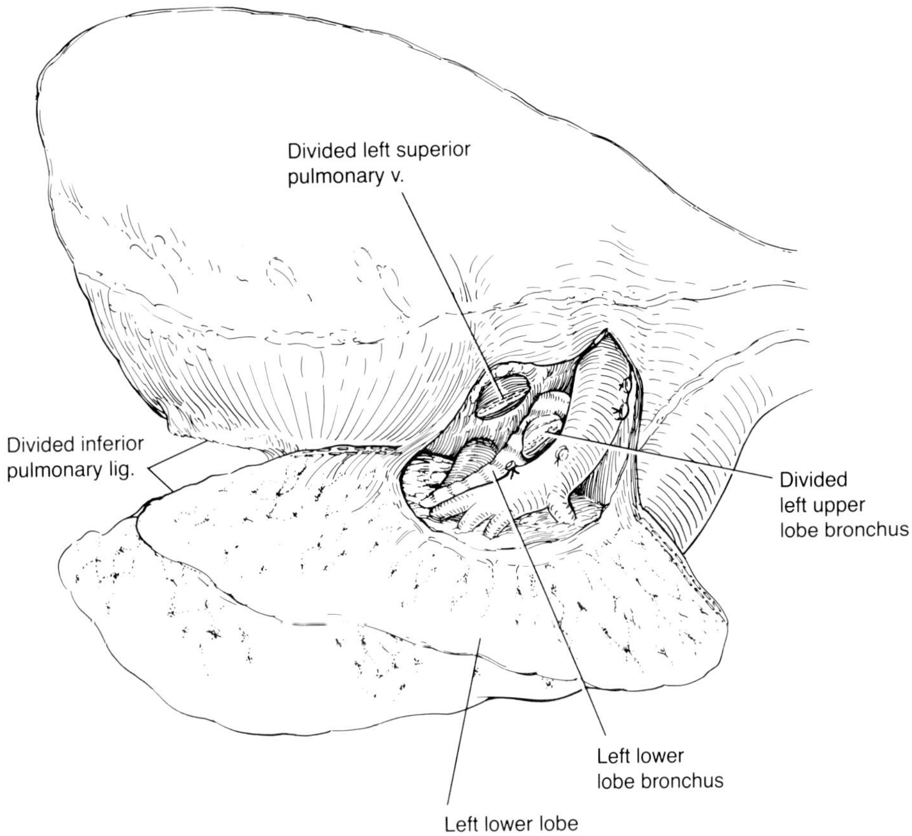

FIGURE 26–5. Completed left upper lobectomy.

W. GLENN YOUNG, JR., M.D.

27
Left Lower Lobectomy

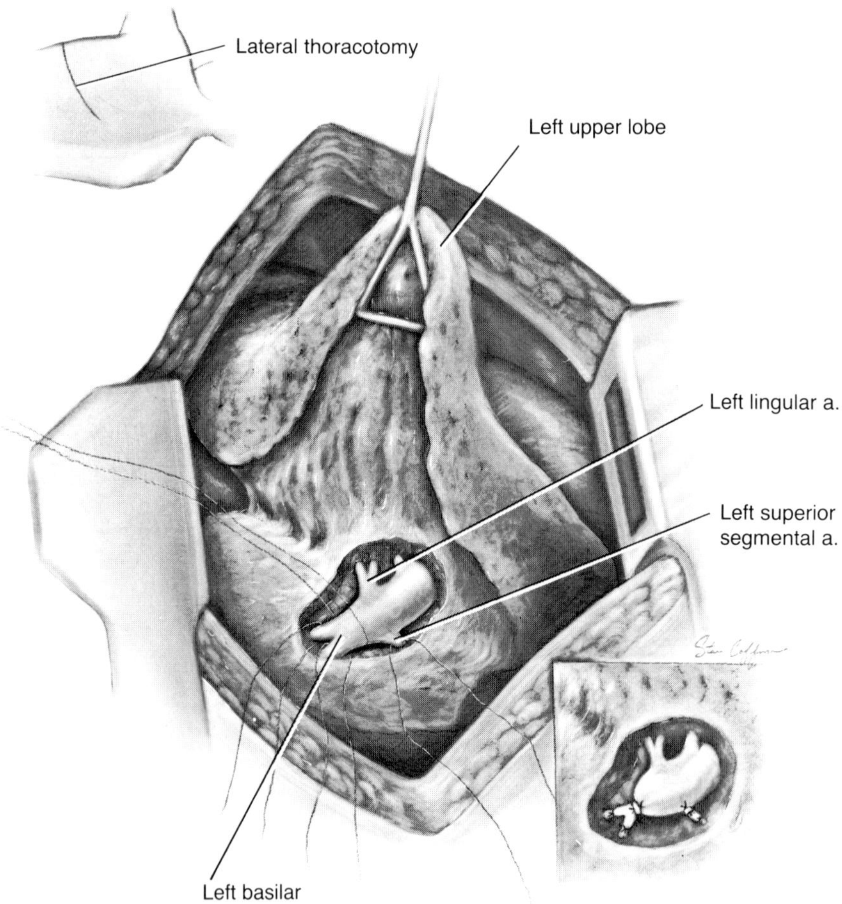

FIGURE 27–1. With the left lung collapsed and the upper lobe retracted anteriorly, dissection is begun in the major fissure, exposing the pulmonary artery.

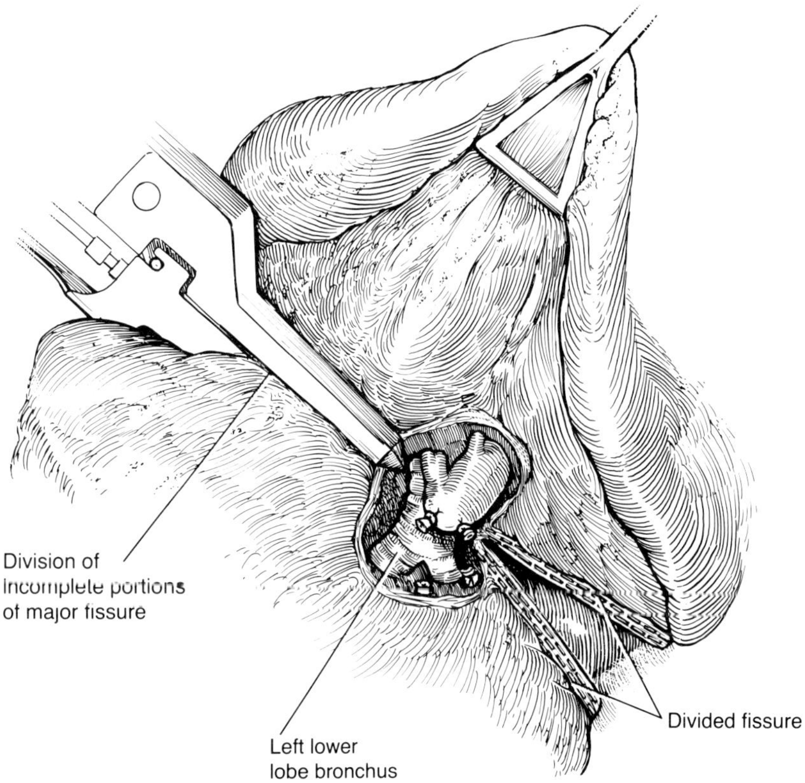

FIGURE 27–2. The arterial branch to the superior segment and the basilar arterial trunk are individually doubly ligated, transfixed, and divided. Incomplete portions of the major fissure are divided using the GIA stapler.

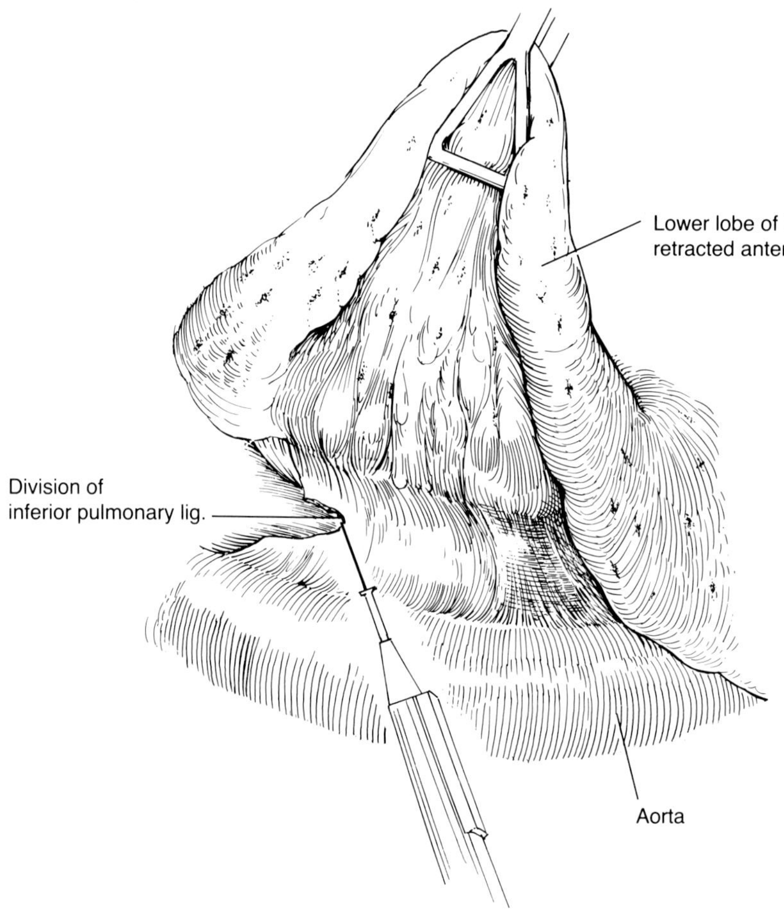

FIGURE 27–3. The lower lobe is retracted anteriorly, exposing the inferior pulmonary ligament adjacent to the aorta and overlying the inferior pulmonary vein.

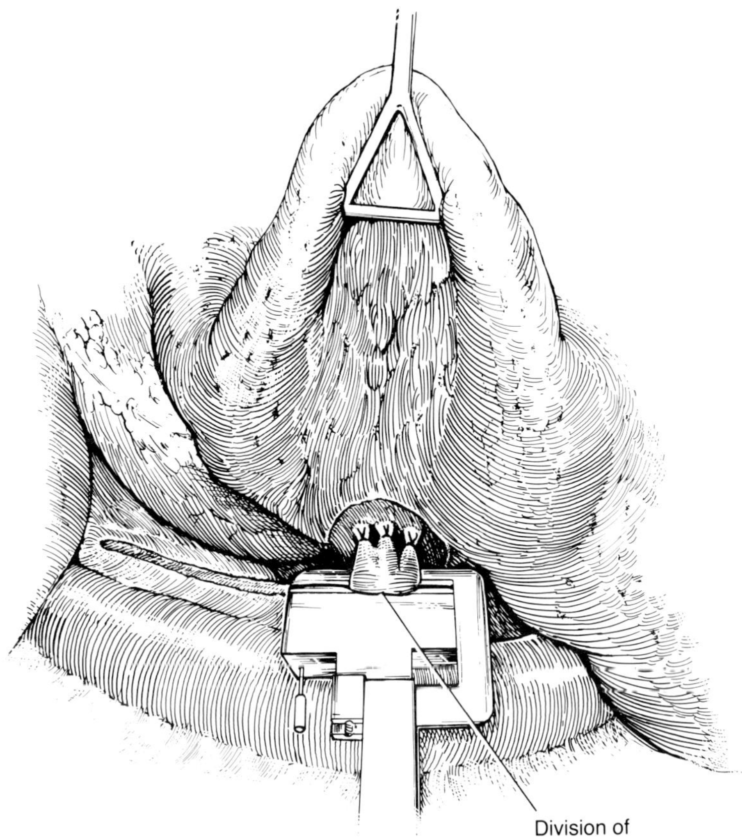

FIGURE 27–4. Division of the inferior pulmonary ligament exposes the inferior pulmonary vein, which is controlled with ligatures distally and the vascular stapler proximally.

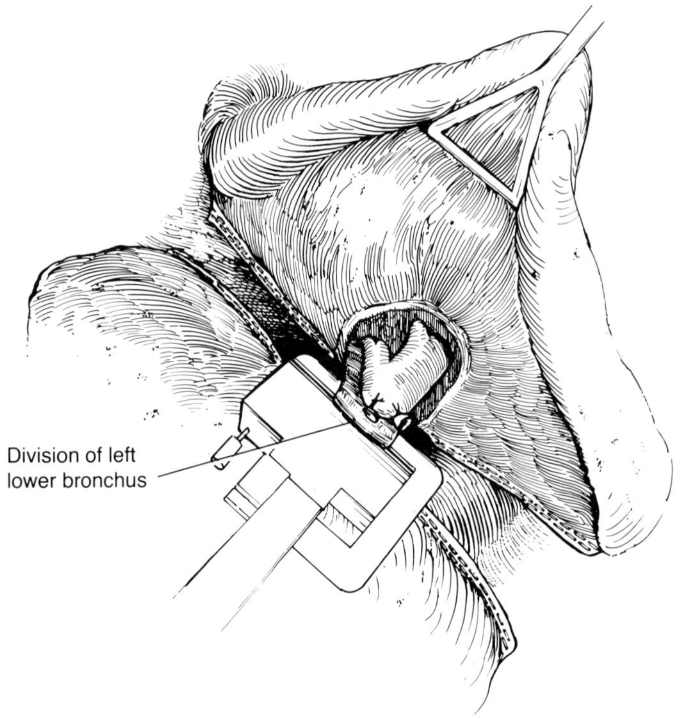

FIGURE 27–5. After the inferior vein is divided, the only remaining attachment of the lower lobe is the bronchus, which is cleared of surrounding tissues, closed with the TA-30 stapler close to the upper lobe bronchus, and divided. Incomplete portions of the major fissure are divided using the GIA stapler.

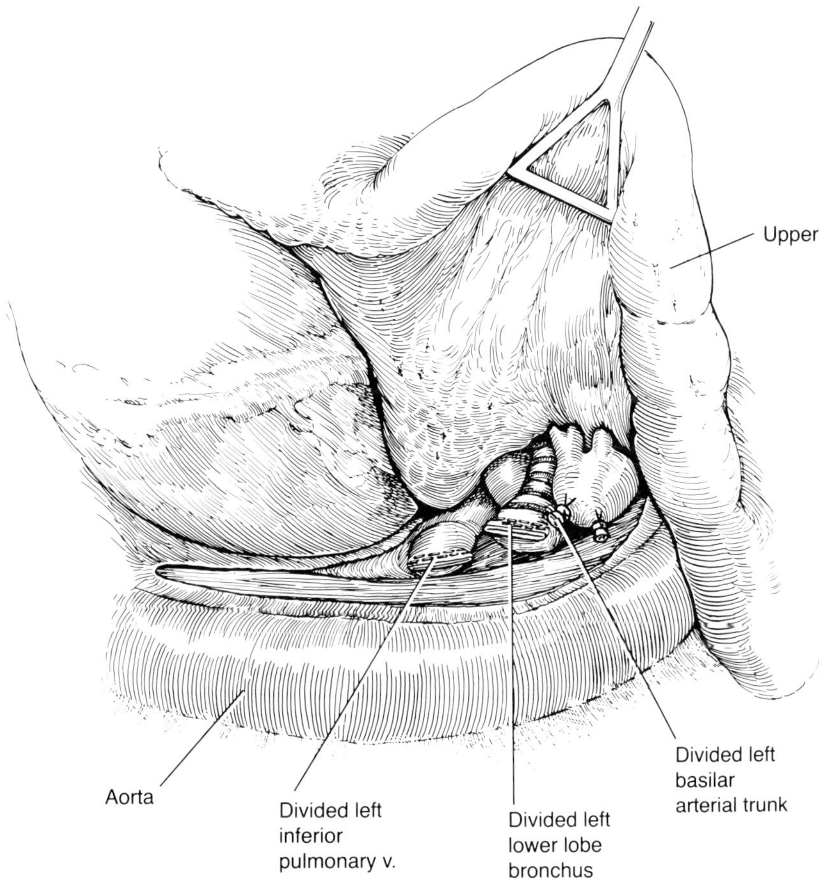

FIGURE 27–6. Completed left lower lobectomy.

WALTER G. WOLFE, M.D.

28

Right Pneumonectomy

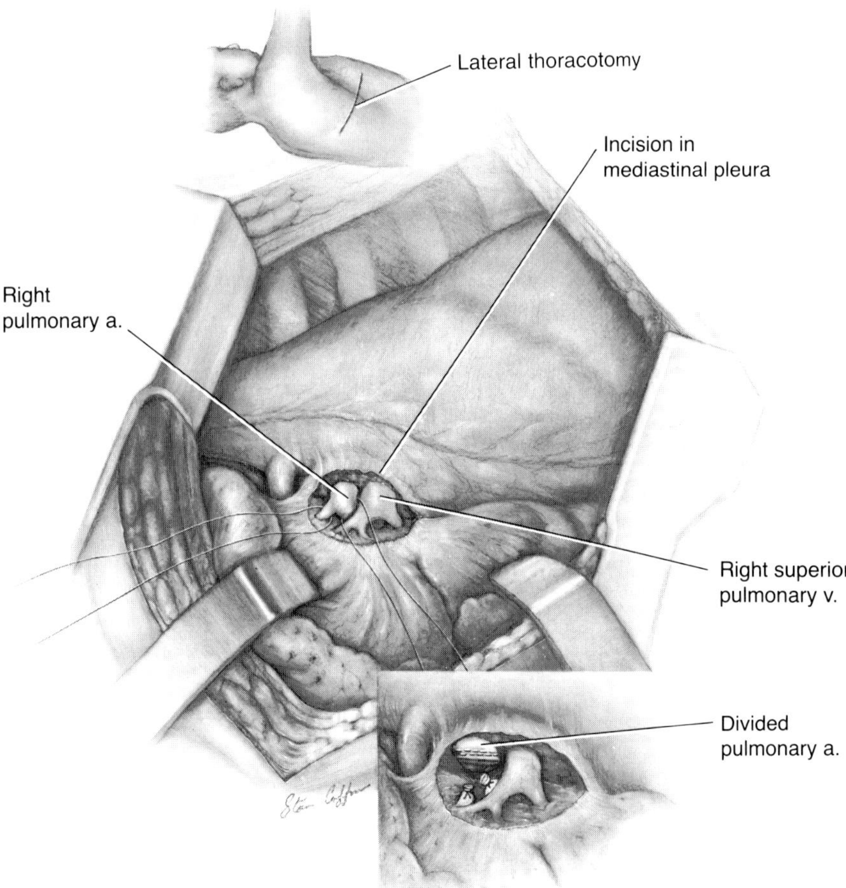

FIGURE 28–1. A right posterolateral thoracotomy incision is performed using a muscle-sparing technique if possible. The chest is usually entered through the fifth intercostal space, and the fifth rib is cut posteriorly. The patient is prepared with a double-lumen tube, and, usually, an epidural anesthetic is to be used postoperatively. The lung is collapsed, the inferior pulmonary ligament is taken down, and the hilum is mobilized. Any lymph nodes in the area of the azygos vein or in the mediastinum superior to the azygos vein are excised for frozen section. Resection is begun around the main pulmonary artery using sharp and blunt dissection, with the right main pulmonary artery being mobilized from the mediastinum with the finger. The vessels are encircled with ligatures. A vascular stapler is placed across the pulmonary artery and closed, the staple line is fired, and the stapler is removed with certainty that the staple line is complete and intact.

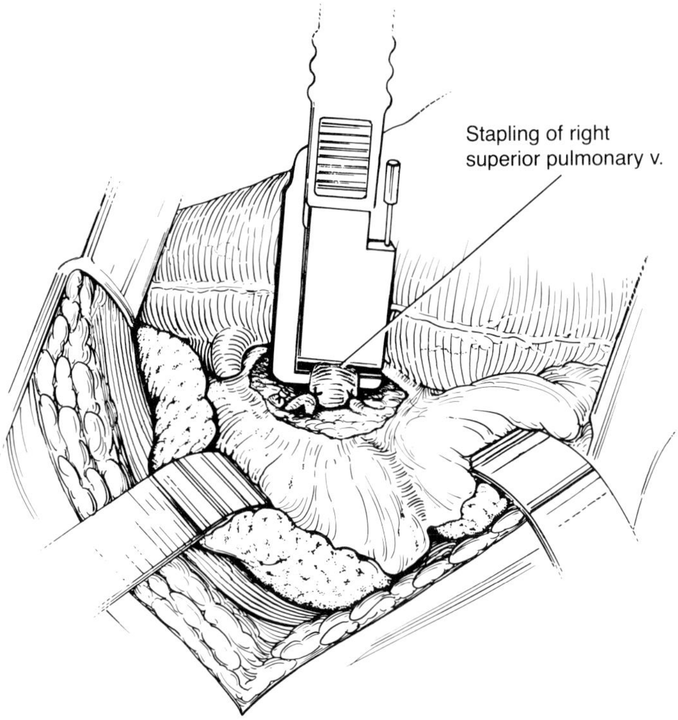

FIGURE 28–2

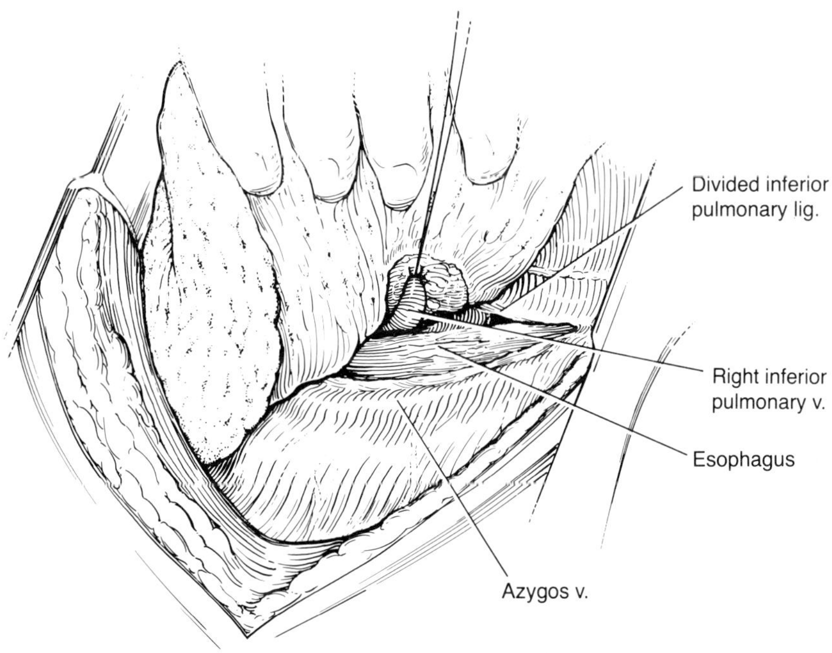

FIGURE 28–3

FIGURES 28–2 and 28–3. The superior and inferior pulmonary veins are dissected free in a similar manner and encircled, with the stapler being fired and then removed to ensure closure before the vessel is divided.

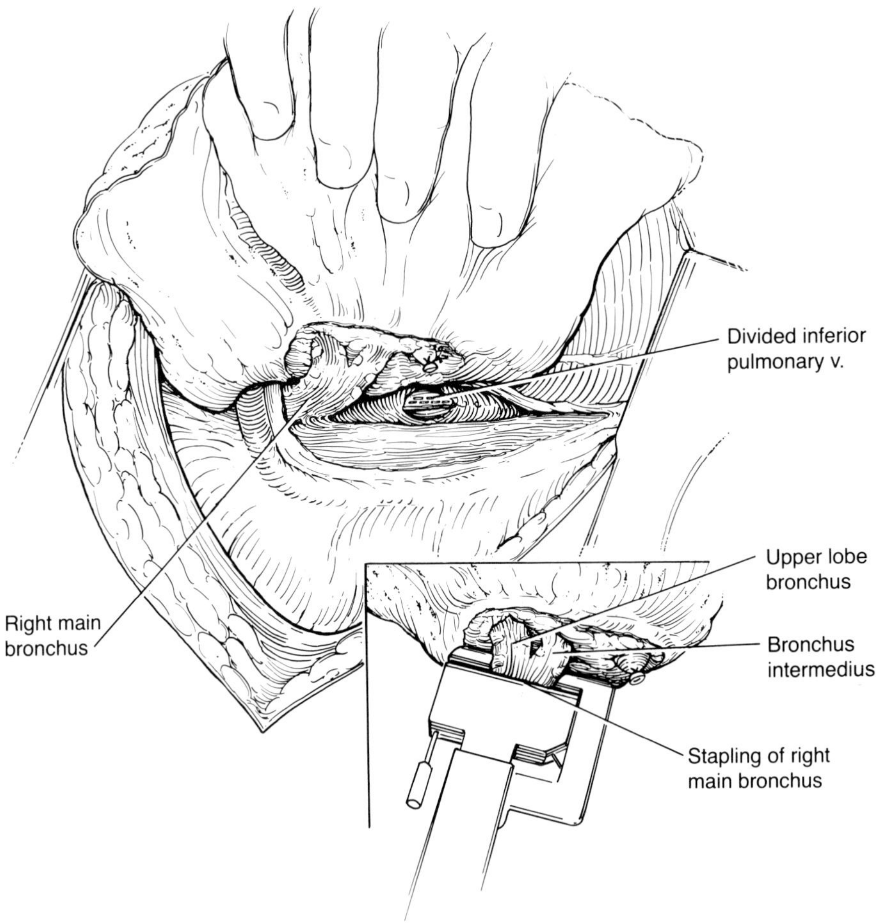

FIGURE 28–4. The right main bronchus is dissected from the remaining structures. The stapler is placed as close to the carina as possible and fired. The suture line is carefully inspected to ensure complete closure, and the specimen is removed.

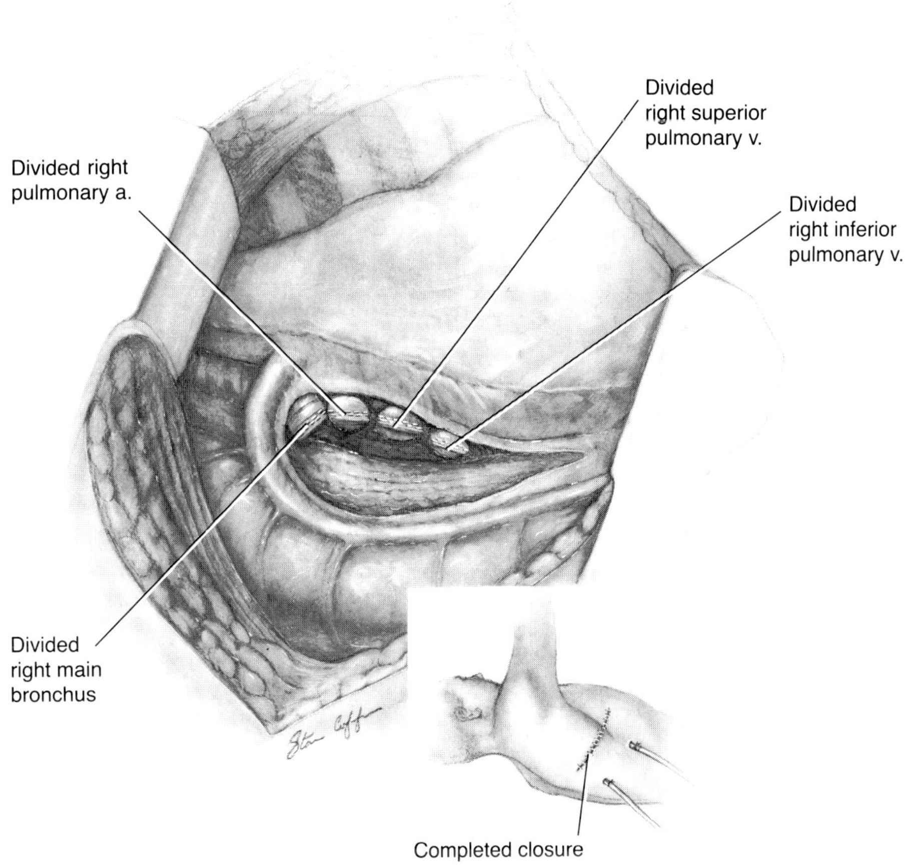

FIGURE 28–5. Once hemostasis is complete and there is no evidence of air leak, the chest is closed in layers. The patient is then positioned supine, and the pressures adjusted in the right hemithorax. A chest film is taken immediately after operation to ensure that the mediastinal position is appropriate. Chest tube drainage is rarely used following pneumonectomy.

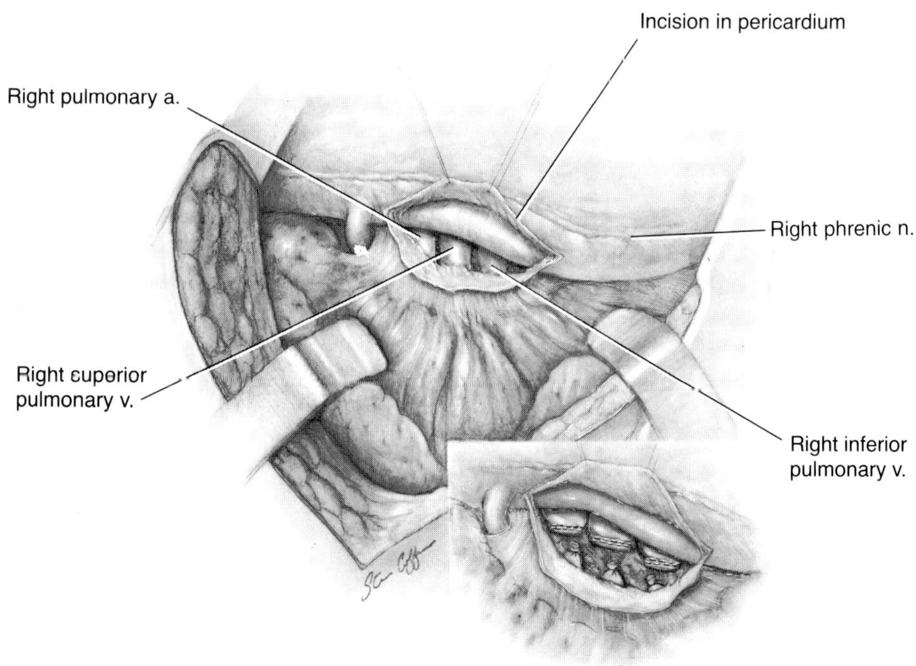

FIGURE 28–6. The approach to the vessels within the pericardium is shown. Generally, the reason for this exposure is to excise a portion of pericardium with the phrenic nerve owing to involvement of these structures with the tumor. This maneuver allows an adequate margin to be obtained.

W. GLENN YOUNG, JR., M.D.

29

Left Pneumonectomy

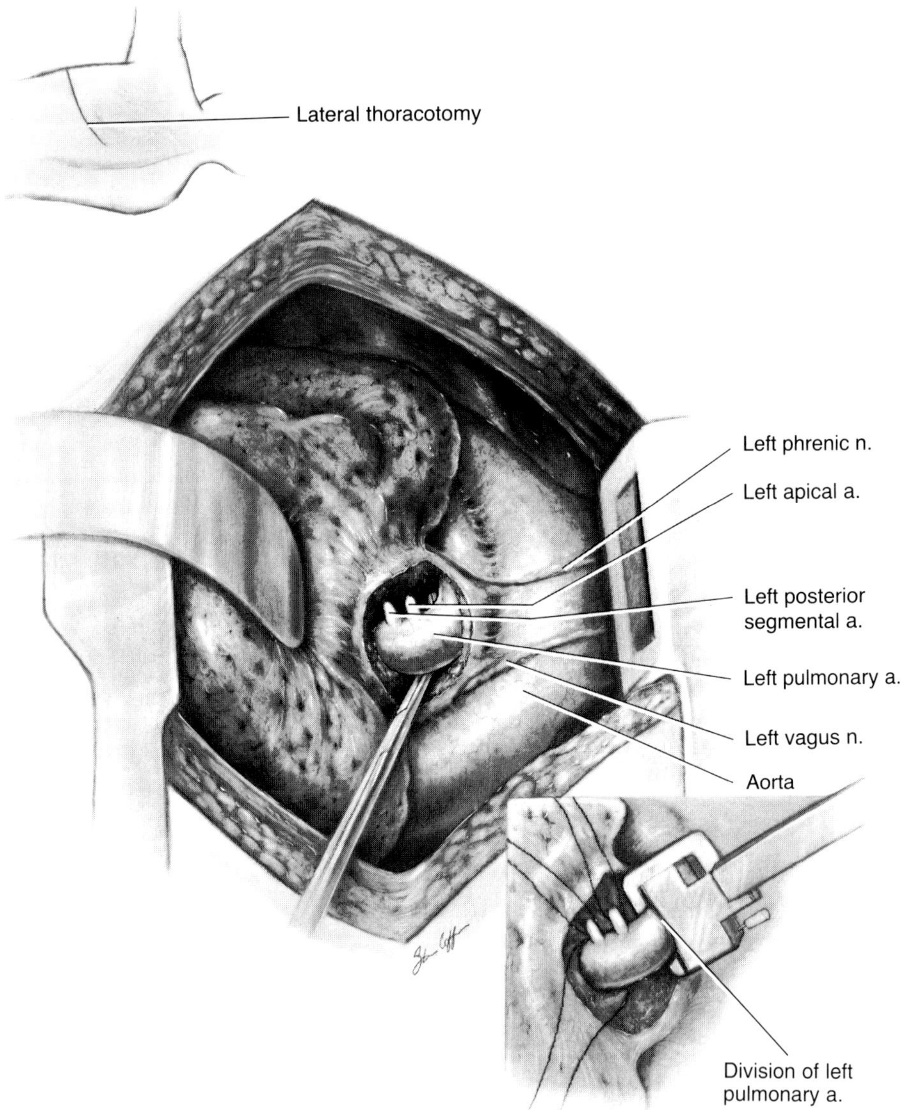

FIGURE 29–1. With the lung collapsed and retracted inferiorly, the pleura overlying the left pulmonary artery is opened with careful dissection of the left pulmonary artery.

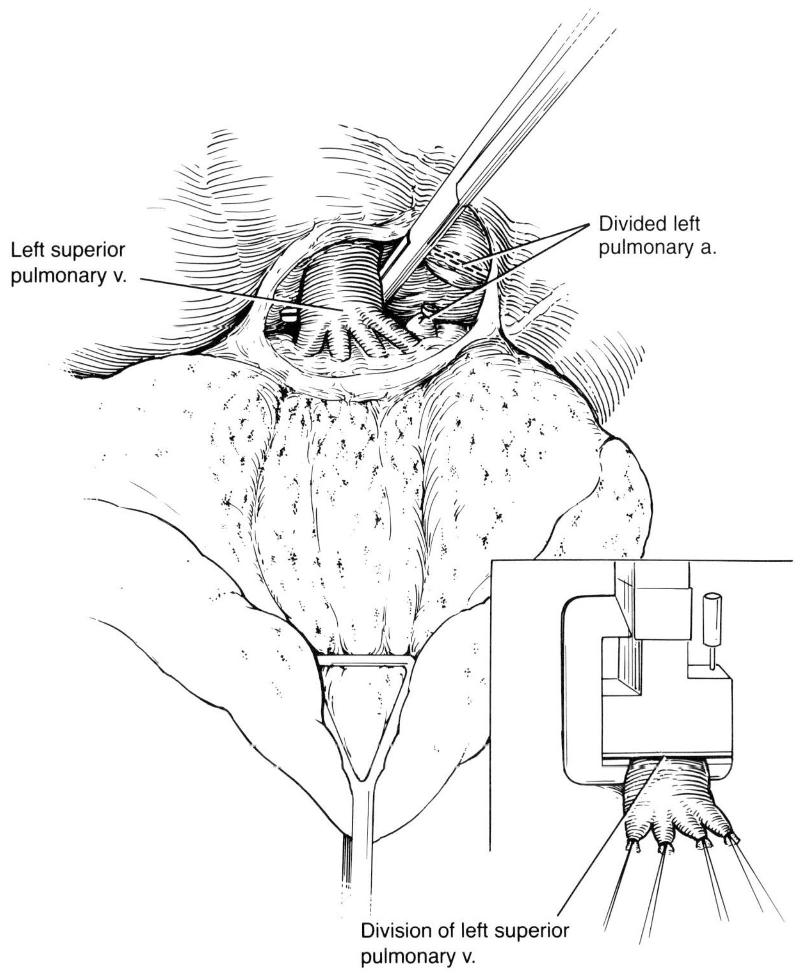

FIGURE 29–2. Ligatures are placed distally on the main arterial trunk and perhaps the first branch or two, and the proximal pulmonary artery is secured with the vascular stapler. The superior pulmonary vein is next divided in a similar manner at its junction with the pericardium. When using the stapler on these large vessels, it is wise to release the device and check the staple line prior to dividing the artery or vein.

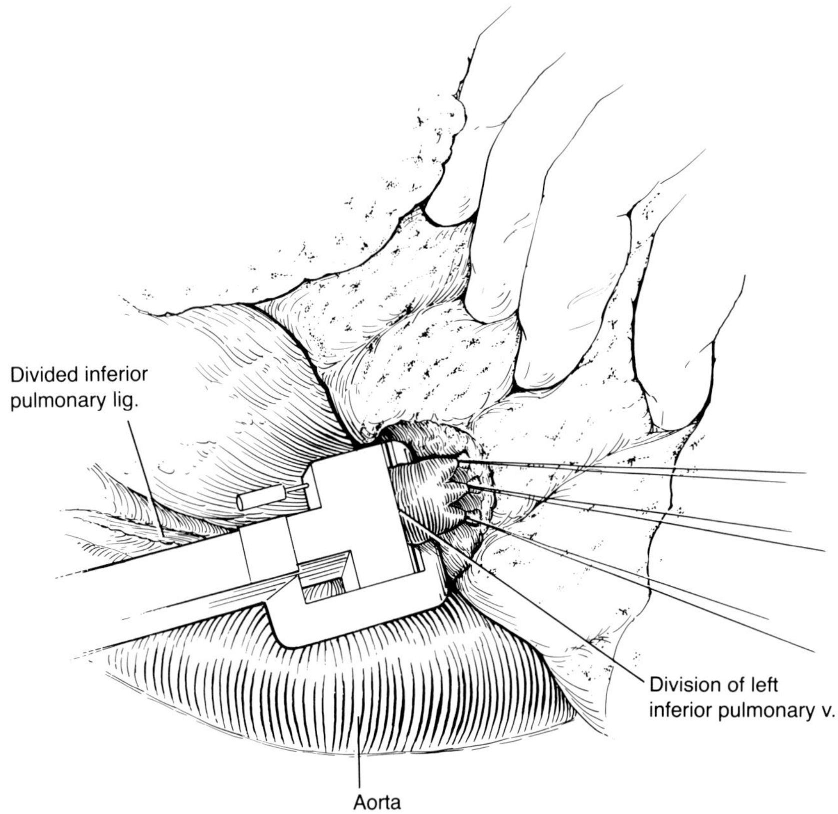

FIGURE 29–3. The lung is elevated superiorly, exposing and dividing the inferior pulmonary ligament. The inferior pulmonary vein is closed with the vascular stapler and divided.

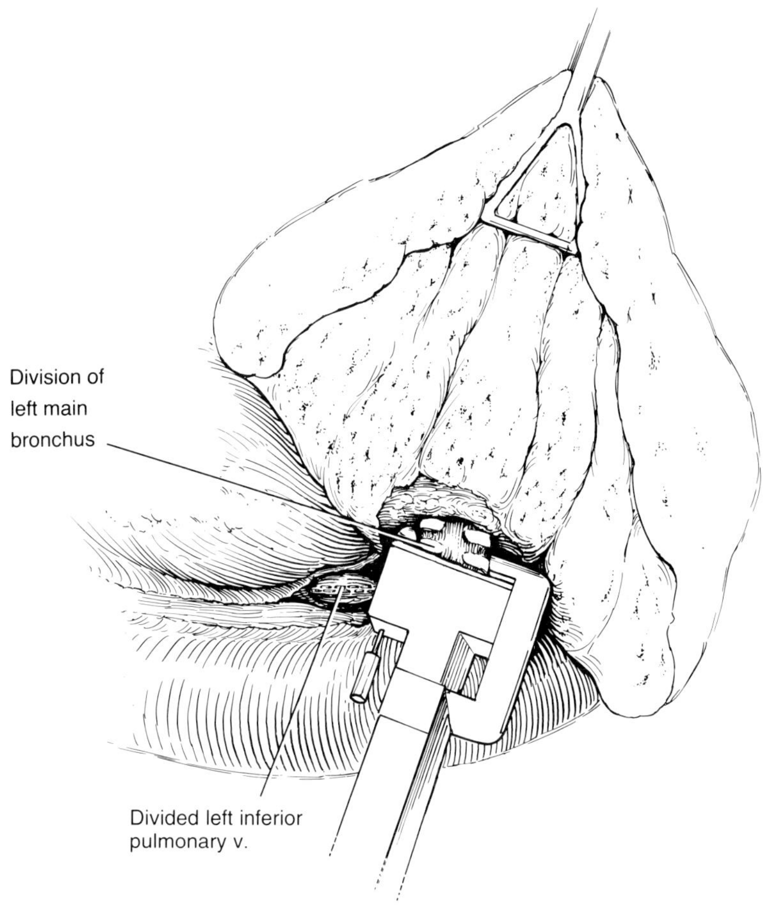

FIGURE 29–4. Individual bronchial arteries are identified and ligated. The left main bronchus is dissected as far superiorly as is feasible and is closed with a TA-30 stapler.

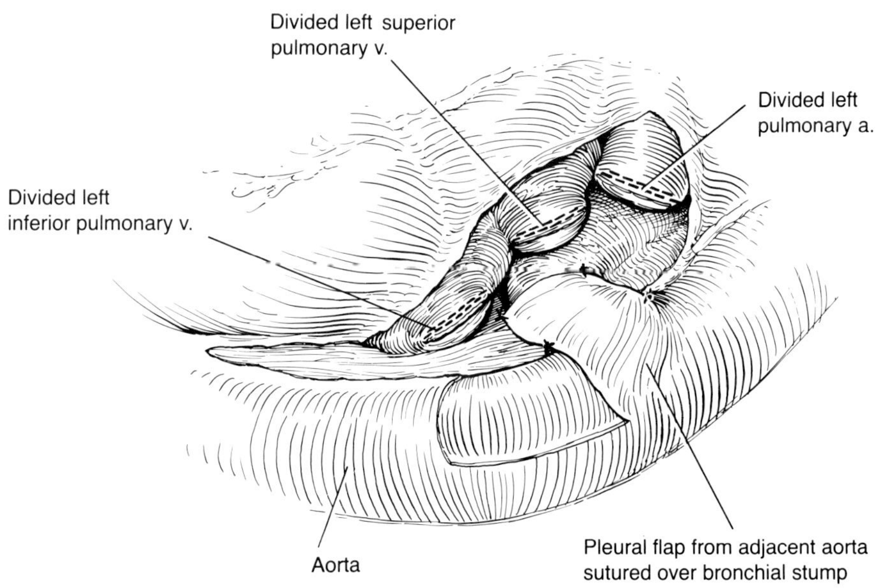

FIGURE 29–5. The bronchial stump is reinforced with a pleural flap obtained from the adjacent aorta. Closure of the chest is accomplished without chest tube drainage.

DAVID C. SABISTON, JR., M.D.

30

Embolectomy for Acute Pulmonary Embolism

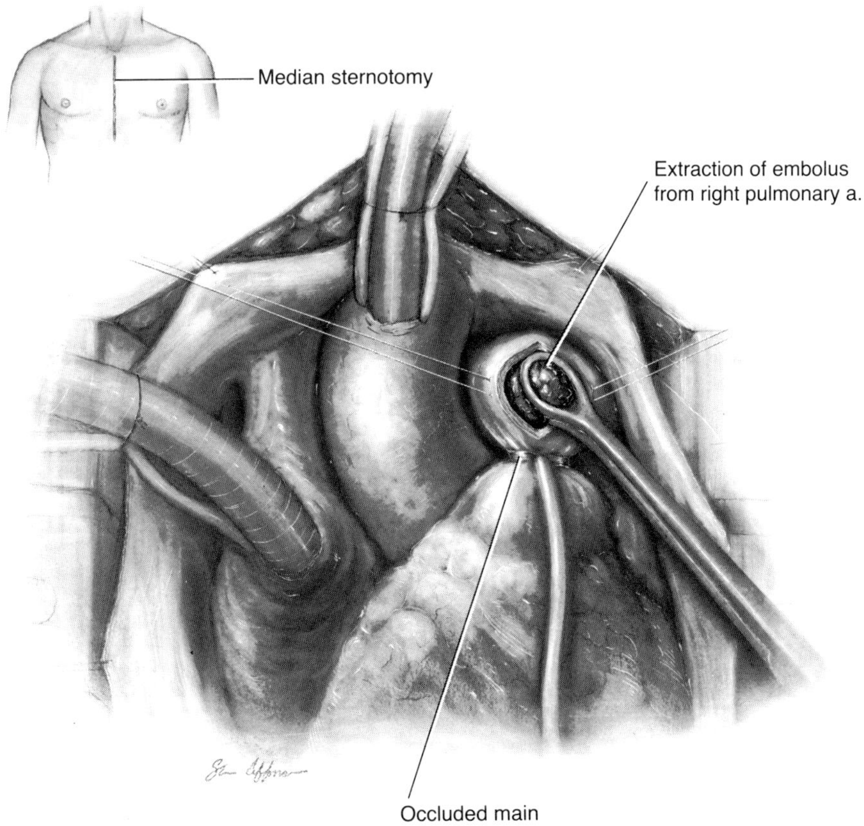

FIGURE 30–1. A median sternotomy is made and provides excellent exposure of the proximal pulmonary artery. The patient is placed on cardiopulmonary bypass with a venous cannula in the right atrium and an arterial cannula in the ascending aorta. The main pulmonary artery is exposed, and a longitudinal incision is made.

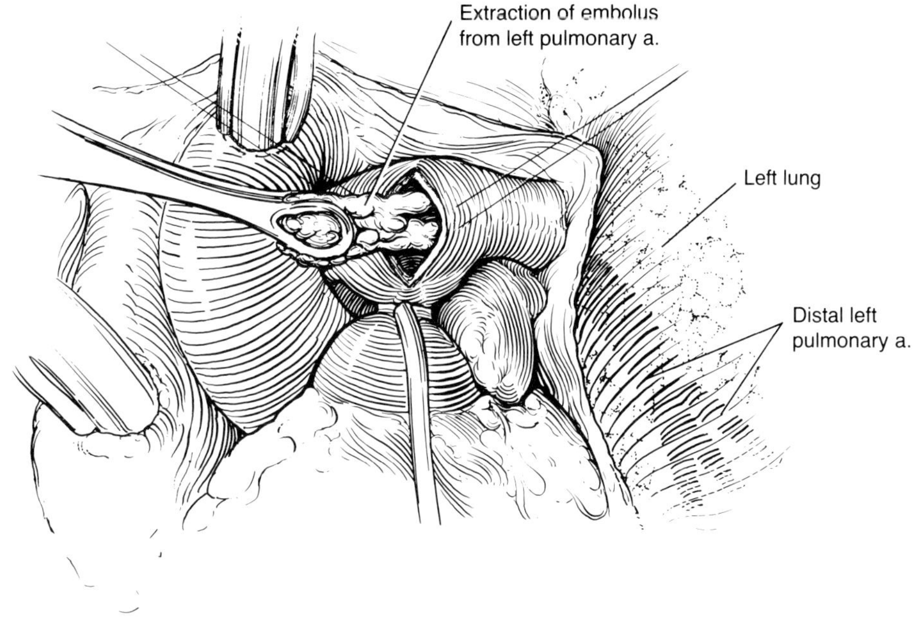

FIGURE 30–2. A long sponge forceps or curved gallstone forceps is inserted into the pulmonary artery and passed into the branches in the *open* position. At various levels, the forceps are closed and the entrapped emboli are withdrawn. The major branches of the pulmonary arteries on both the right and the left are entered with care taken that the forceps are always open during insertion and closed during withdrawal.

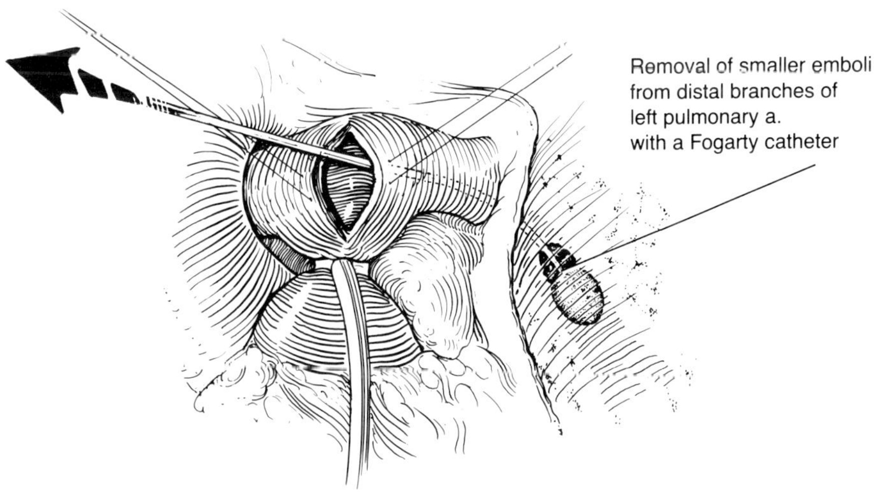

FIGURE 30–3. After each major branch has been thoroughly embolectomized, a Fogarty catheter is passed into the branches as far distally as possible. The balloon is inflated and the catheter withdrawn for removal of smaller emboli. After the Fogarty catheter has been passed into each of the distal arteries in a systematic manner, the entire pulmonary arterial tree is copiously irrigated with saline. While this is being done, general compression of both lungs with the hand directs more peripheral emboli to the central arteries, where they can be flushed with irrigation.

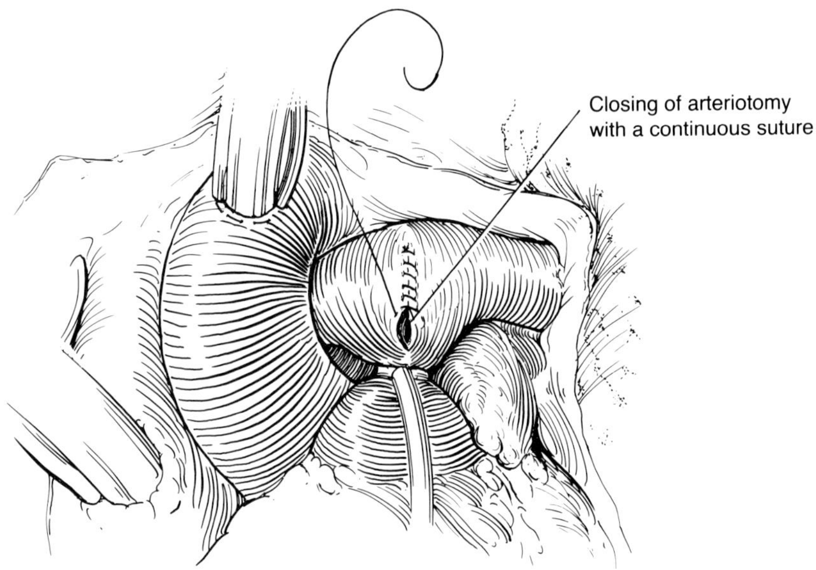

FIGURE 30–4. The pulmonary artery is closed with a continuous nonabsorbable suture, and cardiopulmonary bypass is gradually discontinued, allowing the heart and lungs to resume normal function.

DAVID C. SABISTON, JR., M.D.

31

Embolectomy for Chronic Pulmonary Embolism

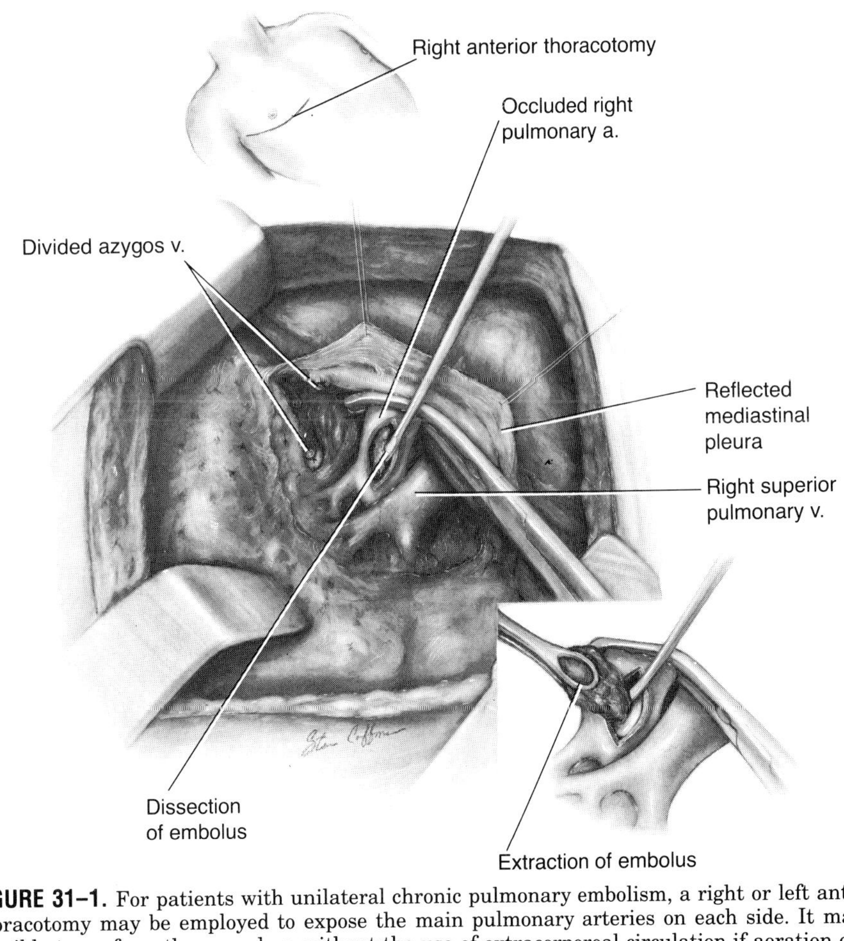

FIGURE 31–1. For patients with unilateral chronic pulmonary embolism, a right or left anterior thoracotomy may be employed to expose the main pulmonary arteries on each side. It may be possible to perform the procedure without the use of extracorporeal circulation if aeration of the opposite lung is sufficient to maintain the patient during the brief periods of occlusion of the opposite pulmonary artery during embolectomy. If cardiopulmonary bypass is necessary, it can be initiated by cannulation of the right atrium for venous return and the ascending aorta (or femoral artery) for arterial inflow. The right pulmonary artery is dissected in the hilus, and an arterial clamp is used to occlude it proximally. An incision is made distally overlying the chronic emboli, and they are dissected from the intima surface of the pulmonary artery. These chronic emboli are then removed with a sponge forceps or a curved gallstone forceps until all have been completely dissected and withdrawn.

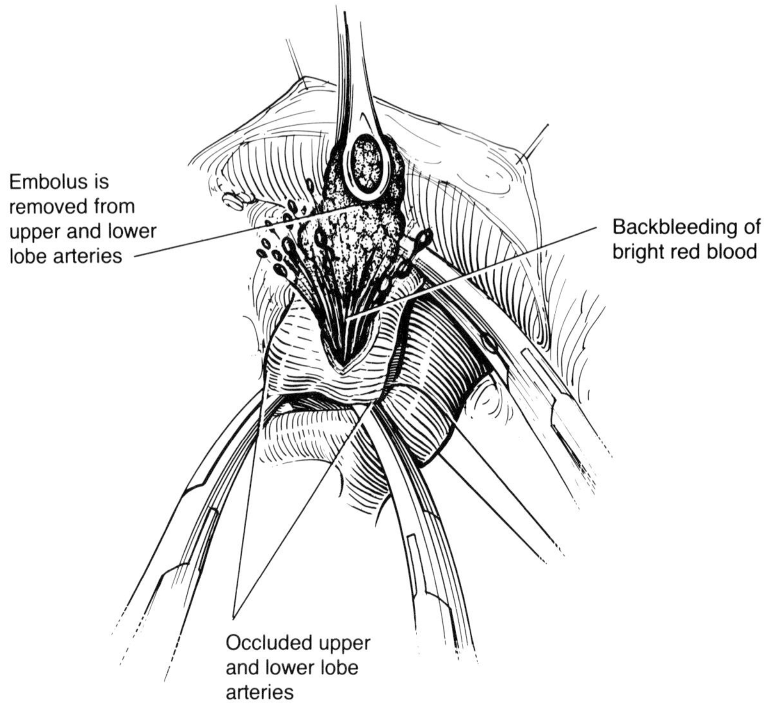

FIGURE 31–2. After the chronic emboli have been removed, vigorous backbleeding of bright red blood can be seen, which signifies that the distal pulmonary circulation is patent and provides firm evidence that the pulmonary artery will remain open, as after embolectomy there is adequate distal runoff of the pulmonary circulation.

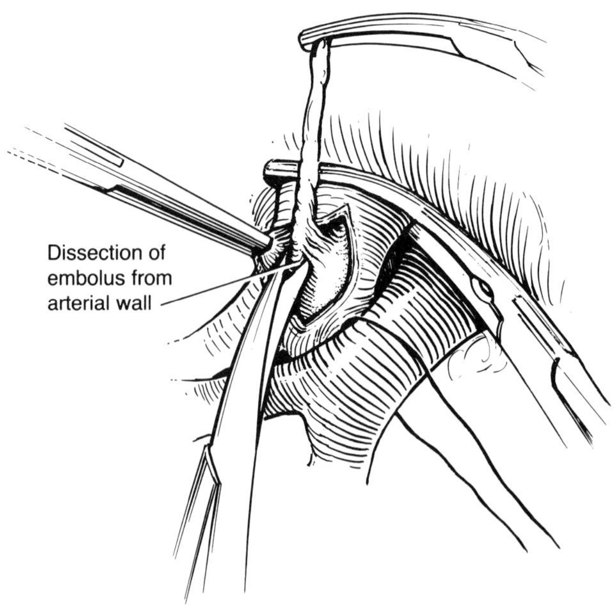

FIGURE 31–3. It is often necessary to make separate arteriotomies in the distal pulmonary vessels to dissect the chronic emboli from the pulmonary arterial wall.

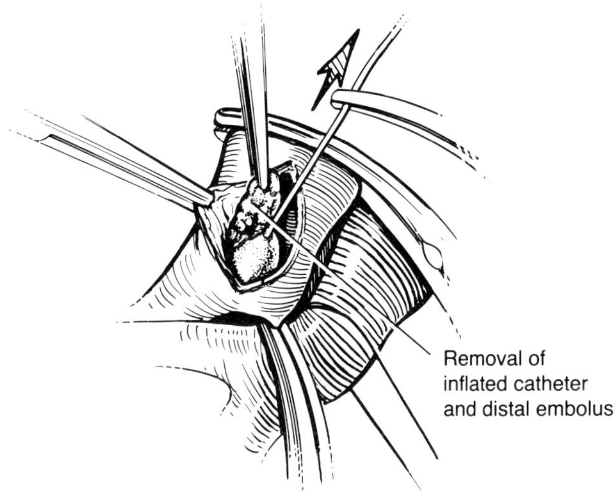

FIGURE 31–4. Fogarty embolectomy catheters are passed distally into the smaller branches of the pulmonary artery, the balloon is inflated, and the catheter withdrawn with retraction of more, smaller emboli.

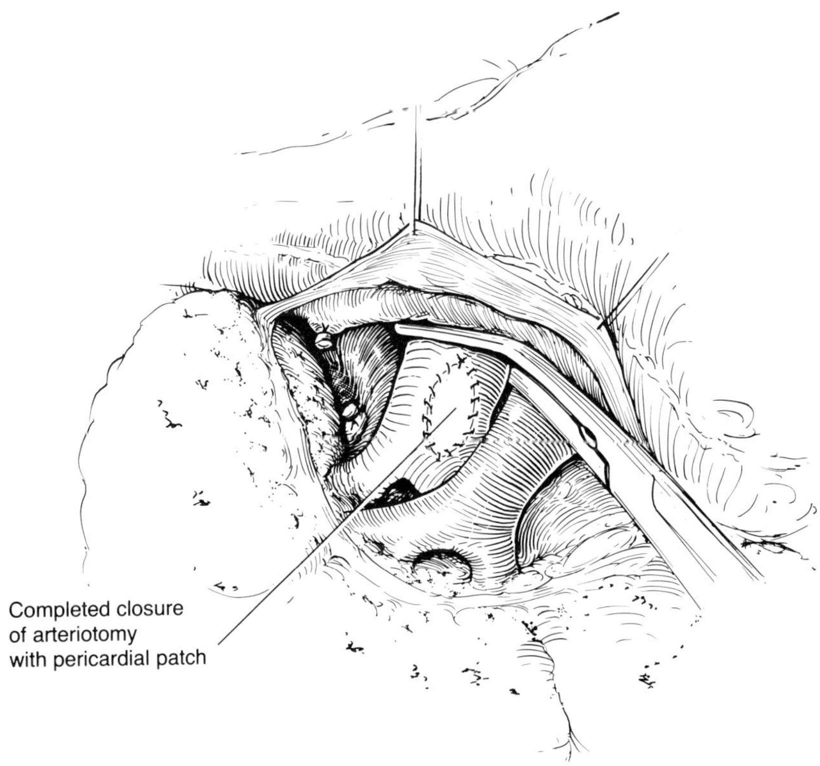

FIGURE 31–5. The pulmonary arteriotomies often are closed with a pericardial patch to prevent pulmonary arterial stenosis.

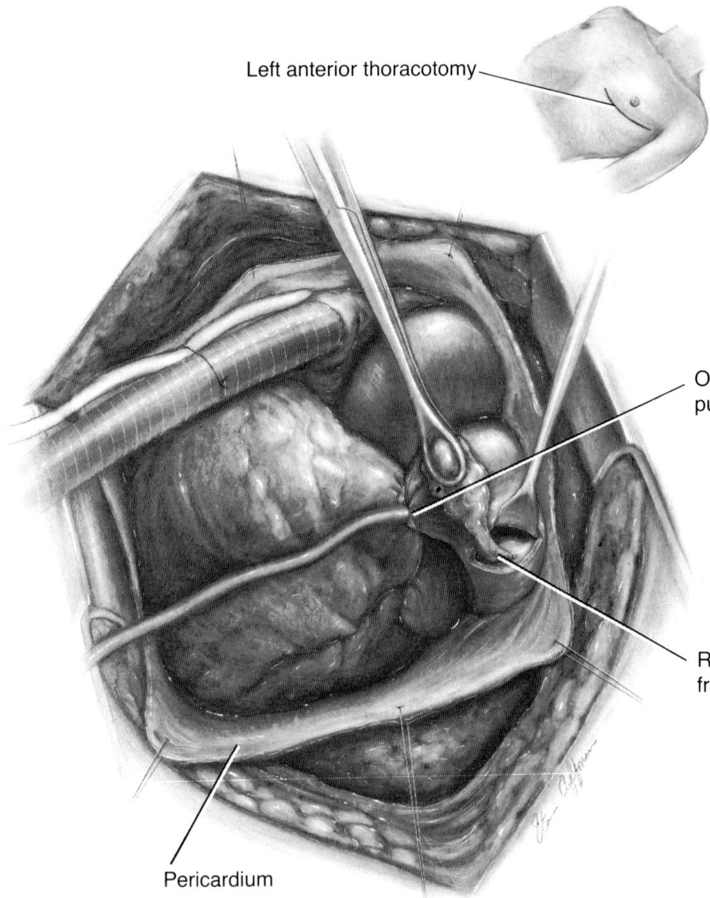

FIGURE 31–6. When the pulmonary embolism is primarily confined to the *left* lung, a left anterior thoracotomy can be made (with or without extracorporeal circulation). The pleural cavity is entered through the third intercostal space, and the venous outflow cannula may be placed into the right atrium or with a pursestring suture into the right ventricle. The main pulmonary artery is usually massively enlarged with significant pulmonary hypertension. A tape is passed beneath the proximal pulmonary artery for control, and if the right pulmonary artery requires exposure for embolectomy, the sternum can be transected and the incision can be extended into the right third intercostal space with entry into the right pleural cavity and dissection of the right pulmonary artery and its branches. Tape around the main pulmonary artery is occluded, and arteriotomy is made distally, exposing the chronic pulmonary embolus. The embolus is dissected from the arterial wall. Considerable tedious dissection is required for this procedure. Bright red backbleeding is encountered when the patent portions of the distal pulmonary arteries are reached, indicating that the distal circulation is open and that the pulmonary embolectomy is apt to be successful.

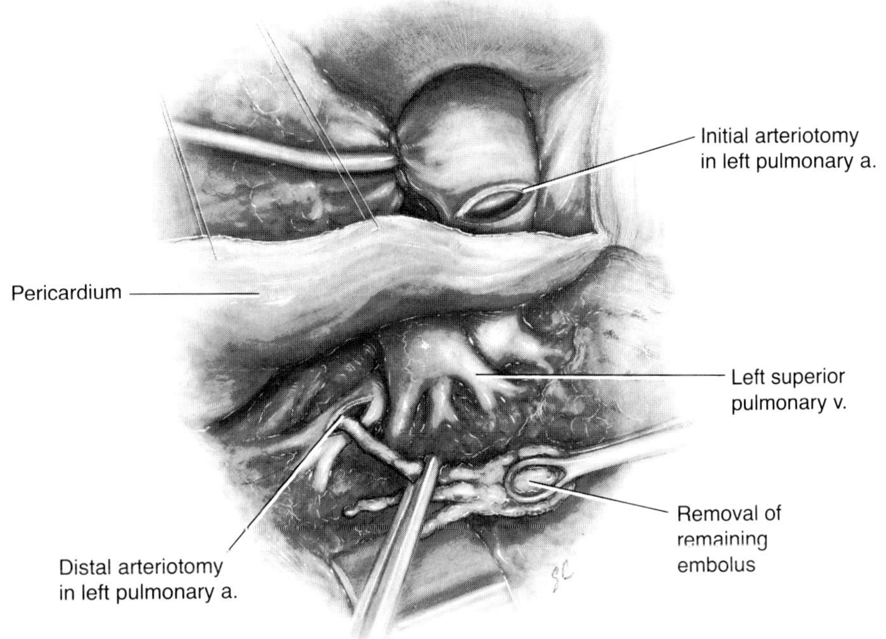

FIGURE 31-7. A Fogarty catheter is passed distally into each of the smaller branches and inflated, and the smaller emboli are withdrawn. The pulmonary arterial tree is copiously irrigated with saline, and further emboli are aspirated. The pulmonary arterial incisions are closed, usually with a pericardial patch to prevent stenosis. The patient is gradually removed from cardiopulmonary bypass, and the incision is closed.

SECTION VIII

The Esophagus

A
Benign Lesions

SAMUEL M. MAHAFFEY, M.D.

32
Esophageal Atresia with Distal Tracheoesophageal Fistula

Congenital tracheoesophageal fistula is an abnormal communication between the trachea and esophagus caused by incomplete septation of the primitive foregut. In most patients, the fistula is associated with esophageal atresia. The most common anatomic configuration is esophageal atresia with a blind proximal esophageal pouch, and the distal esophageal segment connects to the posterior wall of the trachea, usually just above or at the carina. Less commonly, fistulas may form from the proximal esophageal segment, from both the proximal and distal esophageal segments, or without esophageal atresia (H-type fistula). Rarely is esophageal atresia not associated with a fistula. This frequently creates a long gap between the esophageal segments and is often best managed by interposition of colon, stomach, or jejunum.

Esophageal atresia with distal tracheoesophageal fistula occurs in one of 2500 live births. More than half of these infants have associated congenital anomalies, frequently those of the VACTERL association (*v*ertebral, *a*norectal, *c*ardiac, *t*racheo-*e*sophageal, *r*enal, *l*imb). Approximately one fourth of the affected infants have associated structural heart disease.

Primary repair by division of the tracheoesophageal fistula and end-to-end esophagoesophostomy is the preferred operative approach. Routine gastrostomy is not necessary. Infants with associated anomalies or pulmonary insufficiency due to aspiration are often managed best by decompressing gastrostomy and staged repair. Infants with substantial ventilatory requirements may require urgent ligation of the tracheoesophageal fistula owing to the large air leak through the fistula and resultant gastric distention. The fistula should also be ligated if the infant's condition deteriorates as a result of a large air leak after placement of a gastrostomy.

Perioperative mortality is quite low and is usually the result of uncorrectable structural heart disease. Approximately one third of infants develop anastomotic strictures that require dilation on at least one occasion. In addition, the incidence of gastroesophageal reflux is relatively high, often necessitating an antireflux operation.

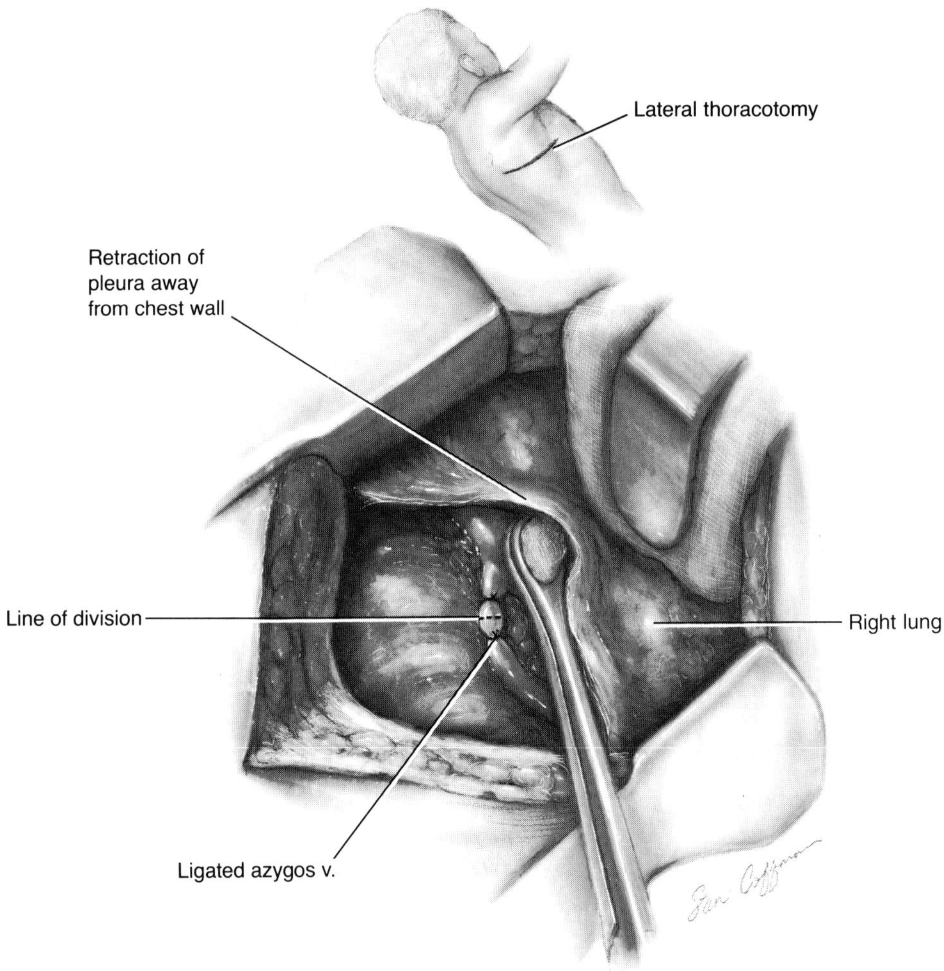

FIGURE 32–1. An extrapleural approach through the periosteum of the fourth rib is preferred. The parietal pleura is swept down by blunt dissection. The azygos vein is ligated in continuity and divided for exposure.

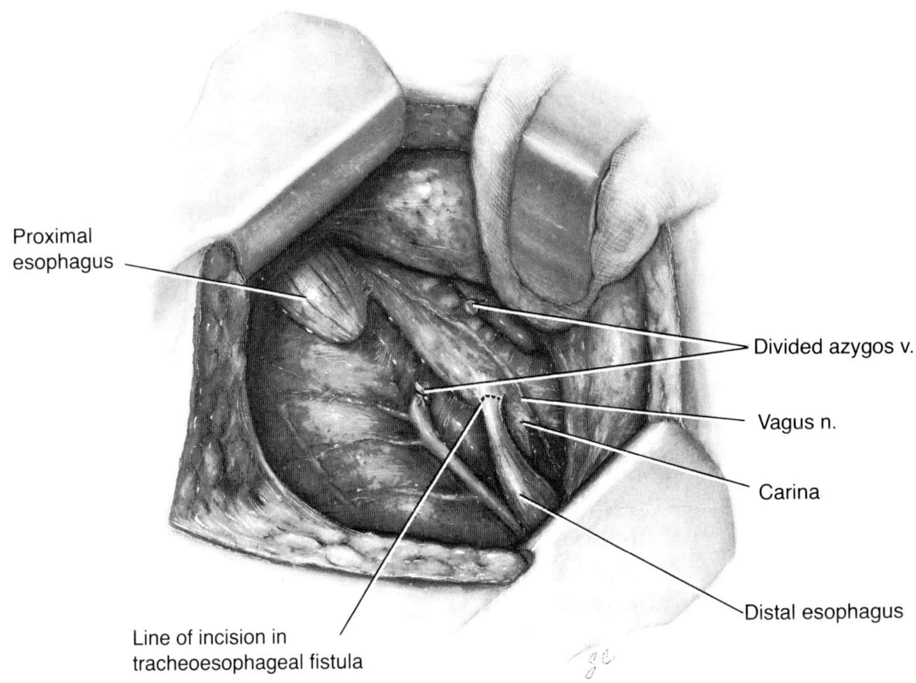

FIGURE 32–2. The proximal esophageal pouch has a longitudinal blood supply and can be mobilized extensively to span the gap between the esophageal segments. The distal esophagus has a segmental blood supply and should not be mobilized. Mobilization of the distal esophagus also tends to pull the gastroesophageal junction into the thorax, promoting gastroesophageal reflux.

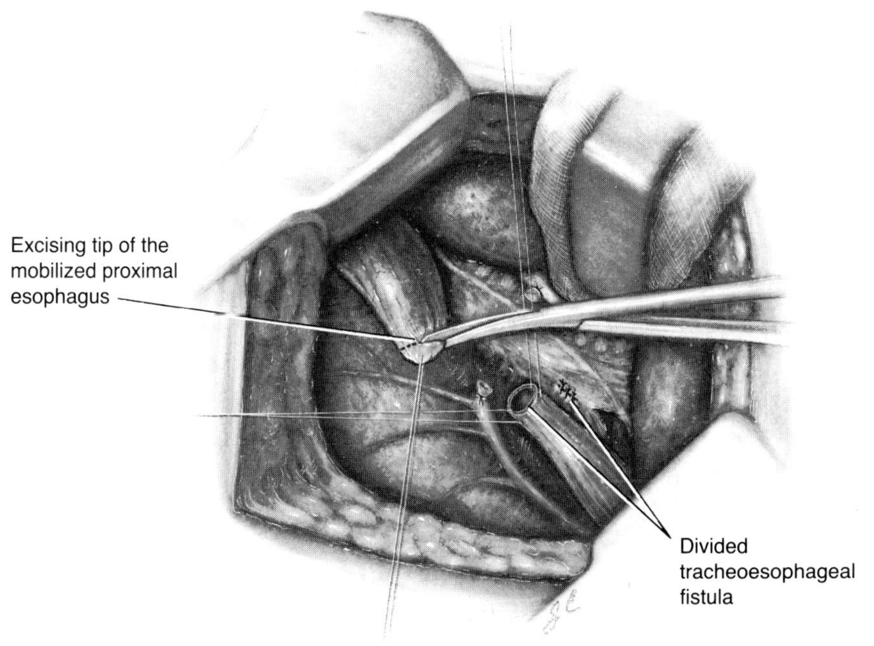

FIGURE 32–3. After division of the tracheoesophageal fistula, the tracheal defect is closed with interrupted sutures. Care should be taken not to compromise the tracheal lumen. The distal tip of the proximal esophageal pouch is opened, and a single-layer end-to-end anastomosis is performed.

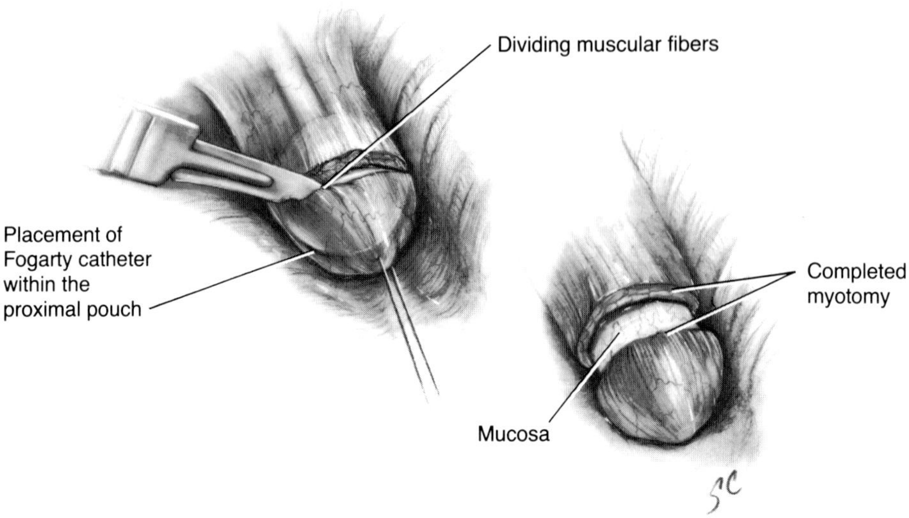

FIGURE 32–4. If the distance between the esophageal segments is too great to allow anastomosis without tension, circular myotomies can be performed on the proximal esophageal segment. This is facilitated by placement of a Fogarty catheter within the proximal pouch. Inflation of the balloon places the wall under some tension and allows clean division of the muscular fibers. Generally, two myotomies can be performed within the chest, and a third myotomy can be performed in the neck if necessary. Approximately 1 cm in length is gained with each myotomy.

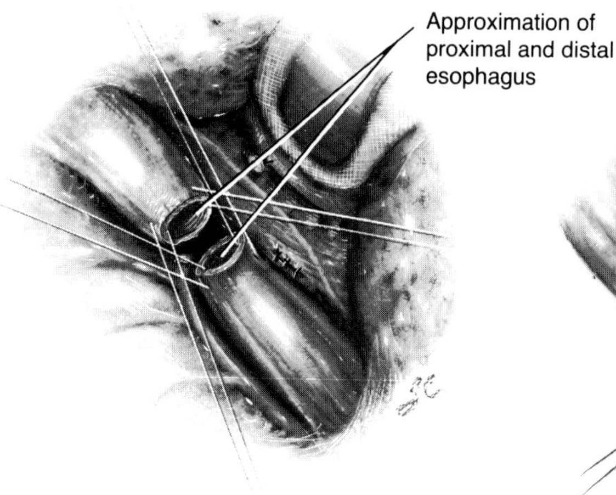

FIGURE 32–5

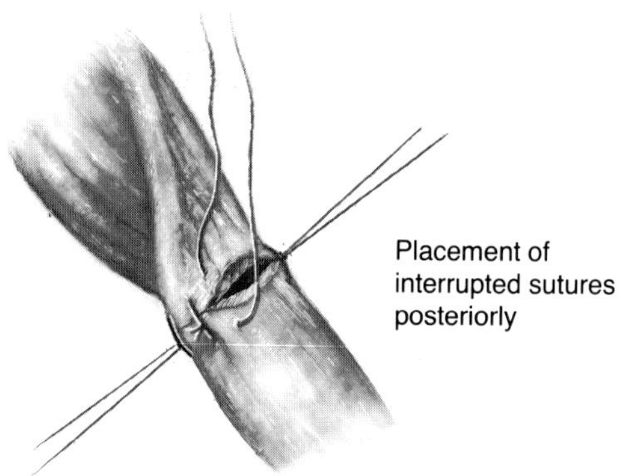

FIGURE 32–6

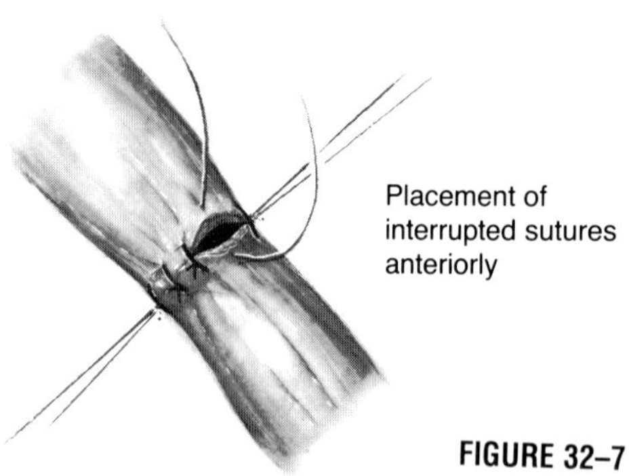

FIGURE 32–7

FIGURE 32–5. The esophageal segments are rotated for completion of the posterior row. A nasogastric tube can be carefully passed through the anastomosis to allow easy completion of the anterior wall.

FIGURE 32–6. Interrupted sutures are placed posteriorly to repair the esophageal segments.

FIGURE 32–7. The anastomosis is completed anteriorly with interrupted sutures.

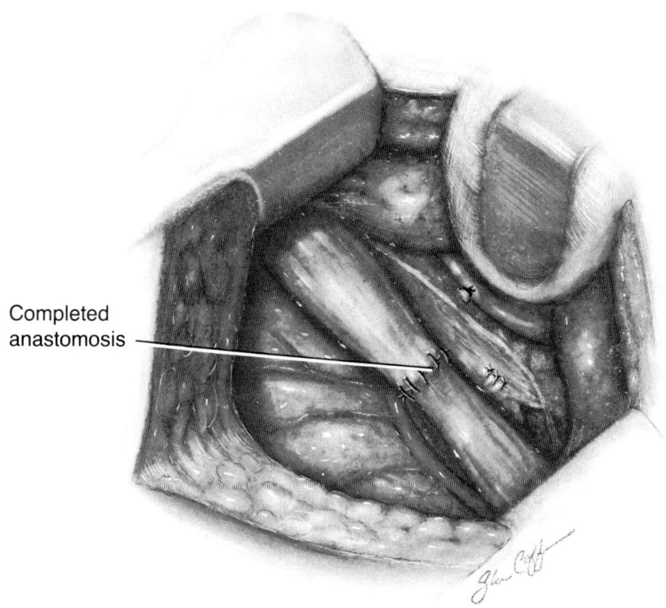

FIGURE 32–8. Tracheal closure and esophageal anastomosis are completed. Local tissue should be placed between the suture lines to prevent reformation of the fistula. Closed suction drains are used to evacuate the extrapleural space. Small anastomotic leaks are not uncommon and usually are self-limited.

WALTER G. WOLFE, M.D.

33
Resection of Zenker's Diverticulum

FIGURE 33–1. A skin incision is made medial to the sternocleidomastoid muscle. The dissection is extended and the vessels are retracted laterally, and the diverticulum is dissected free.

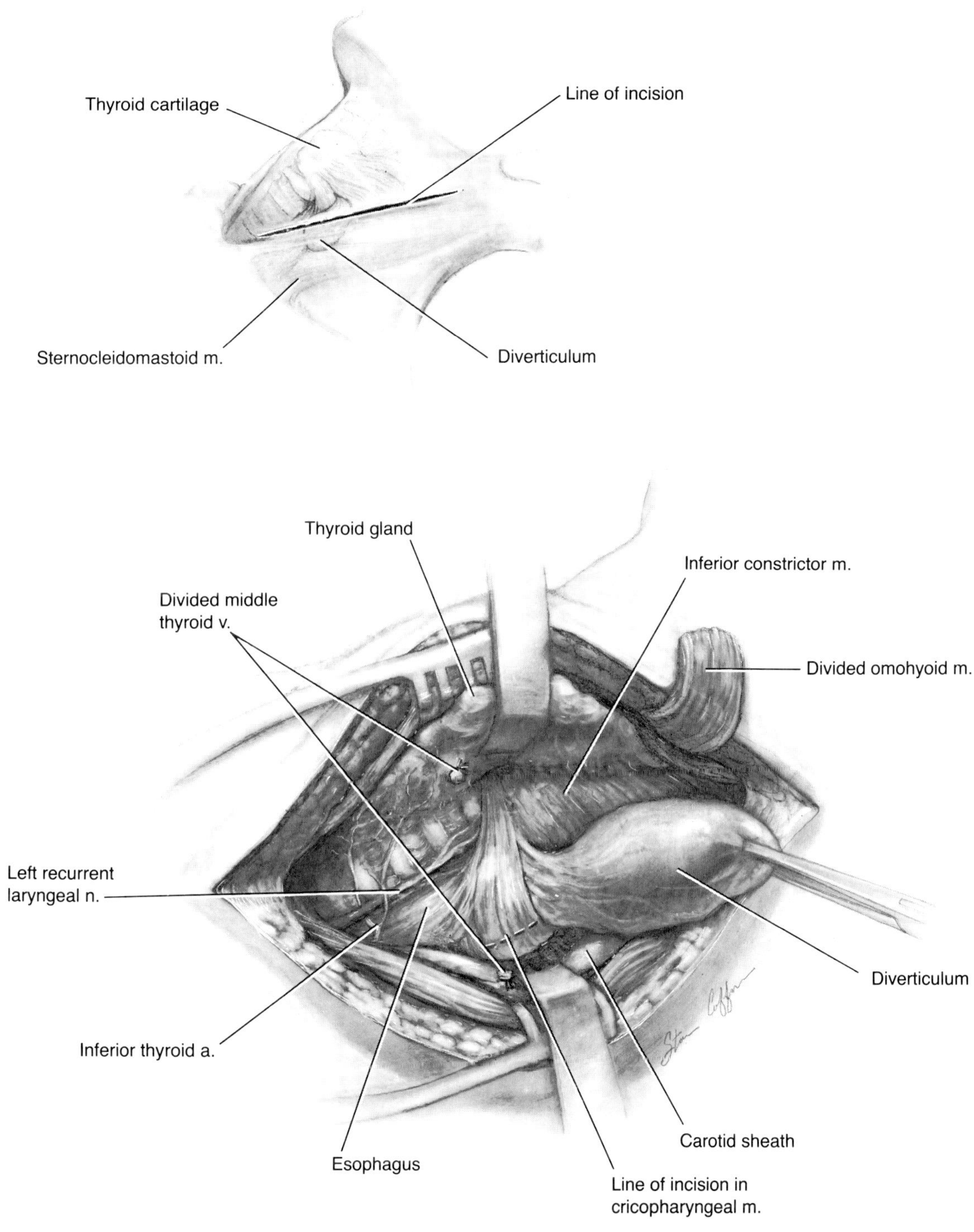

FIGURE 33–1 *See legend on opposite page*

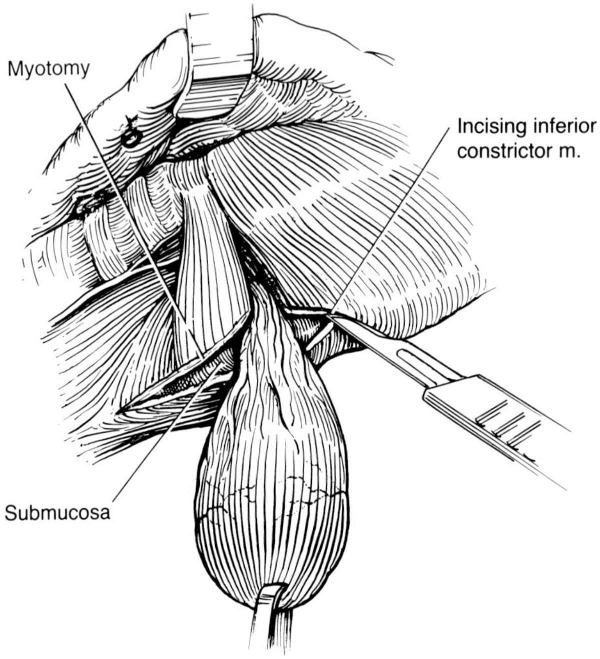

FIGURE 33–2. A myotomy is made across the cricopharyngeal muscle and down onto the esophagus. The myotomy can also be extended slightly above the diverticulum.

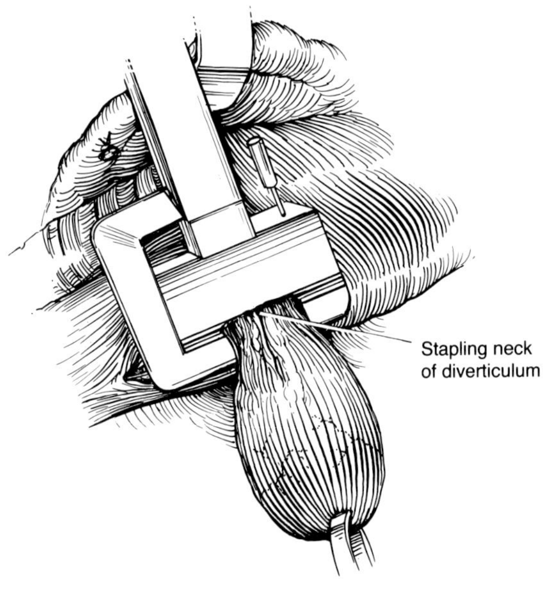

FIGURE 33–3. The neck of the diverticulum can usually be transected and closed with a TA-30 stapling instrument.

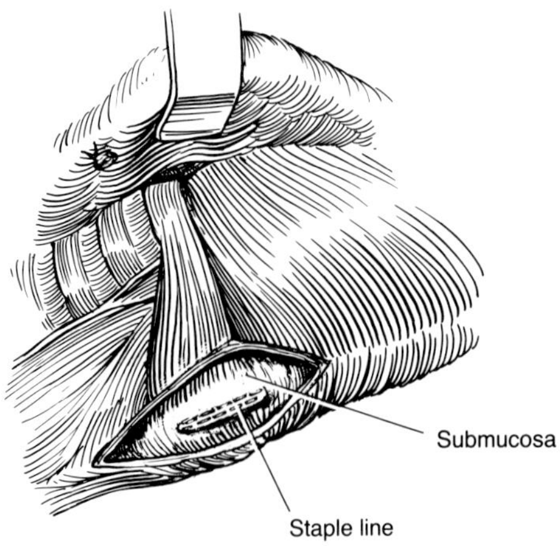

FIGURE 33–4. After the specimen is removed, the staple line is inspected. The submucosa should bulge slightly through the myotomy. The neck of the diverticulum is closed in layers, and a drain is placed near the anastomosis. A contrast swallow is usually obtained on the fifth postoperative day to ensure complete healing before food intake is begun.

WALTER G. WOLFE, M.D.

34
Correction of Hiatal Hernia: Belsey Procedure

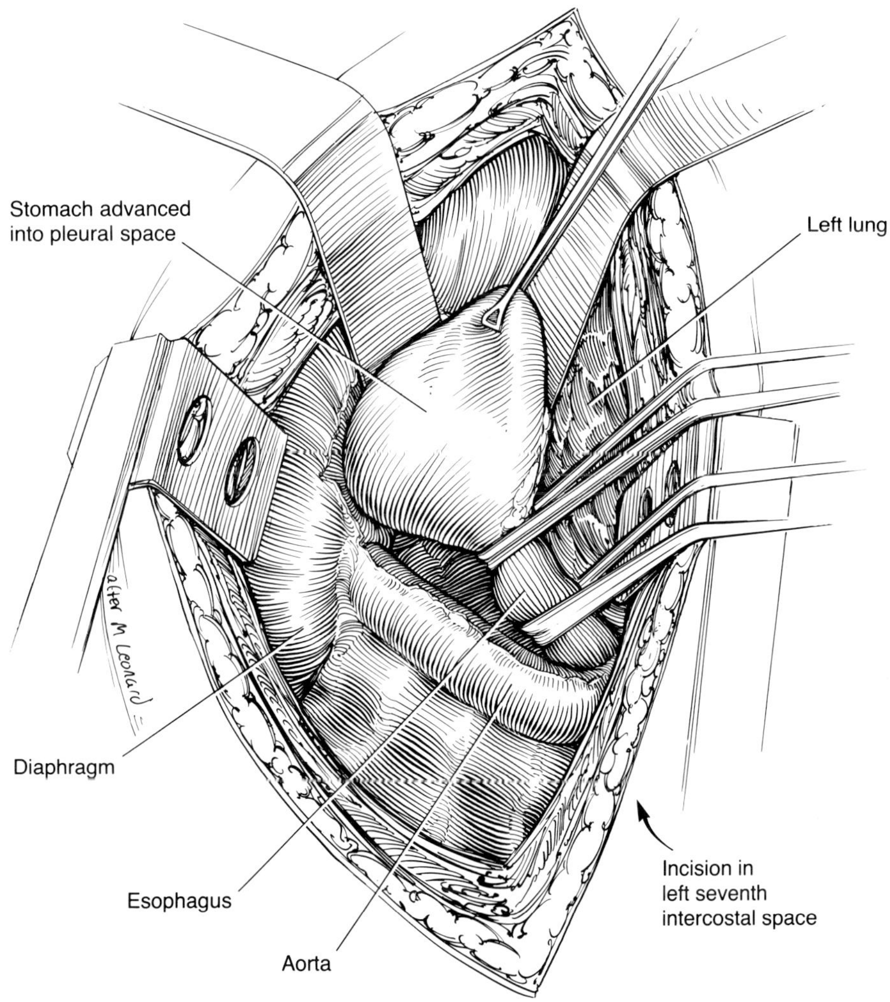

FIGURE 34–1. With the patient in the left lateral position, an incision is made in the left chest. The pleural space is usually entered through the seventh intercostal space, without transecting a rib posteriorly. The mediastinal pleura is opened, and the esophagus is mobilized to the inferior vein and down to the hiatus. The hiatal hernia is mobilized and freed from the crura. The peritoneal cavity is entered, and the stomach is completely freed from all surrounding structures. The amount of esophagus mobilized from the vein up to the arch depends on the extent of the hiatal hernia and whether or not a "short esophagus" is present.

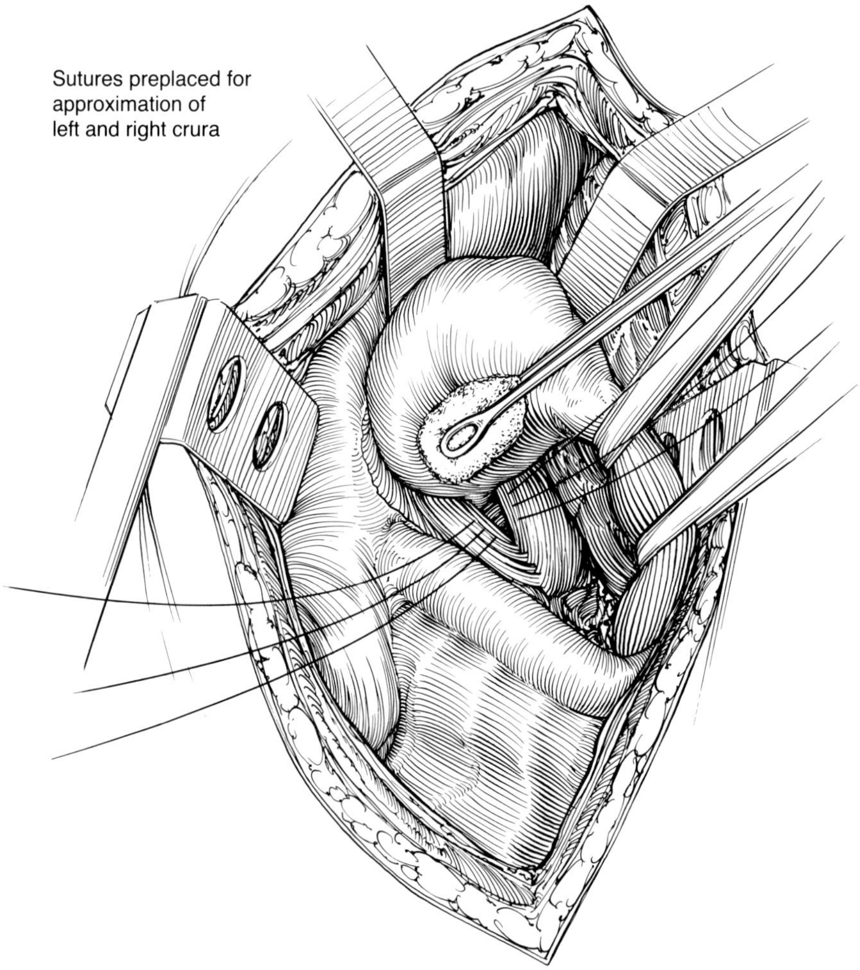

FIGURE 34–2. The crural stitches are placed, marked, and left untied.

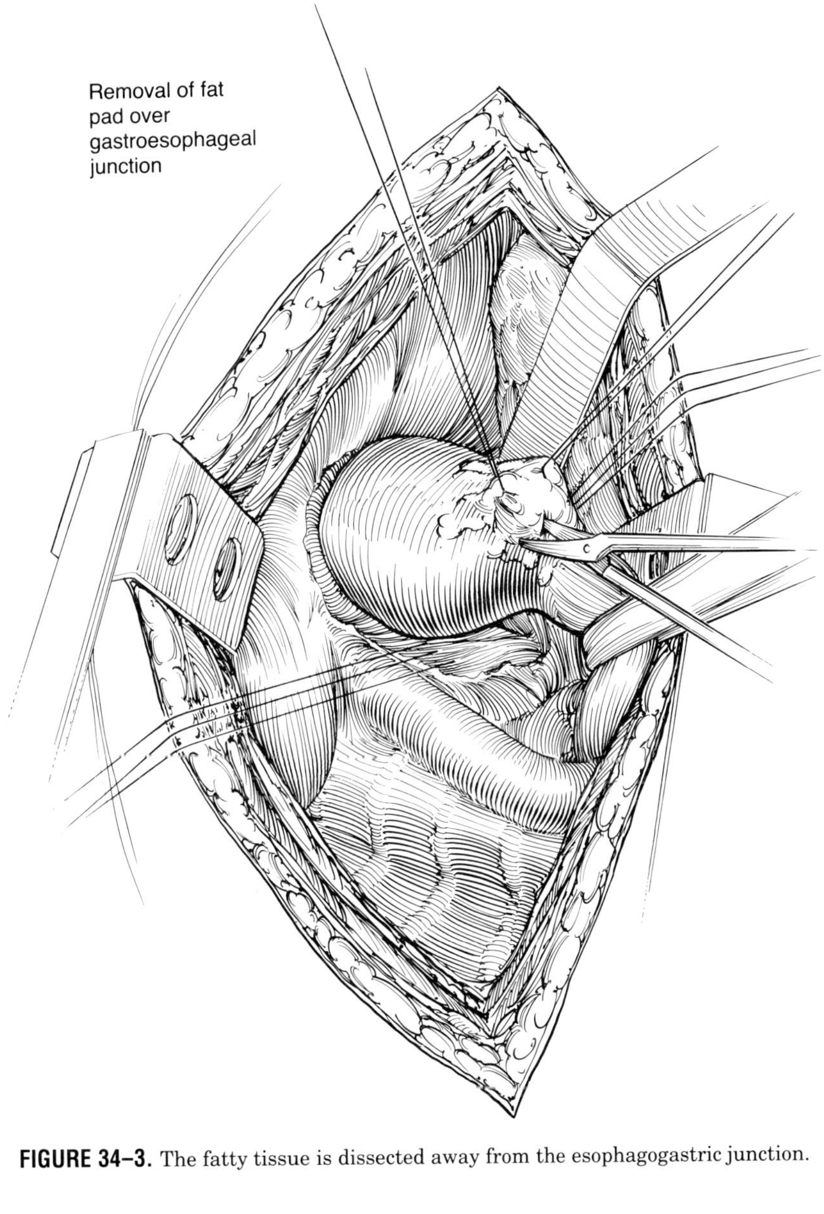

FIGURE 34–3. The fatty tissue is dissected away from the esophagogastric junction.

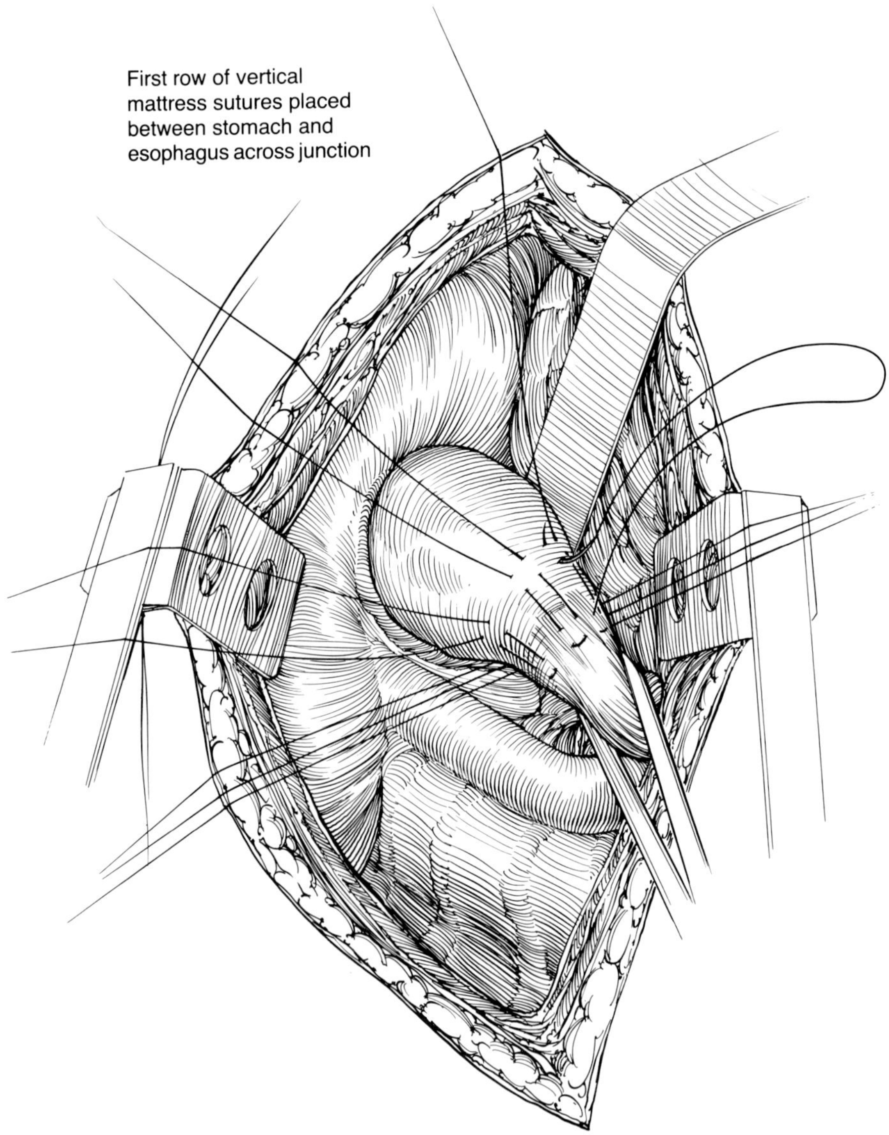

FIGURE 34–4. The first layer of mattress sutures is placed from the stomach to the esophagus across the esophagogastric junction approximately 240 degrees, the circumference of the esophagus.

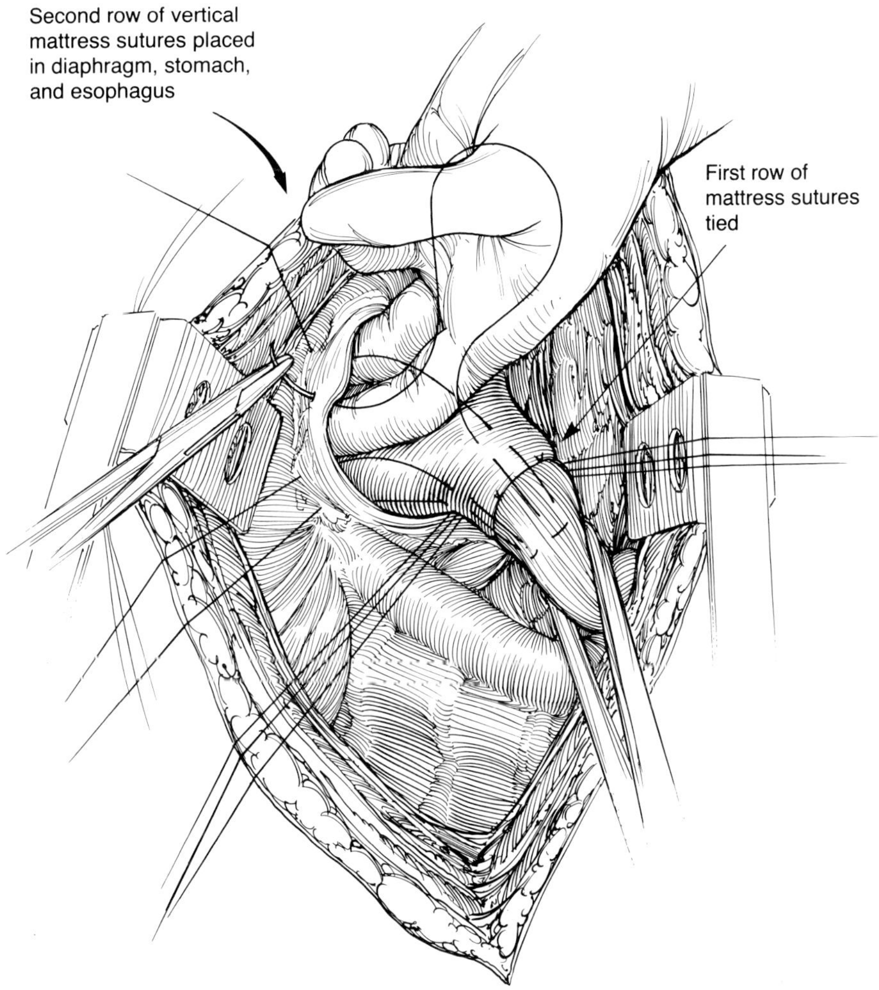

FIGURE 34–5. The first layer of sutures are tied. The sutures of the second layer are then passed through the esophagus, through the fundus of the stomach, and out through the diaphragm and left untied.

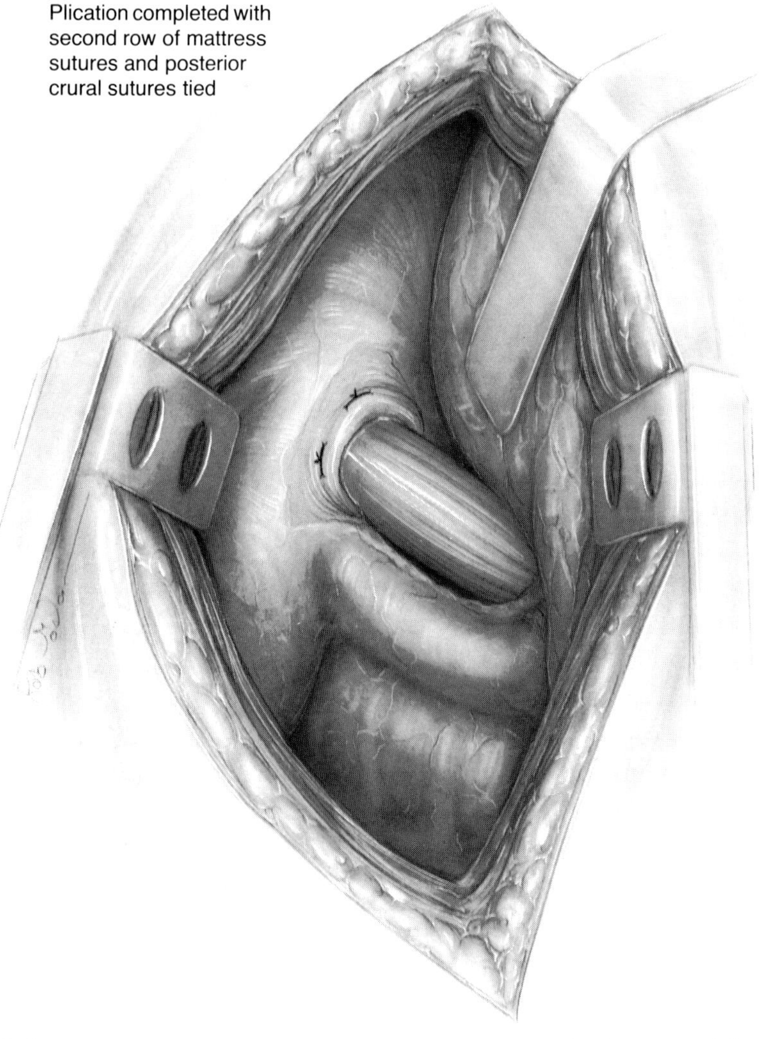

FIGURE 34–6. The esophagogastric junction is reduced below the diaphragm, and the sutures that have been placed through the diaphragm are brought down and tied snugly, completely reducing the gastroesophageal junction below the hiatus.

The crural sutures are then tied, and usually a finger can be knitted through the hiatus, which ensures that the closure is not too tight. A single drainage tube is placed in the pleural space. The ribs are then approximated in the usual manner and the chest is closed in layers.

B
Malignant Lesions

WALTER G. WOLFE, M.D.

35
Left Transthoracic Approach for Esophagogastrectomy (SWEET PROCEDURE)

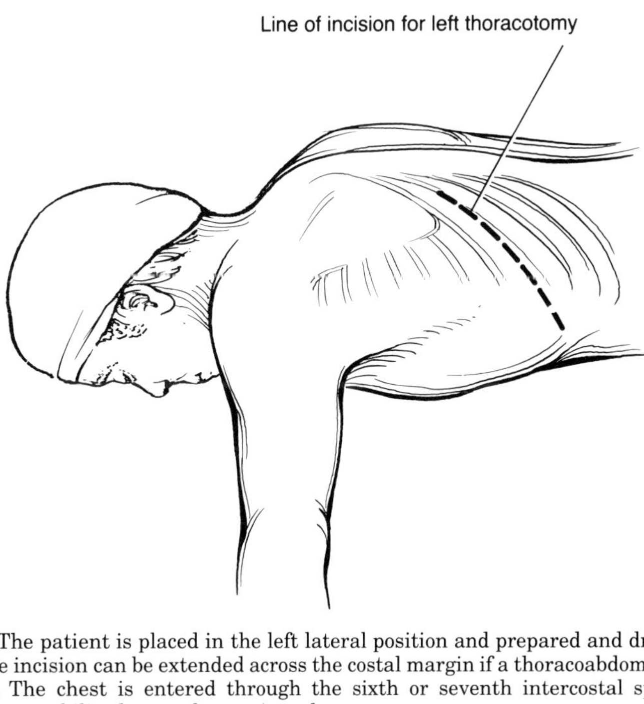

FIGURE 35–1. The patient is placed in the left lateral position and prepared and draped, so that, if necessary, the incision can be extended across the costal margin if a thoracoabdominal operation is appropriate. The chest is entered through the sixth or seventh intercostal space, and the esophagus is then mobilized up to the aortic arch.

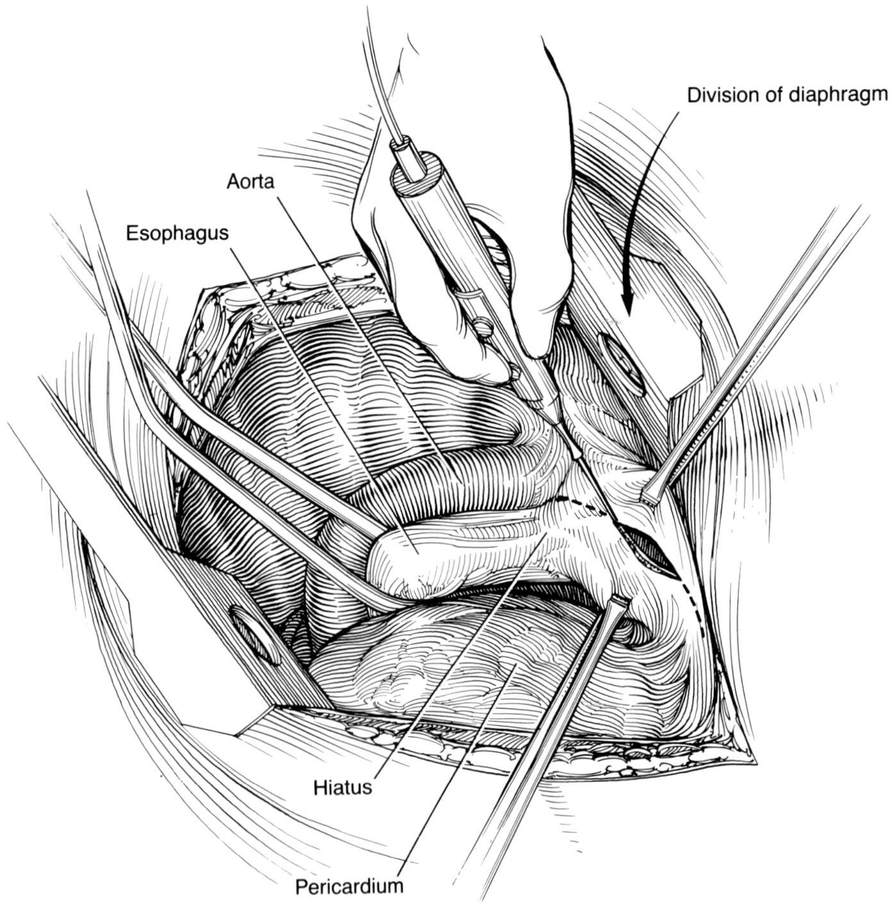

FIGURE 35–2. The diaphragm is split in the tendon to the hiatus, and the stomach is mobilized up to the defect.

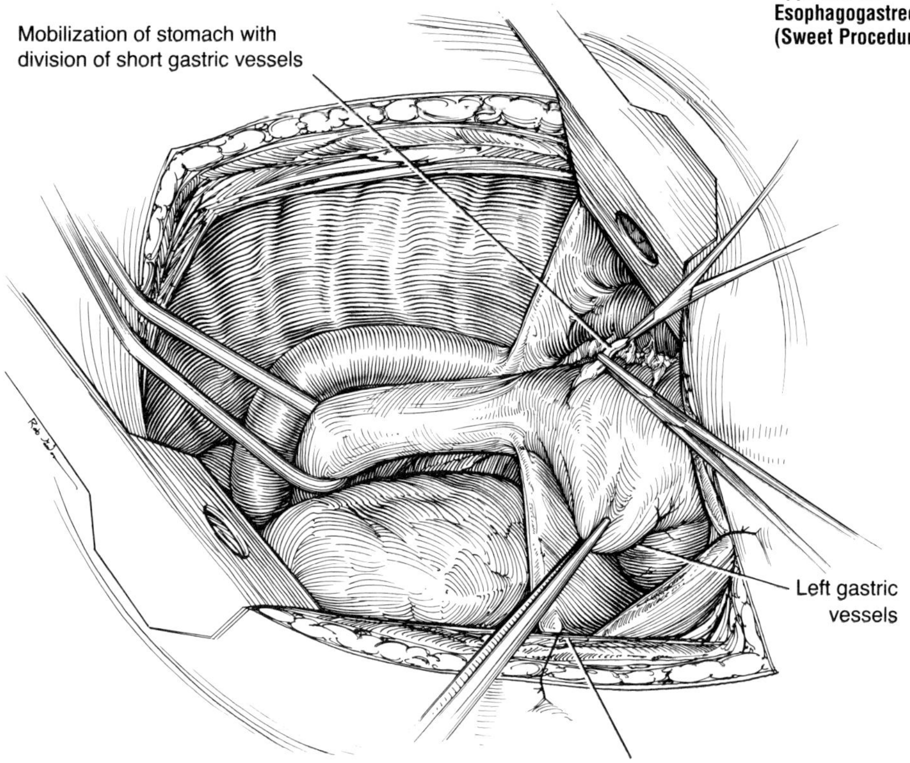

FIGURE 35–3. The short gastric vessels are divided, the spleen is usually preserved, and the stomach is mobilized on the right gastric and right gastric epiploic vessels. The left gastric vessel is then ligated and divided.

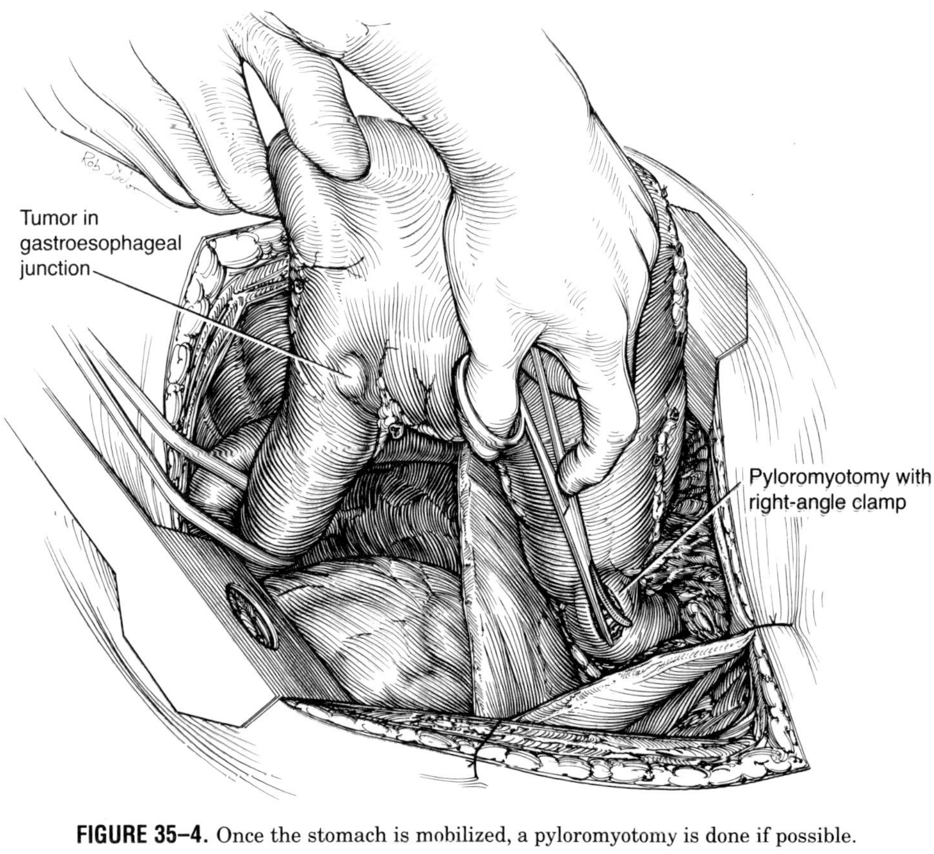

FIGURE 35–4. Once the stomach is mobilized, a pyloromyotomy is done if possible.

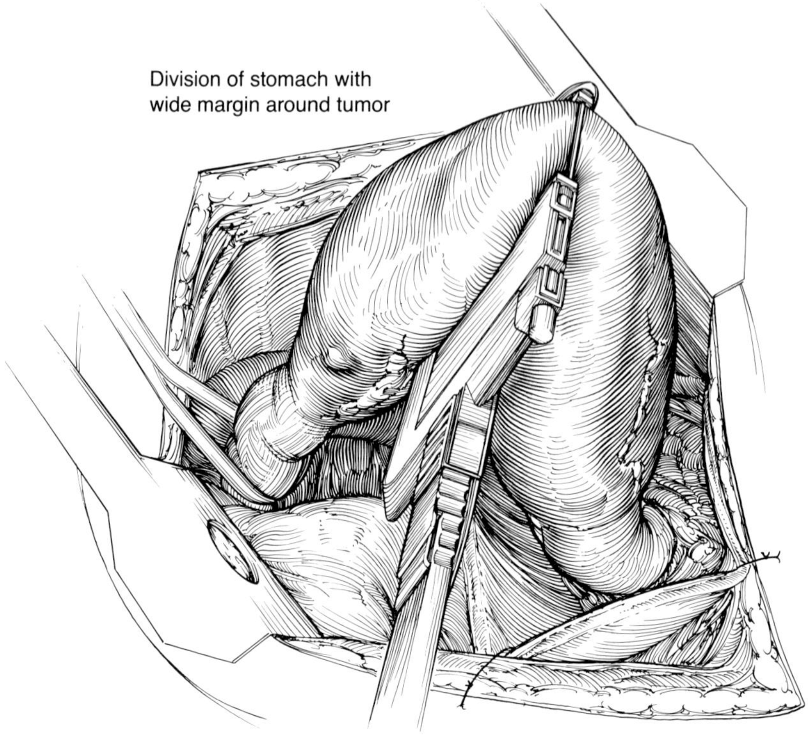

FIGURE 35–5. The stomach is divided with adequate margin on the gastric side of the tumor.

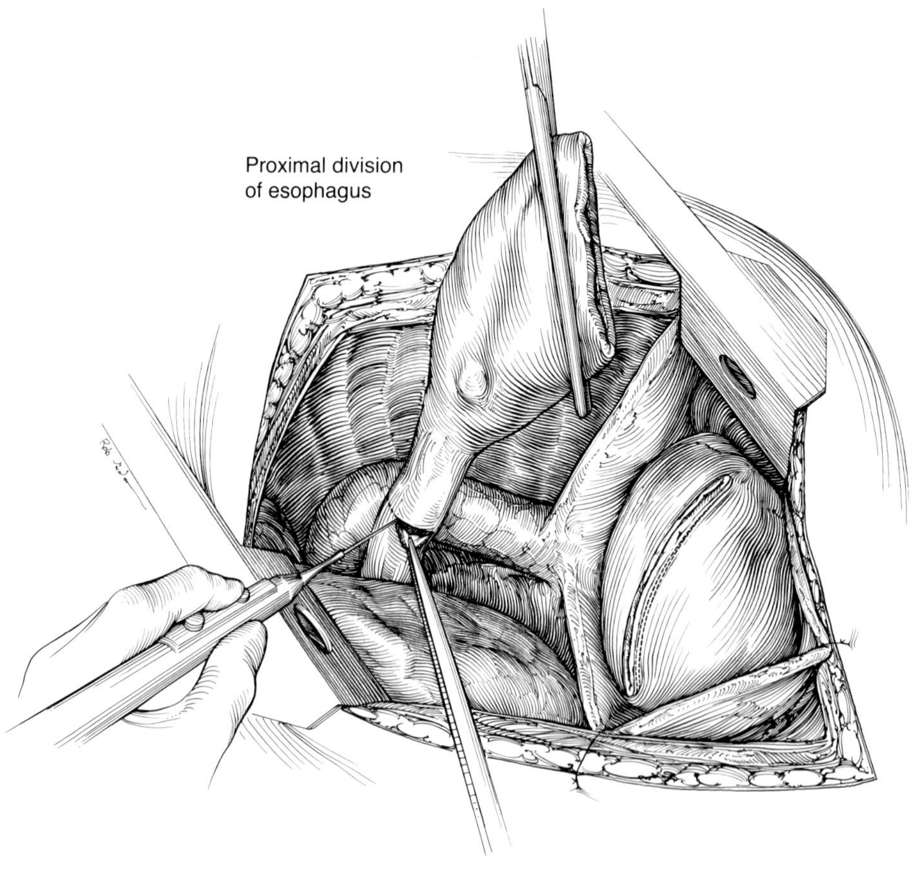

FIGURE 35–6. The esophagus is divided.

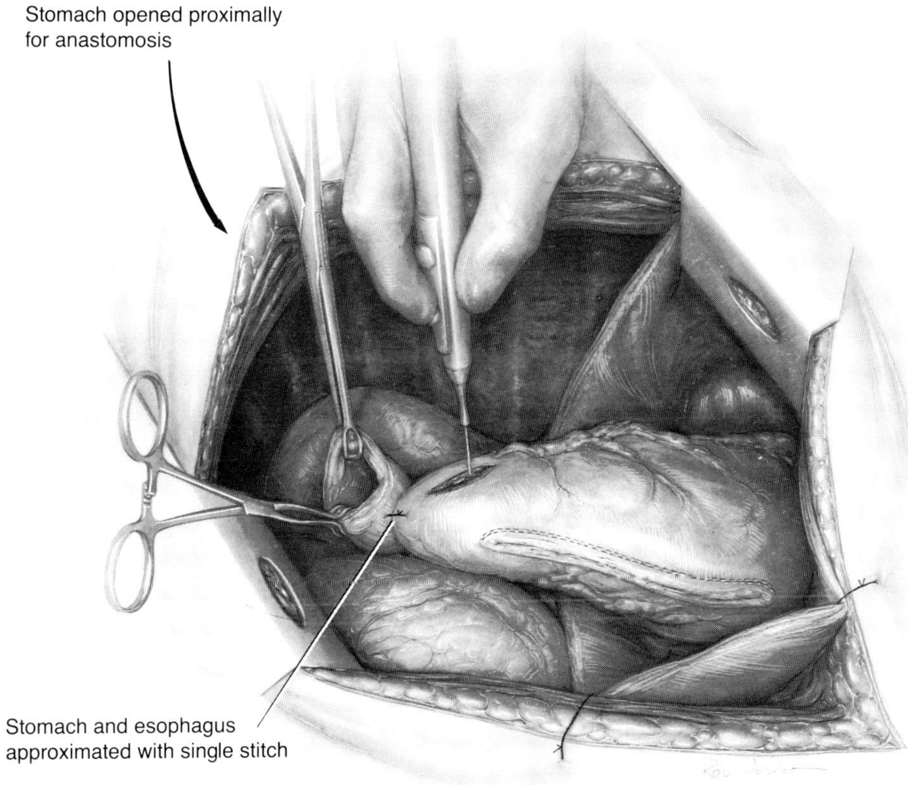

FIGURE 35–7. The stomach is placed within the mediastinum.

FIGURE 35–8

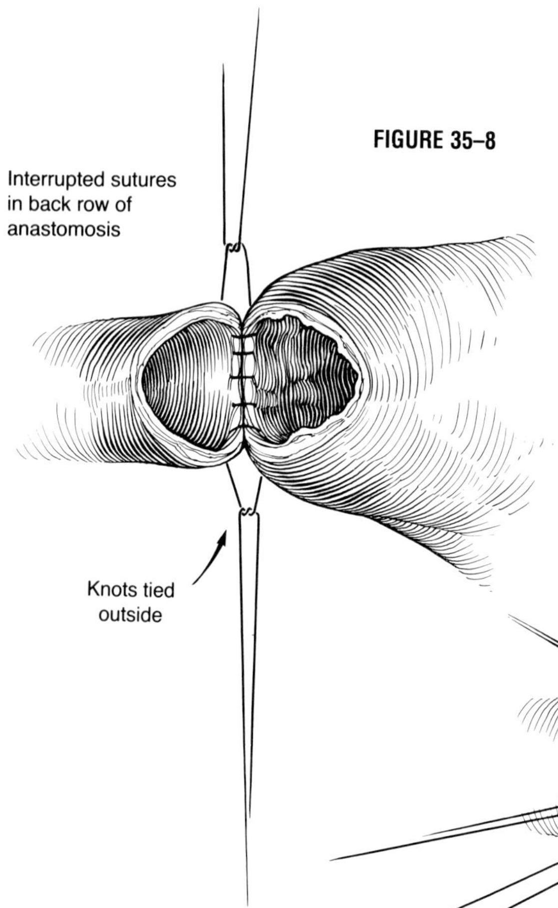

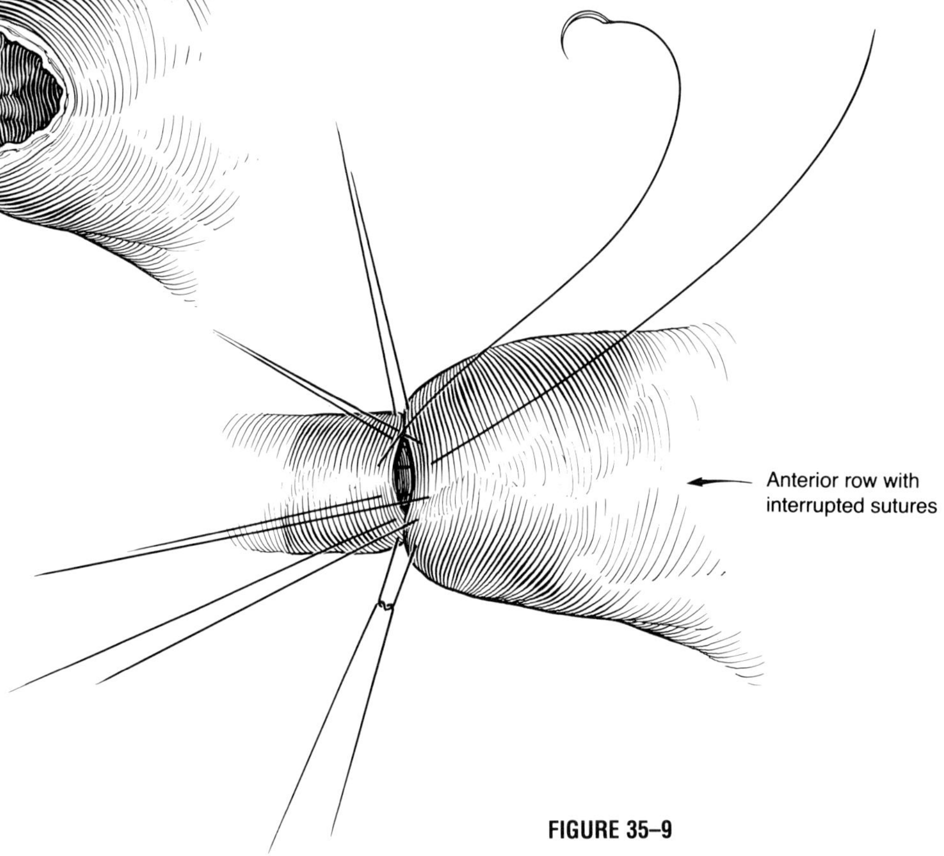

FIGURE 35–9

FIGURES 35-8 and 35–9. The anastomosis is done between the esophagus and the stomach using a single layer of interrupted 3–0 silk sutures.

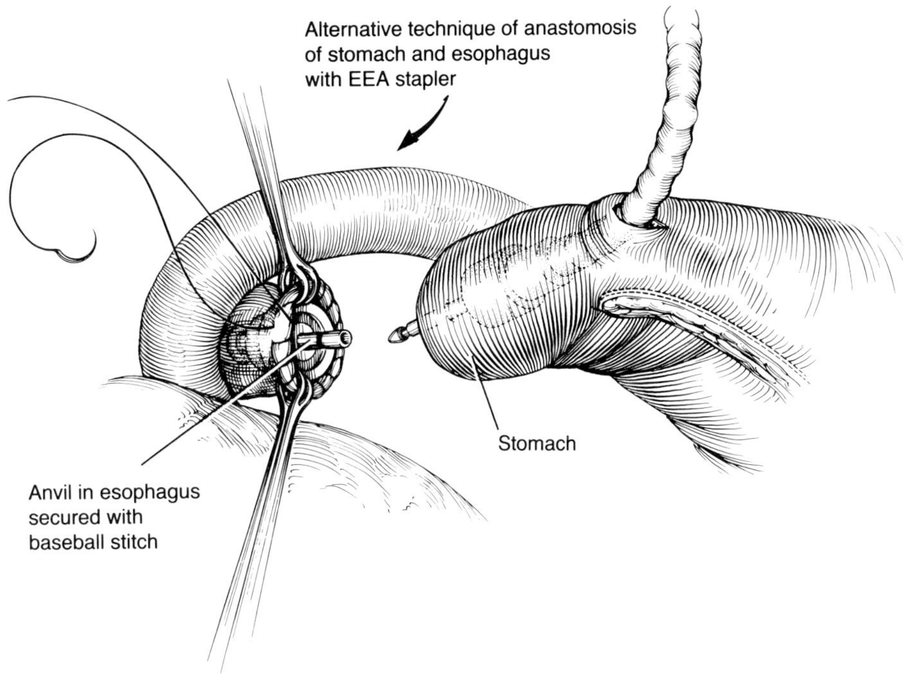

FIGURE 35–10. The anastomosis can be done with the stapling device.

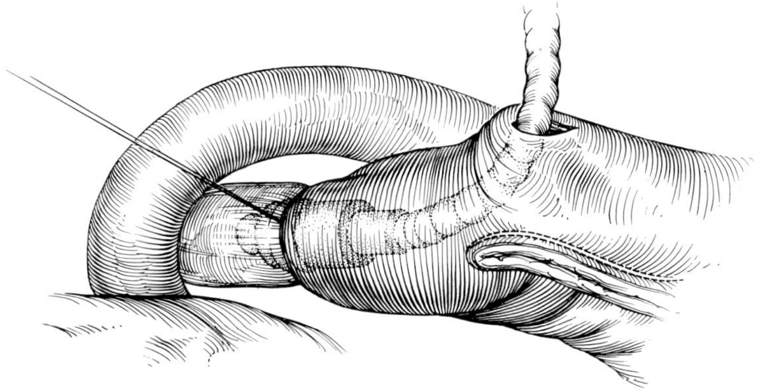

FIGURE 35–11. The incision into the stomach is closed with staples.

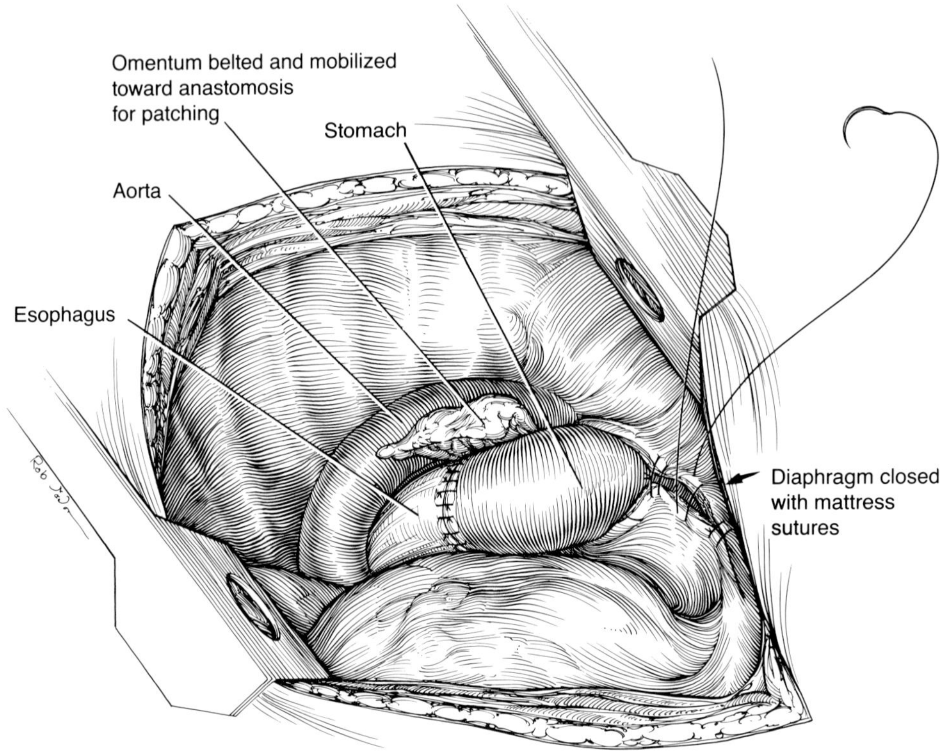

FIGURE 35–12. The stomach is sutured within the mediastinum, and the omentum is readied for use as a patch. The diaphragm is then closed in two layers with interrupted mattress sutures and a running suture.

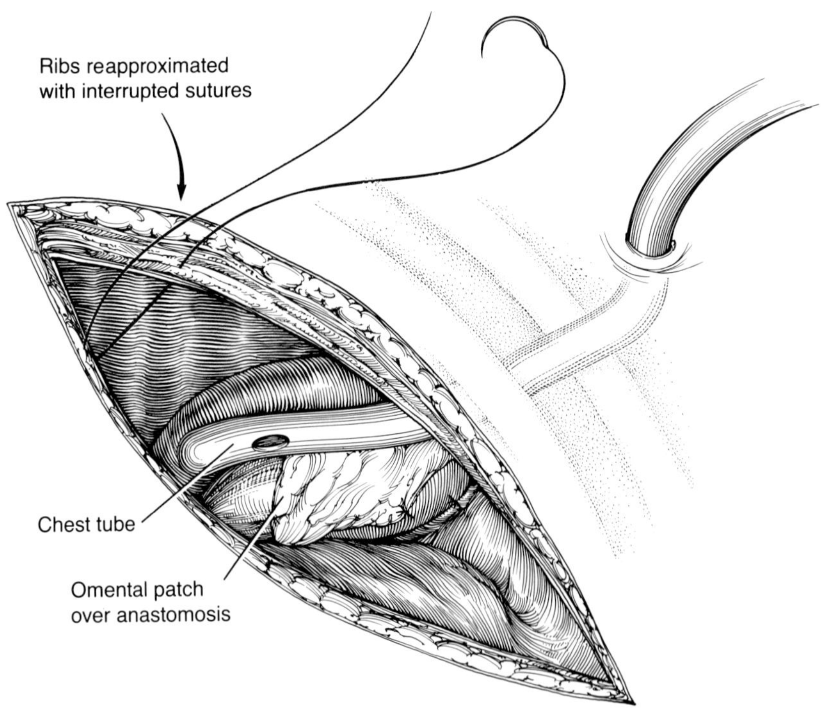

FIGURE 35–13. The ribs are reapproximated with interrupted sutures. The chest and anastomosis are drained, and the incision is closed in the usual manner.

WALTER G. WOLFE, M.D.

36

Ivor Lewis Esophagogastrectomy

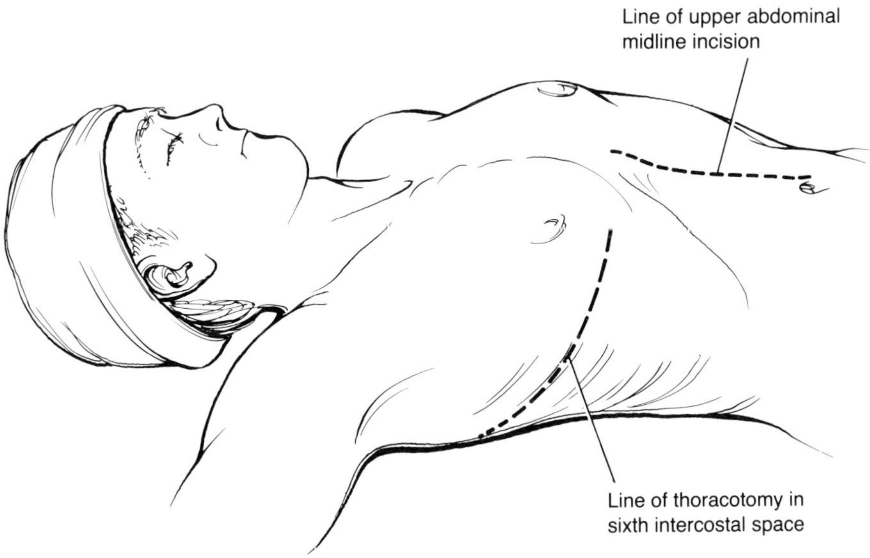

FIGURE 36–1. The patient is placed in a right lateral position such that he or she can be rotated so that the abdominal incision as well as the chest incision can be made in the same field. The abdomen is opened first and exploration performed.

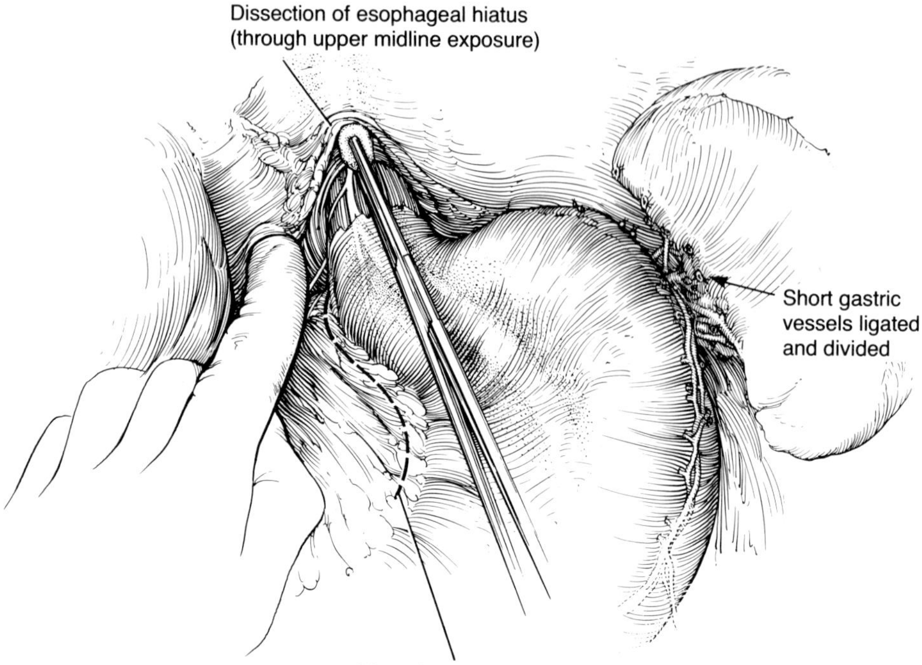

FIGURE 36–2

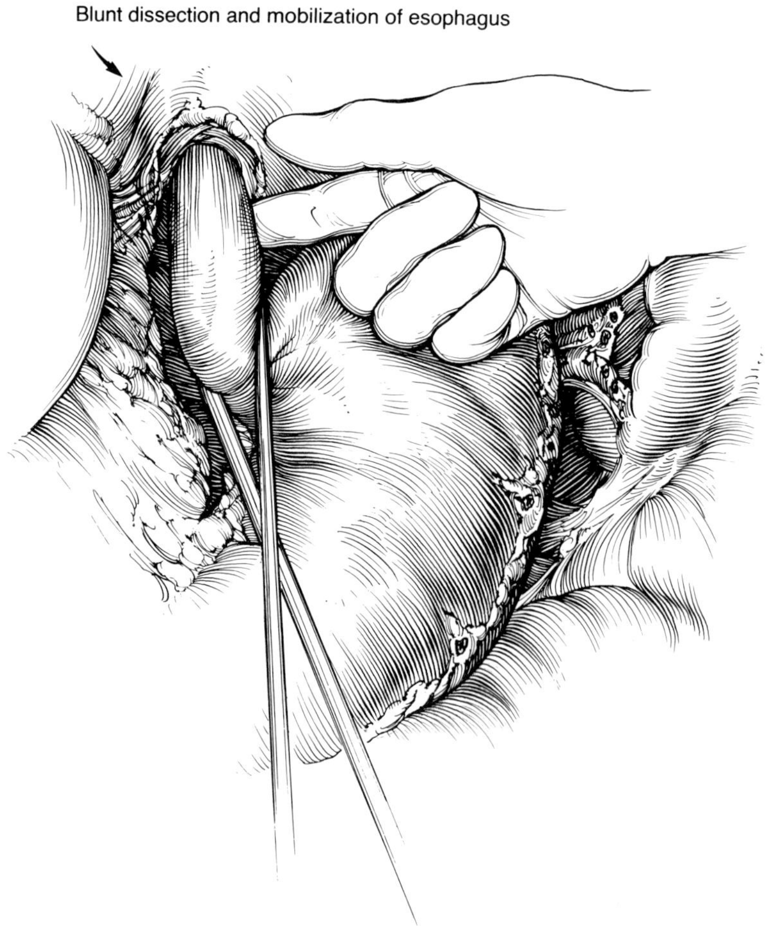

FIGURE 36–3

FIGURES 36–2 and 36–3. If there is no evidence of metastatic disease and the operation continues, the esophageal hiatus is dissected and the stomach is mobilized on the right gastric and right gastric epiploic vessels.

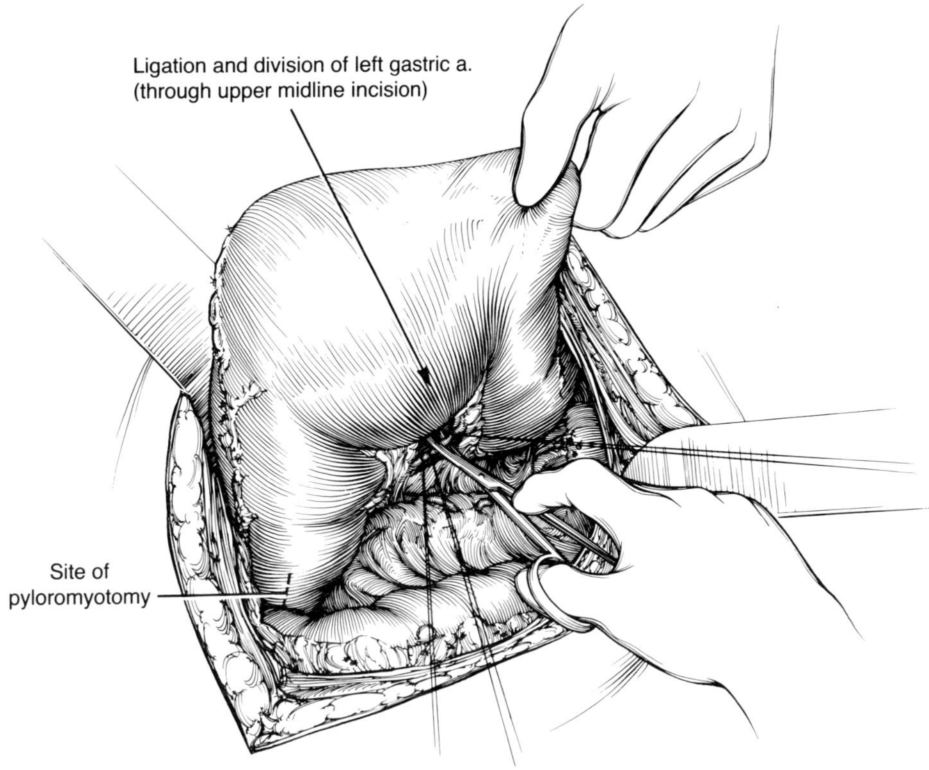

FIGURE 36–4. The left gastric vessels are ligated and divided along with the short gastric vessels.

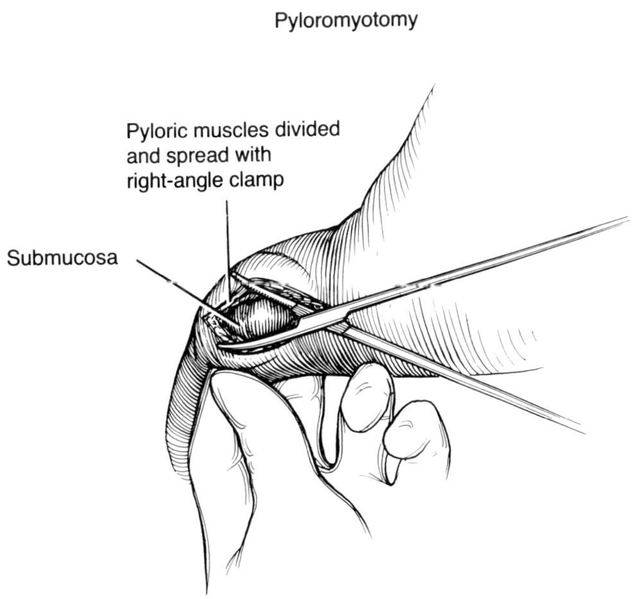

FIGURE 36–5

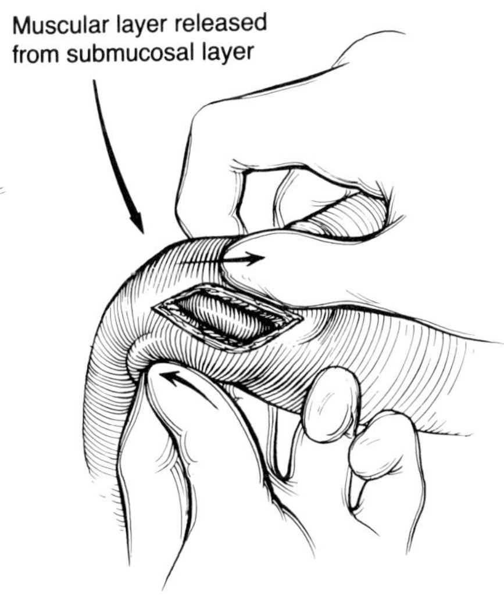

FIGURE 36–6

FIGURES 36–5 and 36–6. A pyloromyotomy is usually done. If the mucosa is entered, then a pyloroplasty is completed.

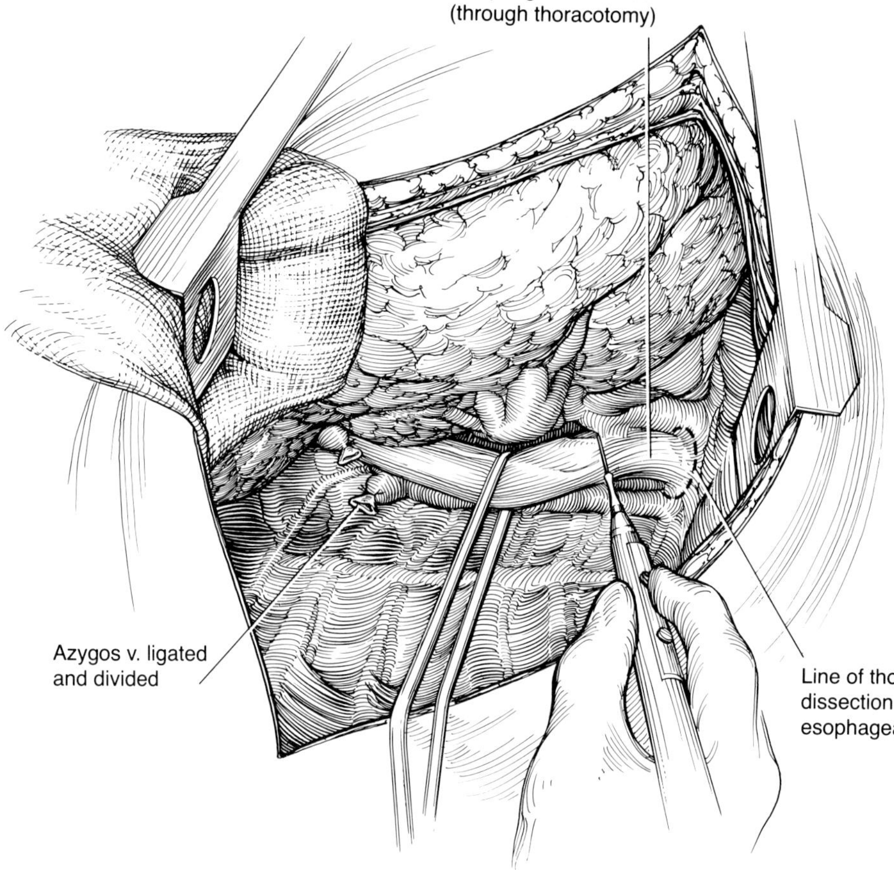

FIGURE 36–7. The thoracotomy is done with the patient rolled to the lateral position, and the chest is entered usually through the fifth or sixth intercostal space. The azygos vein is ligated and divided. The esophagus is then mobilized from the mediastinum.

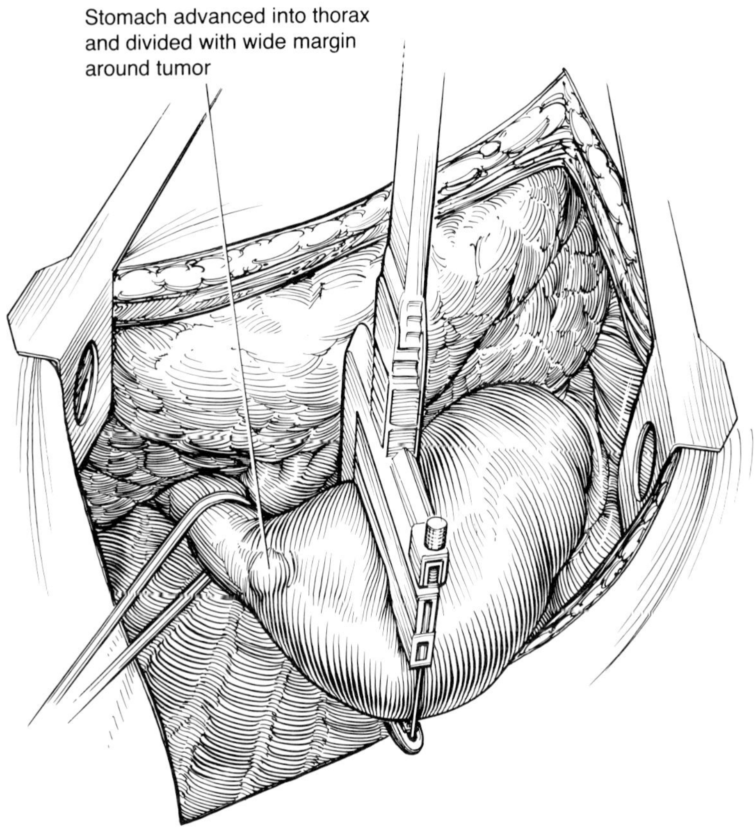

FIGURE 36–8. The hiatus is widened, and the stomach is brought up into the right chest. The stomach is stapled and divided distal to the tumor in the gastroesophageal junction, leaving a safe margin.

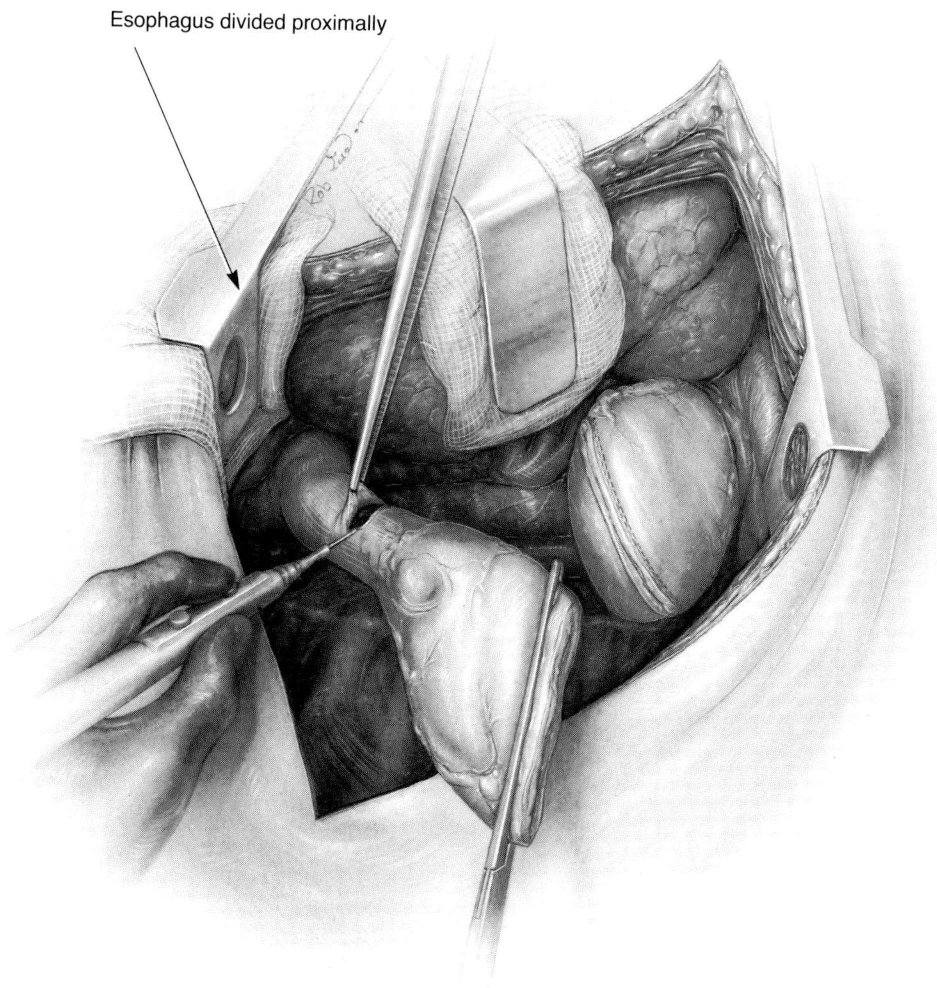

FIGURE 36–9. The esophagus is divided proximal to the tumor.

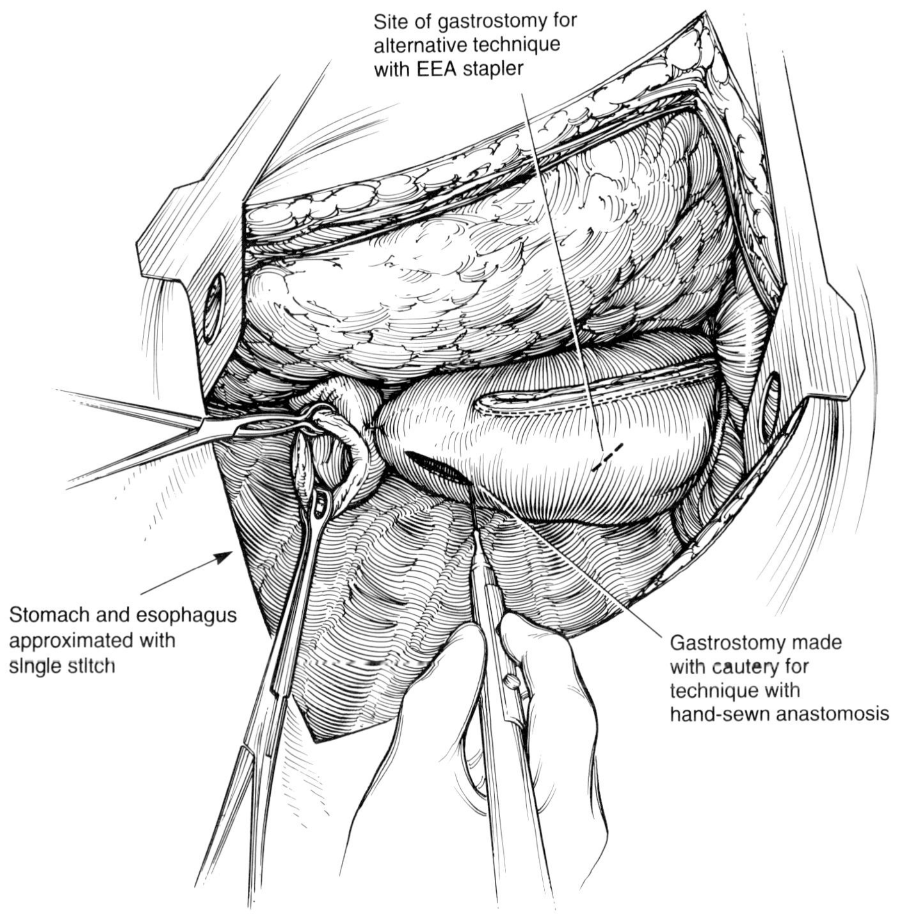

FIGURE 36–10. The anastomosis is done usually above the level of the azygos vein between the stomach and the esophagus.

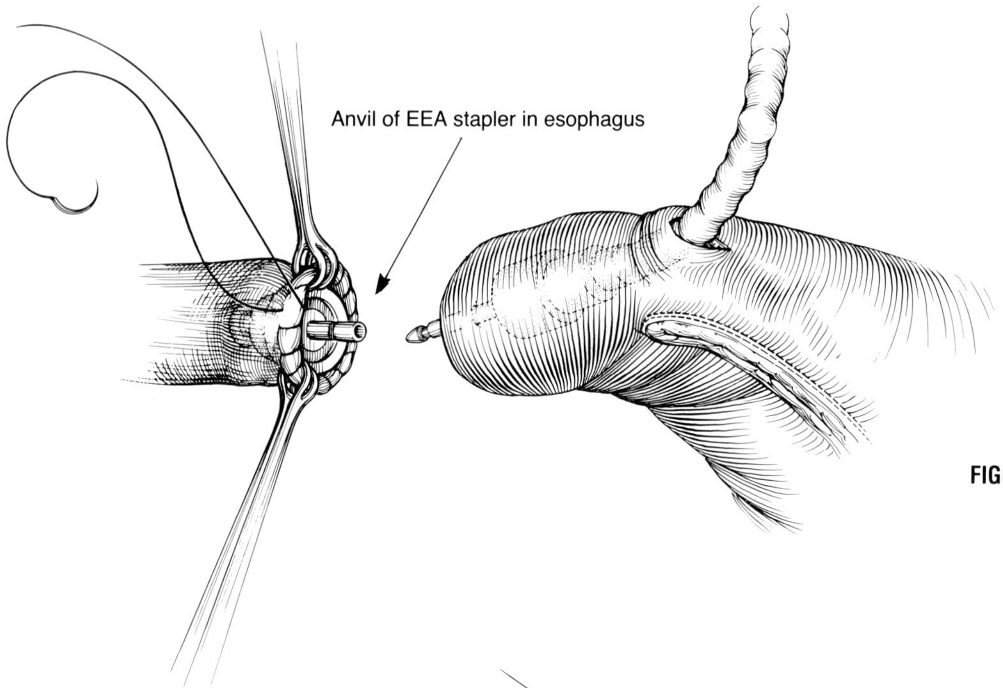

FIGURE 36–11

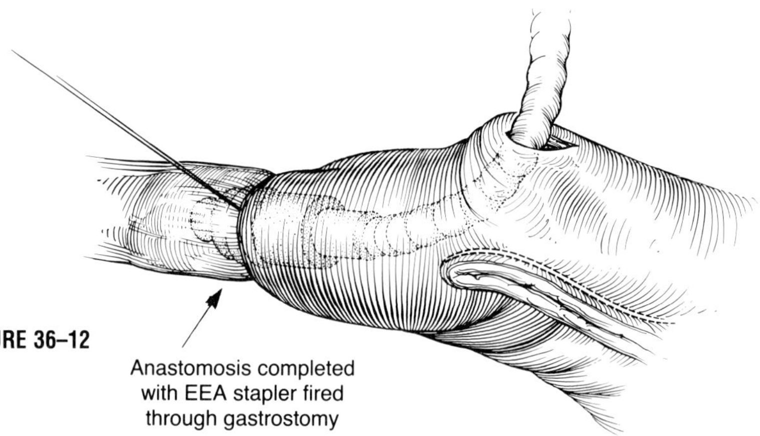

FIGURE 36–12

FIGURES 36–11 and 36–12. A stapling device is used to complete the anastomosis. Alternatively, a single or double layer of sutures can be used to complete the anastomosis.

The stomach is sutured within the mediastinum. The area of anastomosis is drained with a chest tube, and the chest and abdomen are closed in the usual manner.

WALTER G. WOLFE, M.D.

37
Transhiatal (Orringer) Esophagogastrectomy

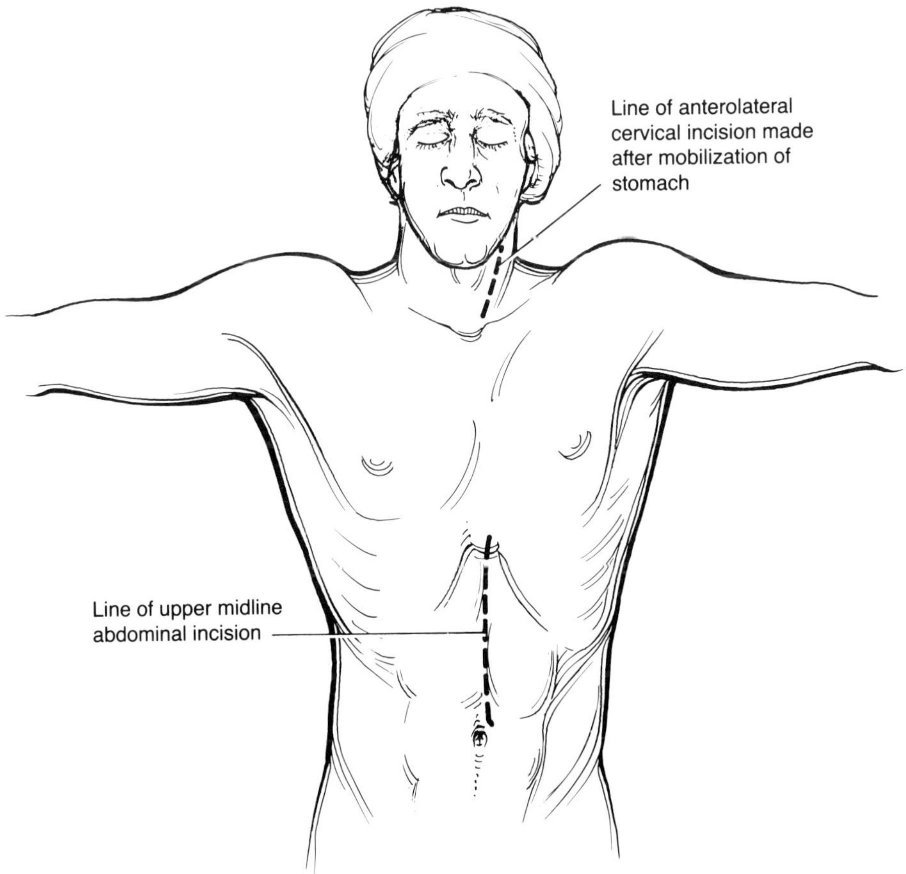

FIGURE 37–1. The patient is placed in the supine position, and the neck, chest, and abdomen are prepared and draped. A midline abdominal incision is made, and a standard cervical incision is made medial to the sternocleidomastoid muscle in the left side of the neck.

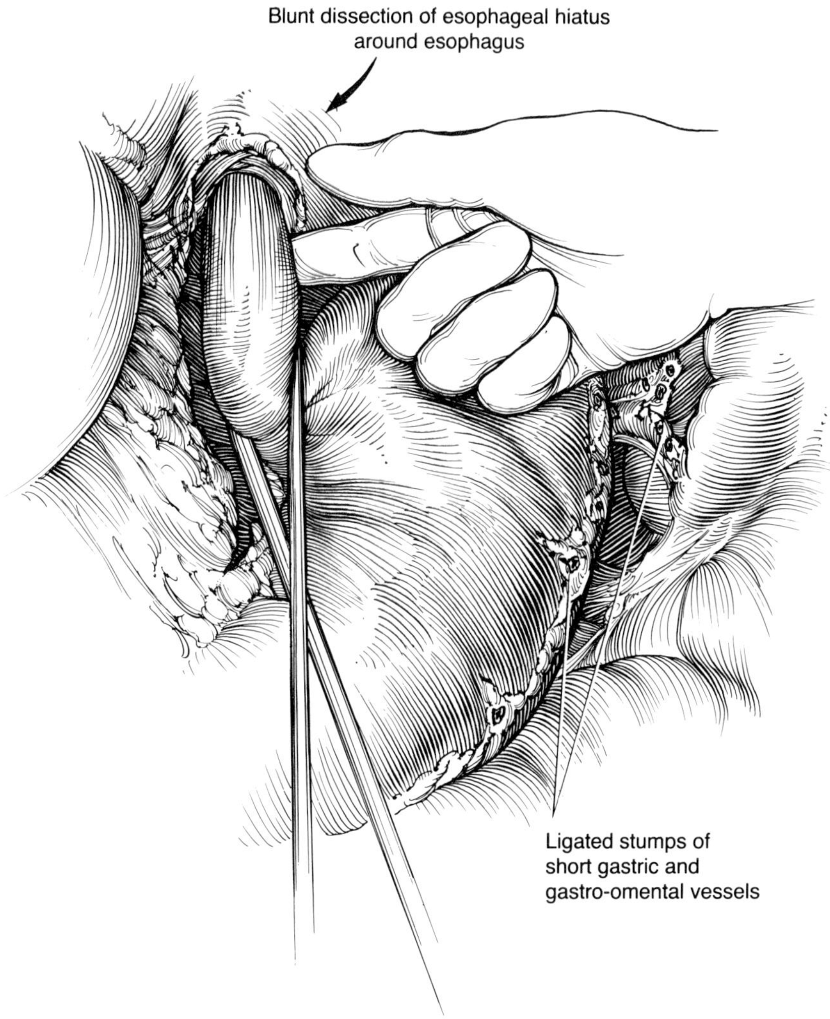

FIGURE 37–2. The hiatus is opened and the esophagus is encircled. The stomach is then mobilized on the right gastric and right gastric epiploic vessels, with the short gastric vessels being ligated and divided, and preserving the spleen in most instances.

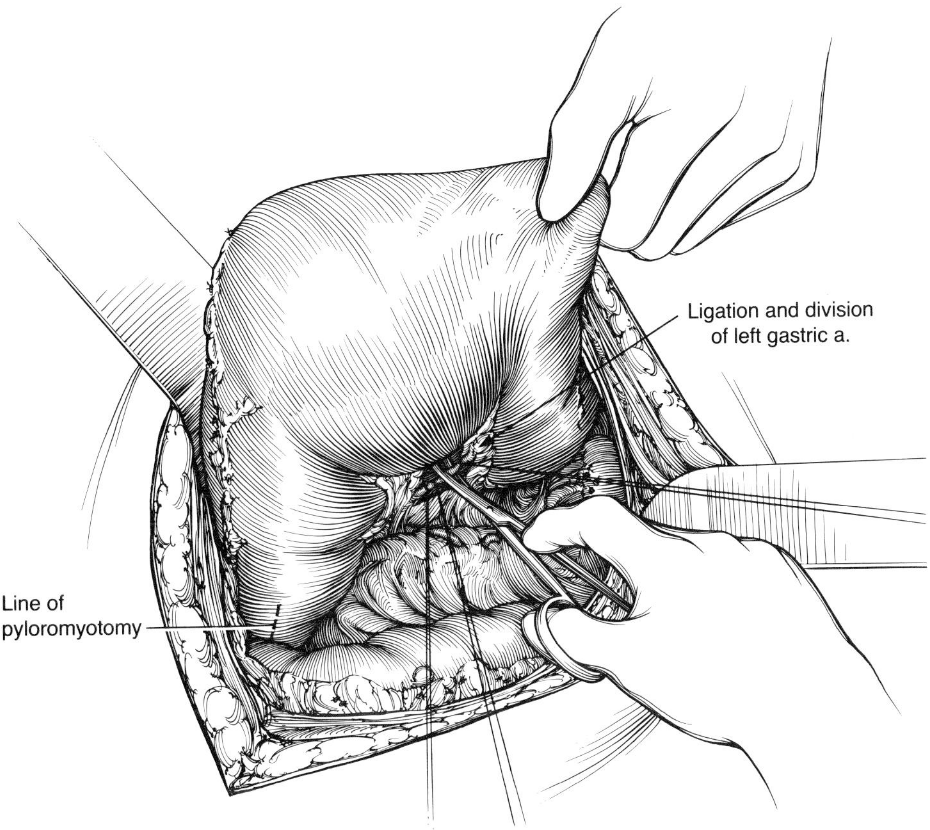

FIGURE 37–3. The left gastric vessel is ligated and divided.

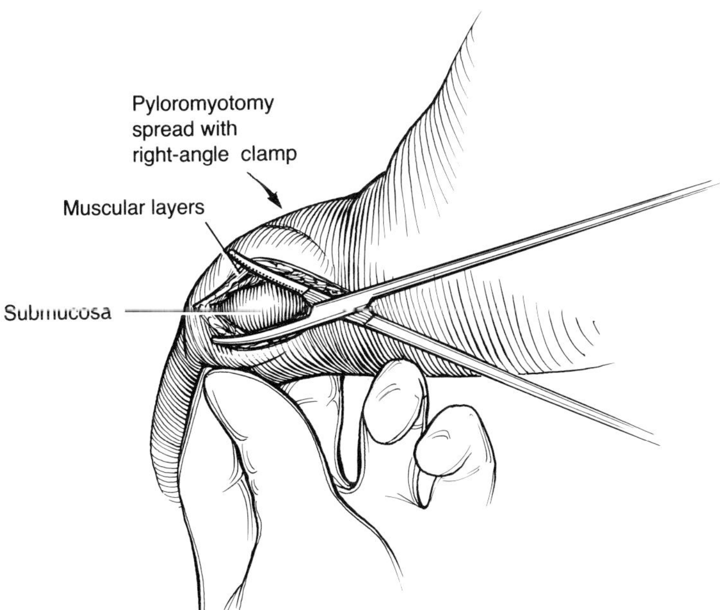

FIGURE 36–4

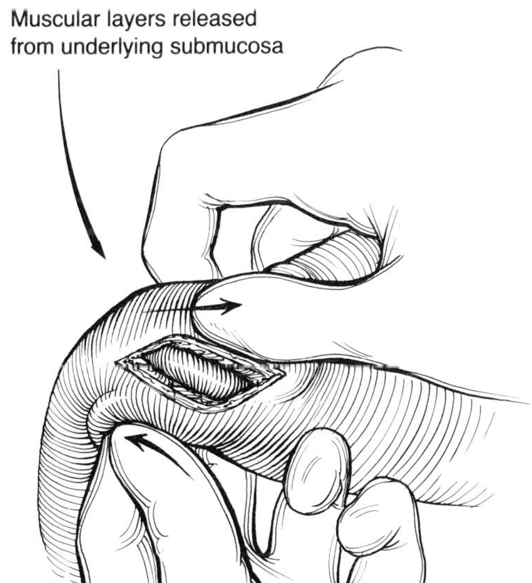

FIGURE 36–5

FIGURES 37–4 and 37–5. In general, the pyloromyotomy is done at this time. If the mucosa is entered, a pyloroplasty is done in the usual manner.

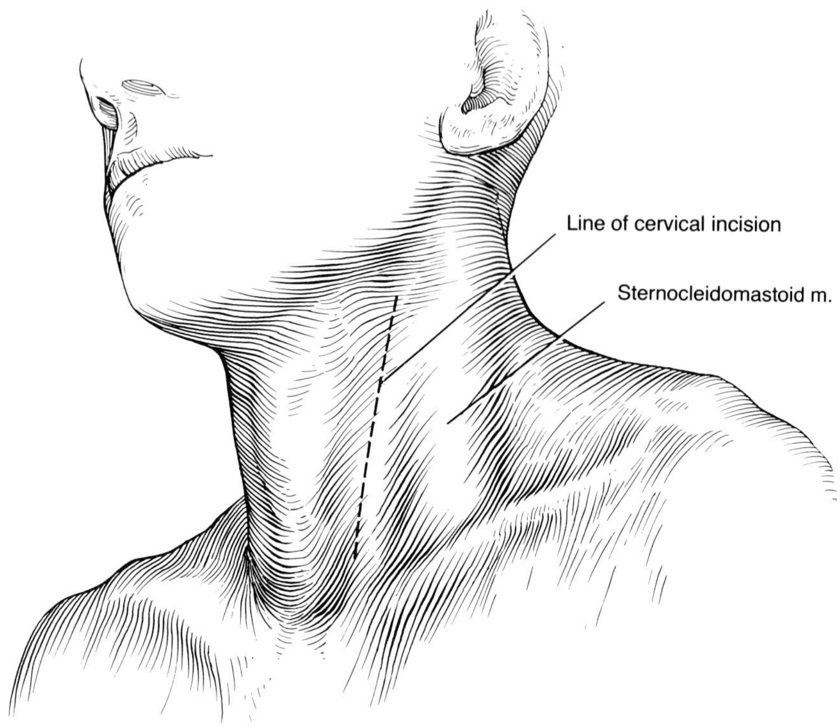

FIGURE 37–6. The neck wound is usually opened simultaneously, or shortly after exploration of the abdomen reveals that there is no metastatic disease.

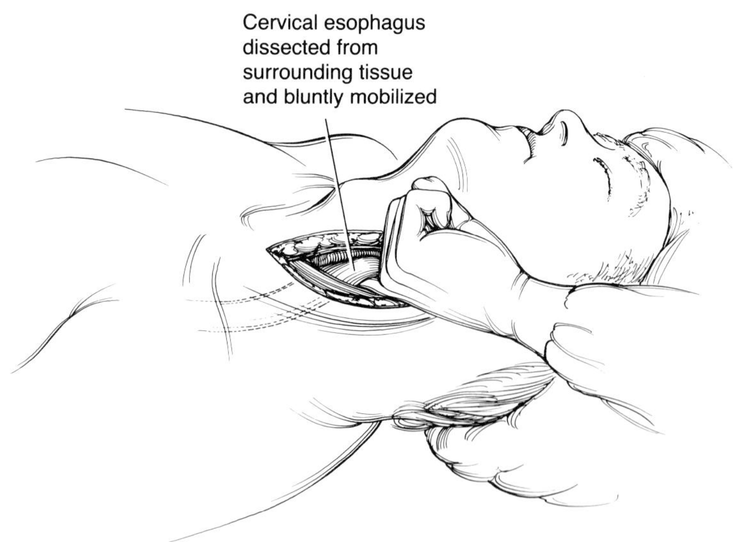

FIGURE 37–7. The esophagus is mobilized, with care being taken to preserve the recurrent laryngeal nerve. The neck dissection is extended, freeing the esophagus from the trachea and surrounding structures, and then the dissection is completed posteriorly.

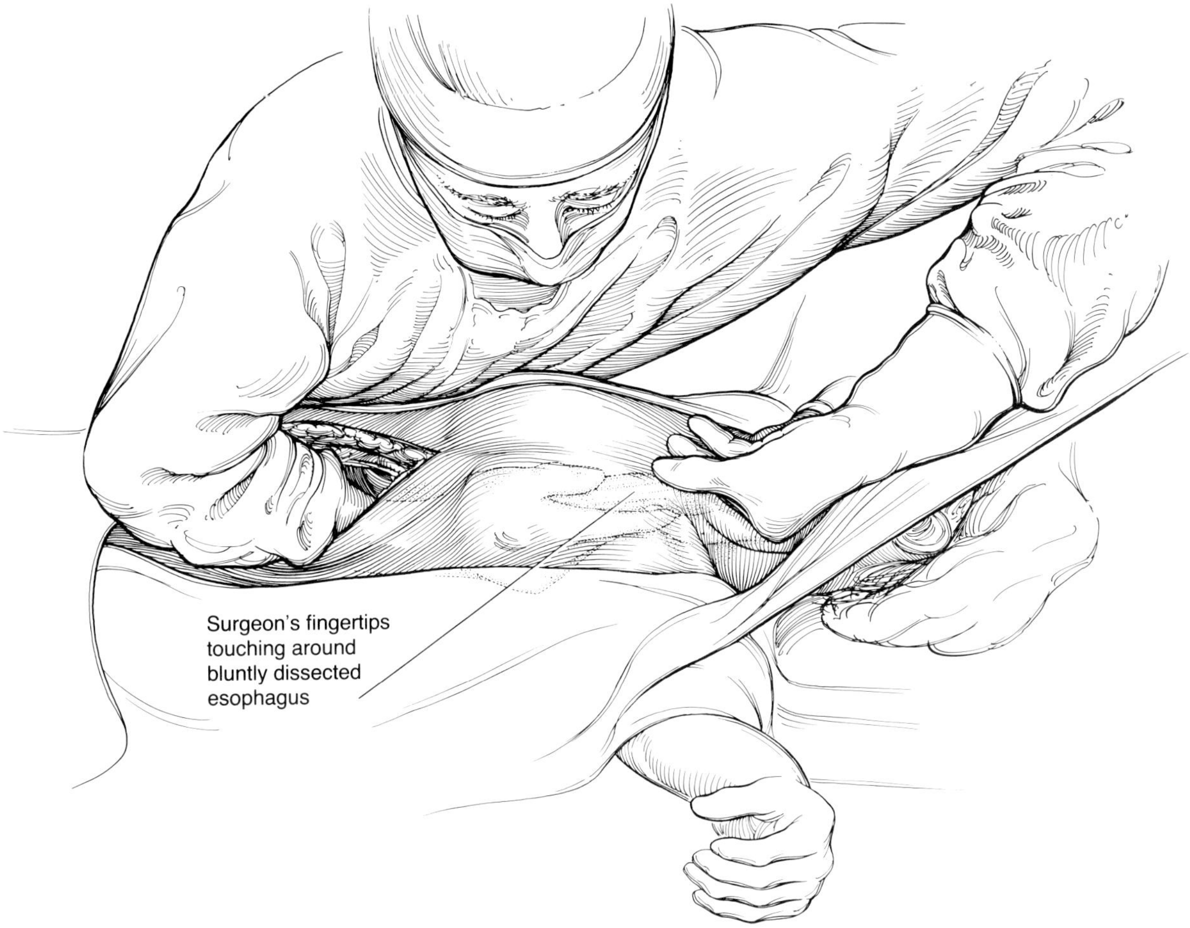

FIGURE 37–8. The most dangerous portion of the dissection is the mobilization of the esophagus from the tracheobronchial tree.

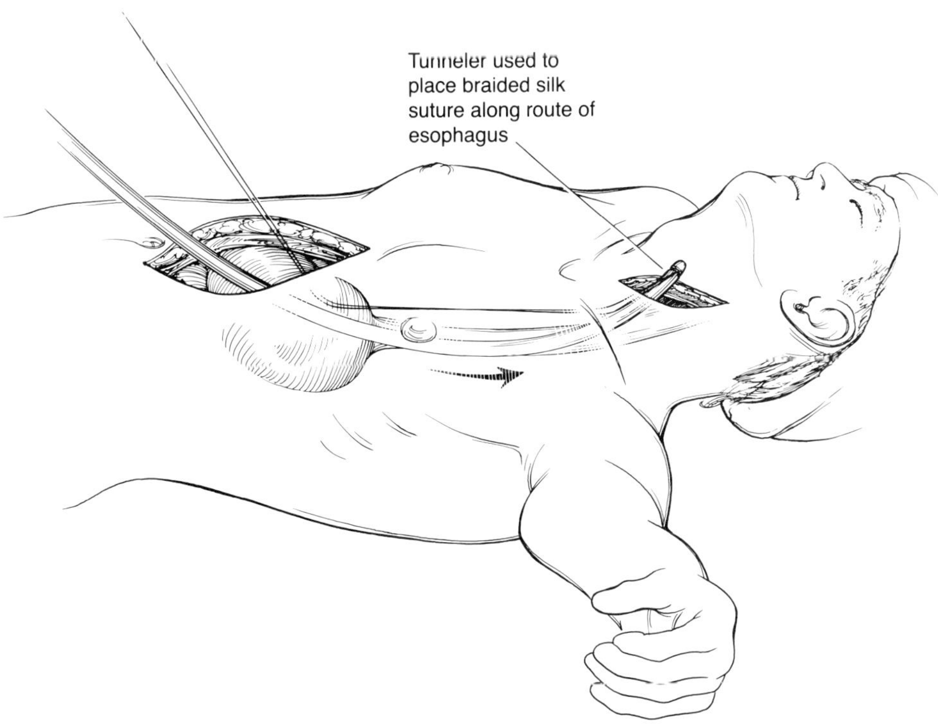

FIGURE 37–9. Once the esophagus is mobilized, a suture is passed into the neck.

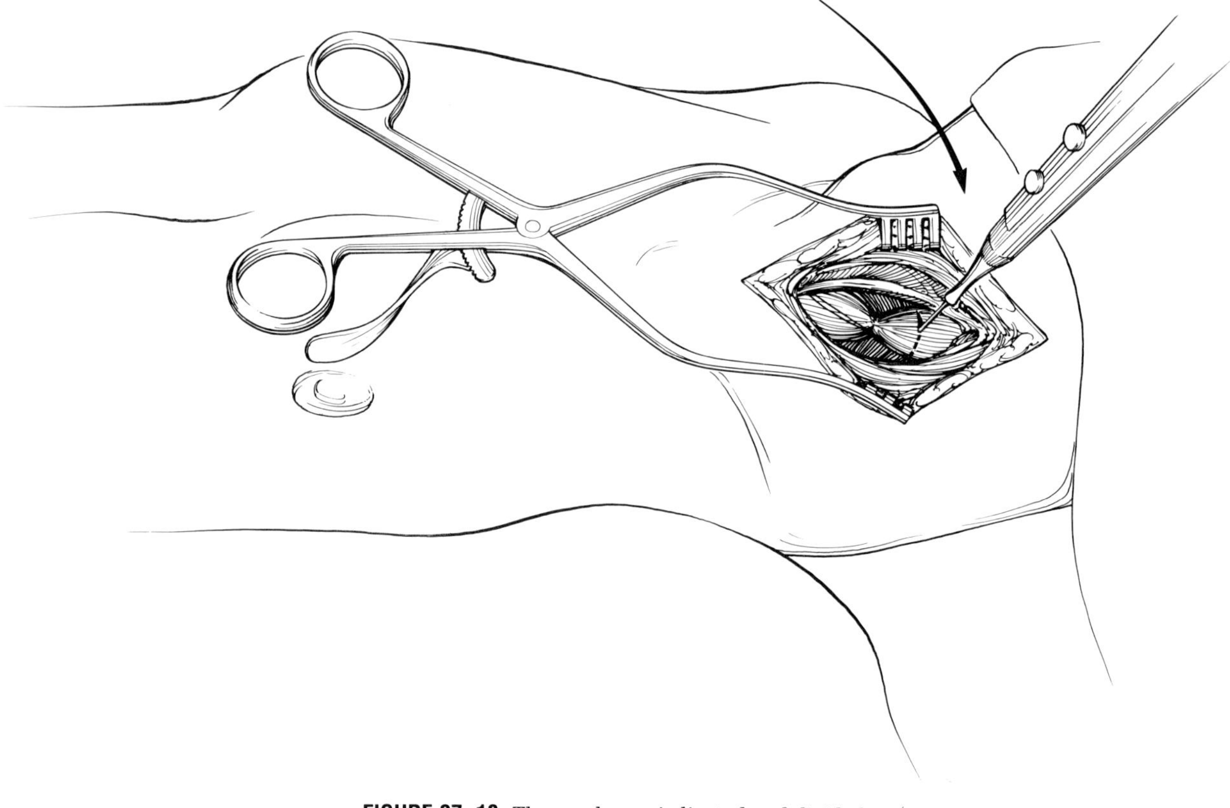

FIGURE 37–10. The esophagus is ligated and divided.

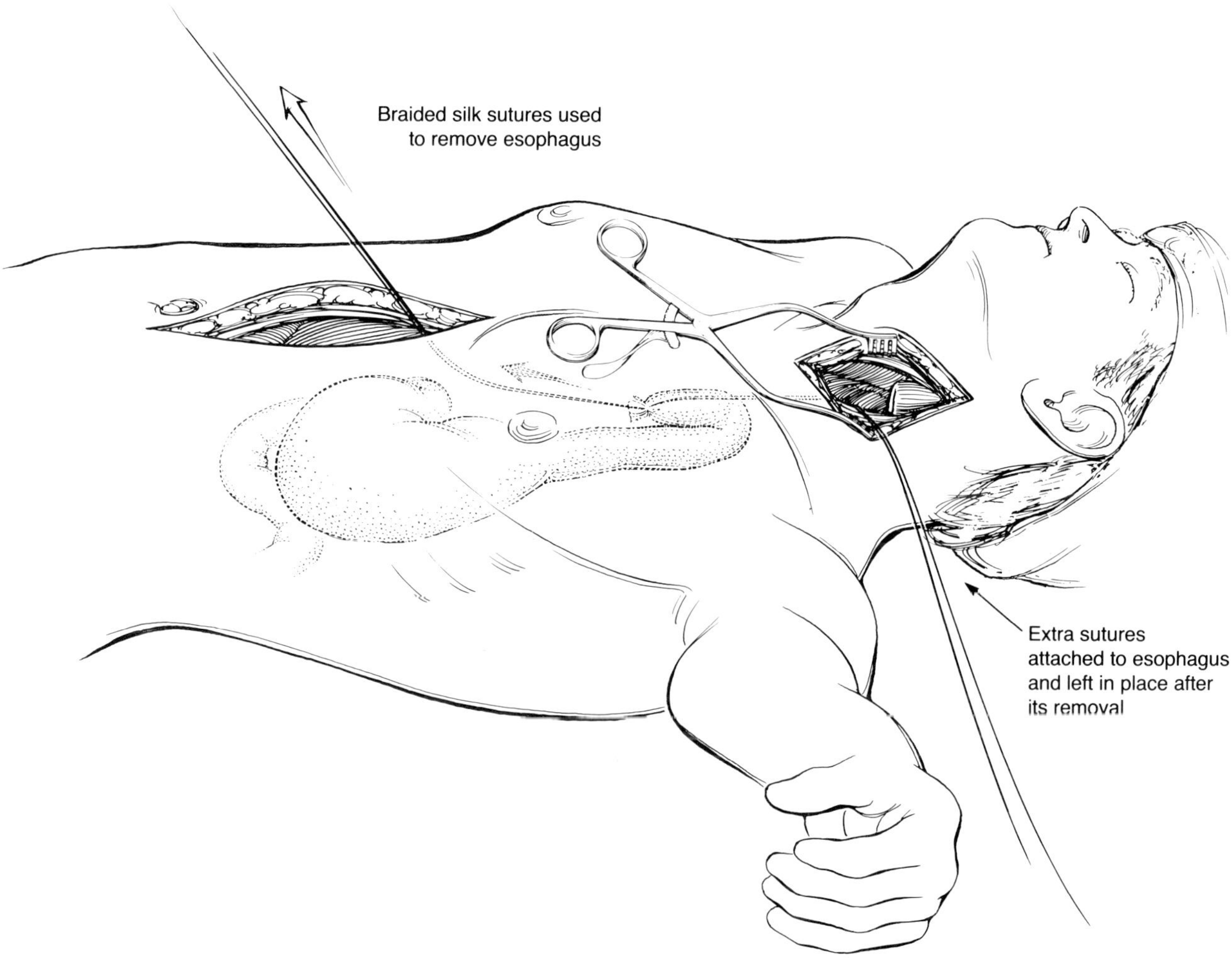

FIGURE 37–11. The esophagus is everted down toward the abdominal incision so that the remaining few attachments, if any, in the area of the tracheobronchial tree can be dissected free and pinched off.

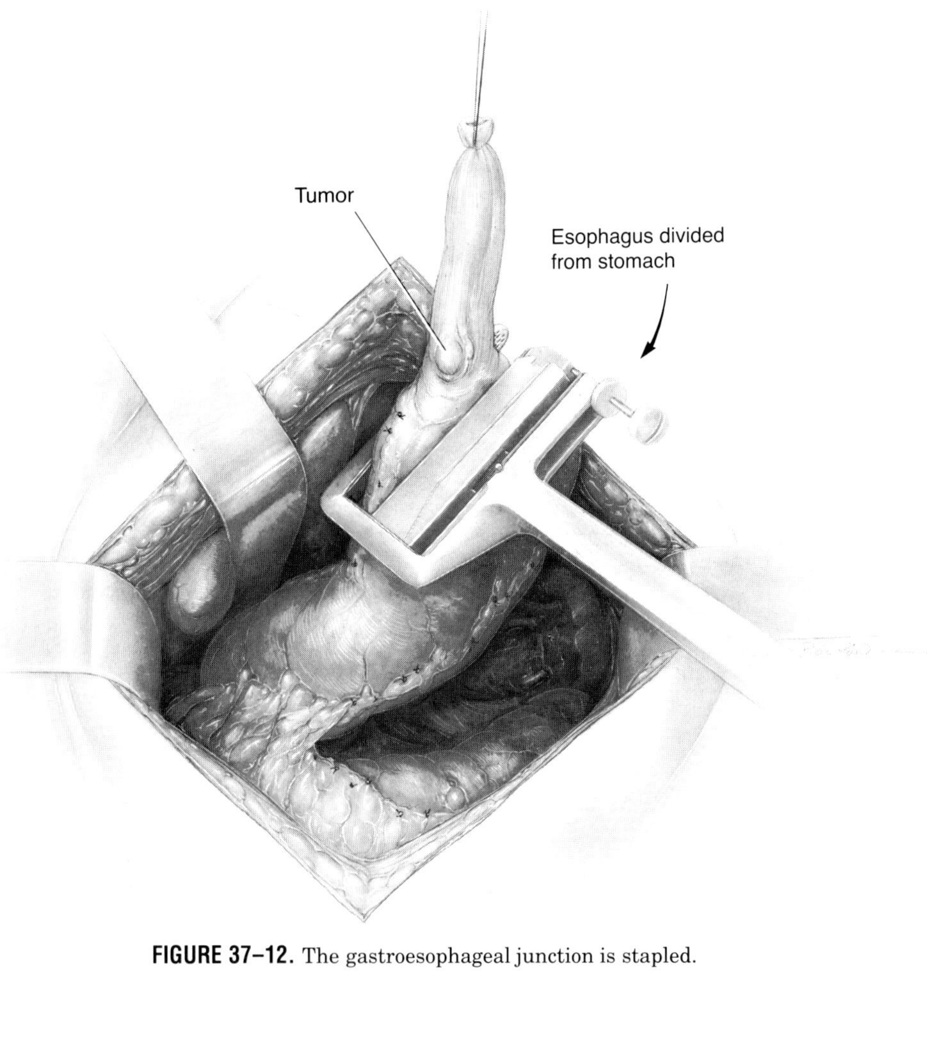

FIGURE 37–12. The gastroesophageal junction is stapled.

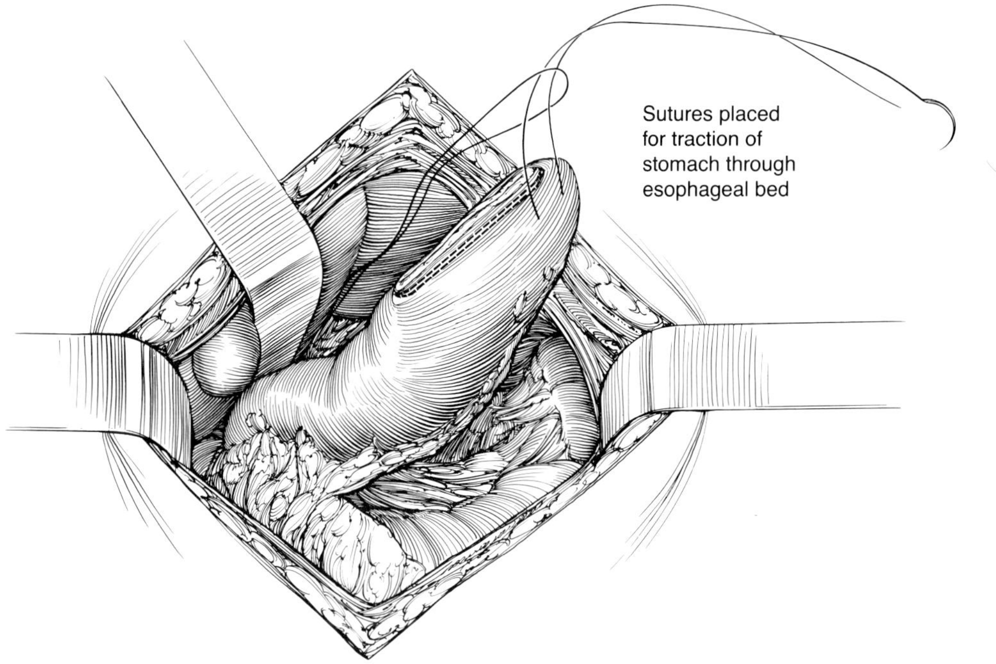

FIGURE 37–13

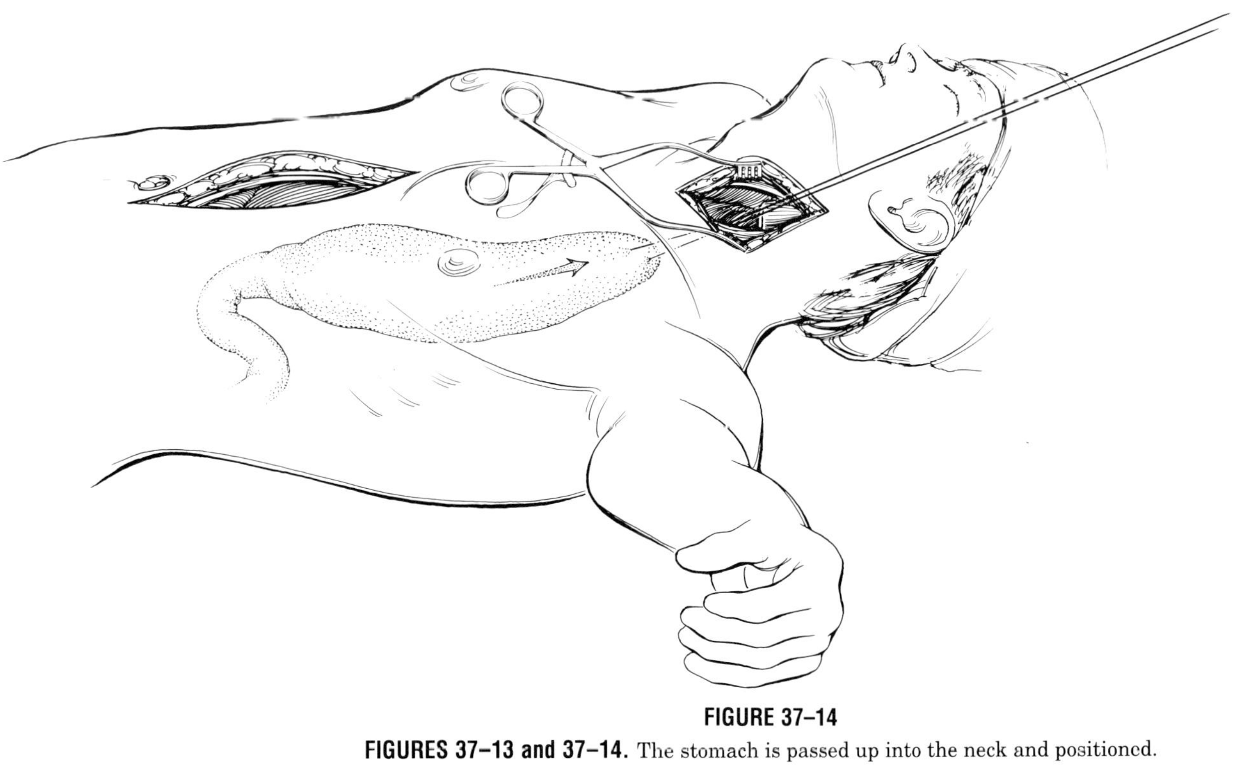

FIGURE 37–14

FIGURES 37–13 and 37–14. The stomach is passed up into the neck and positioned.

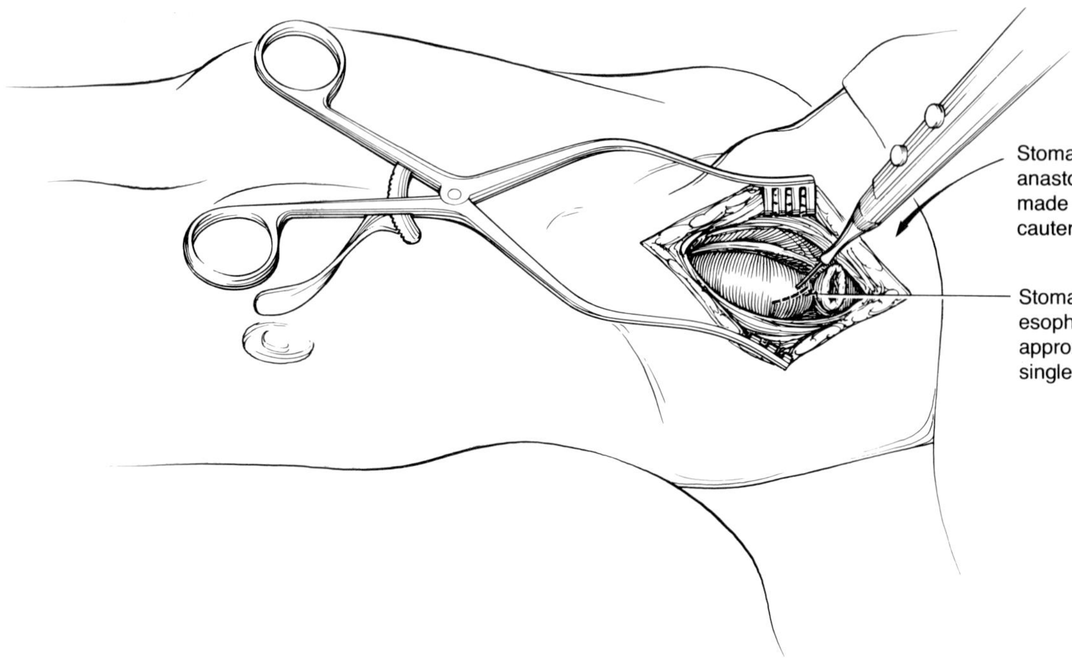

FIGURE 37–15. The stomach is sutured within the neck in preparation for anastomosis.

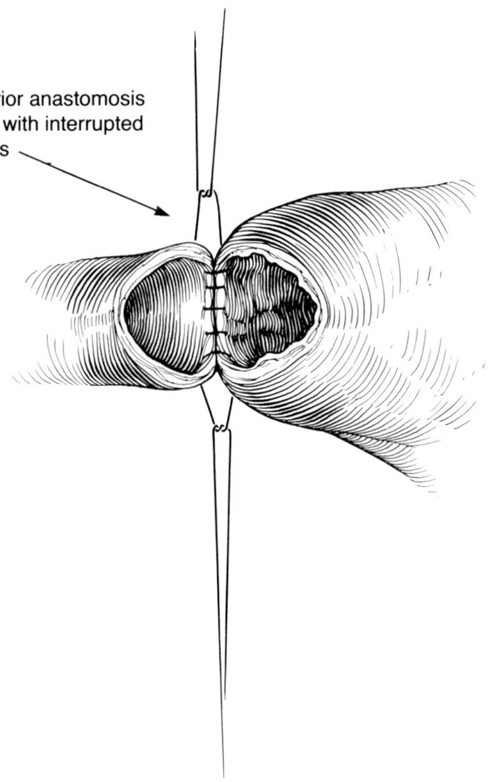

FIGURE 37–16. The anastomosis is done between the esophagus and stomach, usually with a single layer of interrupted 3–0 silk sutures.

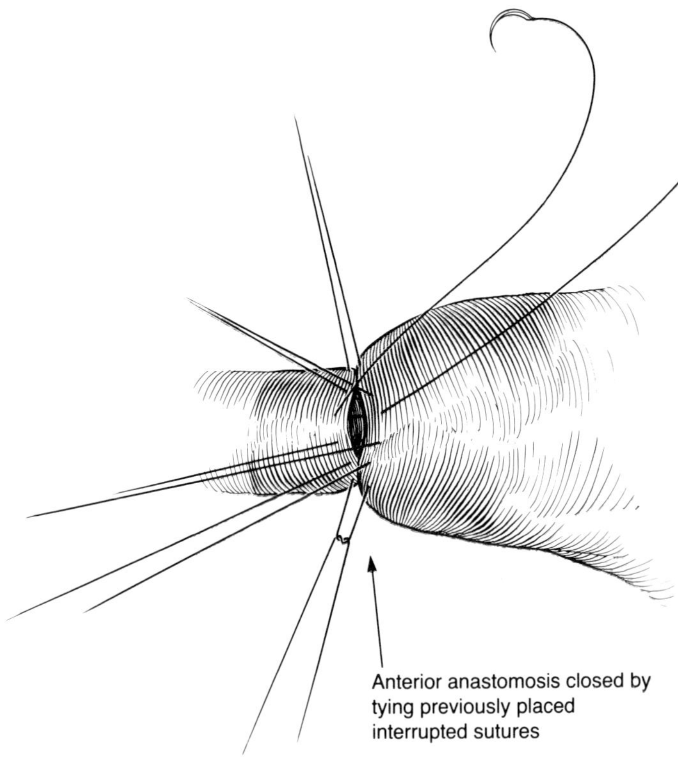

FIGURE 37–17. The anastomosis is joined with interrupted sutures.

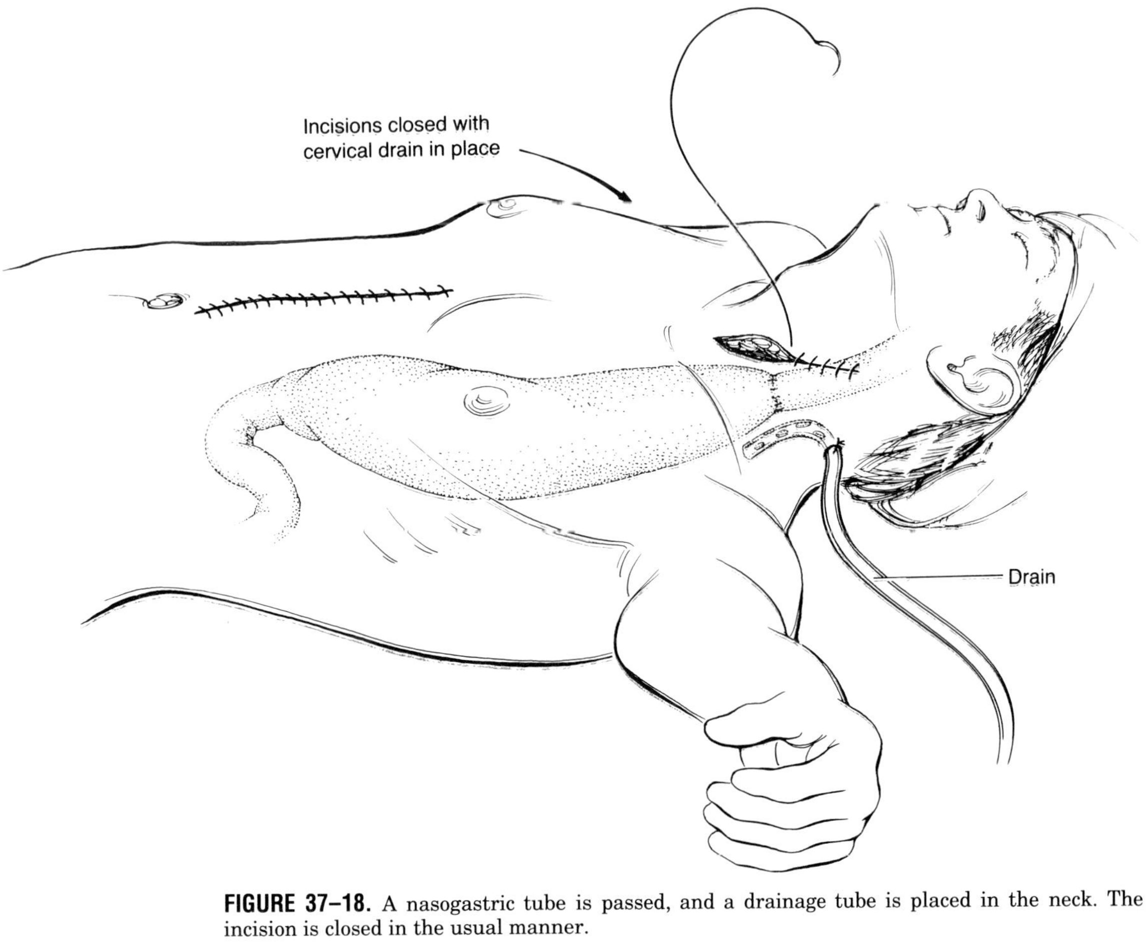

FIGURE 37–18. A nasogastric tube is passed, and a drainage tube is placed in the neck. The incision is closed in the usual manner.

WALTER G. WOLFE, M.D.

38
Correction of Achalasia

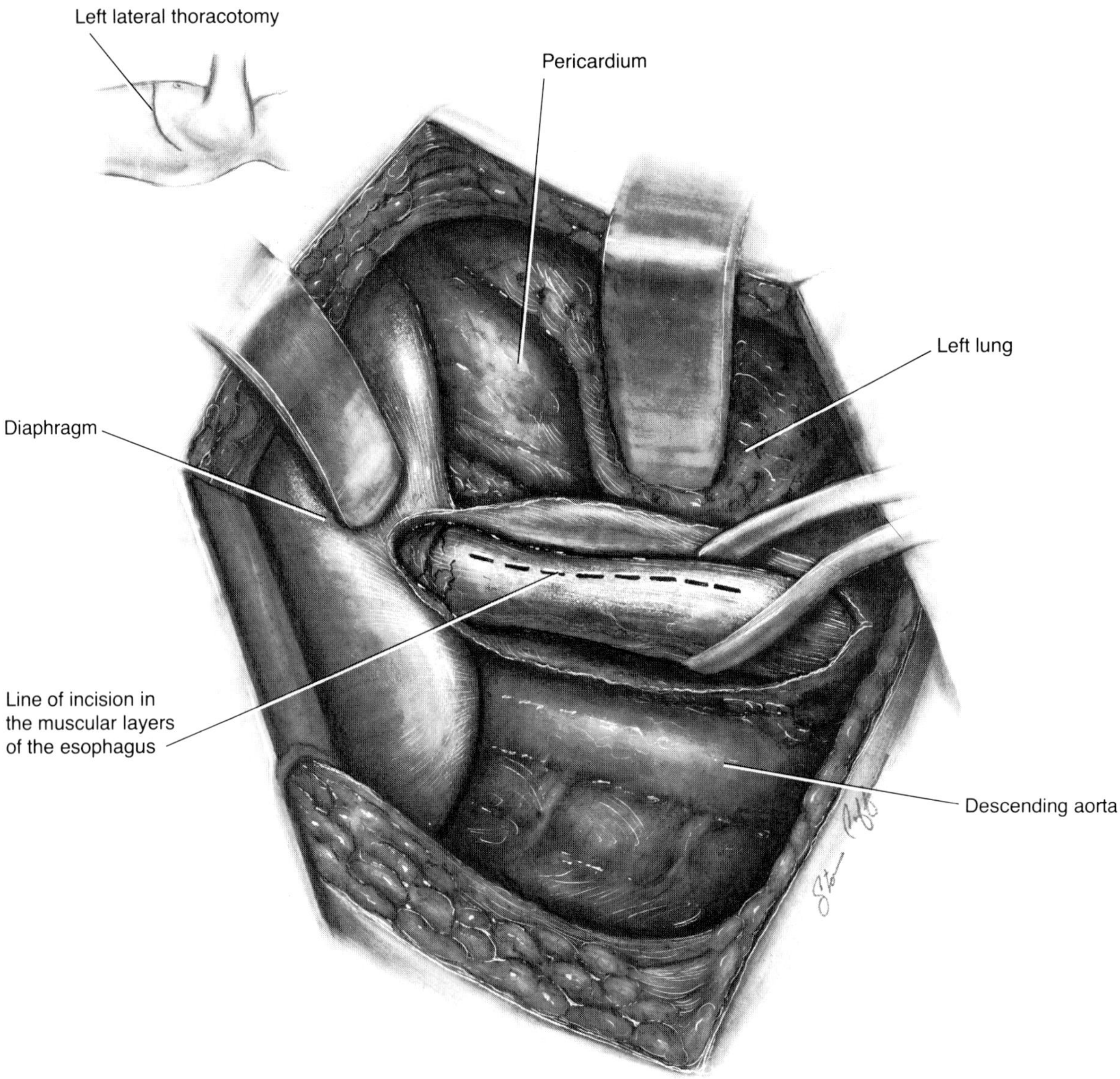

FIGURE 38–1. A small left lateral thoracotomy is made, and the chest is entered through the seventh intercostal space without dividing a rib posteriorly. The mediastinum is opened, and care is taken not to disturb the hiatus. The esophagus may or may not be encircled just below the inferior pulmonary vein.

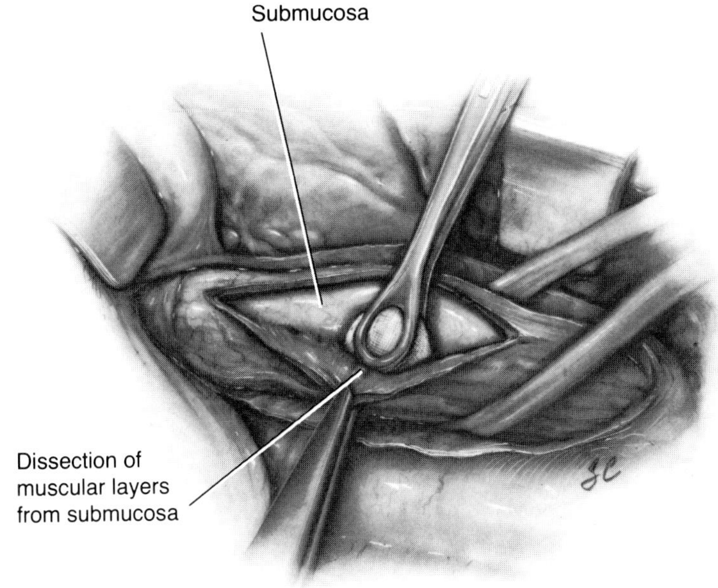

FIGURE 38–2. A myotomy is performed from the inferior vein or from the arch of the aorta, depending on the situation, to the esophagogastric junction, which is identified by the small veins that are present near the stomach in this area. Care is taken not to extend the myotomy onto the stomach more than 9 mm. Muscle is dissected from the submucosa.

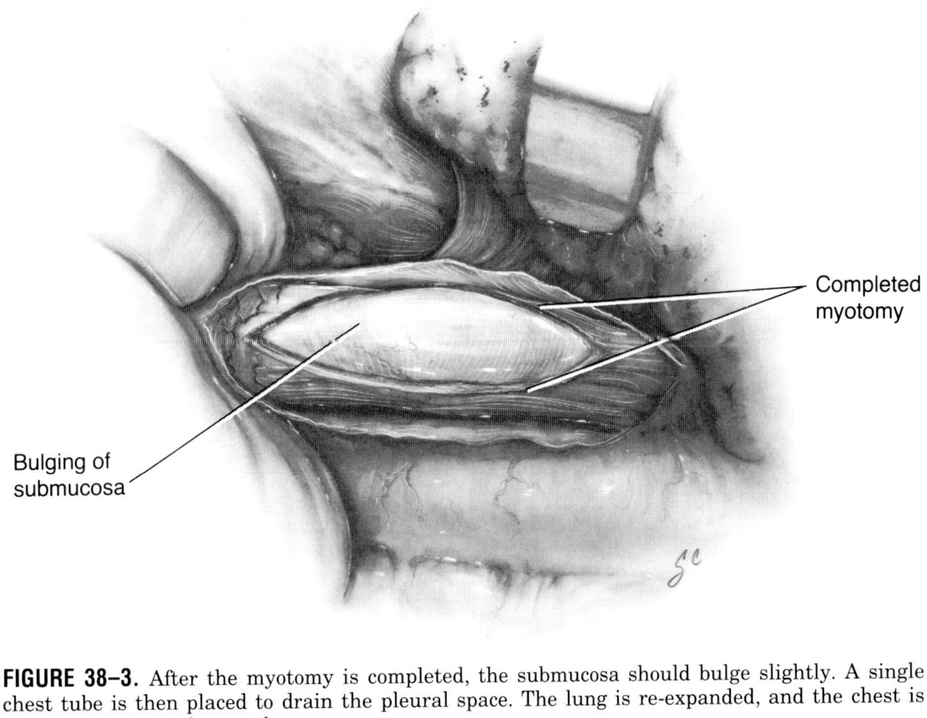

FIGURE 38–3. After the myotomy is completed, the submucosa should bulge slightly. A single chest tube is then placed to drain the pleural space. The lung is re-expanded, and the chest is closed in layers in the usual manner.

SECTION IX

The Diaphragm

SAMUEL M. MAHAFFEY, M.D.

39

Congenital Diaphragmatic Hernia

Until recently, emergent postnatal repair of diaphragmatic hernias was the primary method of management. Despite dramatic improvement in supportive care of infants in recent years, the mortality rate for this lesion remained approximately 60%. Repair of the anatomic defect does not address the underlying pathophysiology, the severe pulmonary hypoplasia. Pulmonary function studies suggest that many infants are actually worse after the repair, owing to marked decreases in total lung compliance. Accordingly, many pediatric surgeons have adopted a protocol of preoperative stabilization, using ventilatory management or extracorporeal life support techniques (extracorporeal membrane oxygenation [ECMO]) to provide adequate gas exchange and oxygen delivery to the tissues. Operative repair is undertaken when the baby has been satisfactorily stabilized. When ECMO has been used for stabilization, the operative repair can be performed while the infant is on ECMO support. Even with these supportive measures, overall mortality for this anomaly remains 40% to 50%. Further improvement in survival will be the result of innovative new strategies that are currently being explored, such as *in utero* repair of the diaphragmatic defect, selective pulmonary vasodilators, and lung transplantation.

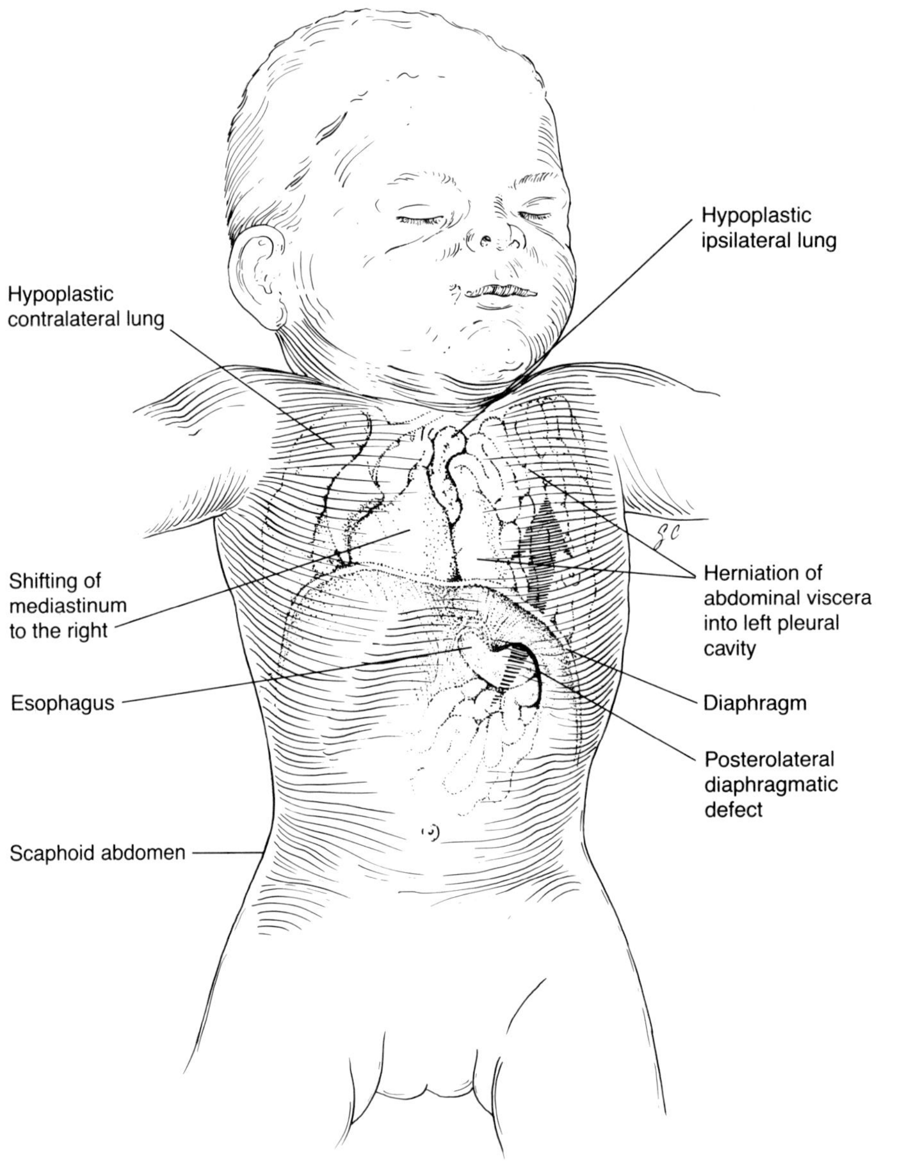

FIGURE 39–1. Approximately 90% of diaphragmatic lesions occur on the left side. A peritoneal sac covering the defect is noted in approximately one third of patients. A marked decrease in volume of the abdominal cavity causes the clinical appearance of a scaphoid abdomen.

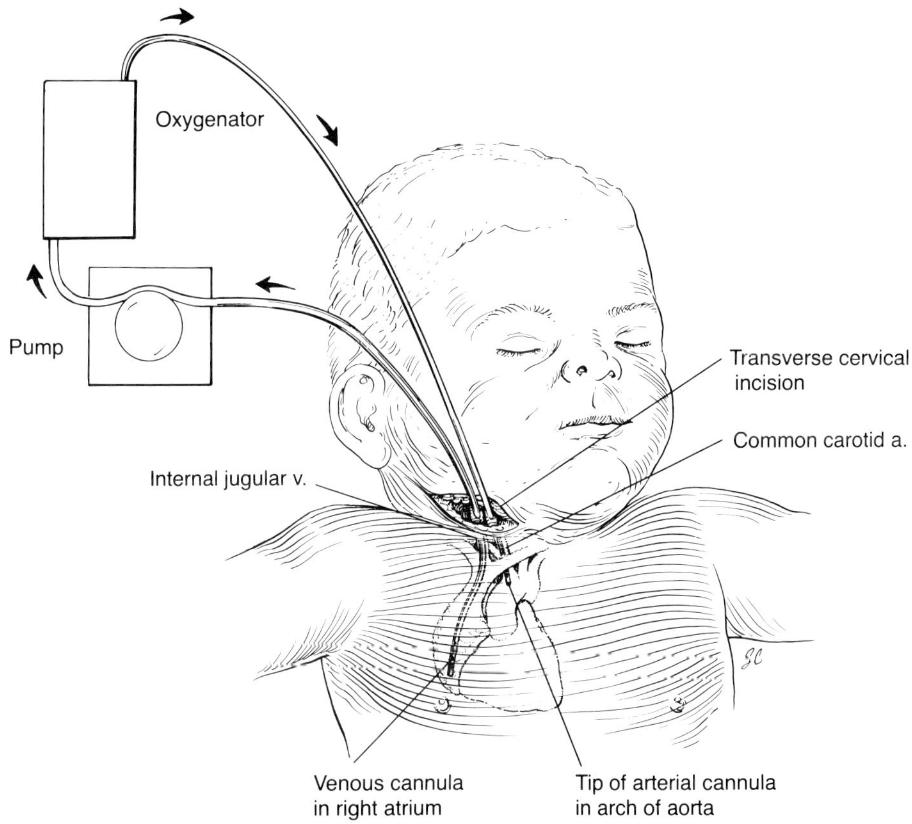

FIGURE 39–2. With ECMO support, unoxygenated blood drains passively from the venous cannula and is then circulated through a membrane oxygenator. The oxygenated blood is rewarmed to the baby's body temperature and returned into the aortic arch. ECMO support may be used preoperatively when the baby cannot be stabilized with conventional ventilatory techniques. ECMO rescue may also be used if severe pulmonary hypertension develops postoperatively.

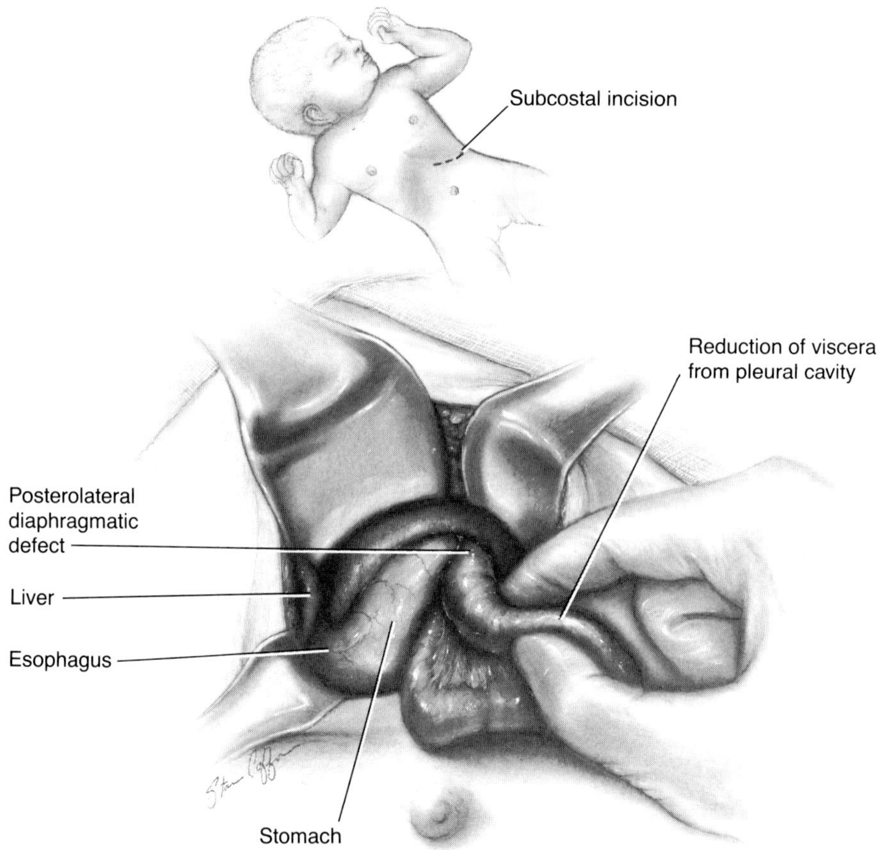

FIGURE 39–3. A transabdominal approach using a subcostal incision is preferred. With gentle traction, the abdominal viscera are reduced from the thoracic cavity. The defect may be enlarged to avoid injury to the abdominal viscera, particularly the spleen.

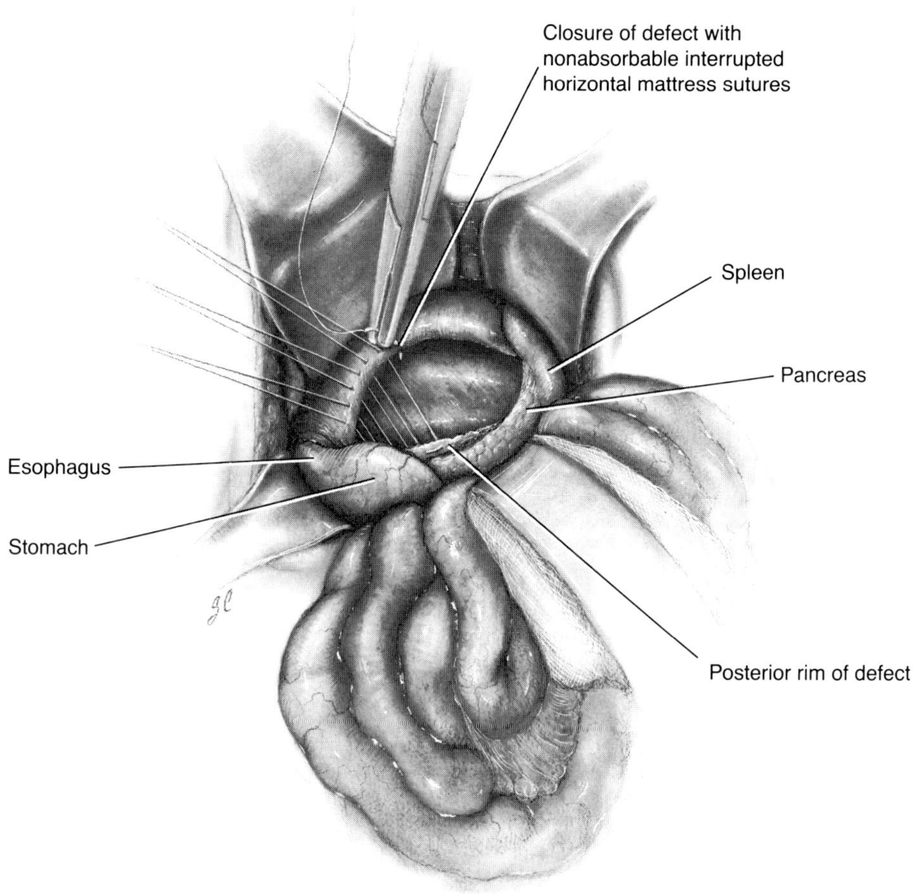

FIGURE 39–4. The small posterior leaflet is mobilized by carefully incising the overlying peritoneum. The medial portion of the defect is closed with nonabsorbable interrupted horizontal mattress sutures. This is an important part of the repair, because inadequate reconstruction of the left crus inevitability leads to significant gastroesophageal reflux. Laterally, the posterior leaflet becomes very small, and the sutures may need to be placed around the ribs to achieve closure of the defect.

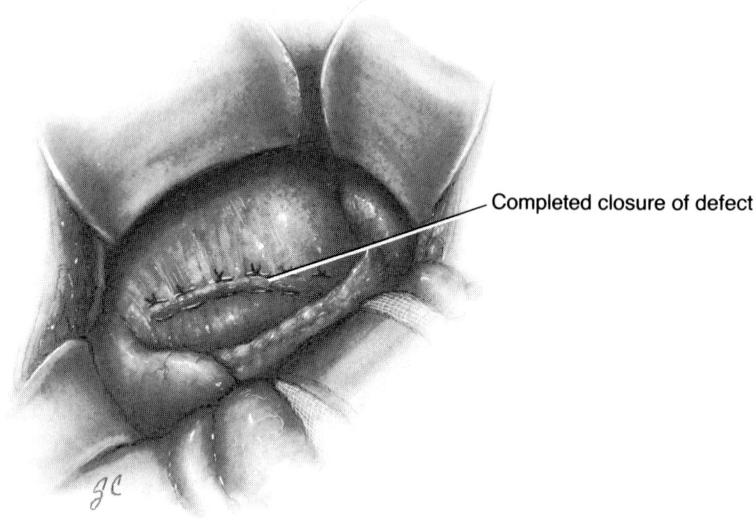

FIGURE 39–5. A thoracostomy tube may be placed at the discretion of the operator. If a thoracostomy tube is placed, it should not be placed to suction; expansion of the contralateral lung slowly shifts the mediastinum back to the midline.

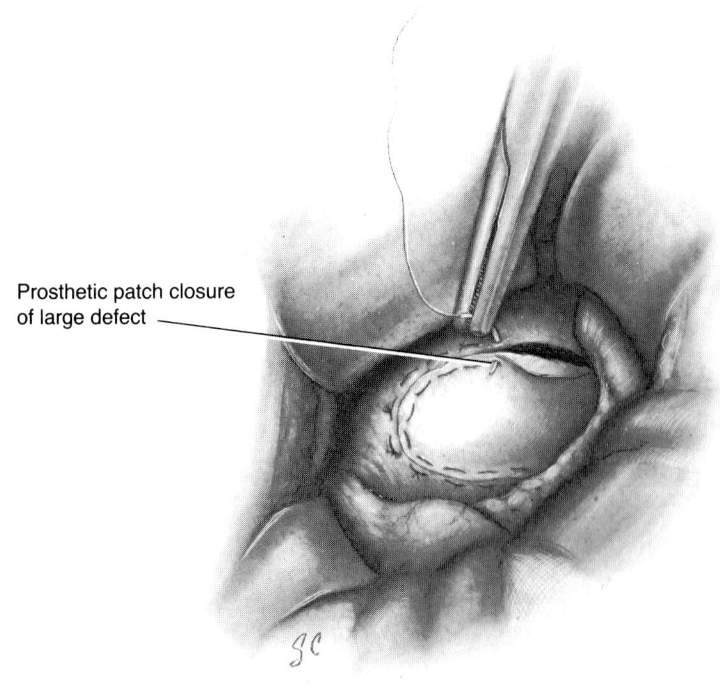

FIGURE 39–6. Large defects that cannot be closed primarily should be closed with tissue or prosthetic material. This can be accomplished with rotation of a tissue flap from the anterior abdominal wall or, more commonly, with a nonabsorbable prosthesis such as PTFE (Gore-Tex).

PETER VAN TRIGT, III, M.D.

40
Placement of Diaphragmatic Pacemaker

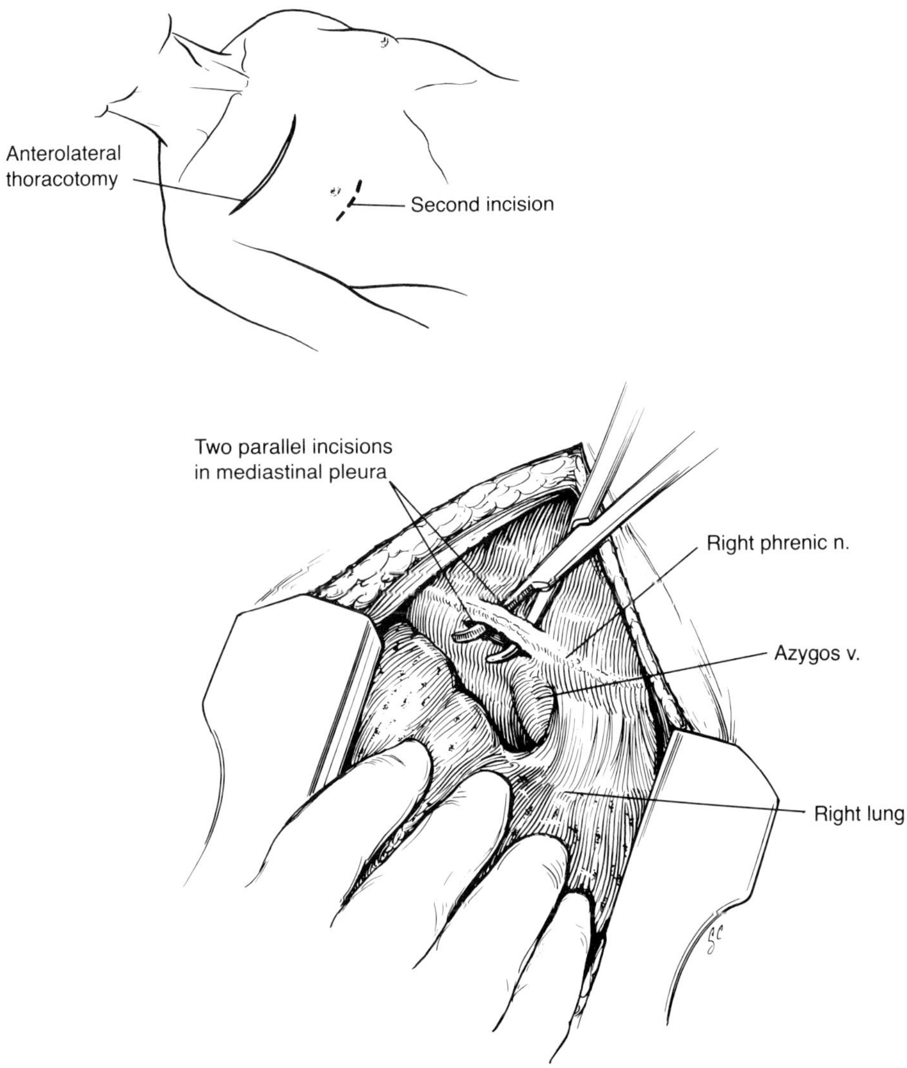

FIGURE 40–1. The thoracic approach to the right phrenic nerve is through an anterolateral thoracotomy in the second interspace. The incision is made from the lateral border of the sternum to just beyond the anterior axillary line, the pectoralis muscles are split in the direction of their fibers, and the chest is entered. The internal mammary vessels are ligated and divided for better exposure, and the ribs are retracted. The lung is retracted laterally, and the phrenic nerve is identified as it passes beneath the mediastinal pleura on the superior vena cava. A site for placement of the electrode is selected so that it lies flat against the mediastinum. Parallel incisions are made through the pleura on each side of the nerve, with preservation of the perineural blood vessels. An angled clamp is passed beneath the nerve, and a tunnel is gently created posterior to the nerve.

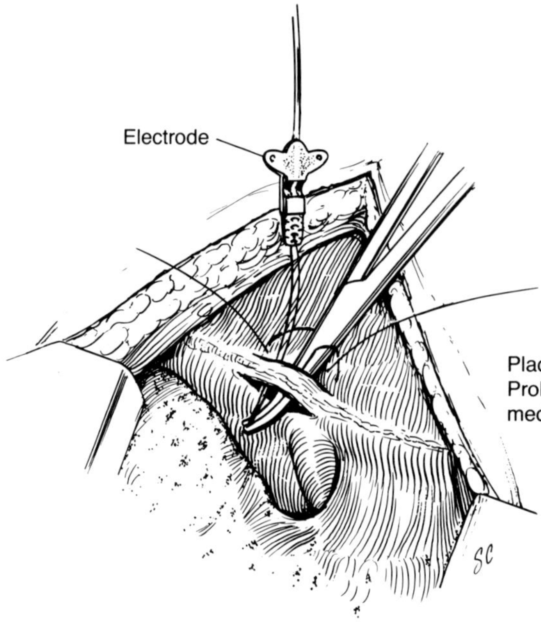

FIGURE 40–2. The toe of the electrode cuff is passed from anterior to posterior beneath the nerve. The heel of the electrode is fixed in position to tissues on the ventral side of the nerve using a previously placed monofilament suture.

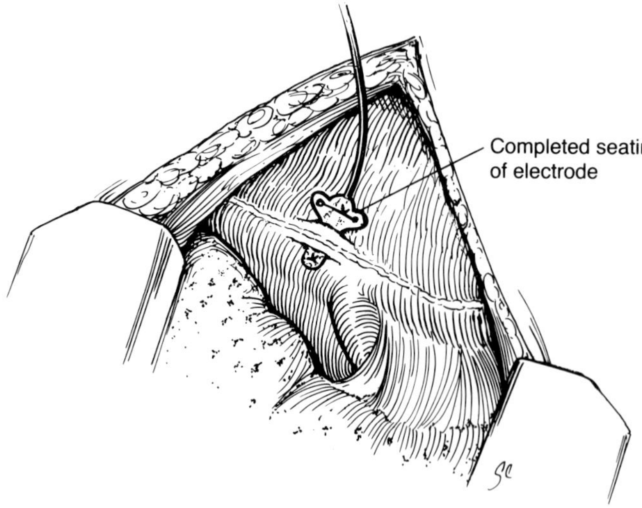

FIGURE 40–3. The toe of the electrode cuff is likewise fixed to the tissues on the dorsal side of the nerve with a second monofilament suture.

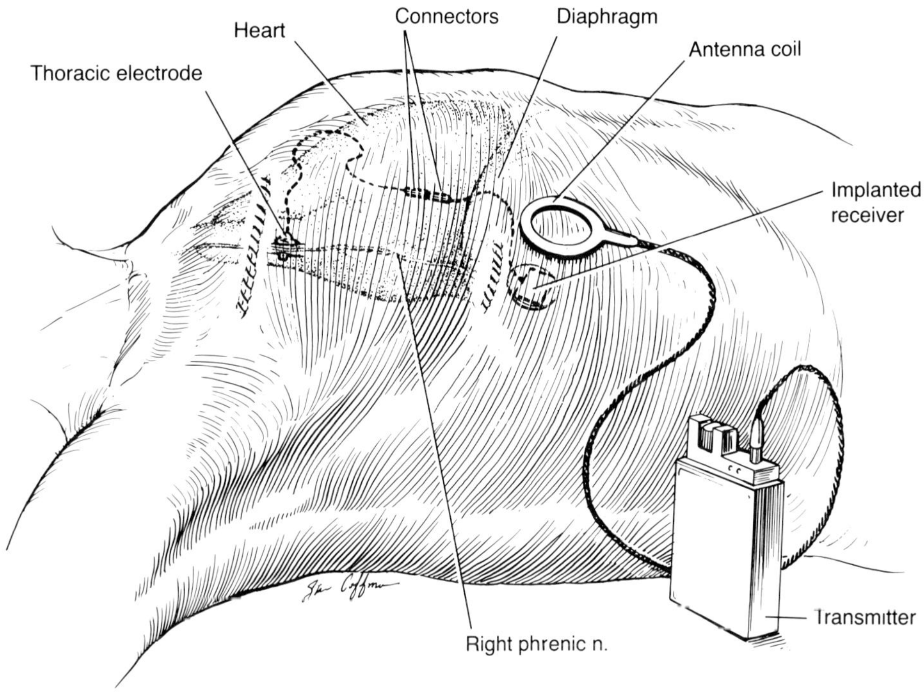

FIGURE 40–4. A subcutaneous pocket is created in the subpectoral fold below the breast to accommodate the radio receiver. The receiver is connected to the electrode by passing the electrode wire from within the thorax through the third or fourth interspace anteriorly into the subcutaneous pocket. A segment of redundant electrode wire is laid anteriorly to prevent tension on the neural electrode.

SECTION X

Pericardium

DONALD D. GLOWER, JR., M.D.

41
Pericardial Window

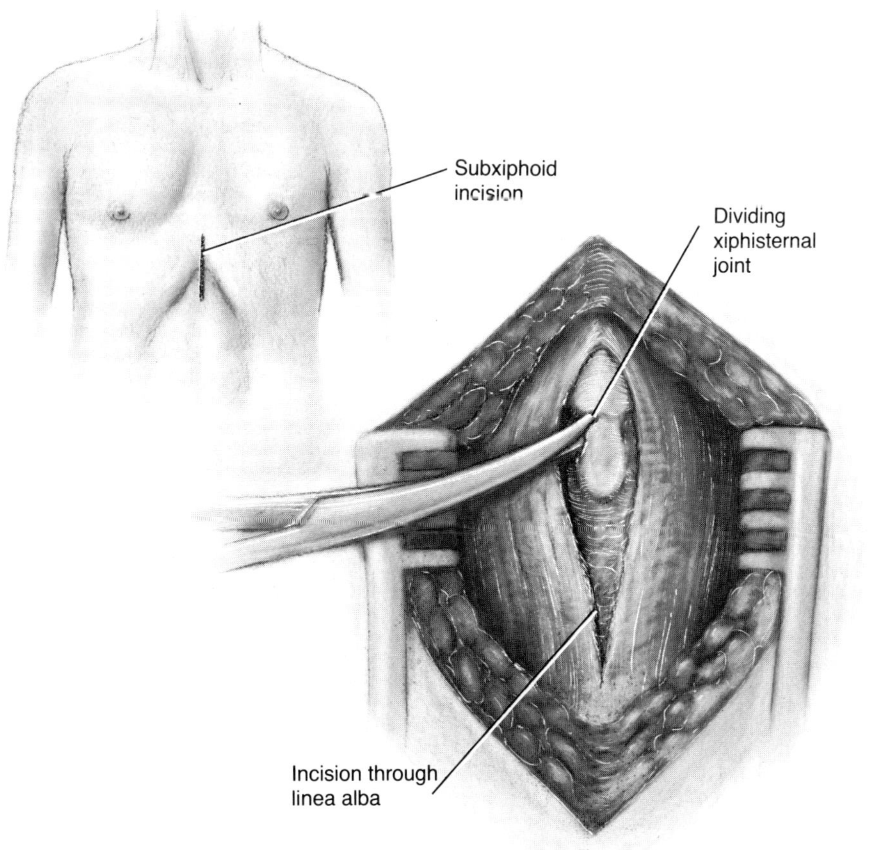

FIGURE 41–1. With use of local or general anesthesia, a 7-cm subxiphoid incision is made. The linea alba is incised 3 cm below the xiphoid, and the xiphoid is excised.

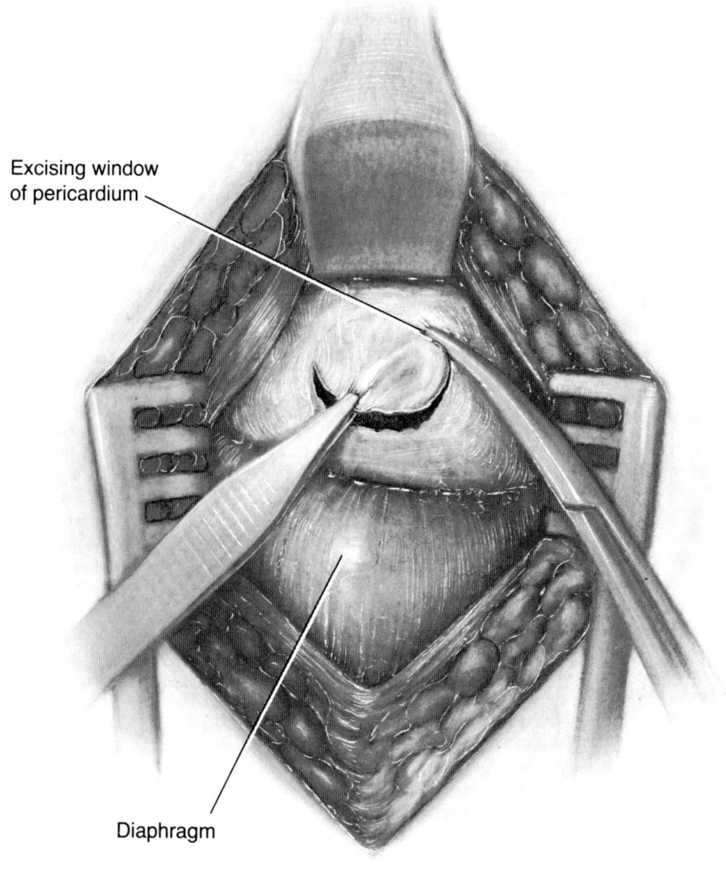

FIGURE 41–2. With the sternum retracted upward, blunt dissection is used to expose the reflection of the anterior pericardium onto the diaphragm. The anterior pericardium is grasped with a clamp, and a 2 × 2 cm piece of pericardium is excised.

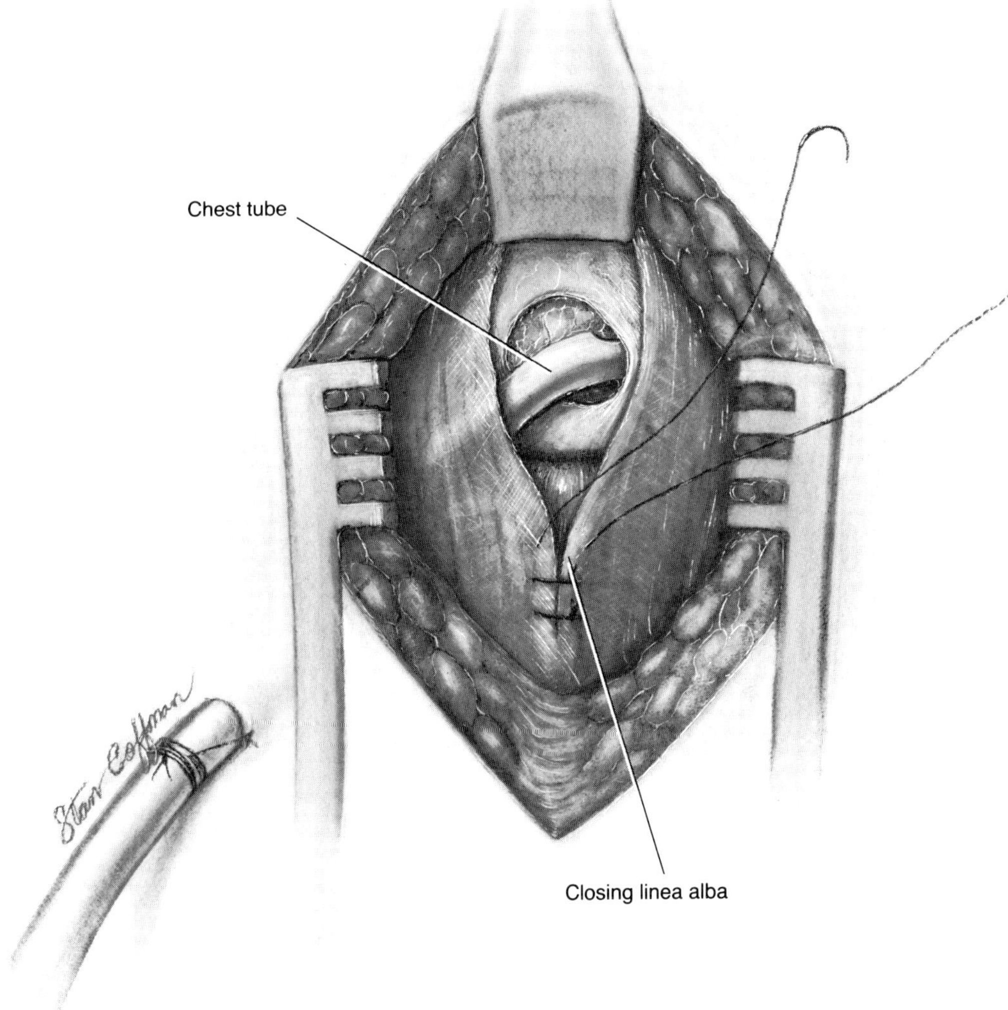

FIGURE 41–3. An angled 32Fr chest tube is placed on the diaphragm in the pericardial space. The tube is placed through the abdominal wall lateral to the incision. The linea alba is closed using interrupted multifilament sutures. The subcutaneous tissue is closed with continuous 2–0 Vicryl suture, and the skin is closed with a skin stapler.

DONALD D. GLOWER, JR., M.D.

42
Pericardiectomy for Effusion

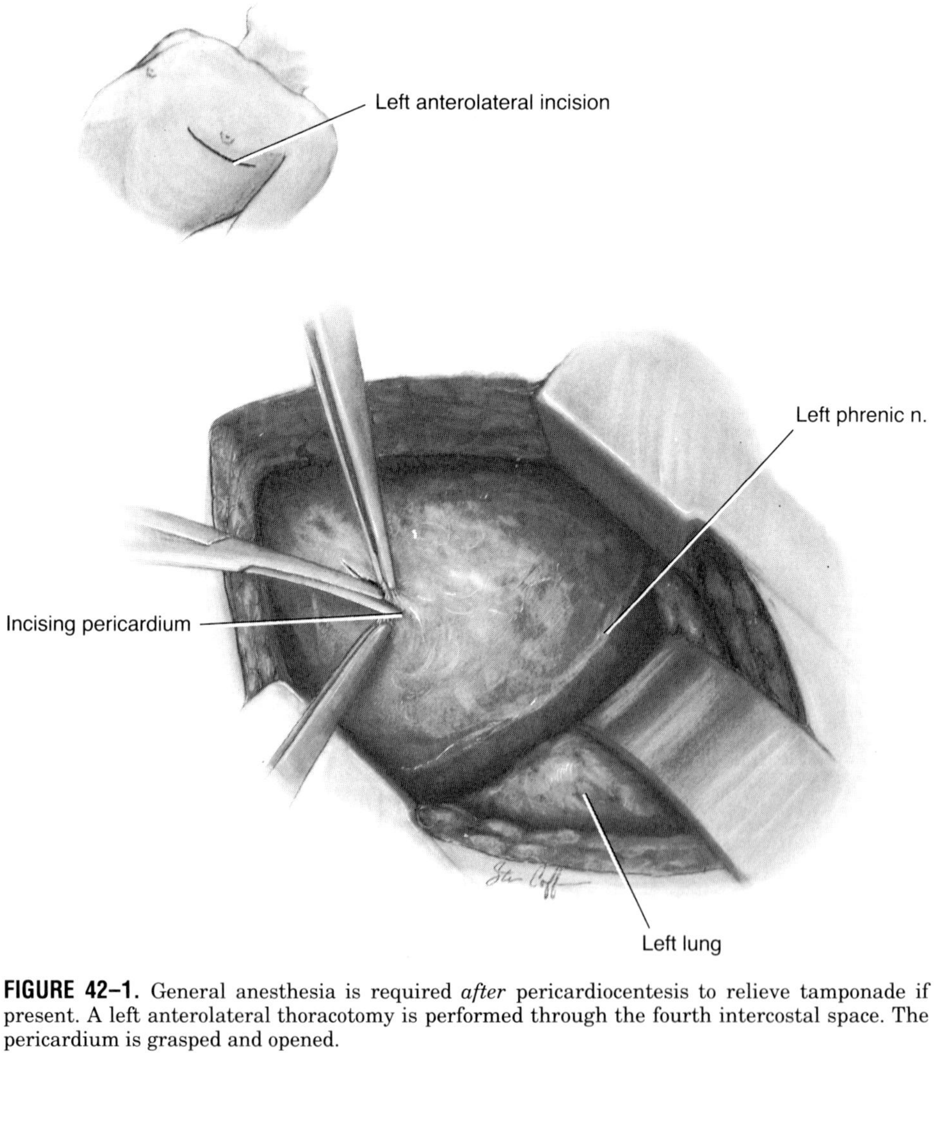

FIGURE 42–1. General anesthesia is required *after* pericardiocentesis to relieve tamponade if present. A left anterolateral thoracotomy is performed through the fourth intercostal space. The pericardium is grasped and opened.

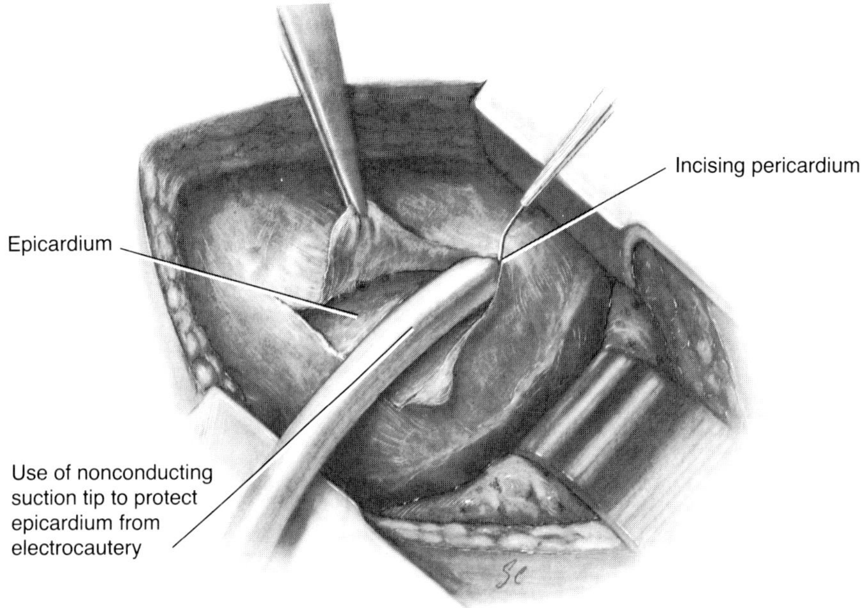

FIGURE 42–2. The pericardium is excised from 1 cm anterior to the phrenic nerve to the substernal area anteriorly and as far superiorly and inferiorly as can be safely done.

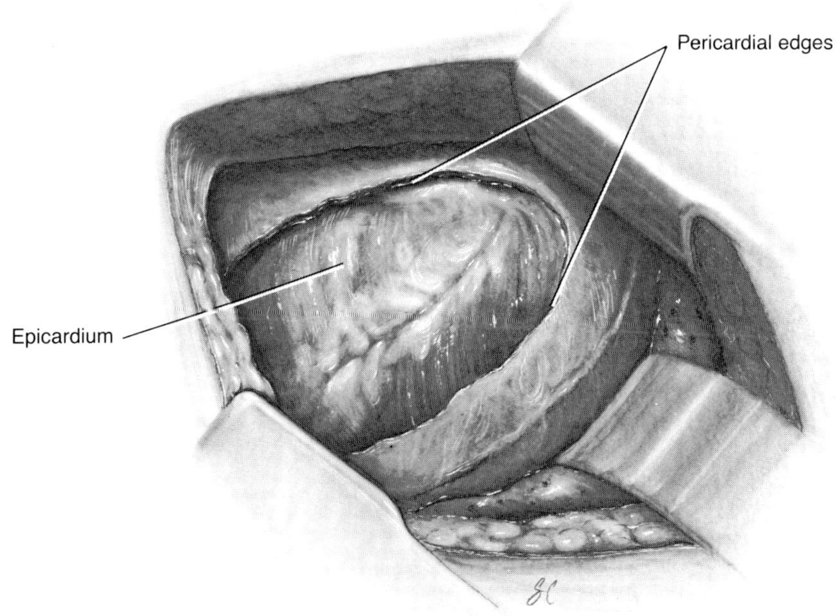

FIGURE 42–3. The pericardial defect should measure at least 4 × 4 cm to minimize the recurrence of pericardial effusion. The chest wall is closed in the standard manner, leaving a single 32Fr chest tube in the pleural space.

DONALD D. GLOWER, JR., M.D.

43

Pericardiectomy for Chronic Constrictive Pericarditis

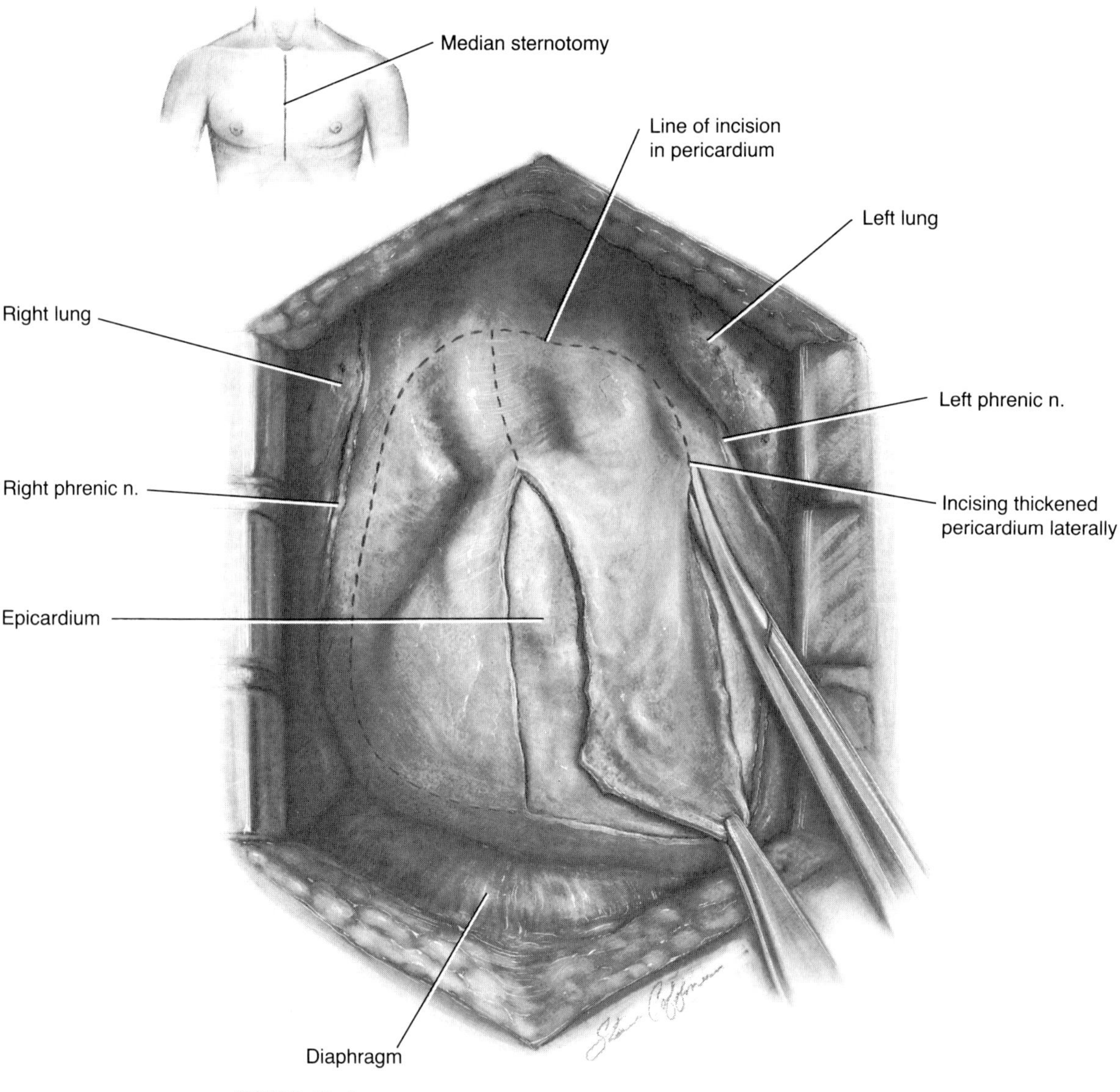

FIGURE 43–1. A median sternotomy is performed, and the pleural space is opened bilaterally to allow identification of the phrenic nerves. The entire anterior pericardium is sharply excised to 1 cm from the phrenic nerves laterally, to the diaphragm inferiorly, and to the great vessels superiorly. If significant constriction of the atria is present, a portion of pericardium posterior to each phrenic nerve may be excised.

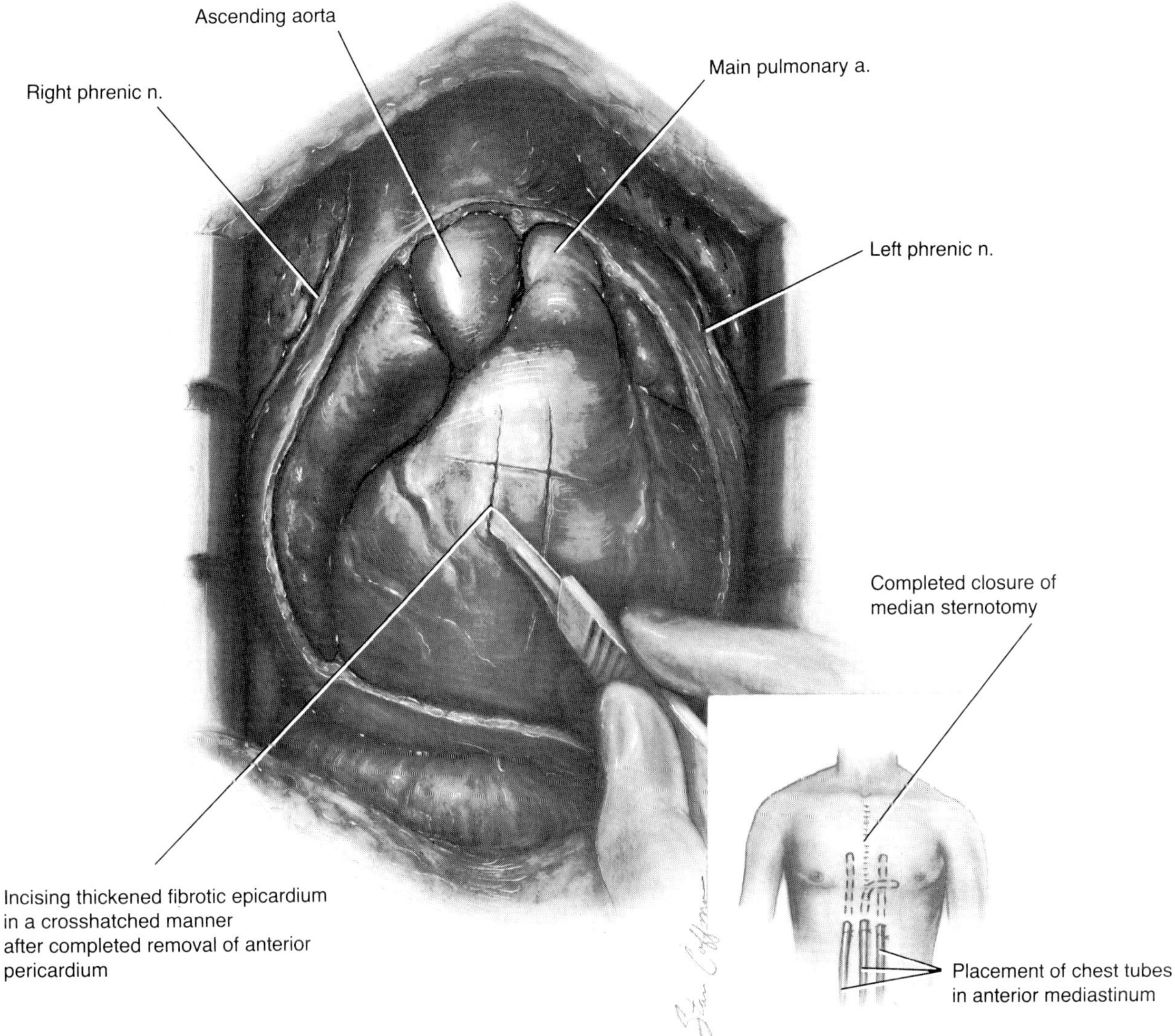

FIGURE 43–2. On rare occasions when a thick, fibrotic epicarditis remains, the epicardium may be incised in a crosshatched pattern, with care taken to avoid injury to epicardial vessels or the atrium.

Inset, Two 32Fr chest tubes are left in the anterior mediastinum, and an angled tube is left on the diaphragmatic surface of the pericardium. The median sternotomy is closed in the standard manner.

SECTION XI

Neoplasms of the Chest Wall

JAMES E. LOWE, M.D.

44

Resection of a Posterior Chest Wall Tumor

Tumors of the chest wall are relatively uncommon but, whether benign or malignant, require excision. The goal of the operation is to excise all tumor-bearing tissue with generous surgical margins. Whether or not to use a prosthetic patch to fill the defect created by resection depends on the size and site of the resection. The following approach is used to resect a posterior malignant chest wall tumor originating from a rib beneath the left scapula.

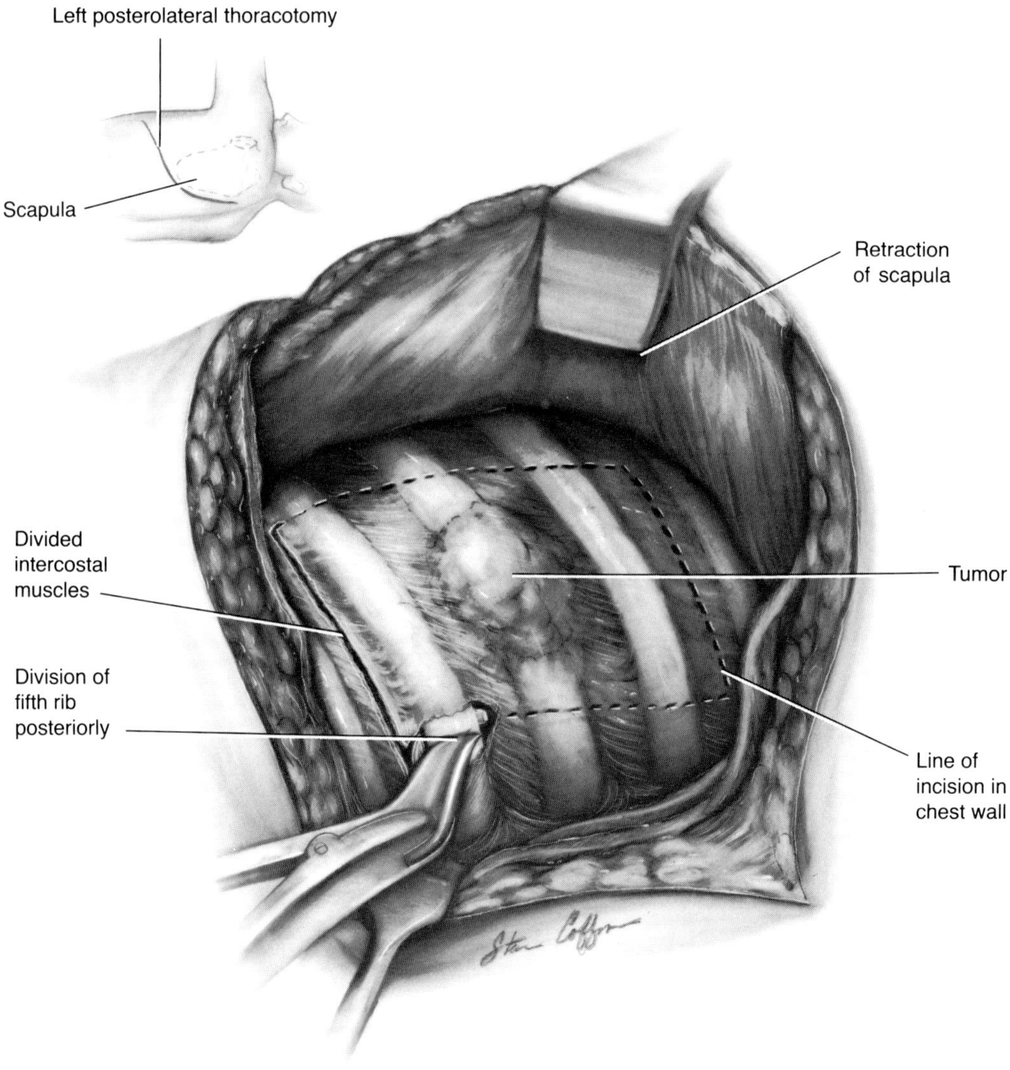

FIGURE 44–1. A standard posterolateral thoracotomy incision is performed. The posterior chest wall muscles and scapula are retracted superiorly. The area of planned resection includes a normal rib above and below the tumor and a minimum of 3-cm margins medially and laterally from the tumor. A rib divider is used to resect three ribs, and electrocautery is used to complete the dissection involving the associated intercostal muscles surrounding the tumor.

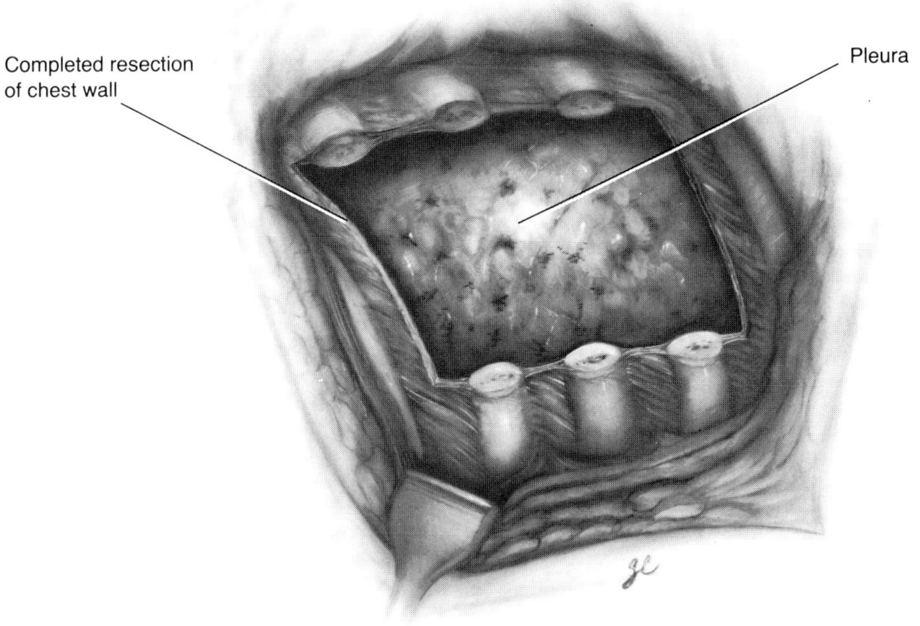

FIGURE 44–2. The typical large chest wall defect is created by adequate tumor resection. In this setting, a prosthetic patch was not required to cover the defect.

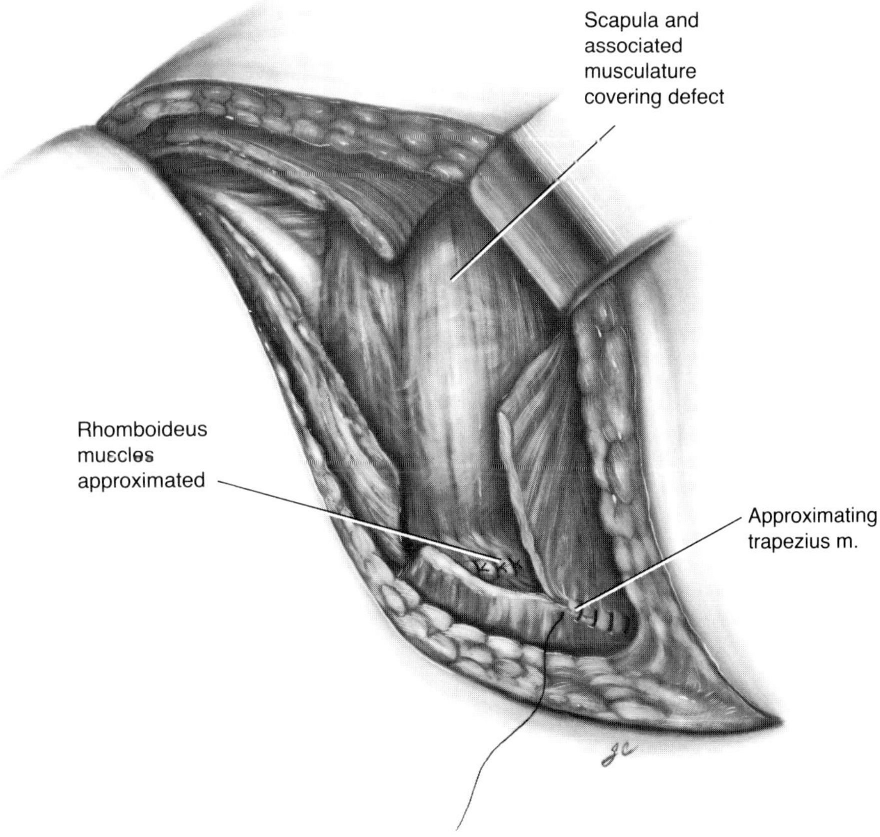

FIGURE 44–3. The scapula covers the posterior chest wall defect.

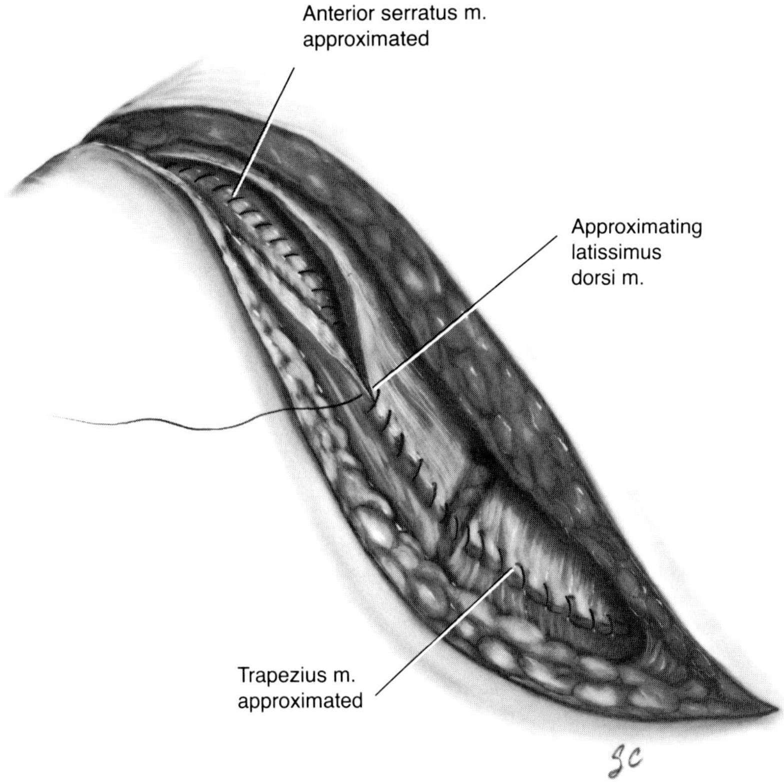

FIGURE 44–4. A single pleural drainage tube is placed, and the chest wall muscles are closed in layers.

JAMES E. LOWE, M.D.

45

Resection and Reconstruction for a Large Anterior Chest Wall Tumor

Adequate resection of a tumor of the anterior chest wall typically creates a large defect requiring a prosthetic patch for an optimal functional outcome and cosmetic appearance.

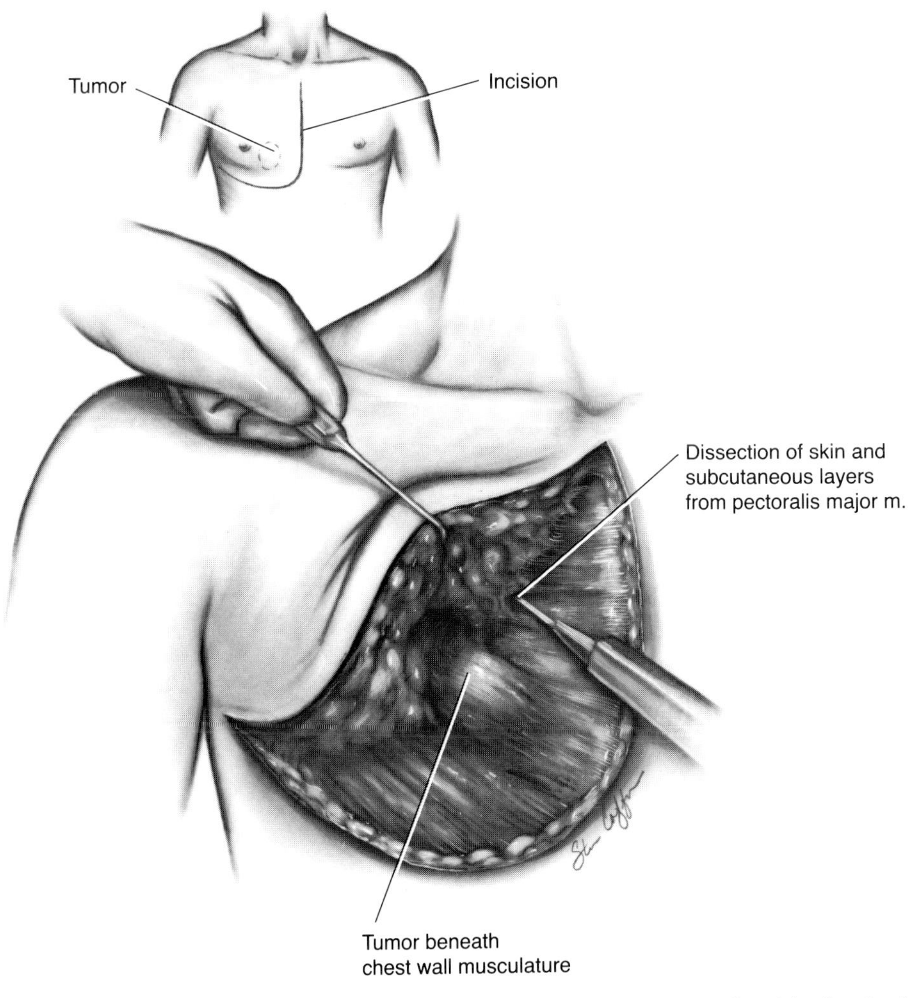

FIGURE 45–1. A malignant chest wall tumor is shown originating from the right fourth rib anteriorly adjacent to the sternum (*inset*). A skin incision is made vertically over the midportion of the sternum and extended inferiorly beneath the right breast. A flap of skin and uninvolved subcutaneous tissue is elevated over the anterior chest wall. The tumor mass is apparent beneath the pectoralis major muscle.

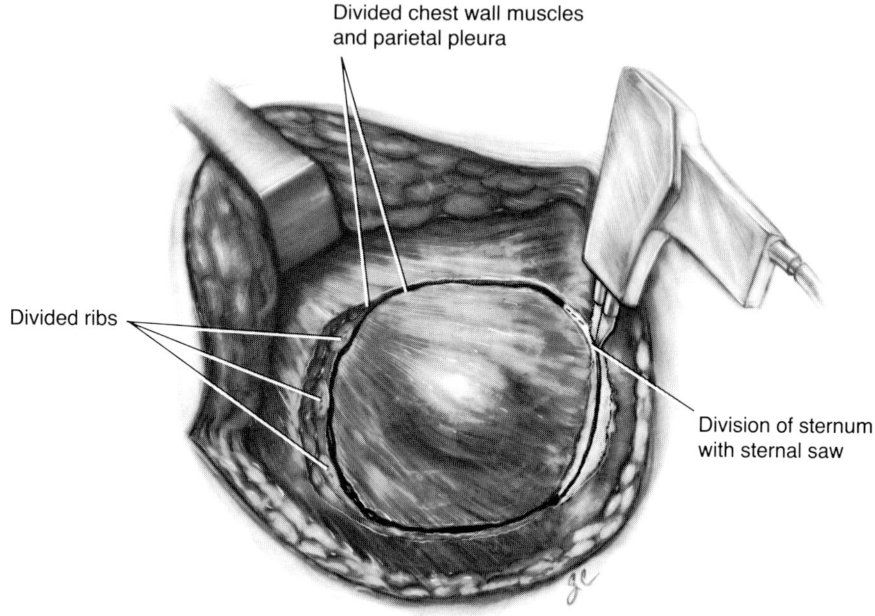

FIGURE 45–2. The involved rib is divided 3 cm lateral to the tumor, as are uninvolved ribs above and below the tumor. Medially, to ensure an adequate surgical margin, a portion of sternum is removed and the right internal mammary artery is ligated at the superior and inferior portions of the sternal resection. The chest wall containing the tumor and overlying pectoralis muscles is then removed *en bloc*.

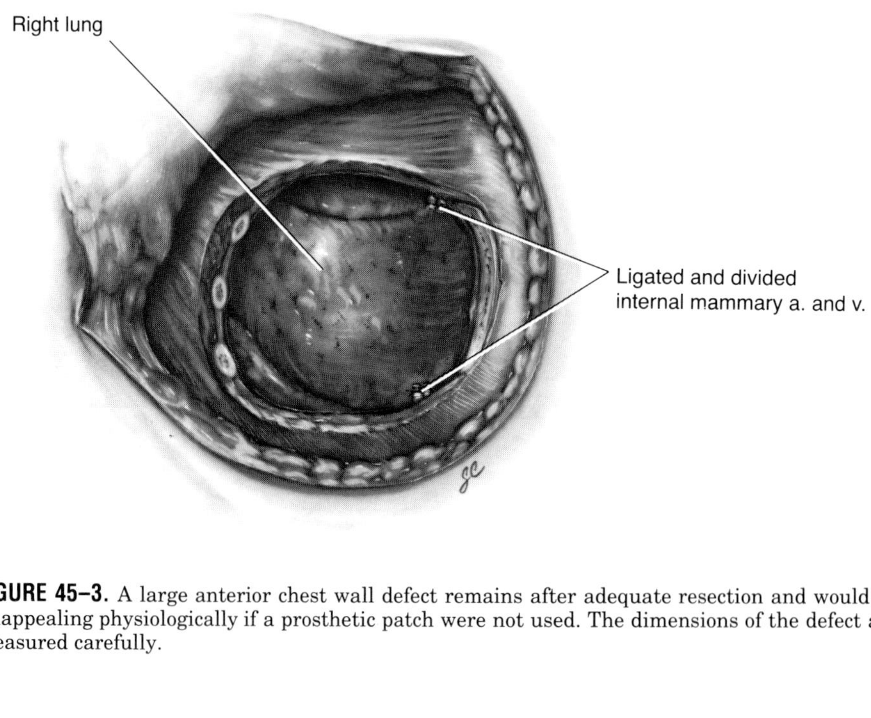

FIGURE 45–3. A large anterior chest wall defect remains after adequate resection and would be unappealing physiologically if a prosthetic patch were not used. The dimensions of the defect are measured carefully.

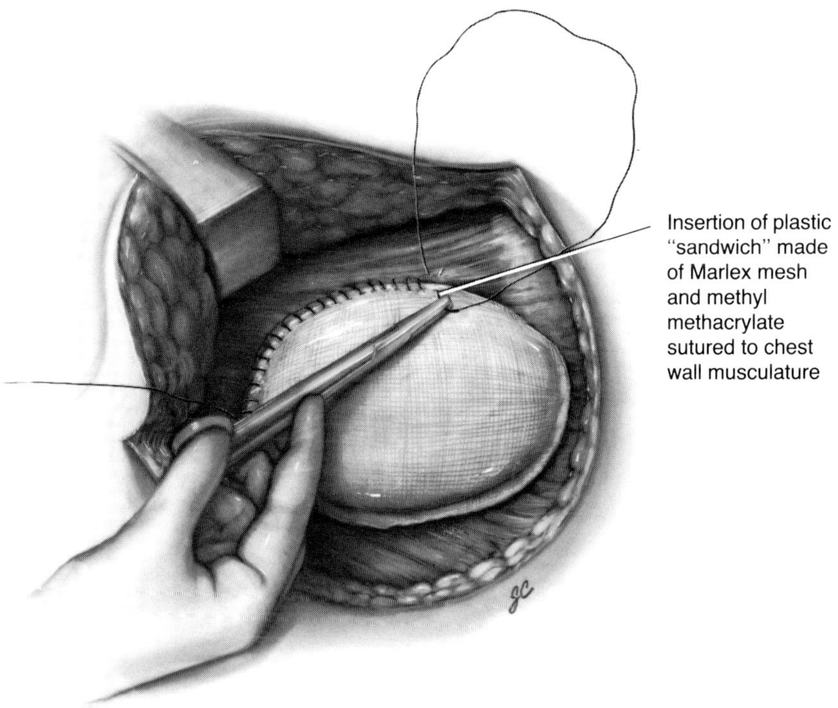

FIGURE 45–4. An appropriate-size prosthetic patch is created using two layers of Marlex mesh sandwiching methyl methacrylate. The prosthesis is allowed to harden after being formed to appropriately fill the anterior chest wall defect. The sandwich of Marlex mesh and methyl methacrylate is then sutured to the pectoralis muscles using a continuous suture of 3–0 Prolene.

SECTION XII

Congenital Heart Disease

ROSS M. UNGERLEIDER, M.D.

46

Patent Ductus Arteriosus

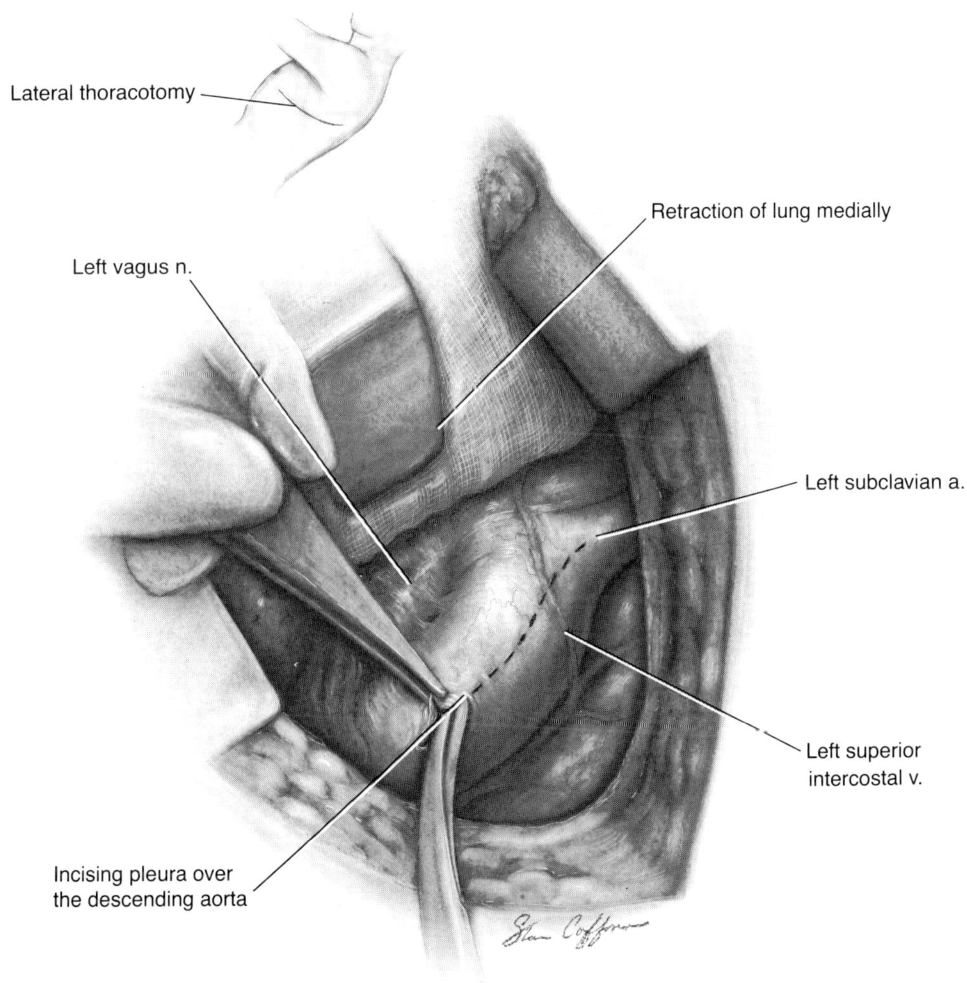

FIGURE 46–1. The ductus arteriosus is exposed through a lateral thoracotomy with the posterior mediastinal pleura being divided and the lung being gently retracted anteriorly. The ductus arteriosus usually underlies the left superior intercostal vein, which in larger patients may need to be divided between ligatures during incision of the mediastinal pleura overlying the aorta.

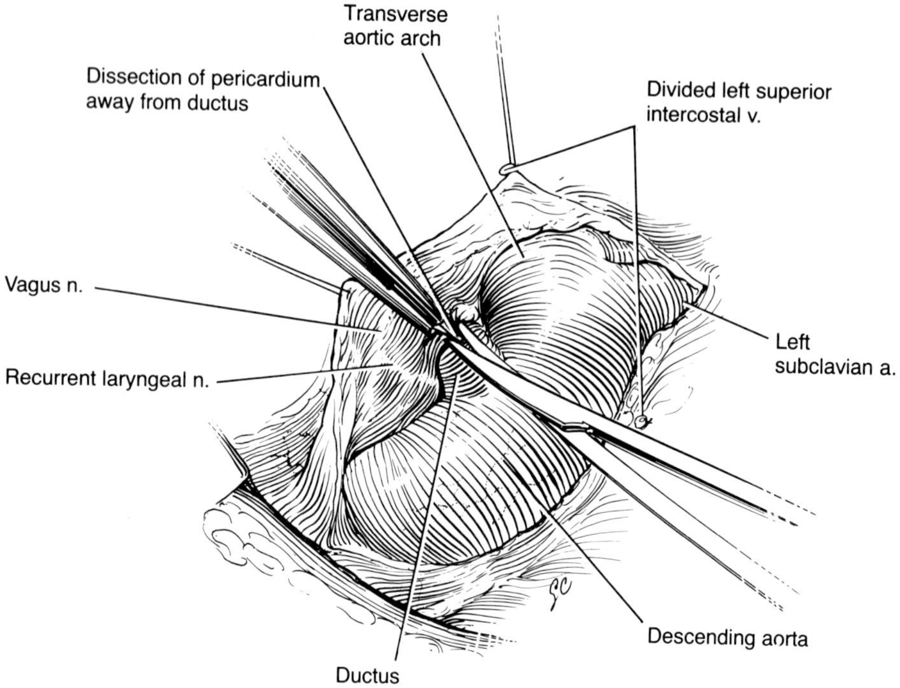

FIGURE 46–2. The adventitia overlying the ductus arteriosus is carefully dissected, and the ductus is positively identified by recognition of the recurrent laryngeal nerve as it passes below the ductus arteriosus in the retracted mediastinal pleura. It is also important to identify the left subclavian artery as well as the transverse aortic arch.

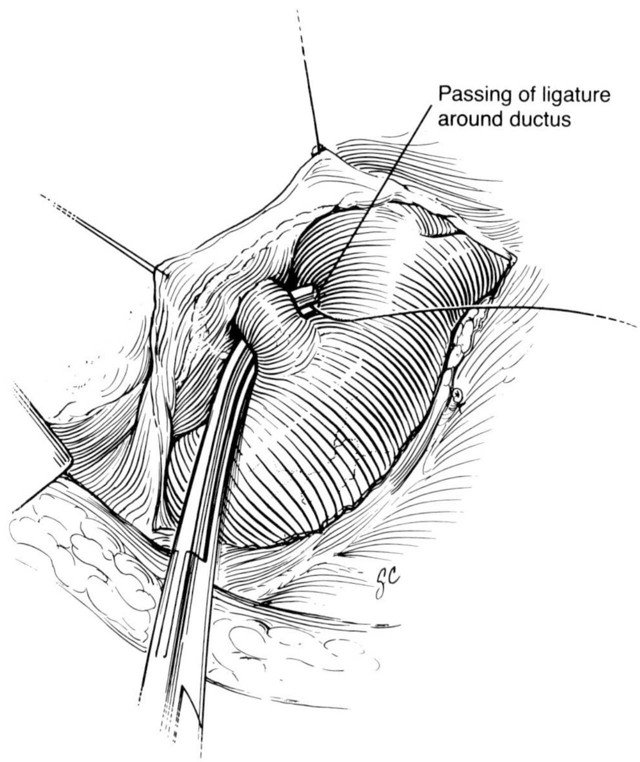

FIGURE 46–3. After the ductus has been freed from adventitial connections with both sharp and blunt dissection, a right-angle clamp is passed below the ductus (usually from inferior to superior) so that the ductus can be encircled with a ligature.

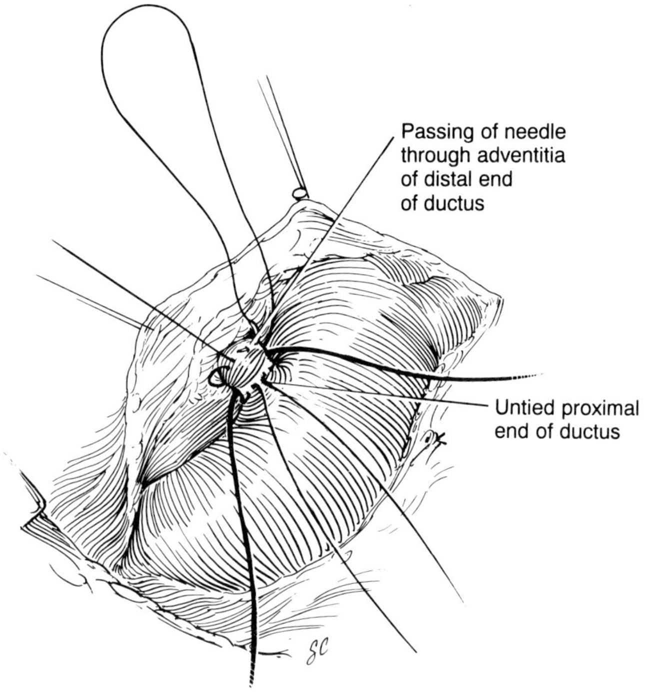

FIGURE 46–4. The right-angle clamp is used to pull an additional suture around the ductus arteriosus at its proximal and distal portion in relation to the aorta. These sutures are attached to a fine needle that is passed through the adventitia (using extremely superficial bites) at the aortic and pulmonary artery ends of the ductus, ensuring that these ligatures remain positioned at either end of the ductus arteriosus.

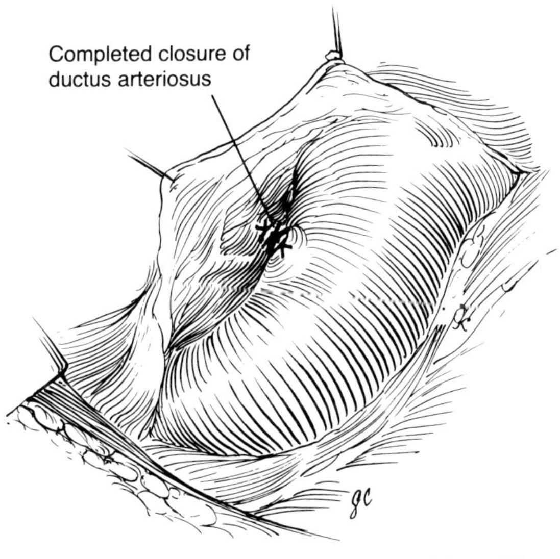

FIGURE 46–5. All three ligatures are tied by tying the aortic end first, followed by the pulmonary end, and finally by tying the central ligature in a manner that occludes the middle of the ductus between the two suture ligatures at either end. This procedure provides complete suture obliteration of the ductus arteriosus, and any previously felt thrill should be obliterated. Diastolic blood pressure should increase noticeably in patients who are being monitored with an arterial line and who have a physiologically significant ductus arteriosus.

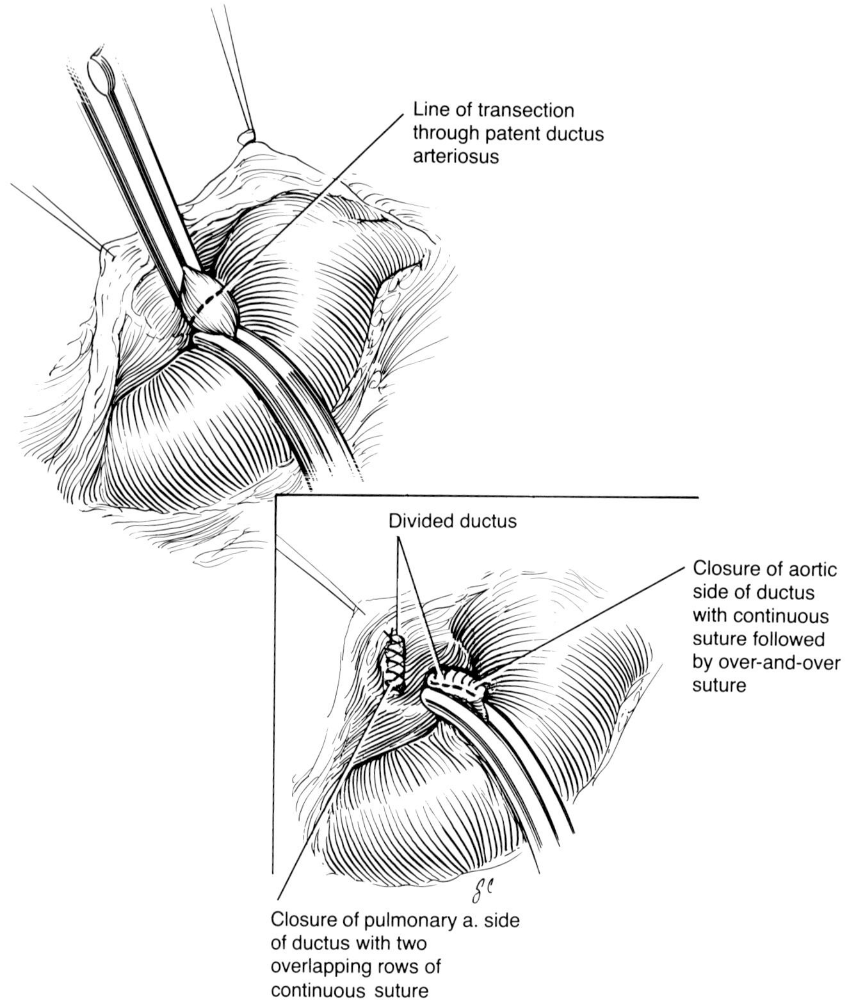

FIGURE 46–6. Rarely, it may be desirable to divide a ductus arteriosus through a lateral thoracotomy. This procedure is more dangerous than ductal ligation and is rarely performed. Performance requires occlusion of both ends of the ductus with a vascular clamp, division of the ductus, and then careful oversewing of each divided end with fine suture material before clamps are removed.

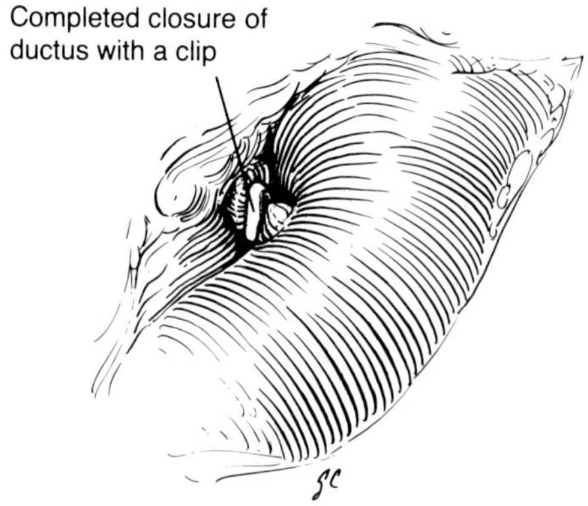

FIGURE 46–7. In premature infants (usually those who weigh less than 1 kg), the ductus arteriosus can be obliterated in the intensive care nursery by a medium-sized hemoclip. This procedure is best performed by dissection of the adventitial tissue on either side of the ductus arteriosus. By carefully retracting the aorta posteriorly, the ductus is easily stretched so that it can be obliterated with a single hemoclip. This procedure is safe, quick, and simple to perform and is recommended for premature infants whose lung disease necessitates an efficient operation.

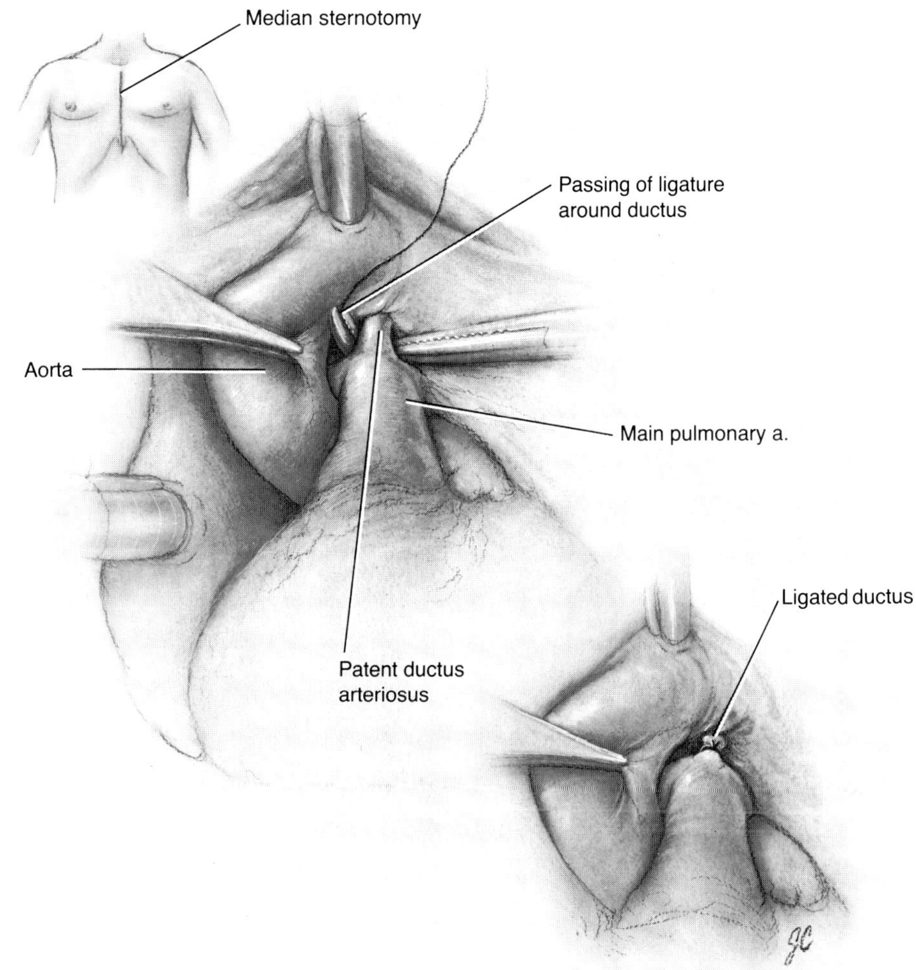

FIGURE 46–8. In some patients with significant intracardiac defects, a ductus arteriosus must be ligated during intracardiac repair. This procedure is easily performed either immediately before or immediately after initiating cardiopulmonary bypass. The main pulmonary artery is dissected distally to expose both the right and left pulmonary arteries as well as the ductus arteriosus, which is usually easily identified, as it appears to be an extension of the main pulmonary artery toward the aorta. By retracting the main pulmonary artery caudad, the ductus arteriosus is easily exposed such that a ligature can be passed around it using a right-angle clamp. This ligature is then securely tied. It is usually unnecessary to divide the ductus in these patients unless subsequent operation requires mobilization of the pulmonary artery from the aorta (such as for a Lecompte maneuver or for mobilization of the pulmonary artery to optimize performance of a conduit or an atriopulmonary connection).

ROSS M. UNGERLEIDER, M.D.

47
Aortopulmonary Window

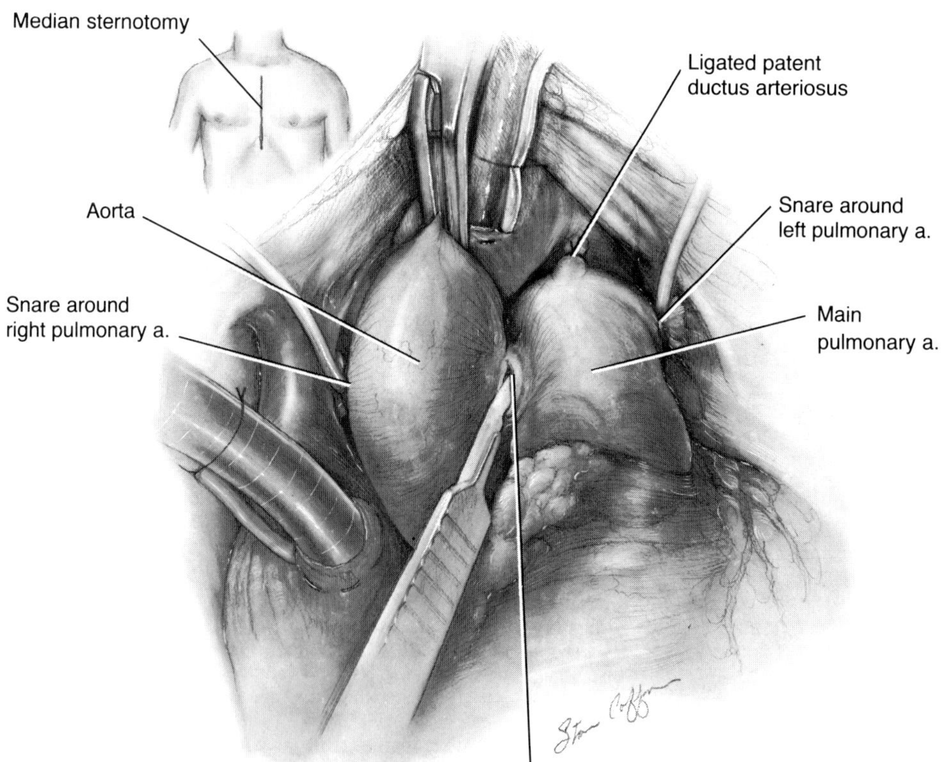

FIGURE 47–1. The aortopulmonary window is exposed through a median sternotomy. After the anatomy is confirmed, the patient is cannulated for cardiopulmonary bypass using a single venous cannula. Control of the right and left pulmonary arteries is achieved, and the ductus arteriosus, when present, is ligated. The patient is then placed on cardiopulmonary bypass, and snares on the right and left pulmonary arteries are tightened. This prevents perfusion of the pulmonary vasculature through the aortopulmonary window. An aortic crossclamp is then applied, and the heart is arrested with cold cardioplegic solution. An incision is made in the aortopulmonary window to separate the aorta from the pulmonary artery. In some patients, the aortopulmonary window is large and involves the right pulmonary artery as well as the main pulmonary artery. The defect produced in the pulmonary artery once the aortopulmonary window is incised can be quite impressive.

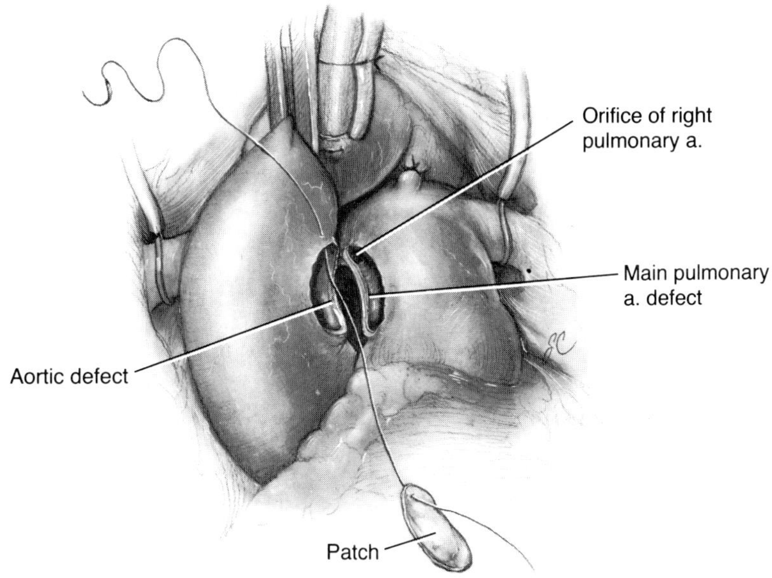

FIGURE 47–2. With the crossclamp still in place, the defect in the aorta is repaired with a patch. This patch can be a homograft or Gore-Tex. Occasionally pericardium is used.

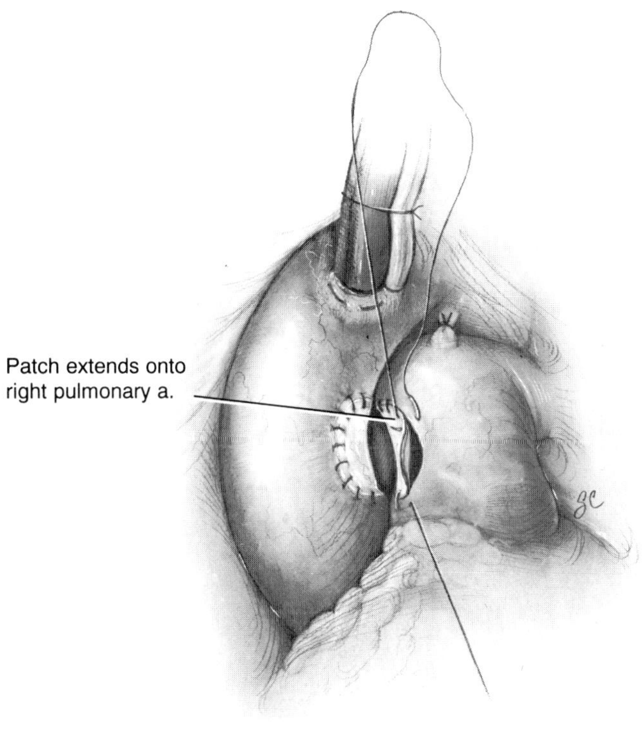

FIGURE 47–3. After the defect in the aorta has been repaired, the aorta is "de-aired" and the crossclamp is removed. The defect in the pulmonary artery is then repaired with a patch during rewarming. In patients with particularly large defects in the pulmonary artery, it may be easier to repair the pulmonary artery with the aortic crossclamp still in place.

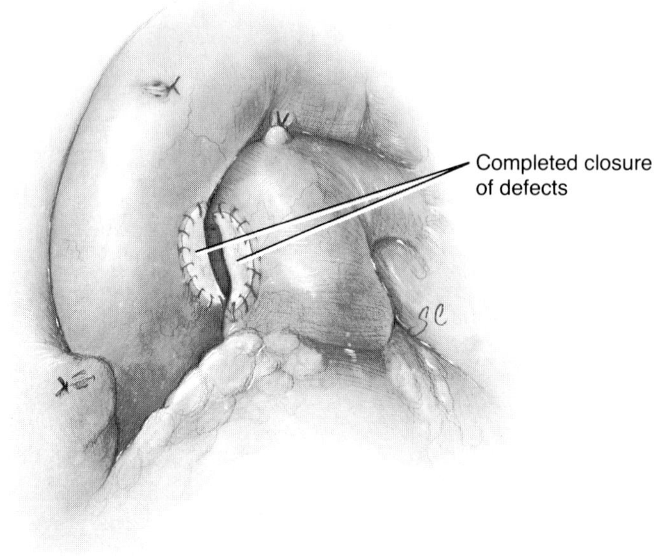

FIGURE 47–4. The completed two-patch repair separates the aorta from the pulmonary artery and limits the potential for the late occurrence of aortopulmonary fistula.

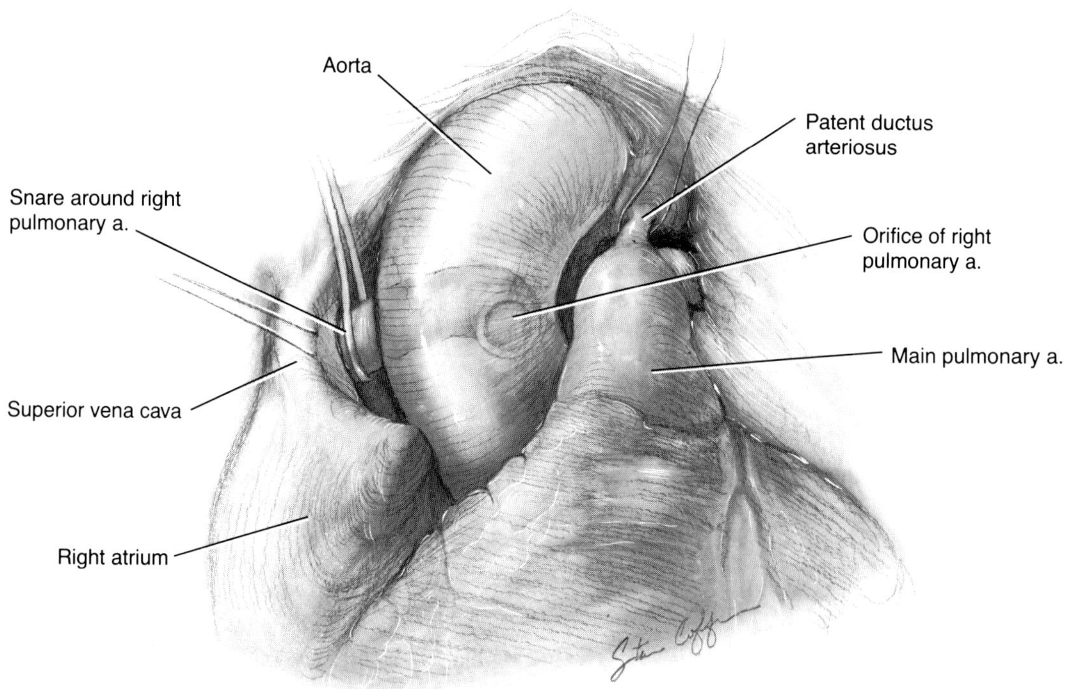

FIGURE 47–5. An unusual form of aortopulmonary window occurs when the right pulmonary artery arises from the posterior wall of the aorta. Although this defect has been referred to as "hemi-truncus," the anatomy and physiology are similar to aortopulmonary window. Preparation for repair is also similar to that for aortopulmonary window. Before initiation of cardiopulmonary bypass, control of the right pulmonary artery is established.

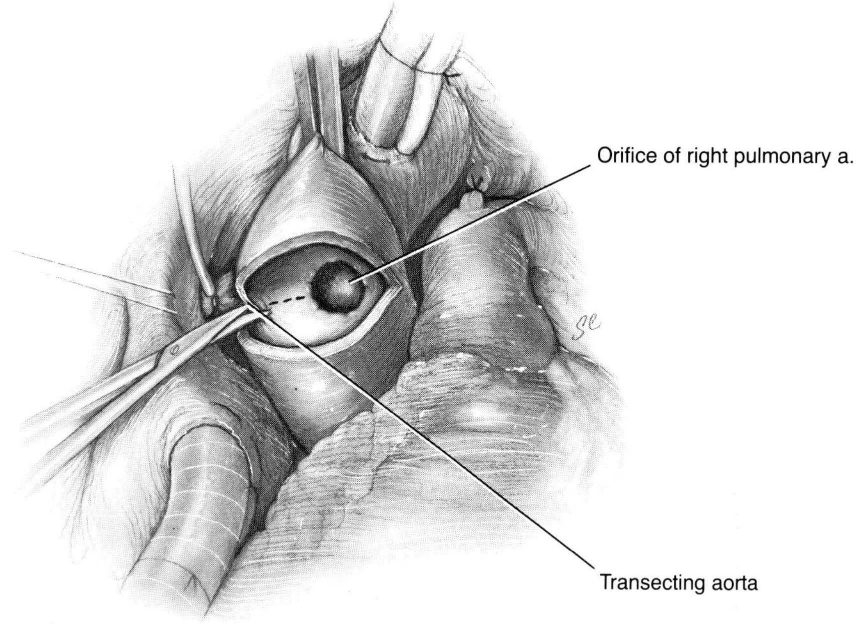

FIGURE 47–6. The patient is placed on bypass using a single venous cannula, and the right pulmonary artery is occluded. When present, a ductus arteriosus is also ligated. The heart is then arrested with cold cardioplegic solution, and an incision is made in the aorta.

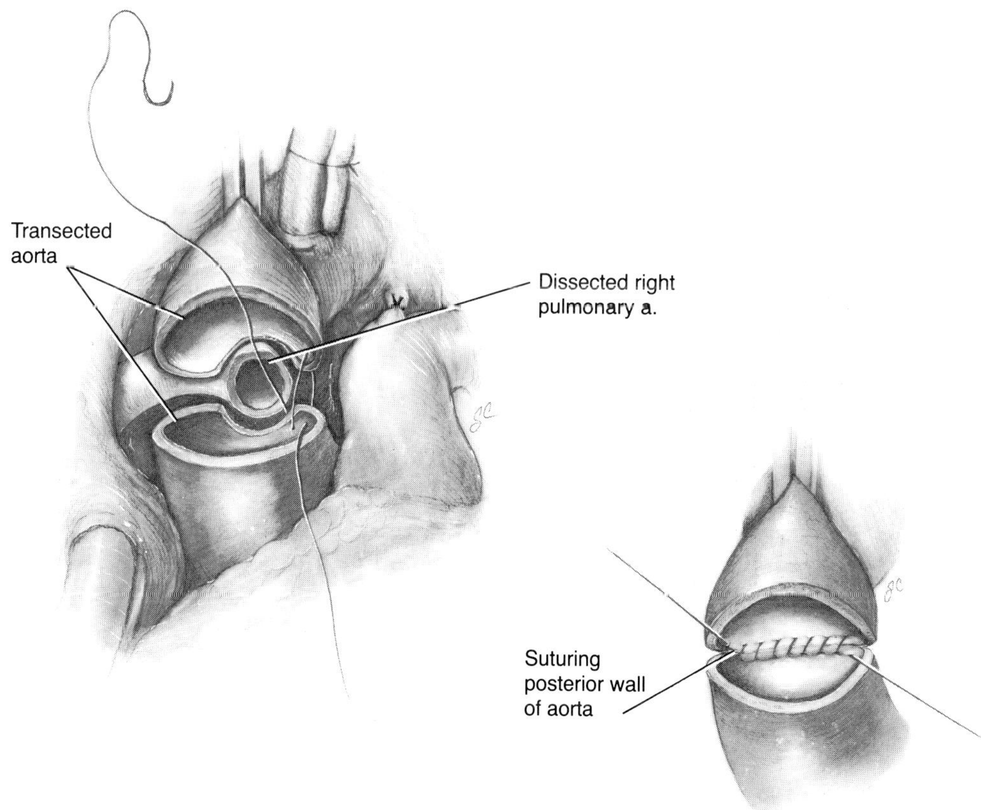

FIGURE 47–7. When the right pulmonary artery arises from the posterior portion of the aorta (as shown), it is usually easiest to remove it by completing the incision posteriorly through the aorta, so that the aorta is transected in a manner that separates the right pulmonary artery from the remainder of the aorta. The aorta is then repaired using a continuous suture technique. When the right pulmonary artery arises from the high, lateral aspect of the aorta (not shown), it is more easily removed by simple excision. The resulting defect in the aorta is then repaired primarily or with a patch.

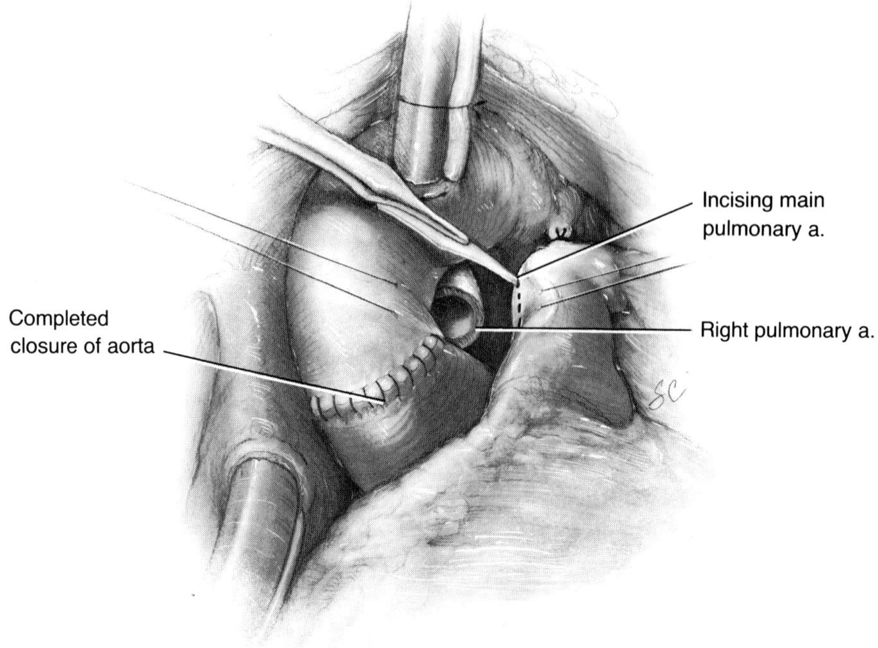

FIGURE 47–8. The right pulmonary artery is brought under the aorta. At this time, the aortic crossclamp can be released, or it can be left in place while the pulmonary artery reconstruction is performed. An incision is made in the main pulmonary artery in a location that appears appropriate for anastomosis of the right pulmonary artery.

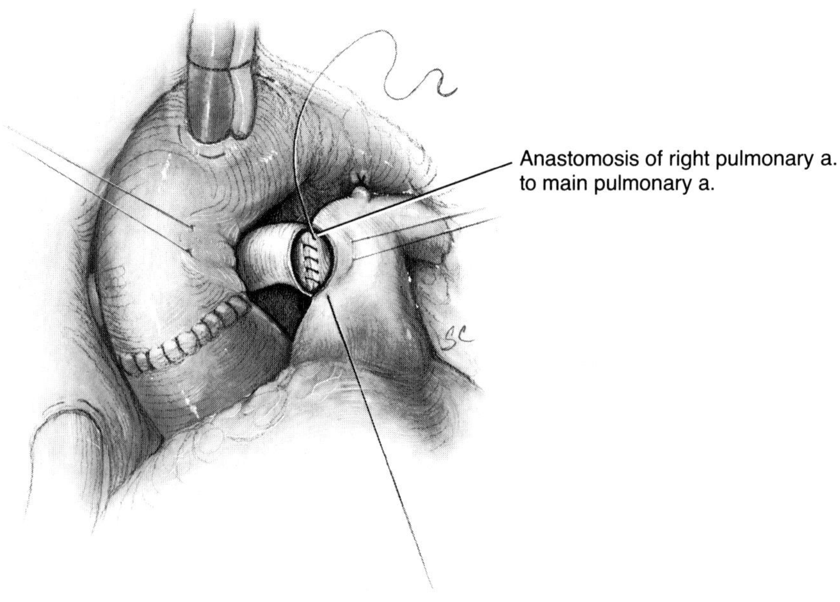

FIGURE 47–9. The right pulmonary artery is connected to the main pulmonary artery using a continuous suture. It is important to perform this anastomosis in a region as close as possible to the usual anatomic location of the right pulmonary artery. In particular, this anastomosis should be on a posterior and lateral portion of the main pulmonary artery.

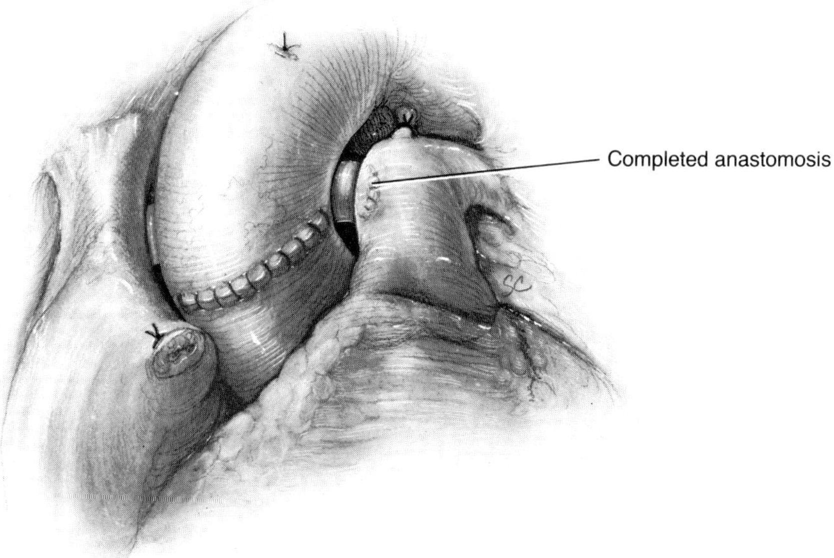

FIGURE 47–10. After completion of this reconstruction, relatively normal anatomy is reestablished.

ROSS M. UNGERLEIDER, M.D.

48

Coarctation of the Aorta

PATCH AORTOPLASTY

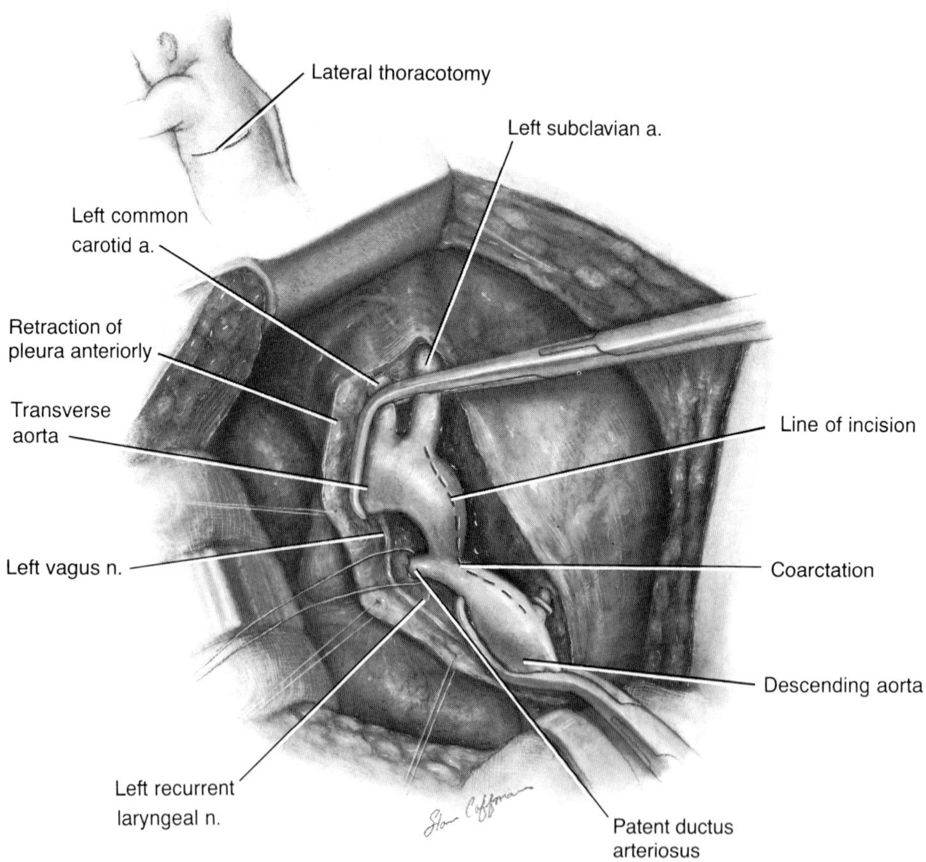

FIGURE 48–1. The aorta is exposed through a lateral thoracotomy. The posterior mediastinal pleura is incised, and the anatomy is inspected carefully so that the transverse aorta, the left common carotid, and left subclavian arteries are identified, enabling clear identification of the descending aorta as well as the ductus arteriosus. The area of coarctation is usually opposite the ductus arteriosus. Vascular clamps are used to control the aorta. Hemoclips can be used to occlude collateral vessels and can be easily removed at the end of the operation.

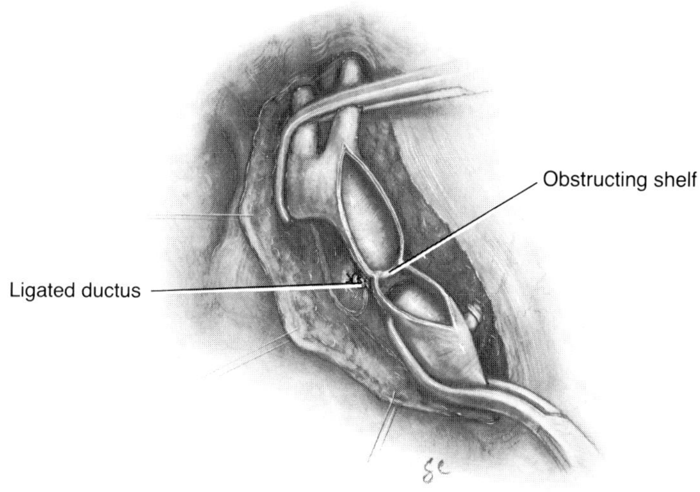

FIGURE 48–2. After the aorta has been controlled with clamps, the ductus arteriosus is ligated, and an incision is made across the area of the coarctation extending well above and below the obstructing ridge of coarctation tissue. Proximal extension of this incision should be onto the subclavian artery. The obstructing shelf should *not* be removed. It is helpful to occlude the descending aorta with a curved clamp, as shown, to control posterior collateral vessels.

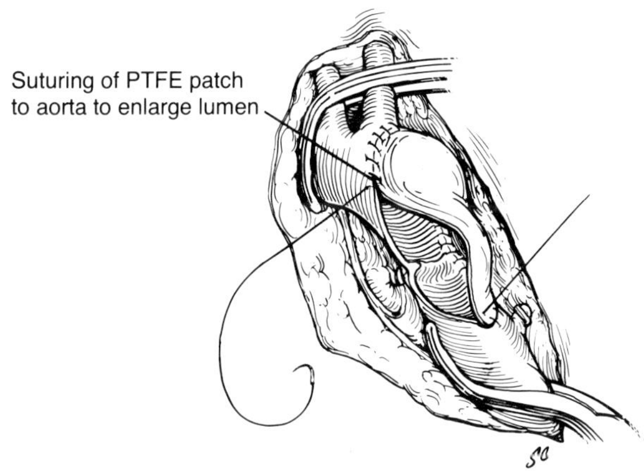

FIGURE 48–3. A *large* patch of PTFE (polytetrafluoroethylene) is used to repair the aortotomy. The patch should be at least one and a half times, and as much as two times, the diameter of the aorta and is sewn into place with continuous nonabsorbable sutures.

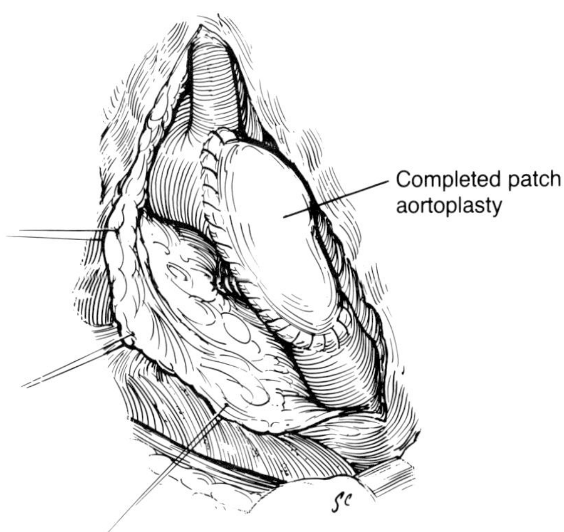

FIGURE 48–4. After completion of the aortoplasty, the clamps are removed. Bleeding should be easily controlled with the use of topical thrombostatic agents and a short period of manual packing. Persistent bleeding should be carefully controlled with interrupted sutures. At the completion of the procedure, there should be a strong pulse below the aortoplasty. The hemoclips on the collateral vessels are removed, and the chest is closed. The posterior mediastinal pleura should *not* be closed over the repair.

SUBCLAVIAN FLAP AORTOPLASTY

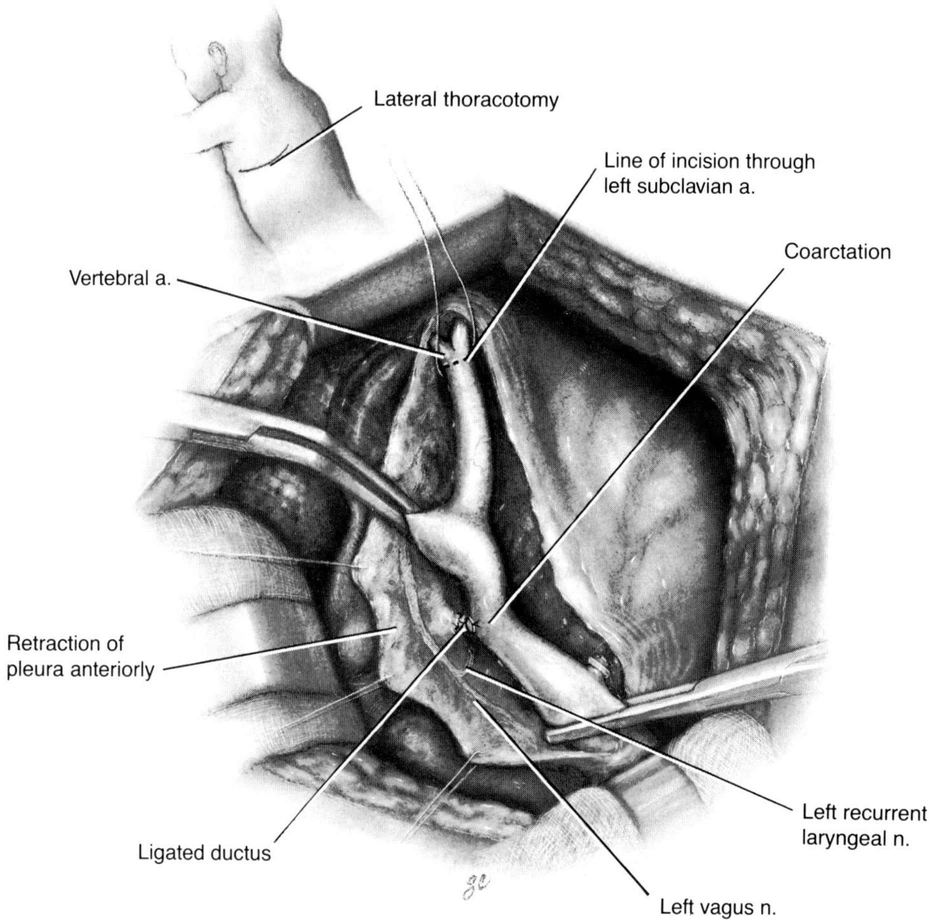

FIGURE 48–5. The aorta is exposed through a lateral thoracotomy, and dissection of the posterior mediastinal pleura is performed so that the left subclavian artery is exposed as far distal as the first branches, which usually includes the vertebral artery. The ductus arteriosus is ligated, and control of the ascending and descending aorta is obtained with clamping. Collateral vessels can be controlled with small hemoclips.

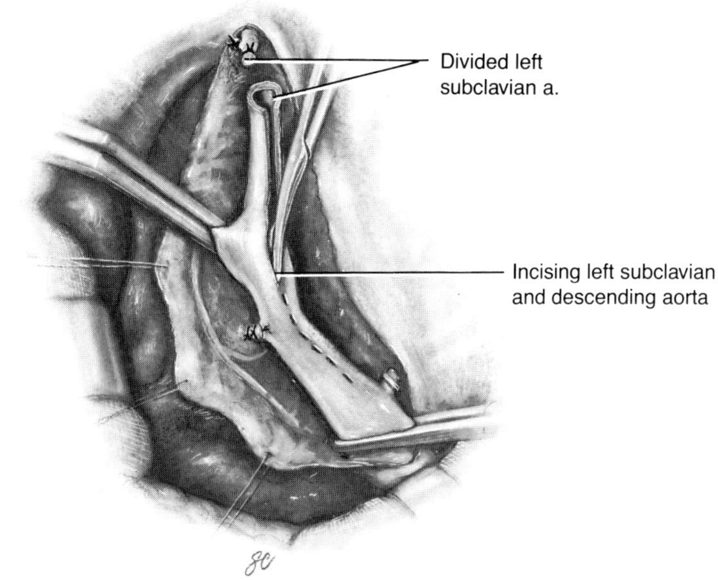

FIGURE 48–6. The subclavian artery is divided proximal to its first branches, with the distal stump being securely tied. A suture ligature placed in the distal subclavian artery is beneficial. The vertebral artery should be ligated to avoid subclavian steal syndrome. The proximal subclavian artery is then incised along its posterior and lateral surface, with the incision extended across the area of coarctation. It is important that the incision extend distally for at least 1 cm beyond the area of coarctation.

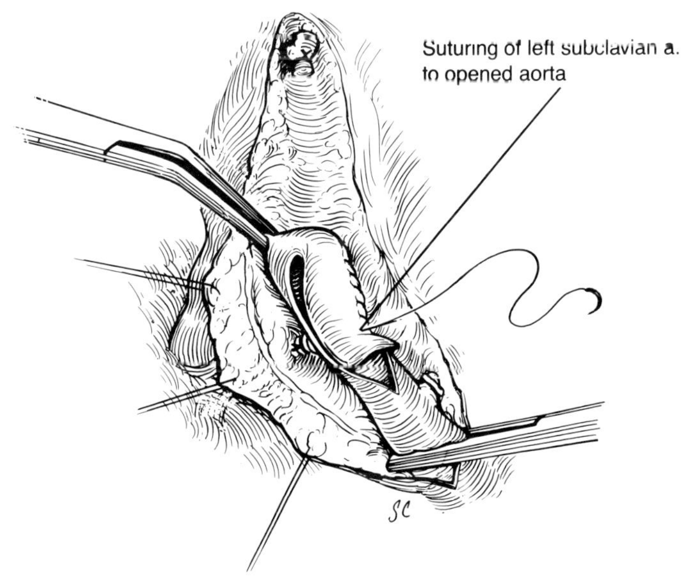

FIGURE 48–7. The flap of subclavian artery tissue that is created is sewn into place over the aortotomy so that the area of narrowing around the coarctation is enlarged. It is probably important not to resect the ridge of intimal tissue in the area of coarctation to limit the potential for aneurysm formation. If the ridge is prominent, it can be excised along with ductal tissue, and the posterior aorta reconnected before patching over the top. This flap aortoplasty is usually easily performed using a continuous suture, although in small infants, the use of occasional interrupted sutures is sometimes helpful to prevent distortion from pursestringing.

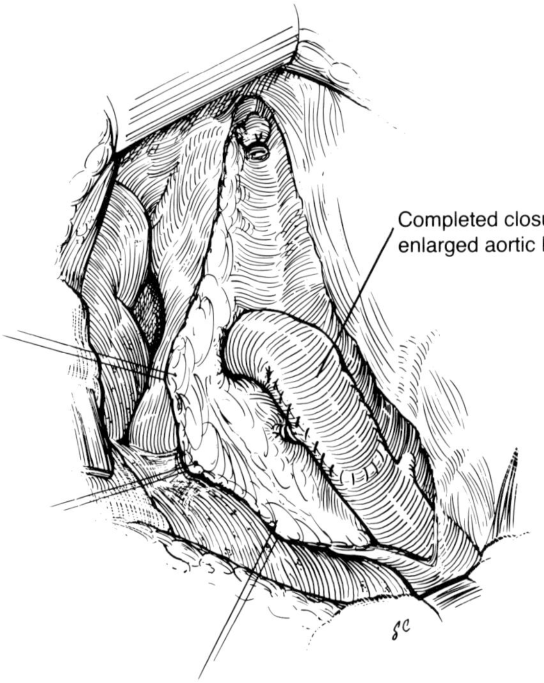

FIGURE 48–8. At the completion of the aortoplasty, the clamps are removed, and a strong pulse should be palpated in the descending aorta. Hemostasis should be achieved with additional sutures, and hemoclips should be removed from the collateral arteries.

END-TO-END ANASTOMOSIS

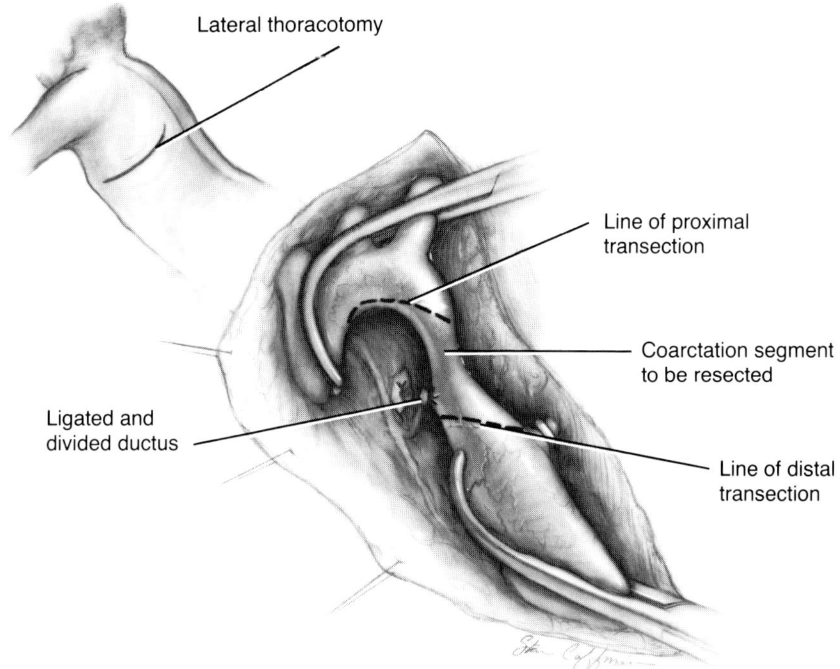

FIGURE 48–9. Patients with long areas of tubular hypoplasia (between the left subclavian artery and ductus arteriosus) or with hypoplasia of the transverse aortic arch may be best treated by extended end-to-end anastomosis. This anastomosis can be accomplished by placement of vascular clamps across the ascending aorta in a manner that occludes the left subclavian and left common artery and that partially occludes the orifice of the innominate artery, thus enabling surgical access to the entire underside of the transverse aorta. It is important to free the descending aorta from adventitial connections as far distally as the diaphragm, and collateral vessels should be controlled with the use of hemoclips. After placement of clamps, the ductus arteriosus is ligated and divided, and the area of coarctation tissue is resected and removed. Alternatively, the ductus arteriosus can be ligated but left in place with the transected segment of coarctation. The procedure then entails reanastomosis of the proximal and distal ends of normal aorta, as shown in Figures 48–10, 48–11, and 48–12.

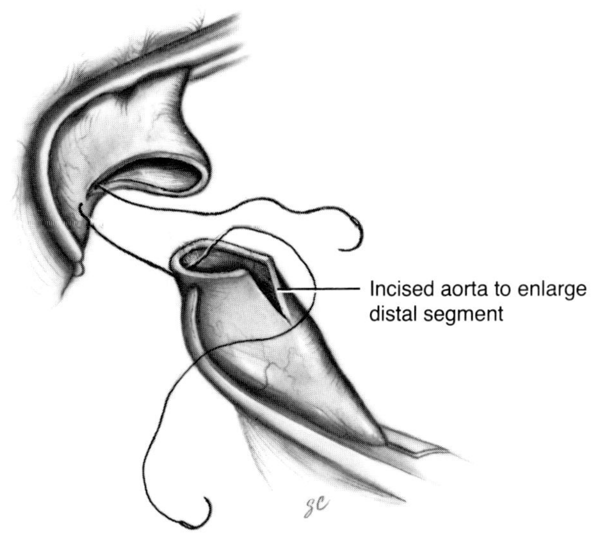

FIGURE 48–10. The anastomosis is begun with a continuous suture at the most proximal point. The distal aorta should easily stretch to cover the "gap" left by removal of ductal and coarctation tissue.

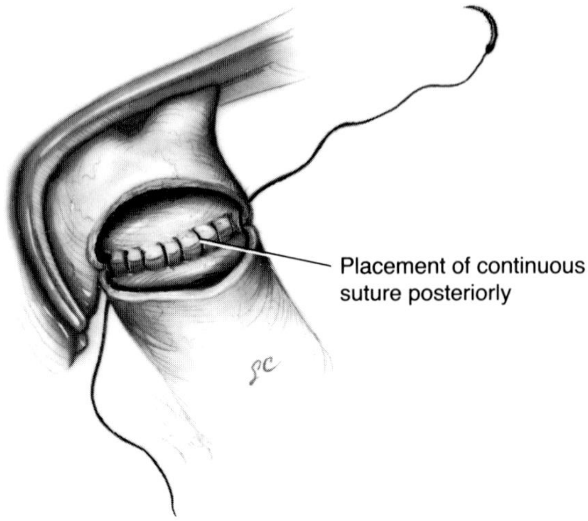

FIGURE 48–11. After the posterior anastomosis has been completed, the clamps are carefully moved toward each other and the suture line is tightened. The anterior anastomosis is then completed by continuing the suture line along the anterior aspect of the aorta.

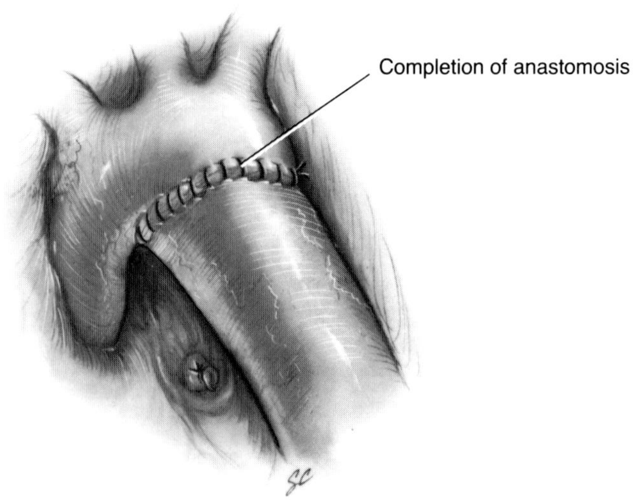

FIGURE 48–12. This anastomosis can be interrupted to prevent pursestringing and stricturing of the coarctation repair, or it can be performed by completion of the continuous suture line (preferred).

VIA STERNOTOMY WITH PATIENT ON CARDIOPULMONARY BYPASS

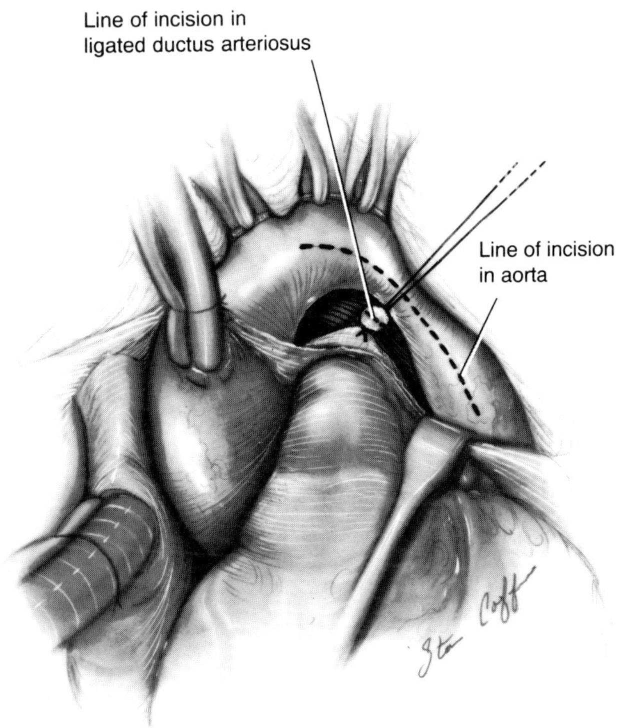

FIGURE 48–13. This procedure is indicated when it is necessary to repair other cardiac defects concomitant with coarctation repair. After sternotomy has been performed and the heart has been exposed by opening the pericardium, the patient is cannulated for cardiopulmonary bypass. Once the patient has been placed on bypass, cooling is begun toward profound hypothermia (18°C). The ductus arteriosus, if present, is ligated unless distal perfusion across the ductus is necessary (as in some cases of severe coarctation). If distal perfusion across the ductus is maintained (by cannulation of the main pulmonary artery with a second arterial inflow cannula), it is important to occlude the branch pulmonary arteries to prevent overcirculation to the lungs. During cooling, the entire aortic arch and head vessels are carefully dissected, and the descending aorta is freed as far as possible from its adventitial connections. After adequate cooling, cardiopulmonary bypass is ceased and the cannulae are removed. With the patient under total circulatory arrest and with the head vessels occluded, the ductus is divided between ligatures. The distal ligature can be used to pull the descending aorta into the surgical field. An incision is then made across the aortic arch and onto the descending aorta.

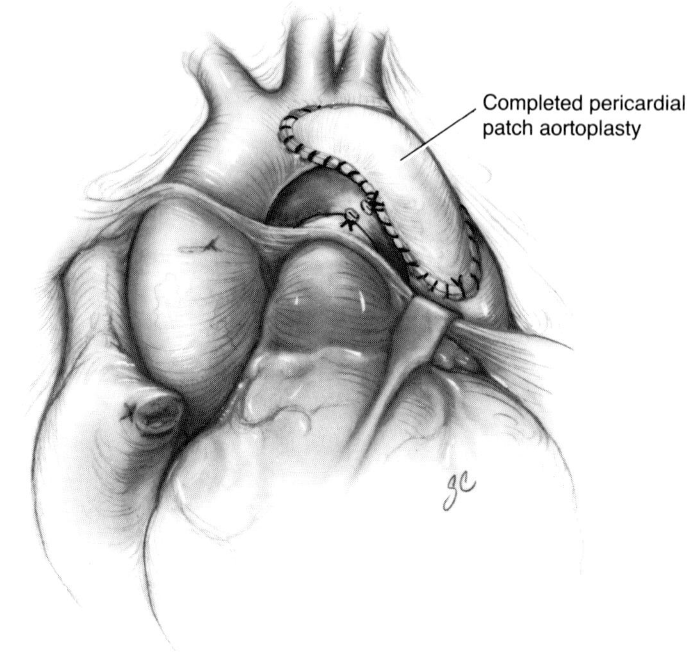

FIGURE 48–14. This incision should traverse the area of coarctation and extend onto the aortic arch as well as onto the distal aorta. This incision can then be patched with PTFE, pericardium, or homograft.

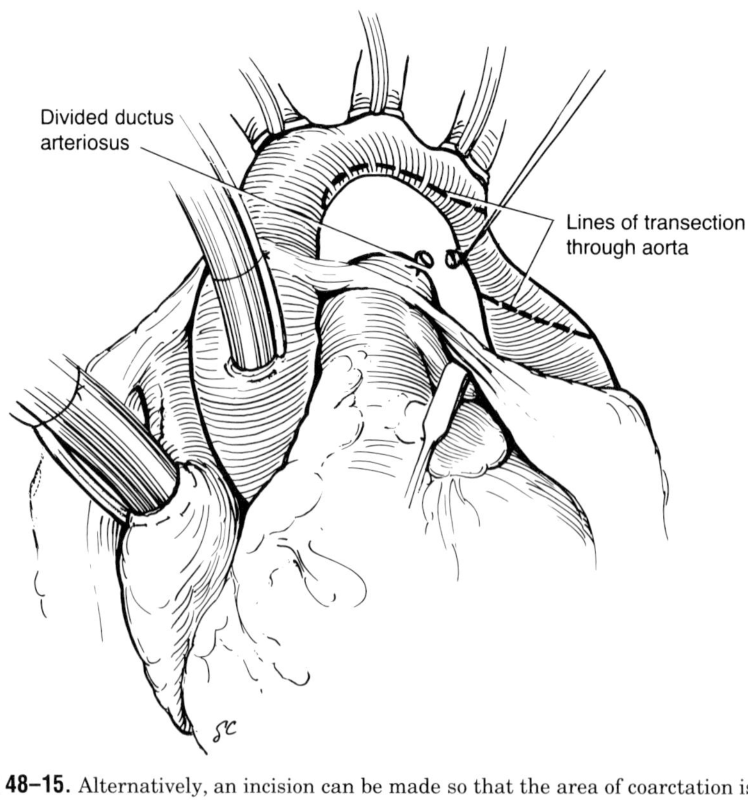

FIGURE 48–15. Alternatively, an incision can be made so that the area of coarctation is excised.

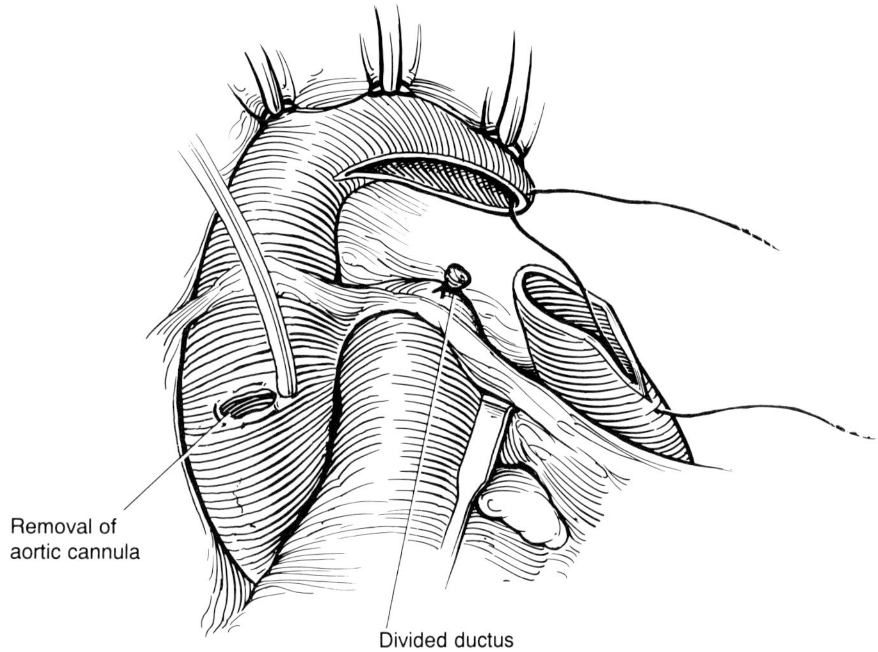

FIGURE 48–16. This technique essentially creates an interruption of the aorta that is repaired using the usual technique of end-to-end anastomosis with continuous fine suture.

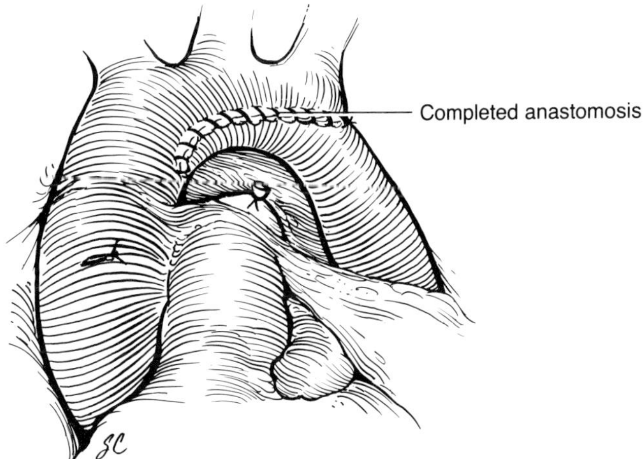

FIGURE 48–17. After the repair is completed, the patient is replaced on bypass; and after any additional cardiac procedures have been completed, the patient is rewarmed and removed from bypass.

ROSS M. UNGERLEIDER, M.D.

49 Aneurysms of the Sinus of Valsalva

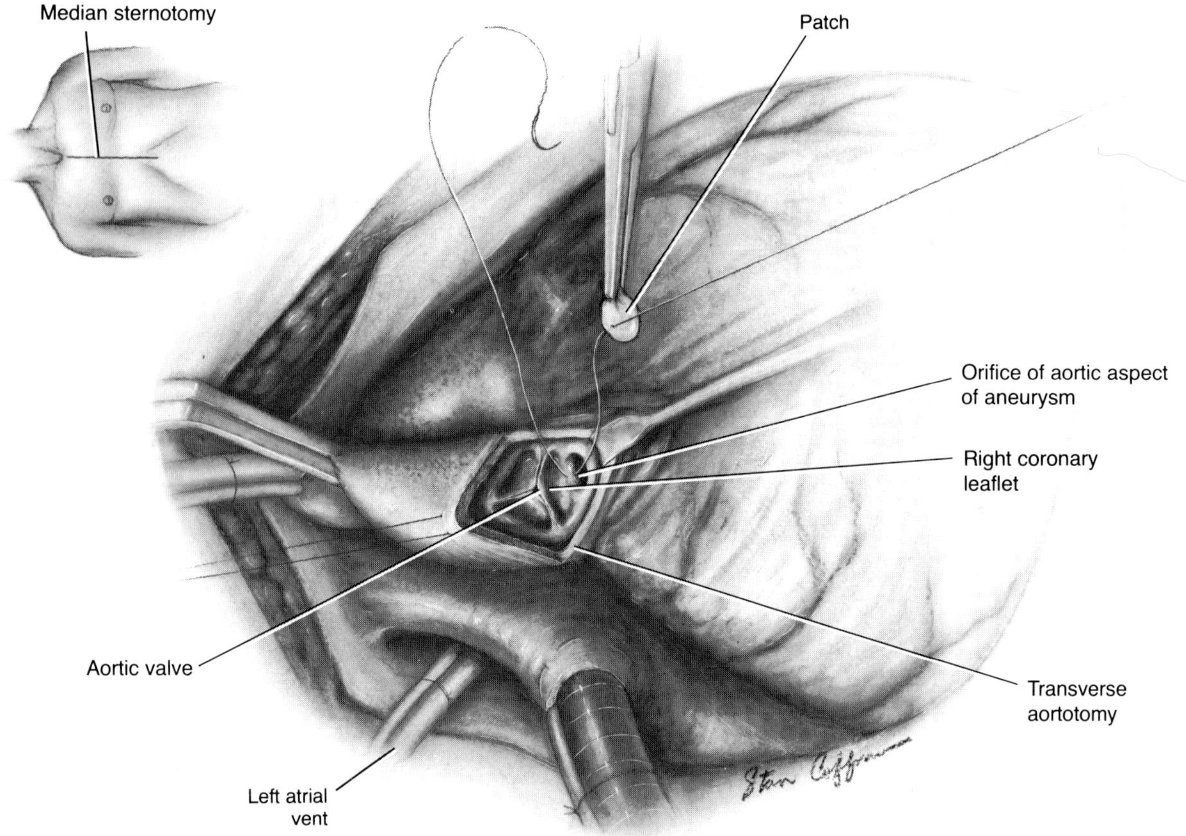

FIGURE 49–1. After median sternotomy, the patient is placed on cardiopulmonary bypass using a single right atrial venous return cannula. The aorta is crossclamped, and the heart is protected with cardioplegic solution. In patients with a large ruptured aneurysm of the sinus of Valsalva, delivery of cardioplegic solution in the aortic root may be ineffective, and it may be more beneficial to deliver the solution either directly into the coronary ostia after aortotomy or retrograde through the coronary sinus. After transverse aortotomy, the sinus of Valsalva aneurysm is usually easily identified in the sinus above the valve leaflet. It is important to distinguish the entrance of the aneurysm from the coronary ostium, and this is usually not difficult.

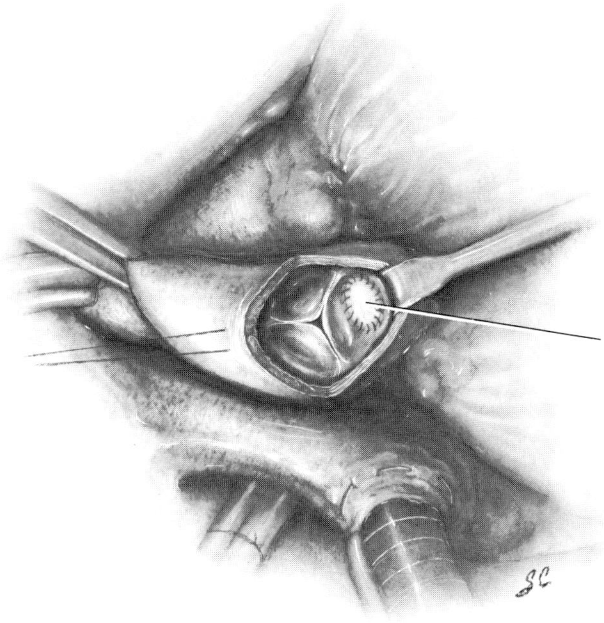

FIGURE 49–2. The entrance to the aneurysm from the aortic side is occluded with a patch (usually PTFE) sewn along the edge of the aneurysm using continuous suture material.

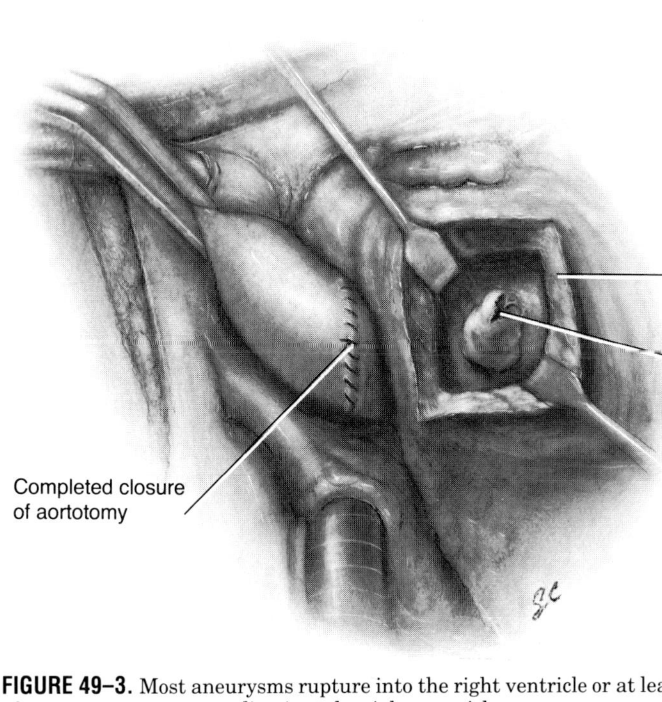

FIGURE 49–3. Most aneurysms rupture into the right ventricle or at least present as a prominence of aneurysm tissue extending into the right ventricle.

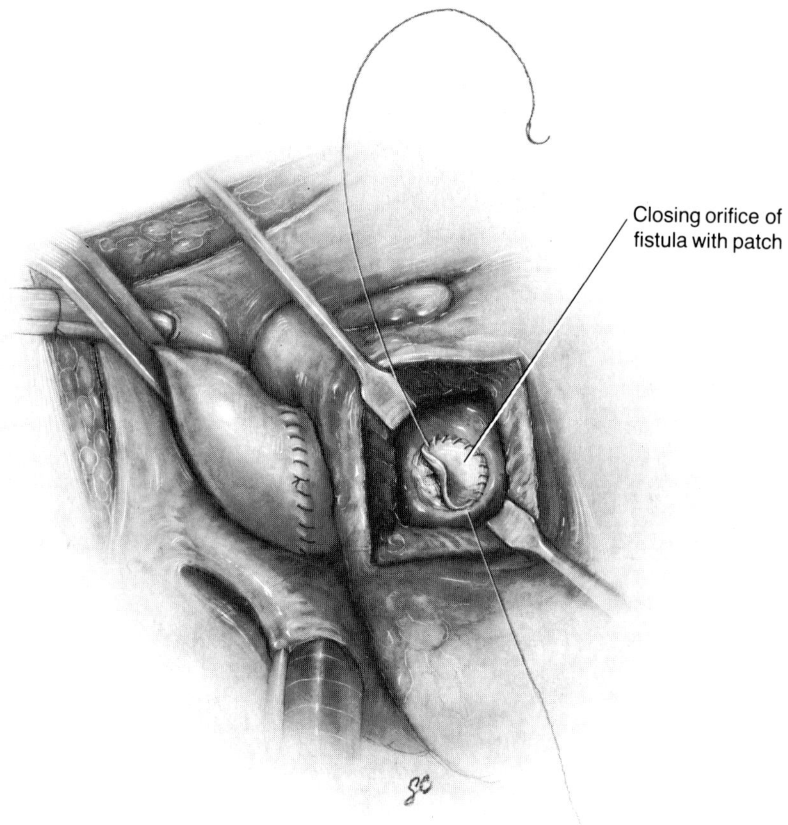

FIGURE 49–4. The aneurysmal tissue can be exposed through a right ventriculotomy, and the intracardiac portion of the aneurysm should be bolstered by placement of a patch at the base of the aneurysm.

ROSS M. UNGERLEIDER, M.D.

50
Atrial Septal Defect, Secundum

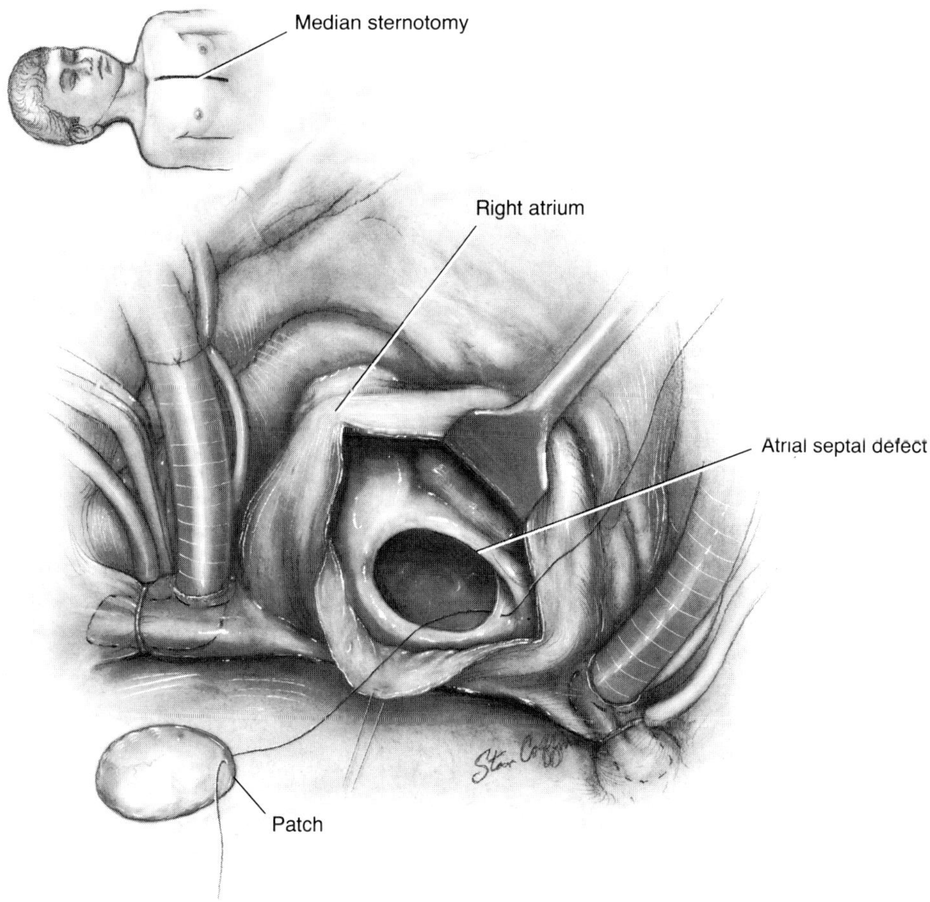

FIGURE 50–1. The heart is exposed through a median sternotomy, the aorta is cannulated in the standard manner, and bicaval venous cannulation is performed. The aorta is crossclamped, and the heart is protected with cardioplegic solution. Caval snares are then secured, and a right atriotomy is performed. The secundum atrial septal defect is identified and should be closed with a patch if the defect is large or if the residual septum primum tissue is fenestrated and poor. In the latter case, the fenestrated septum should be excised to create a uniform large defect. A pericardial or Gore-Tex patch is then constructed and sewn in place using continuous suture material.

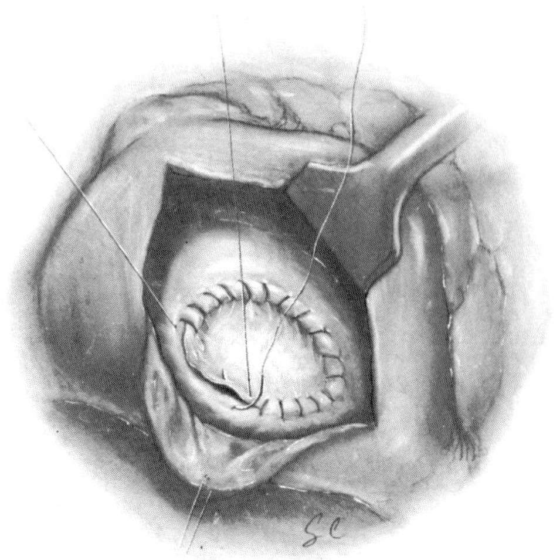

FIGURE 50–2. This suture line should be continued from the inferior portion of the defect toward the superior portion.

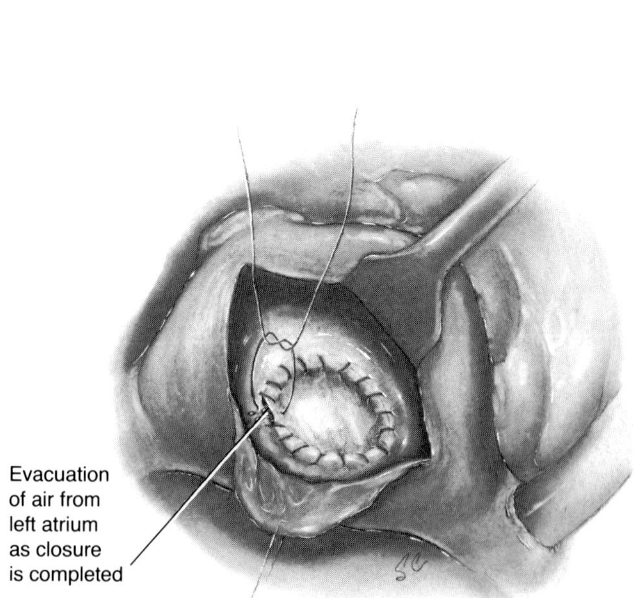

FIGURE 50–3. Before the suture line is tied securely, the lungs should be gently ventilated to fill the left atrium with blood and to remove any residual left atrial air.

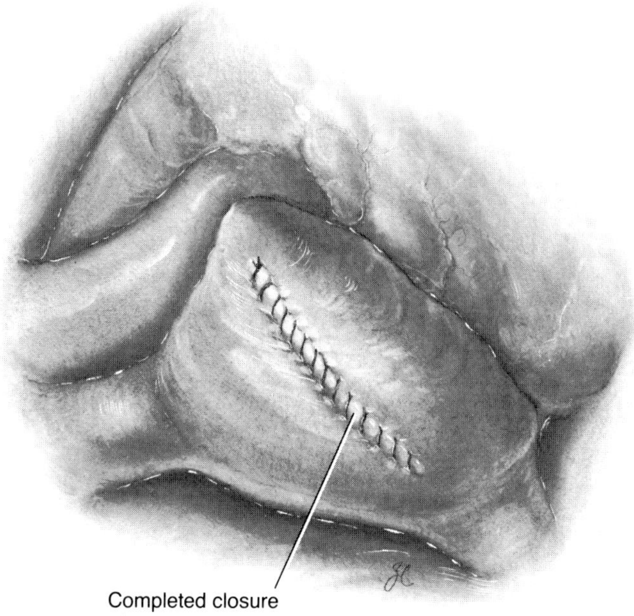

FIGURE 50–4. The aortotomy is closed with continuous suture material. Before this suture line is completed, the snares should be removed on the caval cannulae, and the right side of the heart should be allowed to fill with blood to remove any residual air that might cross tiny communications in the atrial repair.

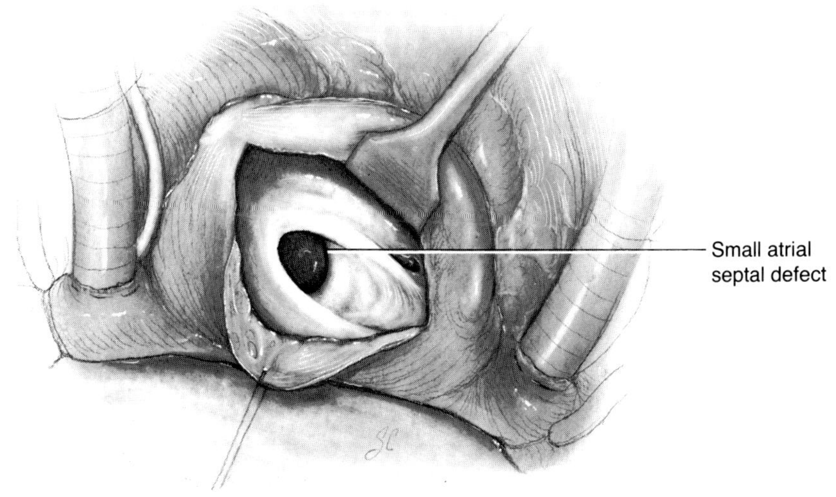

FIGURE 50–5. In patients who have secundum atrial septal defects that either are small or have borders of firm atrial septal tissue, the defect usually can be closed primarily with a continuous suture, as shown in Figure 50–6. Before the suture line is completed, the left atrium should be filled with blood (by gently inflating the lungs) to evacuate residual air.

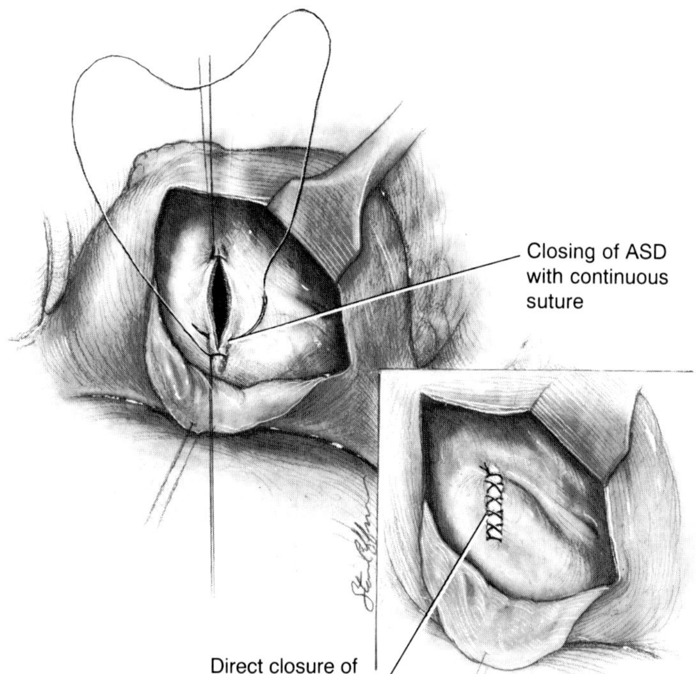

FIGURE 50–6. The atrial septal defect is closed with a continuous suture.

ROSS M. UNGERLEIDER, M.D.

51

Atrial Septal Defect: Repair of Sinus Venosus

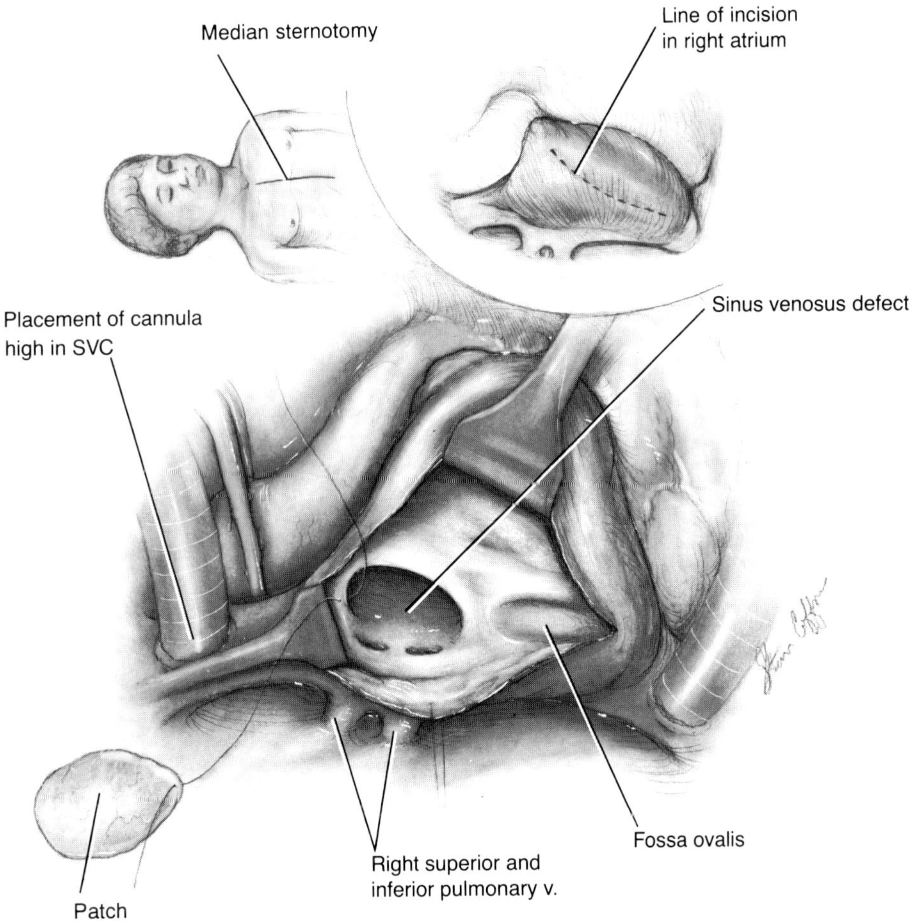

FIGURE 51–1. Exposure of the sinus venosus defect is usually performed through a median sternotomy. The patient is placed on cardiopulmonary bypass using bicaval cannulation. It is usually easiest to place these cannulae directly into the superior vena cava (SVC) and inferior vena cava (IVC). The atrial incision can be made in a standard oblique manner *(inset),* or it can be performed in a longitudinal manner along the posterior aspect of the right atrium so that it can be extended up the SVC if necessary (*inset,* Fig. 51–5). The defect will be easily identified in the sinus venosus portion of the atrium (above the limbus of the septum secundum), and the right pulmonary veins will be seen entering the lateral aspect of this defect. This defect is then closed using a patch (usually pericardium or Gore-Tex) by beginning the suture line at the most superior aspect of the defect. It is also important to examine the fossa ovalis for the presence of a second (secundum) atrial septal defect, which should be repaired when it is present.

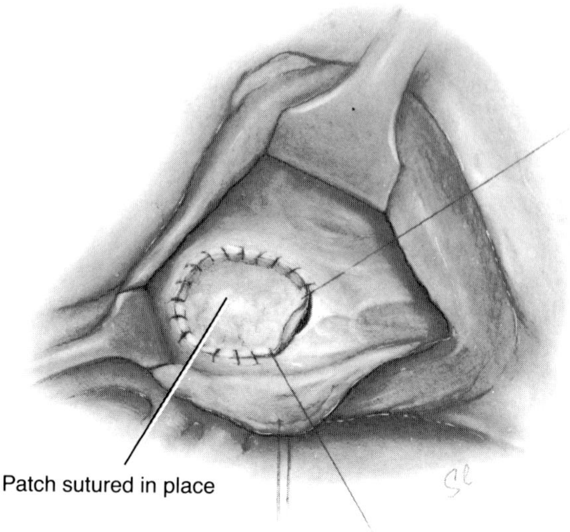

FIGURE 51–2. The patch is placed with continuous suture, and, before the suture line is completed, the lungs are gently inflated to evacuate air from the left atrium.

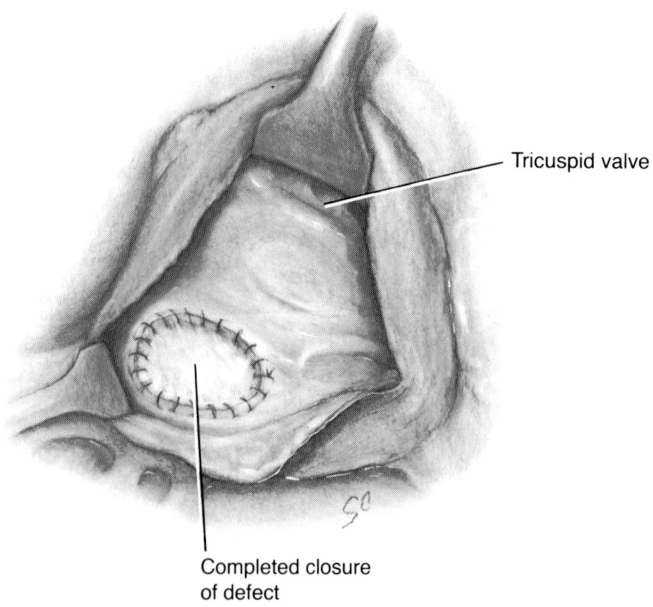

FIGURE 51–3. After the repair is completed, if there are no other atrial septal defects, the atrial incision can be repaired.

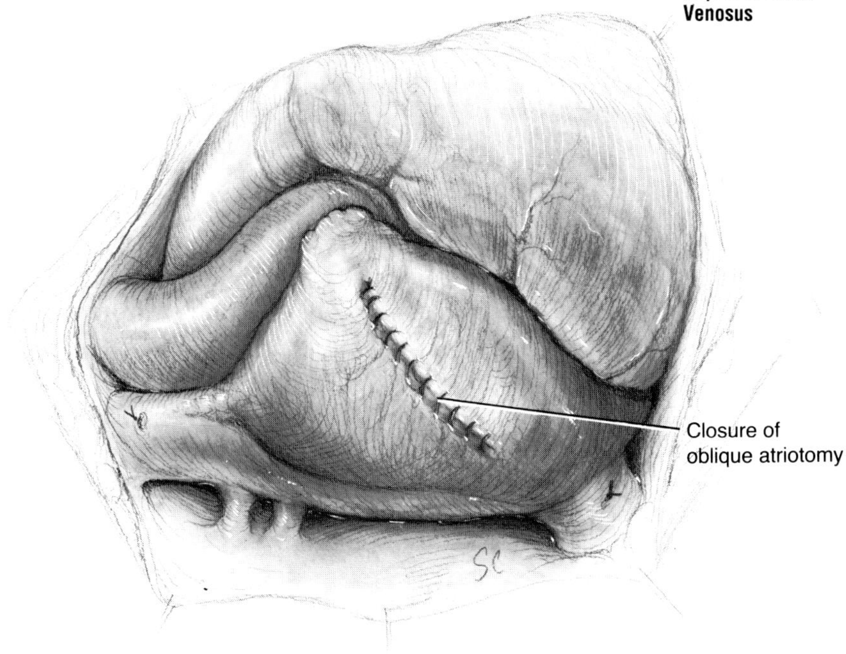

FIGURE 51–4. Atrial incision is repaired.

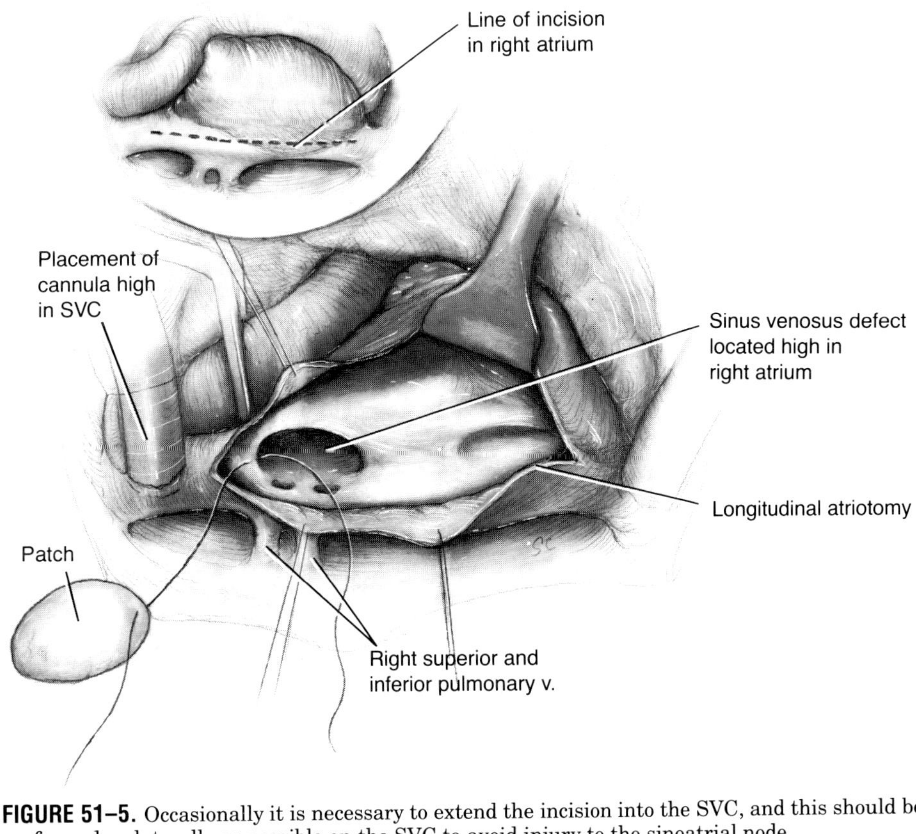

FIGURE 51–5. Occasionally it is necessary to extend the incision into the SVC, and this should be performed as laterally as possible on the SVC to avoid injury to the sinoatrial node.

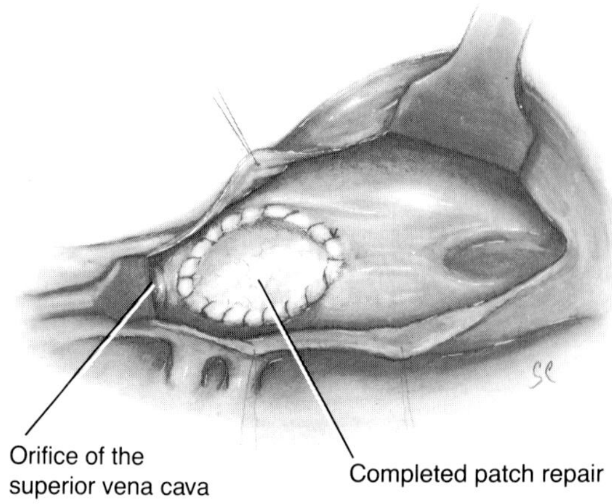

FIGURE 51–6. When this exposure is necessary, a patch can still be placed to close the defect.

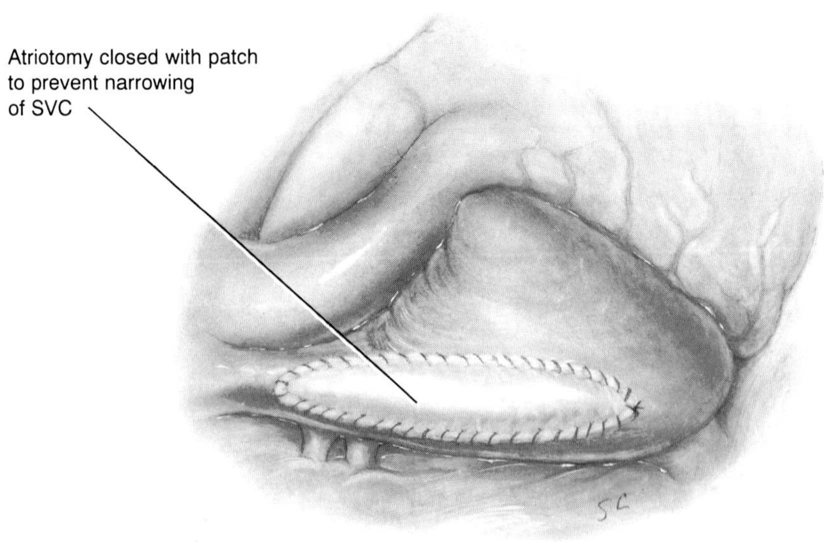

FIGURE 51–7. When the incision is extended onto the SVC, it is helpful to close this incision with a second patch so that the SVC is not narrowed from closure of the incision.

ROSS M. UNGERLEIDER, M.D.

52

Correction of Atrial Septal Defect, Primum

(PARTIAL ATRIOVENTRICULAR SEPTAL DEFECT)

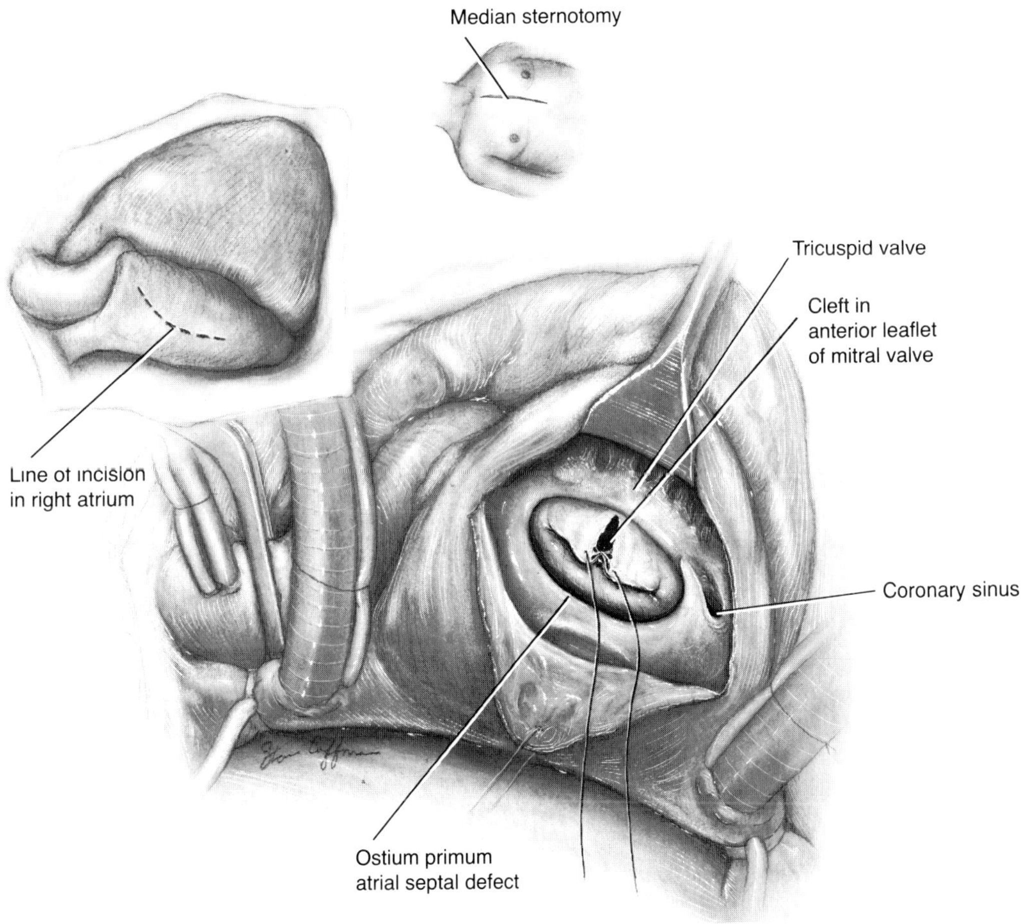

FIGURE 52–1. The defect is viewed through an oblique right atriotomy. The heart has been exposed through a median sternotomy *(upper left inset)*, and the patient has been placed on cardiopulmonary bypass using arterial infusion through an aortic cannula and venous return through separate cannulae placed into the superior and inferior venae cavae directly. The heart has been arrested with cold cardioplegia placed proximal to an aortic crossclamp. The "cleft" in the anterior leaflet of the mitral valve is easily identified, and the "leading edges" of this defect (so defined because this is where leaflet material has chordal attachments) are approximated with a suturc. The borders of the atrial septal defect in the true atrioventricular septum are defined by the annulus between the mitral and tricuspid valves anteriorly, the coronary sinus inferiorly (to the right), and the edge of the atrial septum superiorly (to the left) and posteriorly.

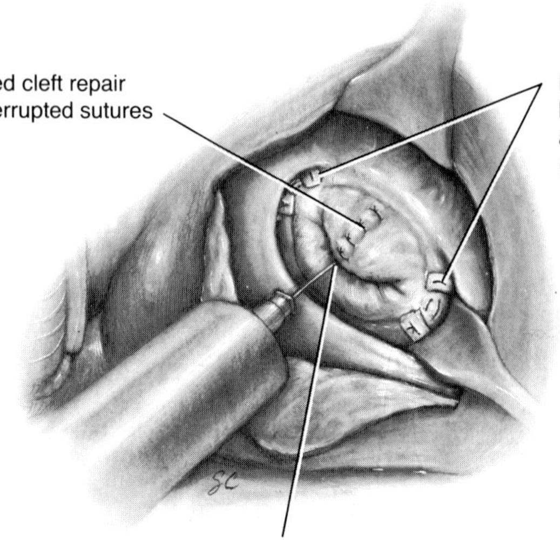

FIGURE 52–2. Cold saline is infused into the left ventricular cavity to delineate the best position for placement of sutures in the "cleft" to provide an optimally competent valve. Usually, interrupted sutures are placed and pledget material is avoided. When pledgets are necessary, those made from pericardium are preferable to those made from Teflon or other synthetic material. Saline is once again infused into the ventricle to demonstrate valve function, and, if necessary, residual insufficiency at the central area of leaflet coaptation can be repaired with carefully placed annuloplasty sutures.

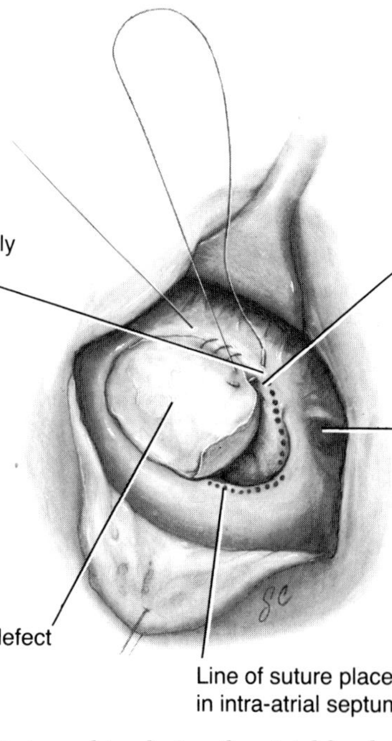

FIGURE 52–3. Attention is turned to closing the atrial level defect. If (as is recommended) the coronary sinus is positioned on the right atrial side, the suture line near the coronary sinus should be carefully placed in the mitral valve leaflet material *(dashed line)*, as opposed to the intra-atrial septum, to avoid injury to the conduction system. The anterior suture line can be placed in the annulus between the mitral and tricuspid valves, and after the suture line passes the coronary sinus, the sutures can be easily placed in the substantial tissue of the intra-atrial septum.

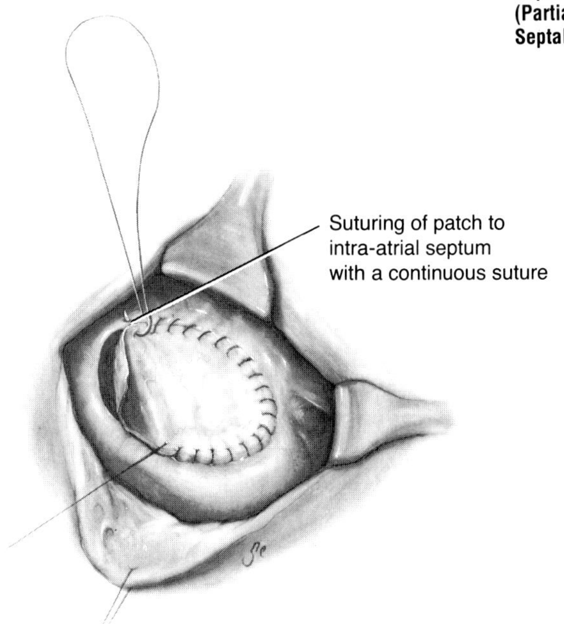

FIGURE 52–4. The patch used for closure of the defect is usually pericardium, but PTFE is an acceptable substitute.

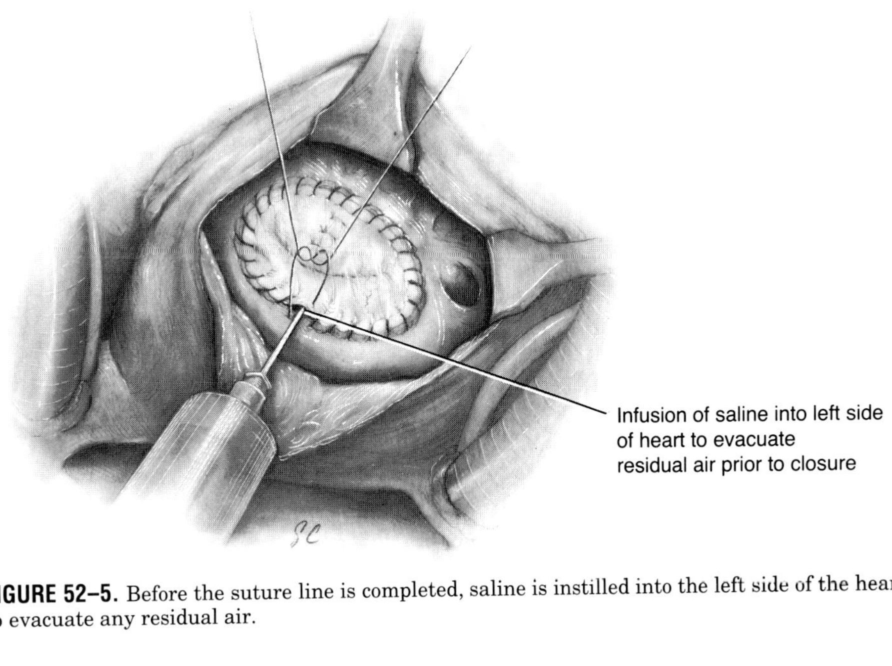

FIGURE 52–5. Before the suture line is completed, saline is instilled into the left side of the heart to evacuate any residual air.

ROSS M. UNGERLEIDER, M.D.

53

Correction of Anomalous Pulmonary Venous Return

FIGURE 53–1. In patients with total anomalous pulmonary venous return (TAPVR), the heart is exposed through a median sternotomy and cannulated for cardiopulmonary bypass with an aortic infusion cannula and a single right atrial cannula for venous return. The patient is then cooled toward 18°C, and the aorta is crossclamped and the heart arrested with cold cardioplegic solution. Although several approaches are described for this procedure, the easiest in our experience is for the surgeon to operate from the patient's left side. The apex of the heart is elevated and retracted (sometimes a pledgeted suture placed through the left ventricular apex provides an excellent "handle") toward the patient's right shoulder. The vertical vein is identified and doubly ligated. The pulmonary veins and the confluence behind the left atrium should be exposed easily through an incision in the posterior pericardium. An incision is then made in the left atrium and matched to an incision in the pulmonary venous confluence.

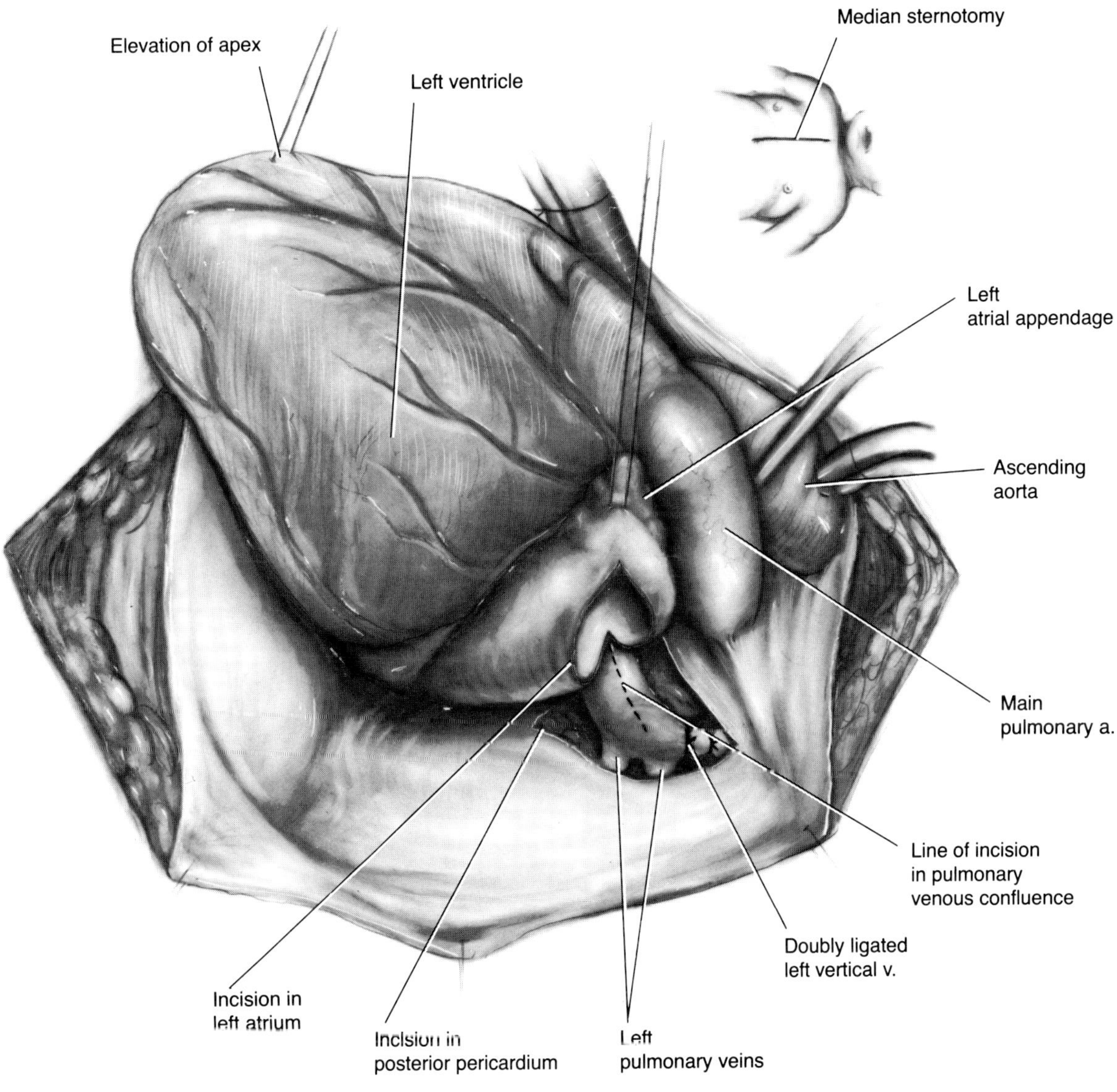

FIGURE 53–1 *See legend on opposite page*

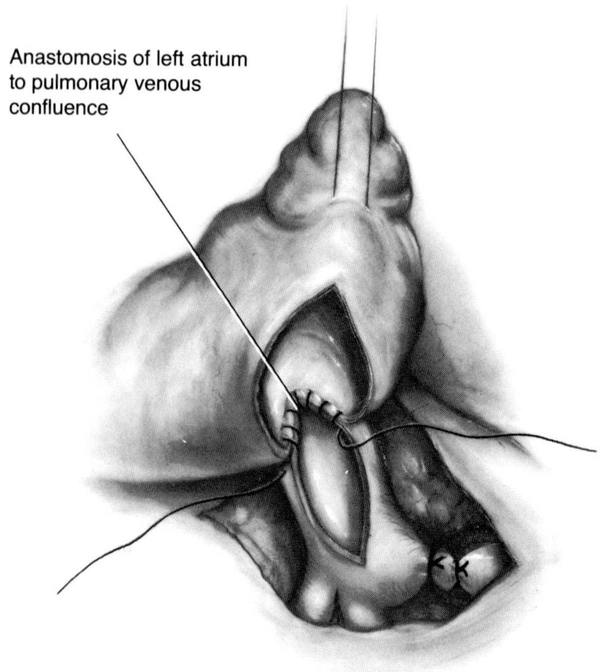

FIGURE 53–2. The left atrium is carefully anastomosed to the pulmonary venous confluence using continuous suture material. If desired, this suture line can be interrupted at occasional points to avoid a "pursestringing" effect. It may also be desirable to use suture material that will chronically absorb. Since most of these patients have an atrial septal defect (ASD), it is often possible to close the ASD through the opening in the left atrium. Alternatively, a small incision can be performed in the right atrium for closure of the ASD.

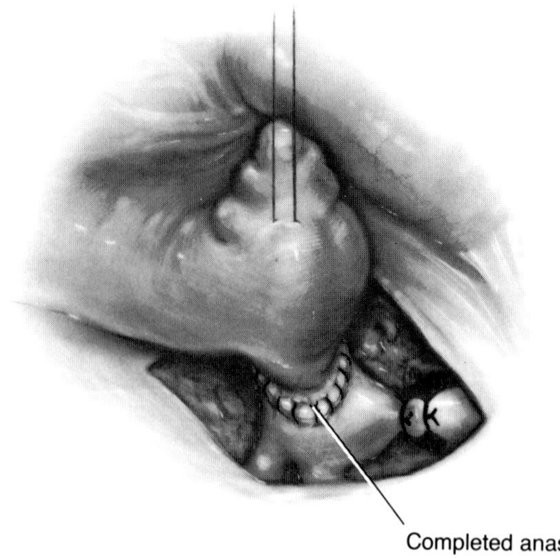

FIGURE 53–3. As the anastomosis is completed, the left atrium must be lowered gently toward the pulmonary venous confluence. When the anastomosis is completed, a right atriotomy can be performed to close the ASD (if the ASD was not closed through the left atrial incision). If a right atriotomy is performed, it is possible to inspect the completed left atrial/pulmonary venous confluence anastomosis through the ASD before the latter is closed. The patient is then rewarmed and weaned from cardiopulmonary bypass. Because these patients may have postoperative pulmonary hypertension, a pulmonary arterial catheter should be left in place for monitoring.

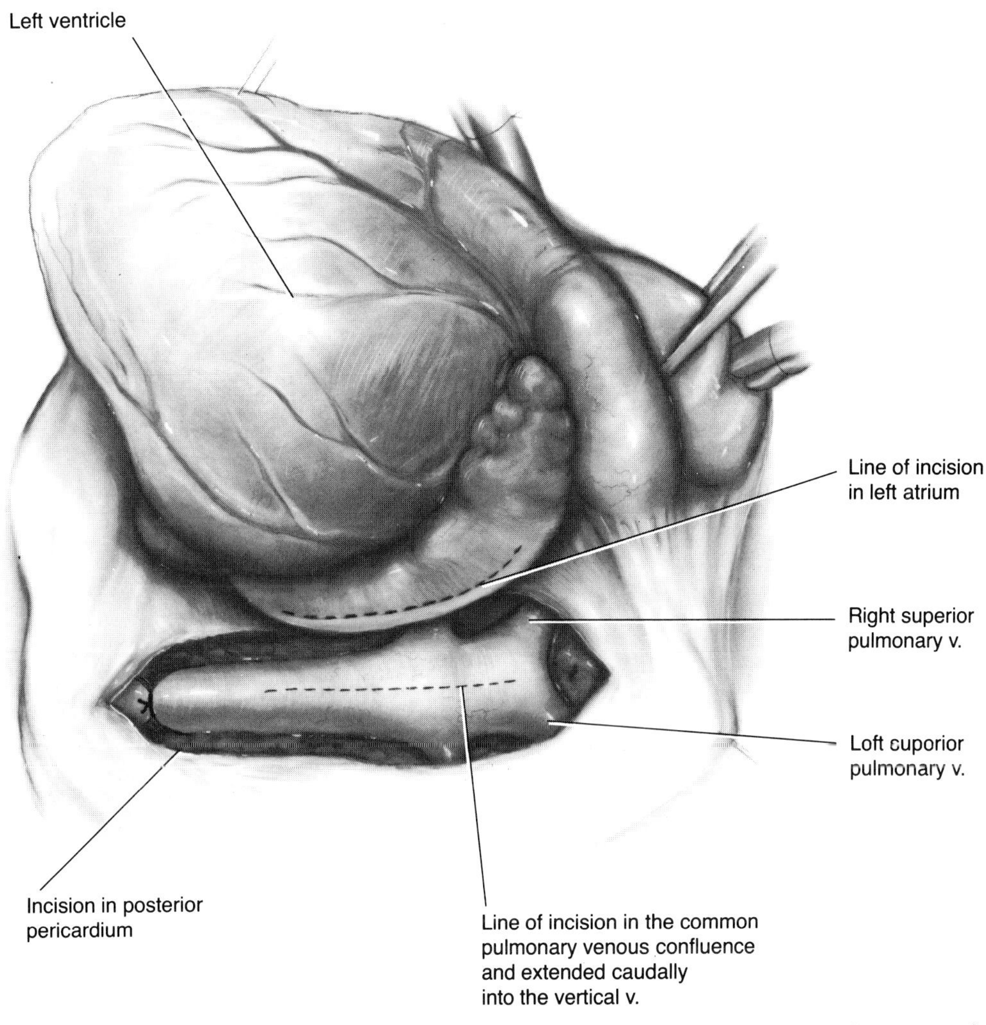

FIGURE 53–4. In patients with subdiaphragmatic pulmonary venous connection, the anatomy is exposed by placing the patient on bypass. After the aorta has been clamped and the heart arrested with cardioplegic solution, the apex of the heart is elevated toward the patient's right shoulder. An incision in the posterior pericardium allows exposure of the pulmonary venous confluence and the descending pulmonary vein. This vein can be ligated just above the diaphragm, and an incision can be made in the confluence opposite a similar incision in the left atrium.

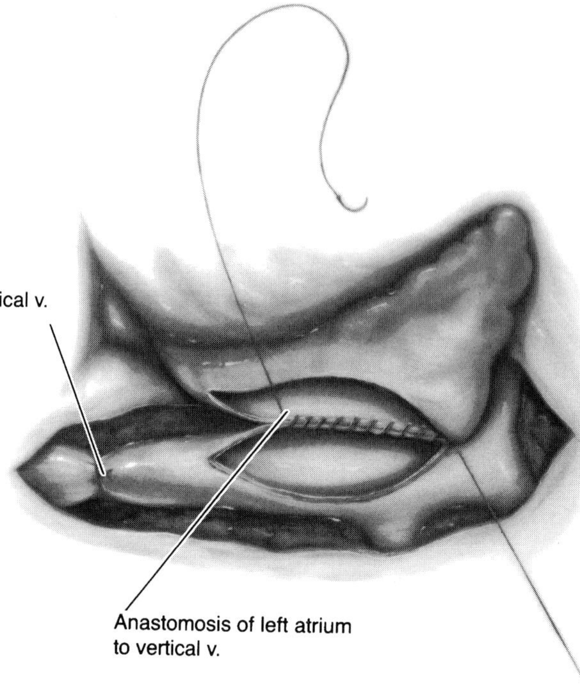

FIGURE 53–5. The left atrium is anastomosed to the pulmonary venous confluence using a continuous suture.

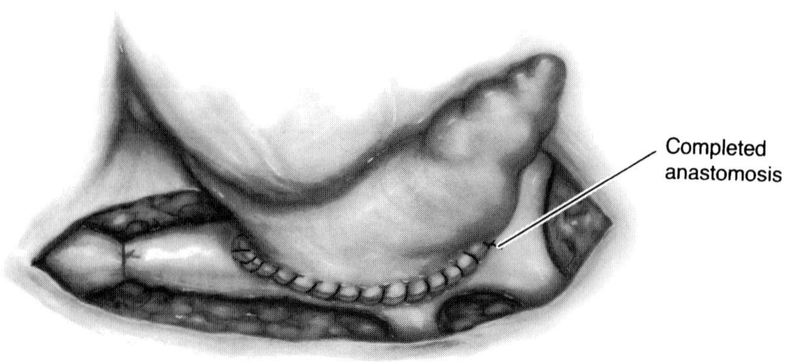

FIGURE 53–6. As this anastomosis is being completed, the left atrium must be lowered gently toward the pulmonary venous confluence. An ASD can be closed through the left atriotomy or through a right atriotomy before bypass is resumed and the patient is rewarmed.

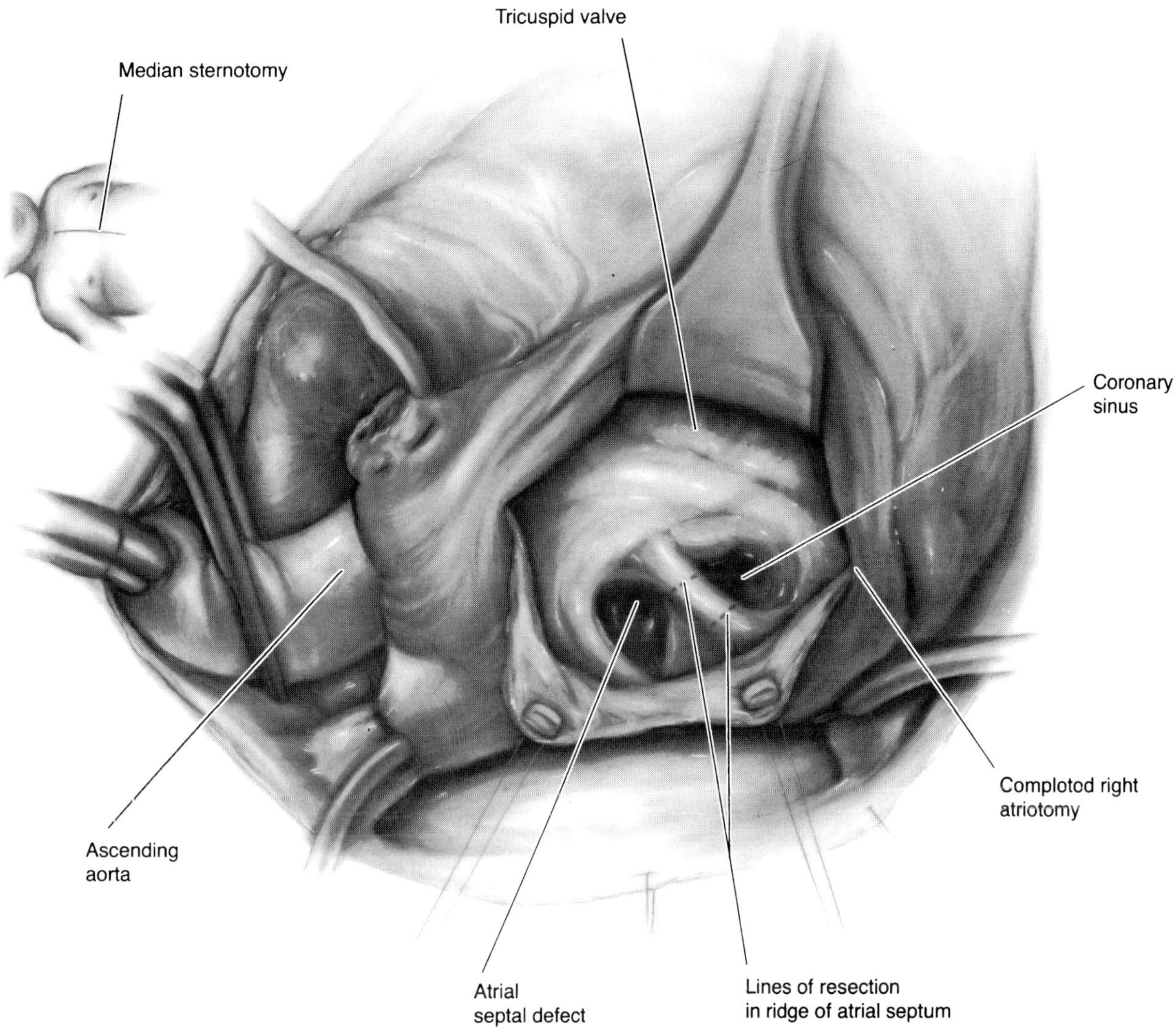

FIGURE 53–7. Anomalous pulmonary venous return to the coronary sinus usually presents with an enlarged coronary sinus separated from a small opening (through an ASD) to the left atrial appendage and mitral valve. The heart is exposed through a median sternotomy, and the patient is placed on cardiopulmonary bypass and cooled toward 18°C. The heart is protected with cold cardioplegic solution placed proximal to a crossclamp, and the right atrial anatomy is exposed during circulatory arrest (as shown with caval snares occluded to prevent venous blood in the cavae from obscuring the field) or with dual cannulation on continuous cardiopulmonary bypass. The ridge of tissue separating the coronary sinus from the ASD is excised to provide unobstructed communication between the two regions.

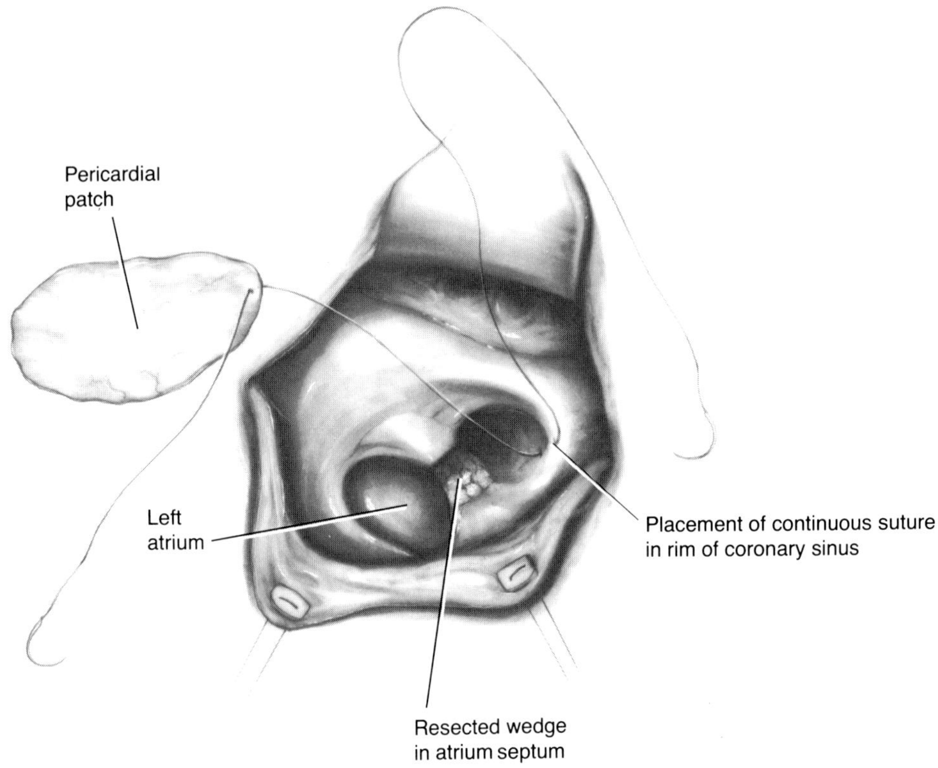

FIGURE 53–8. A patch of pericardium or Gore-Tex is placed over the defect so that the coronary sinus is diverted into the atrial septum. This patch must be large such that it balloons over the defect. Likewise, a substantial amount of tissue must be resected to provide unobstructed communication between the coronary sinus and the ASD.

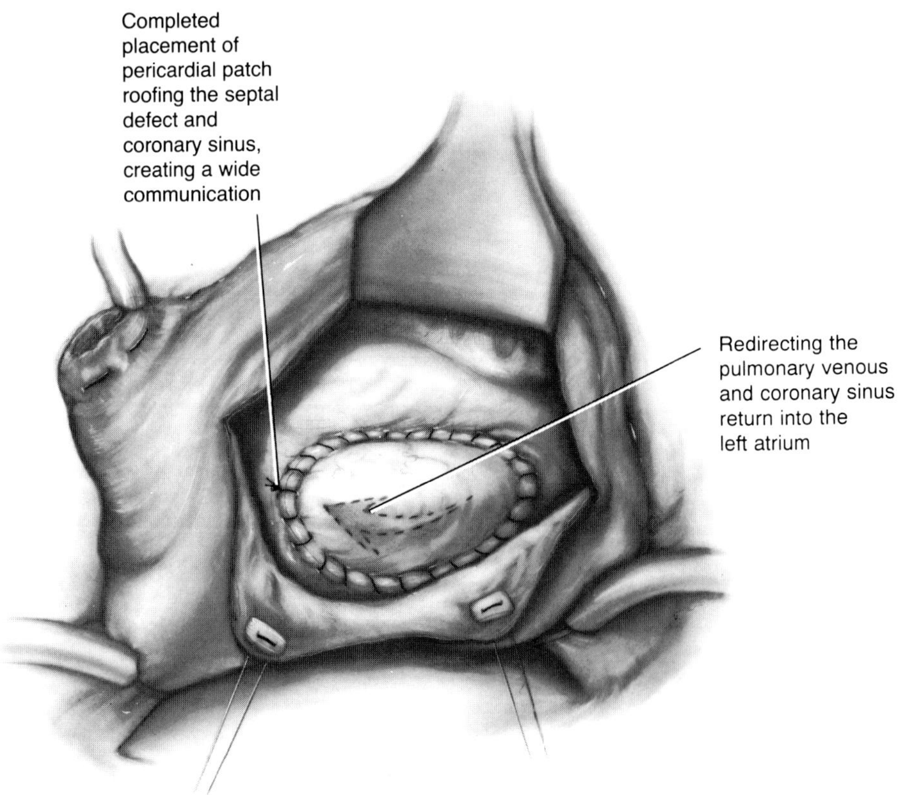

FIGURE 53–9. Once the completed patch is in place, pulmonary venous return, along with coronary sinus return, is directed below the patch toward the left atrium and mitral valve.

ROSS M. UNGERLEIDER, M.D.

54

Correction of Complete Atrioventricular Septal Defect (AV Canal)

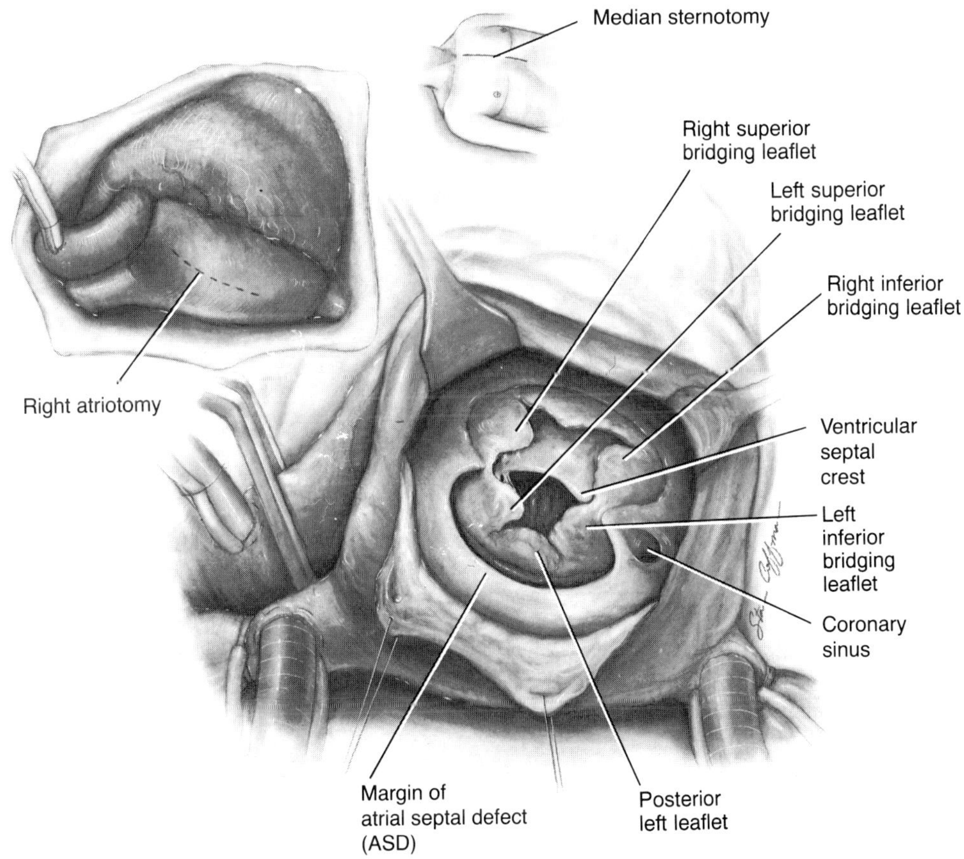

FIGURE 54–1. A complete atrioventricular septal defect (AVSD) viewed through a right atriotomy. The approach has been through a median sternotomy *(upper right inset)*, and the patient has been placed on cardiopulmonary bypass with an aortic infusion cannula and separate caval venous return cannulae. The aorta has been crossclamped and the heart arrested with cold cardioplegic solution. Exposure through an oblique incision in the right atrium (with the edges retracted) (*upper left inset*) demonstrates the anatomic features of the lesion. The coronary sinus and margin of the AVSD delineate the boundaries of the atrial level defect. There is a prominent cleft between the left and right superior bridging leaflets consistent with Rastelli type A classification. Repair of this type of defect occasionally can be accomplished using a single-patch technique without interfering with the normal attachments of the superior bridging leaflets.

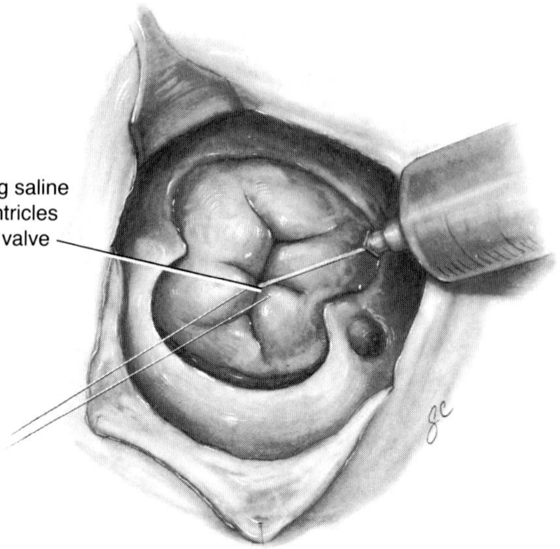

FIGURE 54–2. It is useful to distend the common atrioventricular (AV) valve by injecting cold saline into the ventricular cavities. This enables the surgeon to best delineate the optimal coaptation point of the left superior and inferior bridging leaflets (indicated by the approximation suture), as well as to determine any abnormalities in valve coaptation that require attention during valve reconstruction.

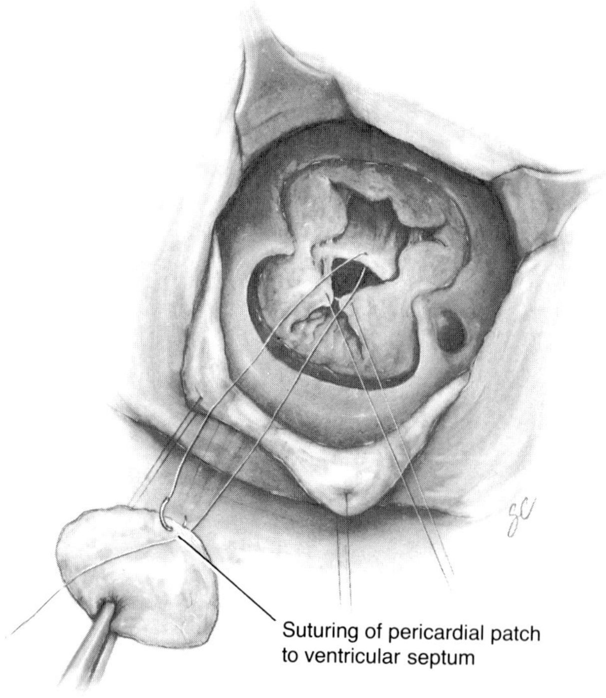

FIGURE 54–3. The suture line in the ventricular septum for the single pericardial patch (a patch of PTFE can also be used) usually is begun at the midpoint of the ventricular septal crest. At this location, sutures can be placed full thickness through the ventricular septum, and it is advisable to take good bites of tissue.

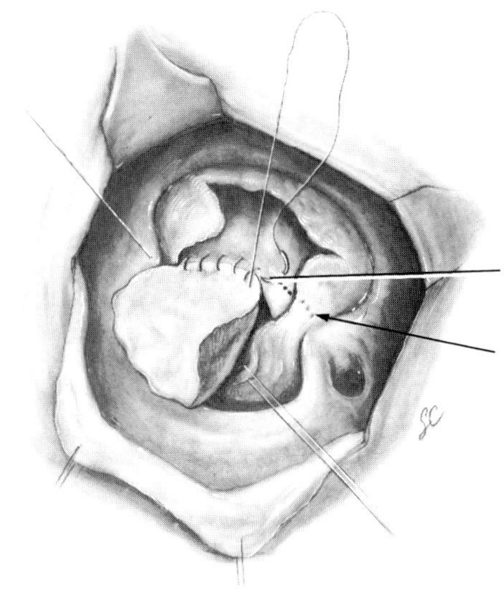

FIGURE 54–4. This suture line is continued toward the superior aspect of the defect and eventually brought out the annulus below the cleft between the left and right superior bridging leaflets. This cleft can be slightly incised toward the annulus, if necessary, to prevent a residual defect where the patch is tucked into the annulus. In this way, the patch is sandwiched between the left and right superior bridging leaflets and completely closes the underlying ventricular septal communication. Attention is then turned to the inferior portion of the ventricular septal defect (VSD). In this portion, the suture line cannot be placed through the full thickness of the ventricular septum, because this will risk injury to the penetrating conduction system. Therefore, these sutures are kept on the right ventricular side of the VSD, and the suture line is directed quickly away from the edge of the defect to avoid further risk of injury to the conduction tissue.

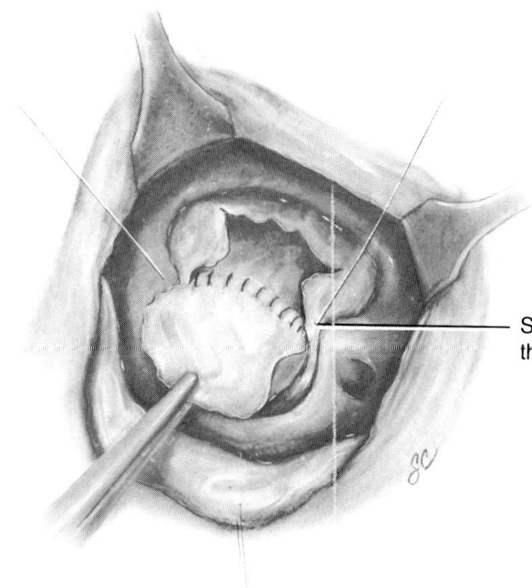

FIGURE 54–5. When the suture line meets the inferior bridging leaflet, it is brought through the substance of the leaflet material near the annulus. Often there are numerous chordal attachments of the inferior bridging leaflet in this region, so it may be necessary to tuck the patch below some of these chordae and weave the suture line so that the chordae are left untethered. In difficult cases, this often can be accomplished more easily by placing some interrupted pledgeted mattress sutures in this location and securing them to the continuous suture line.

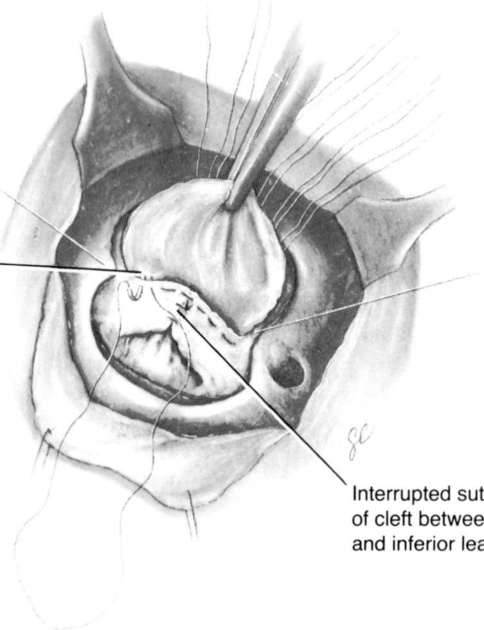

FIGURE 54–6. With the ventricular septal defect now repaired, attention is turned to the left AV valve. In some cases, the left AV valve does not require approximation of the superior and inferior bridging leaflets. However, it is usually best to place a few interrupted sutures between the left superior and inferior bridging leaflets in order to repair the cleft of this newly created mitral valve. When there is prominence of the posterior mitral valve leaflet and deficiency of the commissure between the posterior leaflet and the newly created anterior leaflet, this cleft sometimes may best be left unrepaired. Regardless, the left inferior and superior bridging leaflets must be suspended from the pericardial patch at a level that provides coaptation between the newly created anterior mitral valve leaflet and its posterior leaflet. Often this can best be checked by infusing saline into this newly created "mitral" valve. If significant insufficiency occurs in the central portion, it often can be repaired with carefully placed annuloplasty sutures (see Fig. 52–2).

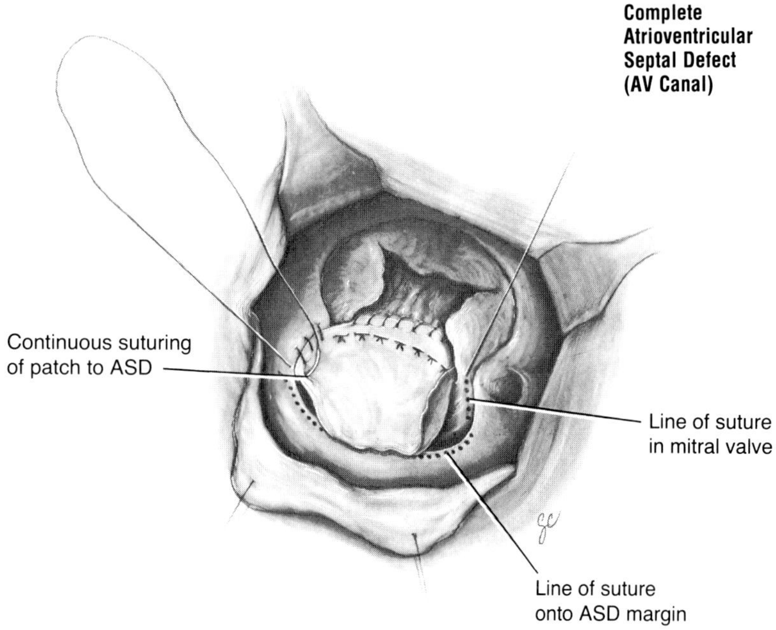

FIGURE 54–7. After the newly created left AV valve competence has been ensured, and the valve suspended at the appropriate point on the patch, the previously placed sutures at either end of the annulus are then used to continue the suture line of the patch around the atrial level defect. This suture line can be placed so that the coronary sinus is retained on the right atrial side of the repair, as long as the sutures near the coronary sinus are placed through the substance of the left inferior bridging leaflet and not into the septum behind the coronary sinus (which might risk injury to the AV node). This technique has been used by the author in more than 70 patients without creating permanent heart block in any patient. This technique is especially useful in patients with a persistent left superior vena cava that necessitates retention of the coronary sinus on the right atrial side.

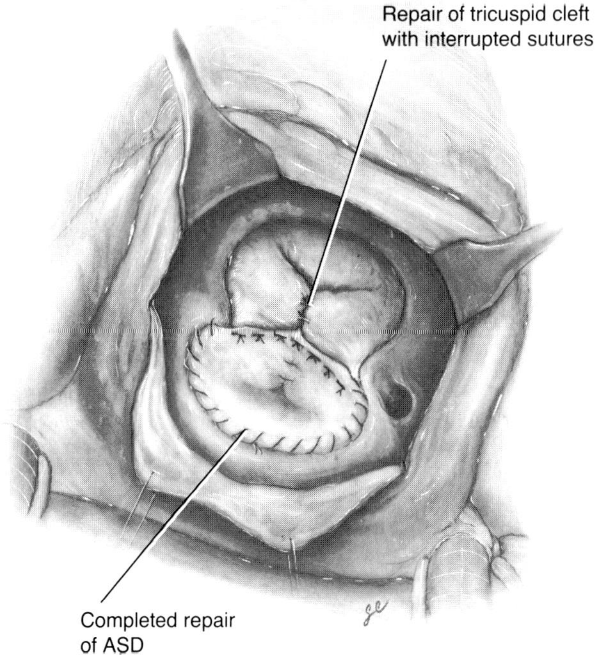

FIGURE 54–8. The tricuspid valve should also be inspected. Occasionally a few additional sutures in the cleft of the tricuspid valve can be used to enhance competence of this valve. This valve can also be checked with infusion of cold saline.

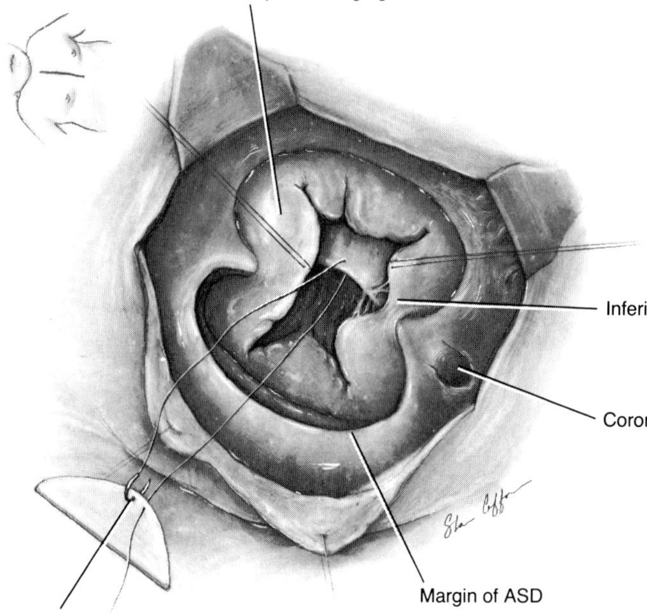

FIGURE 54–9. A Rastelli type C complete atrioventricular septal defect viewed through an atriotomy demonstrates a prominent superior bridging leaflet without a cleft over the ventricular septum or chordal attachments to the ventricular septum. This type of defect is best repaired using a two-patch technique in order to limit incision of the leaflet material, which could potentially result in severe valvar incompetence. After distention and inspection of the leaflet material with infusion of cold saline into the ventricular cavity (see Fig. 54–2), in order to delineate the optimal place for suspension of the valves from the ventricular level patch, a patch of PTFE is placed using a suture line similar to that shown in Figures 54–3 through 54–5. In patients with this anatomy, it is convenient to retract the superior bridging leaflet so that the suture line can be continued along the ventricular septum until it reaches the point where the septum meets the annulus, at which point the suture is brought through the annulus above the superior bridging leaflet.

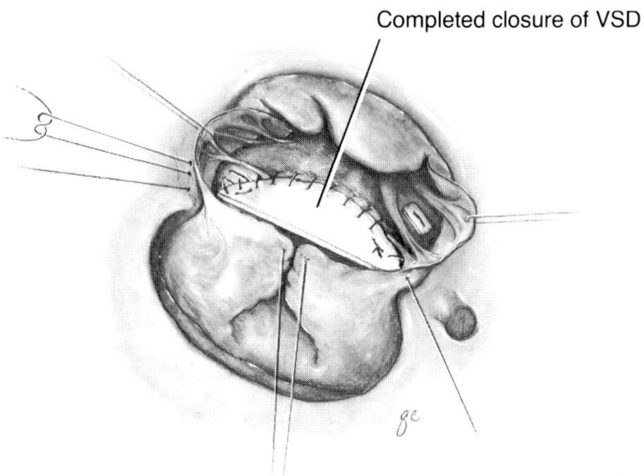

FIGURE 54–10. Because of an increased risk that residual ventricular septal defects may occur at this junction, an additional mattress suture can be placed. With this technique, the incidence of residual ventricular septal defect in this location approaches zero. The suture line is then continued on the superficial aspects of the right ventricular surface along the inferior margin of the ventricular septal defect until it can be brought through the substance of the inferior bridging leaflet. As discussed for Figure 54–5, interrupted pledgeted sutures are best used when there are numerous chordal attachments to prevent residual ventricular septal defects in this location. The left superior and inferior bridging leaflets are then approximated at their best point of coaptation.

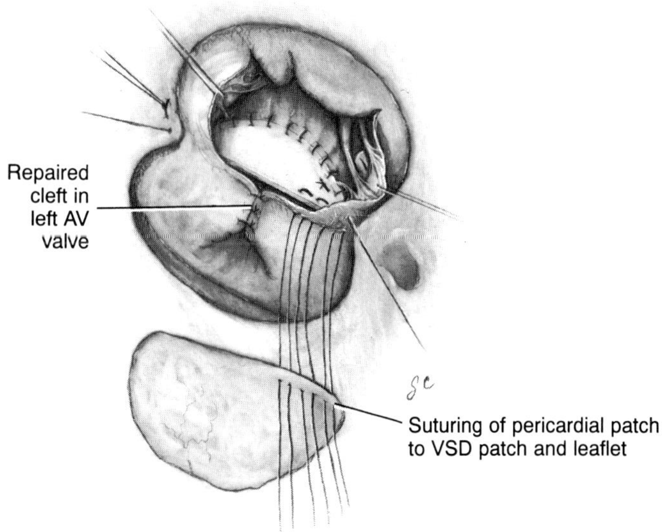

FIGURE 54–11. If appropriate, a few additional sutures are placed to repair the cleft in the left AV valve. The left AV valve is then "sandwiched" between the top of the ventricular septal patch and a second patch for the atrial level defect (which can be pericardium or a second piece of PTFE).

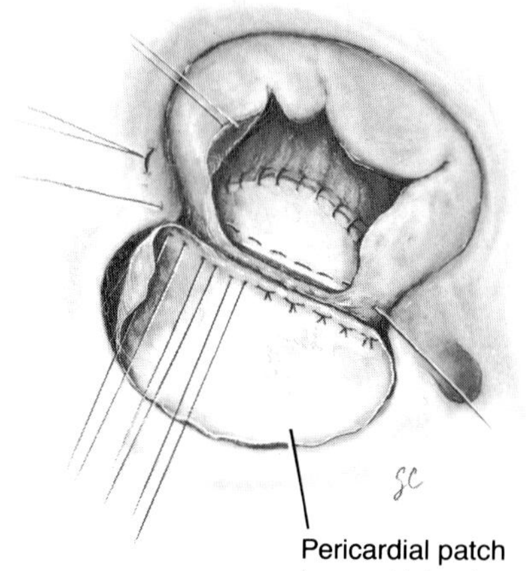

FIGURE 54–12. These sutures are best placed as interrupted mattress sutures, and careful attention must be given to those sutures along the superior portion of the defect to make certain that the ventricular septal patch is brought into the corner of the superior bridging leaflet and then along its border so as not to leave any residual defects.

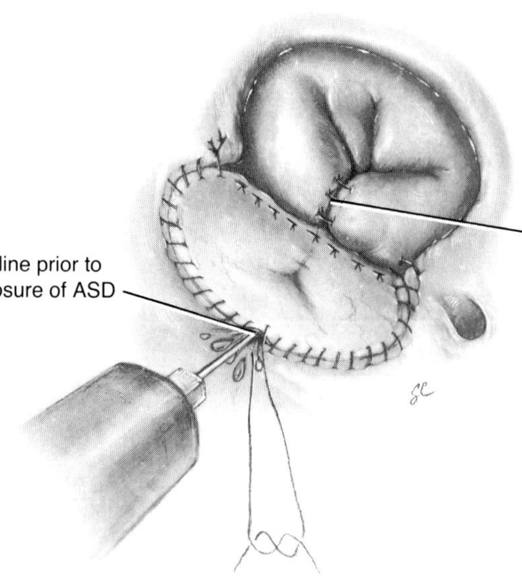

FIGURE 54–13. The remaining portion of the suture line for the atrial level patch is completed, and, before the suture line is completed, the left side of the heart is filled with iced saline to evacuate residual air. Once again, additional sutures can be placed to approximate the cleft of the tricuspid valve to enhance its competence.

ROSS M. UNGERLEIDER, M.D.

55
Ventricular Septal Defect

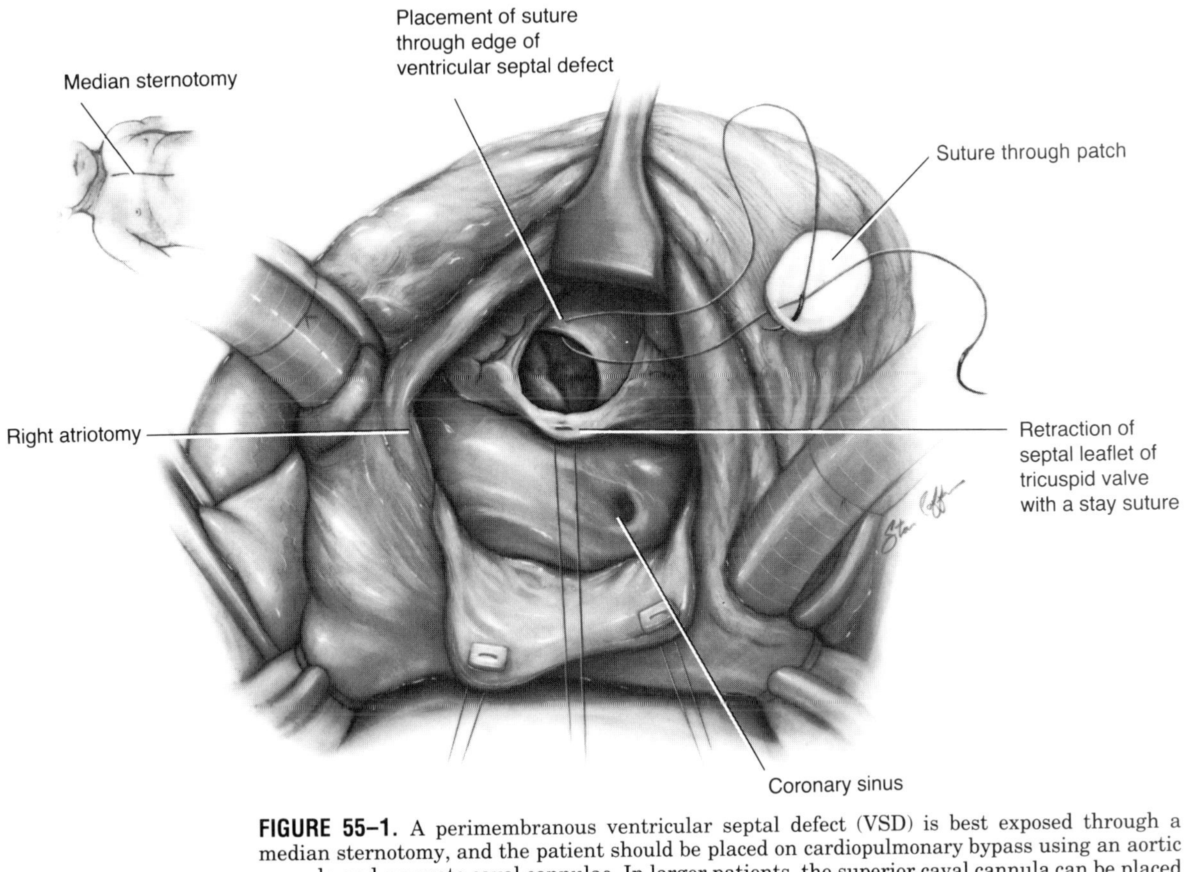

FIGURE 55–1. A perimembranous ventricular septal defect (VSD) is best exposed through a median sternotomy, and the patient should be placed on cardiopulmonary bypass using an aortic cannula and separate caval cannulae. In larger patients, the superior caval cannula can be placed through the right atrial appendage; but in smaller patients and in infants, it is more convenient to place the superior cannula directly into the superior vena cava. A single atrial cannula can be used when the defect is to be repaired through a ventricular incision in small infants or whenever a period of circulatory arrest is going to be used to repair the defect through any incision. The heart is protected with cardioplegic solution, and if a transatrial approach is used, as shown here, the defect usually can be exposed through the leaflets of the tricuspid valve, which can be retracted gently with sutures or with small vein retractors. It is most convenient to begin the continuous suture line at the superior and medial aspect of the defect along the infundibular septum. These defects should almost always be closed with a patch.

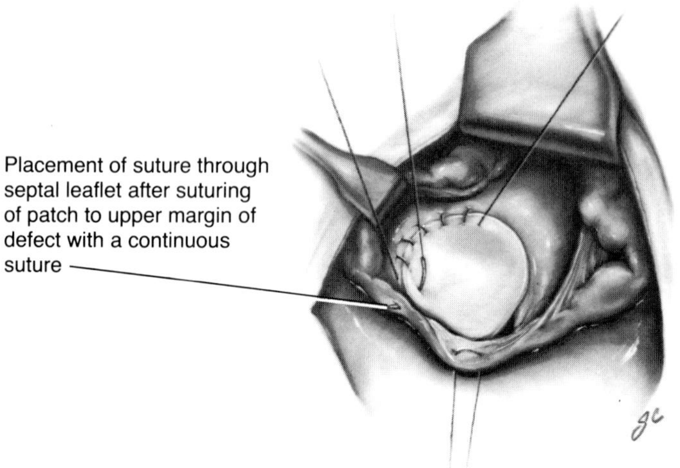

FIGURE 55–2. The suture line is continued along the superior and medial aspect of the defect, and exposure can be enhanced by retraction of the anterior leaflet of the tricuspid valve and by having the assistant gently retract the sutures toward the patient's right side. The suture line is continued until the most medial aspect of the defect is encountered. At this point, the suture can be brought through the base of the tricuspid valve.

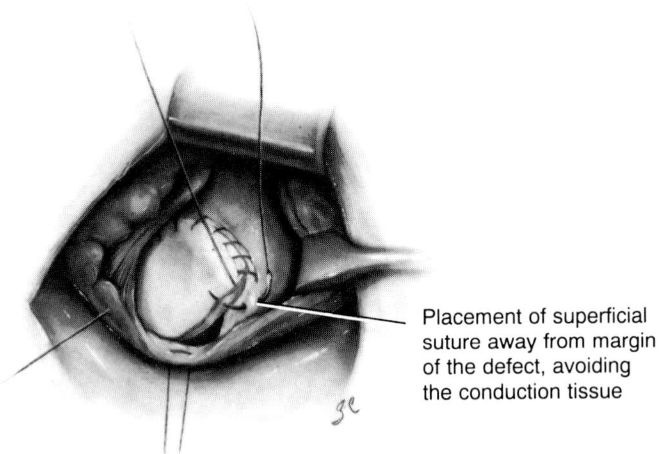

FIGURE 55–3. The inferior portion of the suture line is continued along the defect, and, if necessary, it can be brought below any chordal attachments of the tricuspid valve so that the patch lies below the tricuspid valve apparatus. Along the most lateral portion of the defect, the suture line should be superficial and kept off the edge of the defect to avoid injuring the conduction tissue.

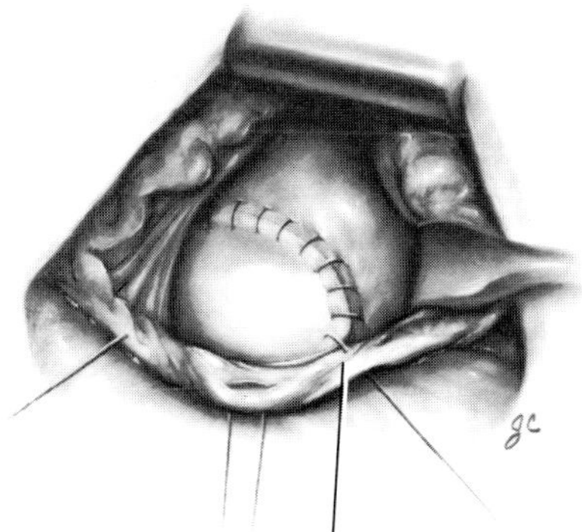

FIGURE 55–4. The suture line is brought through the base of the septal leaflet of the tricuspid valve.

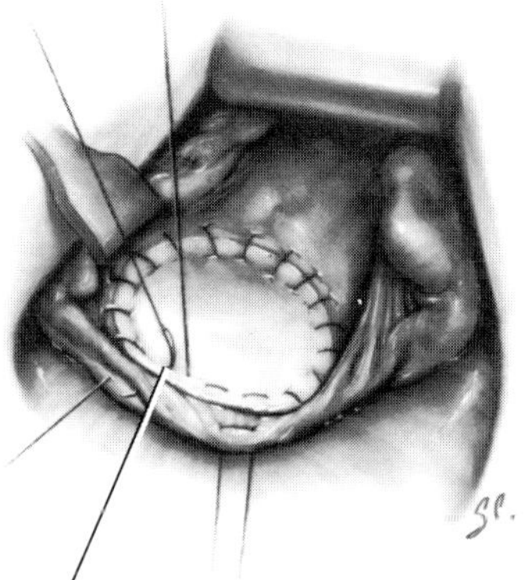

FIGURE 55–5. The suture line is completed by performing a horizontal mattress suture through the base of the septal leaflet of the tricuspid valve.

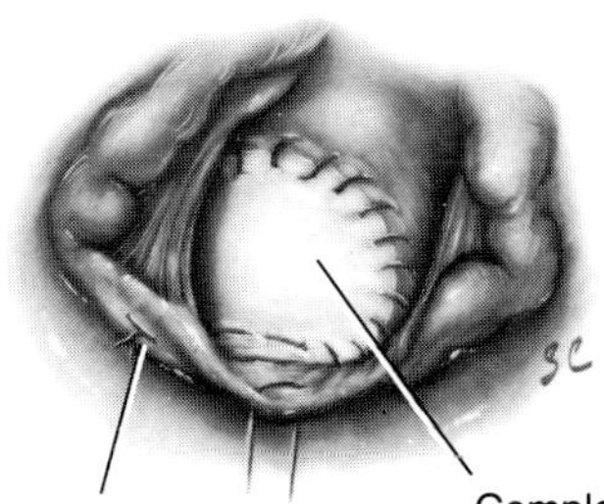

FIGURE 55–6. Sutures can be tied over a small pledget of pericardium, if desired.

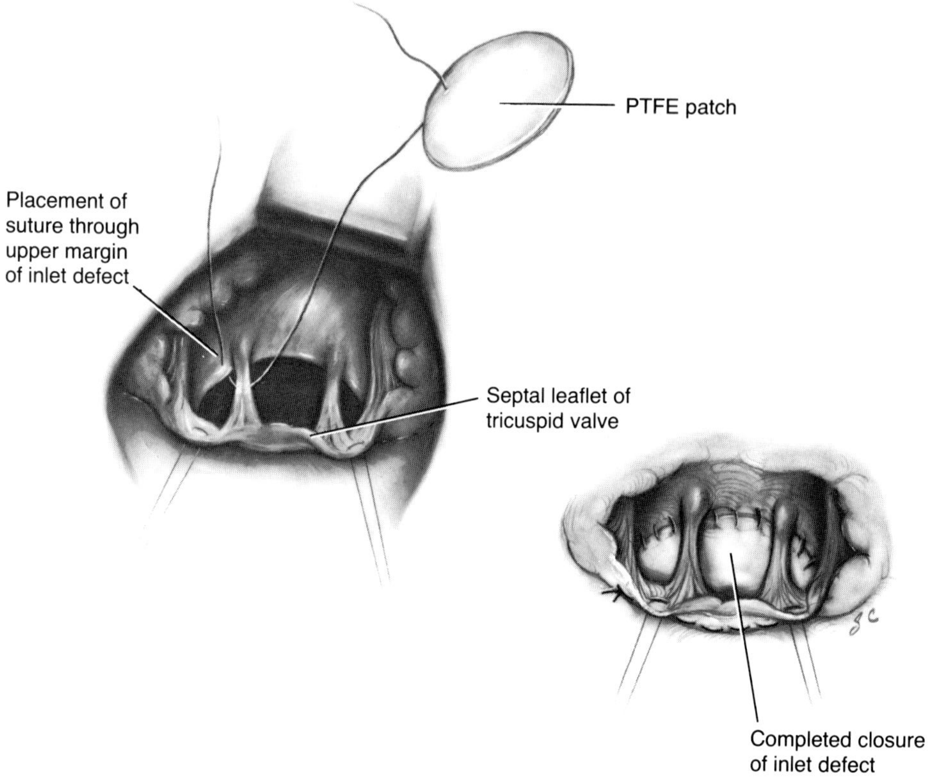

FIGURE 55–7. In patients with inlet ventricular septal defects, there are often more prominent chordal attachments of the septal leaflet of the tricuspid valve extending across the defect. The same suture technique can be used to repair these defects through the right atrium as that described in Figures 55–1 to 55–6, except that it is important to place the patch below the chordal attachments of the tricuspid valve. It is usually easiest to begin the suture line along the infundibular septum and to complete the superior aspect of the suture line before beginning the inferior portion. If the chordal attachments are too thick or numerous, it may be easier to detach the septal leaflet of the tricuspid valve at the annulus and retract it medially, thus exposing the underlying VSD, which is then easily patched. The septal leaflet is reattached to the annulus over the patch with fine suture.

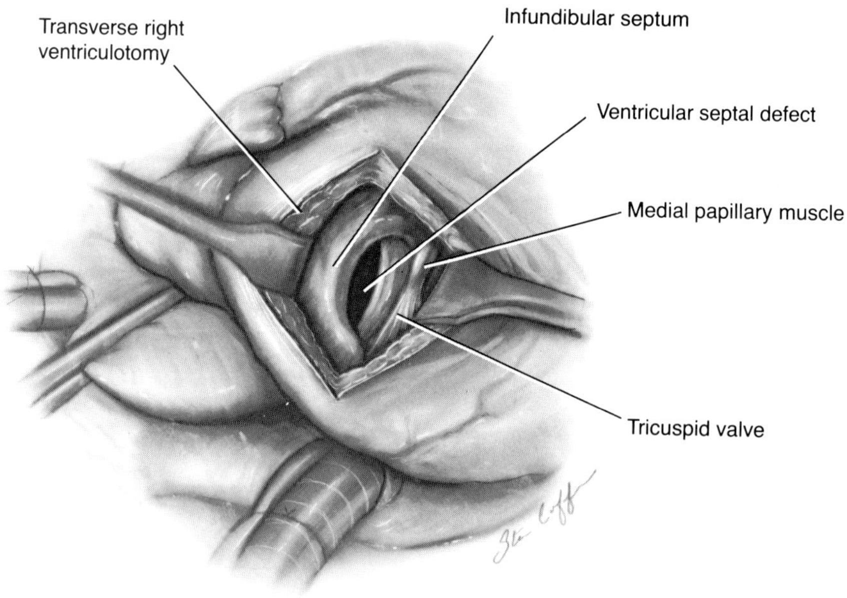

FIGURE 55–8. A perimembranous ventricular septal defect also can be closed through a transverse right ventriculotomy, where it will be easily visualized below the infundibular septum. The advantage of a ventricular incision is that the chordal attachments of the tricuspid valve appear to lie below the defect, and in some instances this may make the defect easier to close.

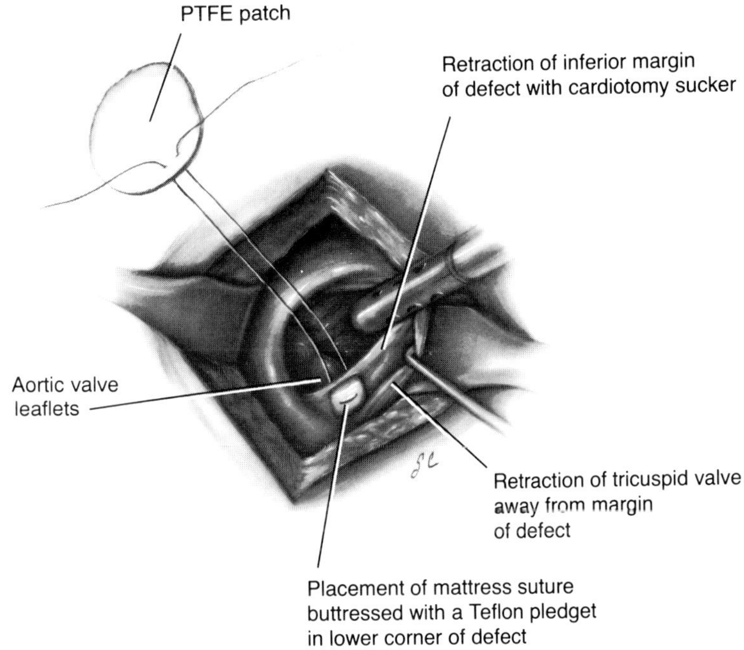

FIGURE 55–9. The suture line is begun along the posterior portion of the defect near the ventricular infundibular fold. The defect can be easily exposed by placing a cardiotomy sucker through the defect. This technique works very well in small patients on continuous bypass with a single atrial cannula.

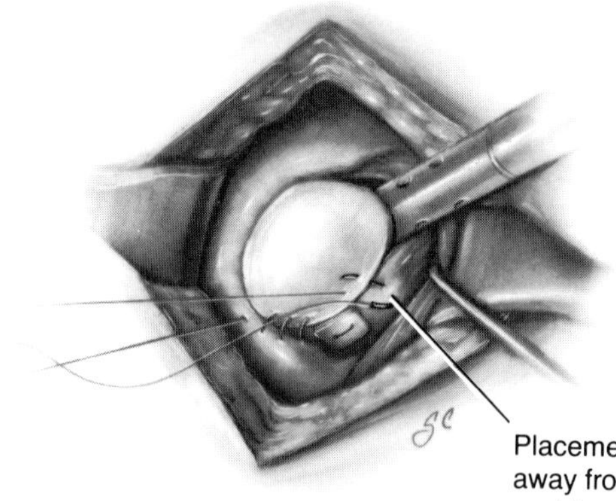

FIGURE 55–10. The superior portion of the defect is closed first with continuous suture, until the suture is brought out through the infundibular septum. Next, the posterior and inferior portion of the defect is closed, with care taken to keep the sutures that are along the inferior border of the defect superficial and away from the edge of the defect, to protect the conduction tissue.

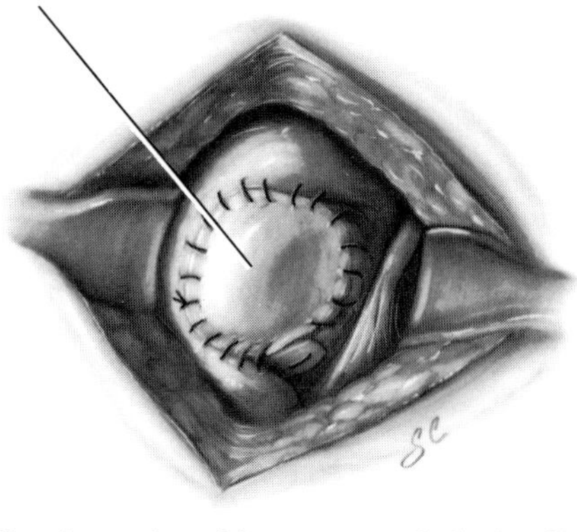

FIGURE 55–11. The suture line is continued in a counterclockwise direction until the defect is completely closed. The ventriculotomy can then be closed with a double line of continuous suture material.

ROSS M. UNGERLEIDER, M.D.

56
Tetralogy of Fallot

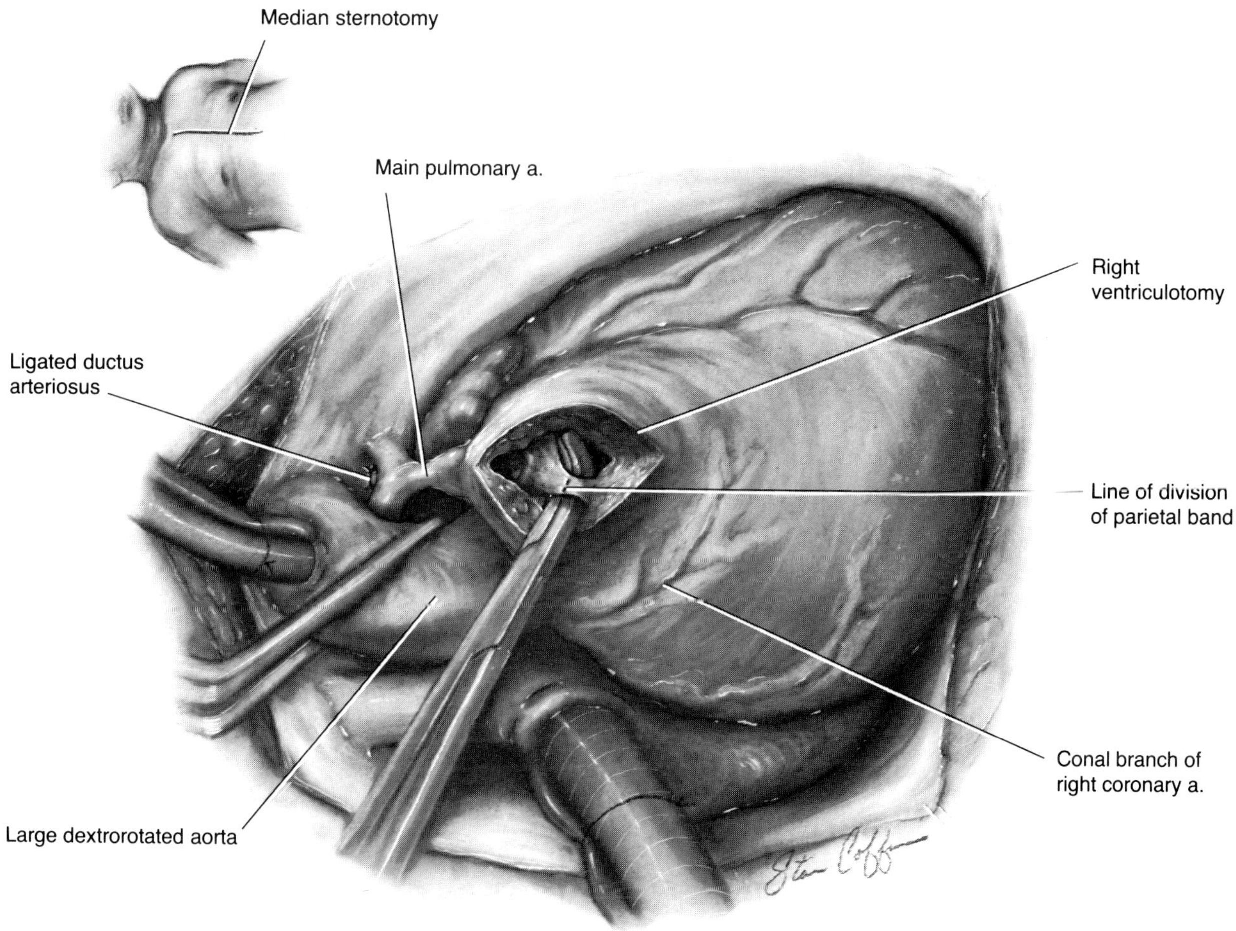

FIGURE 56–1. The heart is exposed through a median sternotomy, and the anatomy should be carefully inspected. In particular, the presence of a persistent left superior vena cava, an anomalous coronary artery crossing the right ventricular (RV) outflow tract, or anomalies of the pulmonary artery that might interfere with complete repair should be noted. After it has been determined that the patient has no contraindication to complete repair, he or she can receive heparin, and cannulae are placed for cardiopulmonary bypass. Venous return can be accomplished through bicaval cannulation or with a single atrial cannula. The latter can be used during continuous flow on small infants if the ventricular septal defect (VSD) is to be closed through a ventriculotomy, or for any approach to the ventricular septal defect if a period of circulatory arrest is to be used. After the patient has been cooled on cardiopulmonary bypass, the aorta is crossclamped and the heart is arrested with cardioplegic solution. Even when a transannular patch may be necessary, the initial incision is made in the infundibular portion of the right ventricular outflow tract, and the parietal band of the infundibular septum is divided over a right-angle clamp. This ventriculotomy should be limited in its extent to the RV outflow portion of the heart.

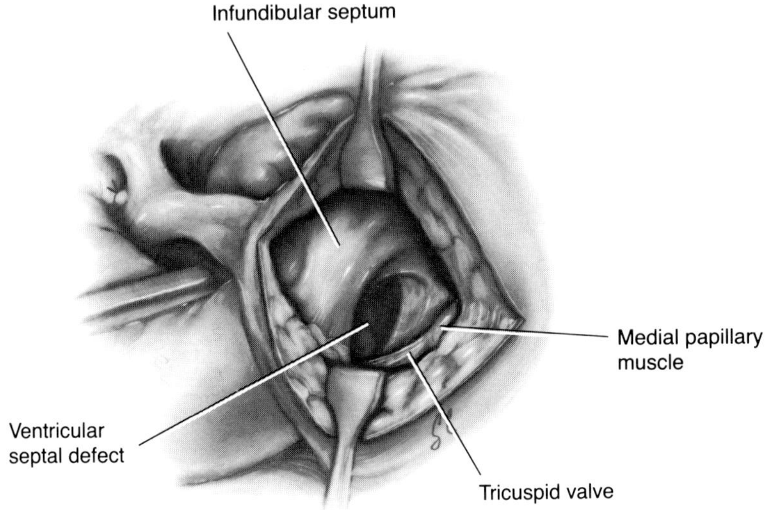

FIGURE 56–2. With the parietal band resected, it is possible to visualize the ventricular septal defect through the small ventriculotomy incision. In many cases, and especially if there is no concomitant large atrial septal defect, it is convenient to close the ventricular septal defect through this limited ventriculotomy.

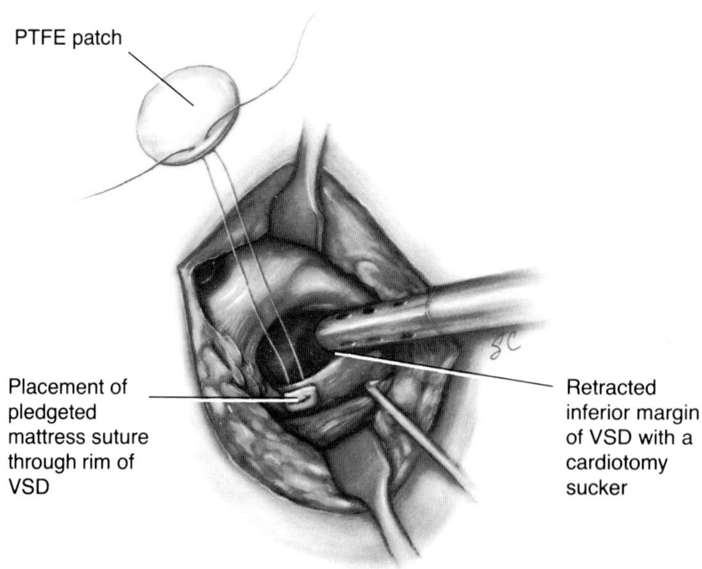

FIGURE 56–3. A cardiotomy sucker is placed through the ventricular septal defect to help expose the borders of the defect. The defect should be closed with a prosthetic patch (usually Gore-Tex), and the suture line can be placed either with continuous monofilament suture material or with interrupted sutures placed around the border of the defect.

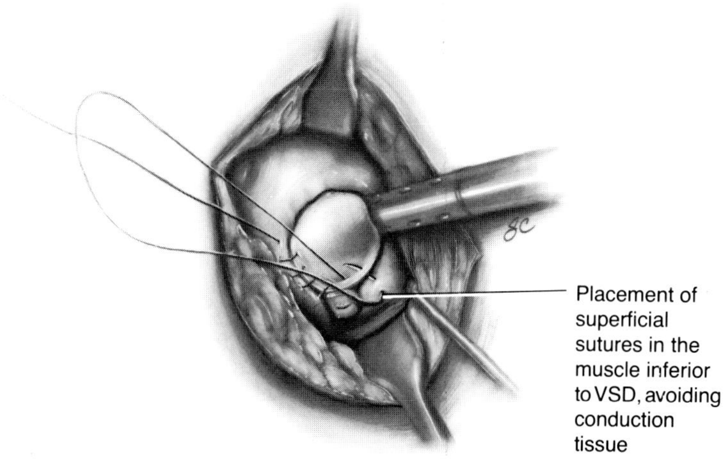

FIGURE 56–4. A continuous suture line has the advantage of efficiency and avoids the difficulty of tying multiple sutures through the small incision, which might tear the fragile muscle around the ventricular septal defect. This suture line is usually continued superiorly up the ventricular infundibular fold until it reaches the infundibular septum, and then posteriorly and inferiorly along the superficial right ventricular surface of the defect (to avoid injuring the conduction tissue).

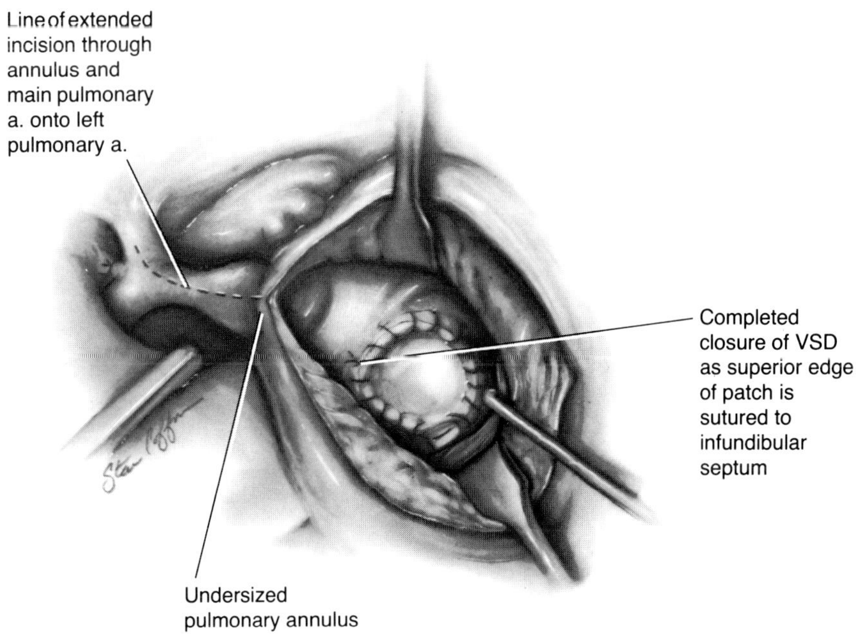

FIGURE 56–5. This inferior suture line is brought around the border of the defect in a counter-clockwise direction until the defect is closed. The pulmonary annulus is then inspected, and if it is felt that the annulus and valve restrict adequate RV outflow, the ventricular incision can be extended *(dashed line)* across the pulmonary valve annulus and on to the main pulmonary artery, extending past the pulmonary bifurcation toward the left pulmonary artery.

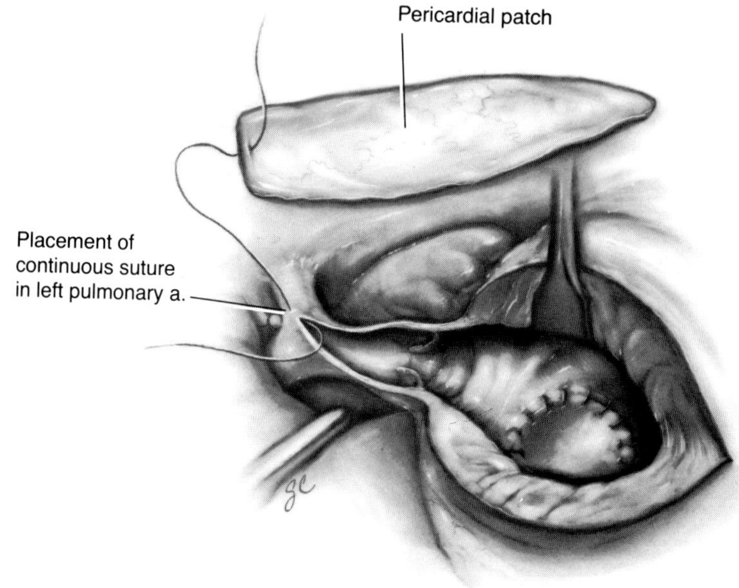

FIGURE 56–6. The transannular incision is repaired with a patch of pericardium (or Gore-Tex) placed with continuous suture material. The distal extent of this patch should be broad, so as not to produce narrowing of the left pulmonary artery origin.

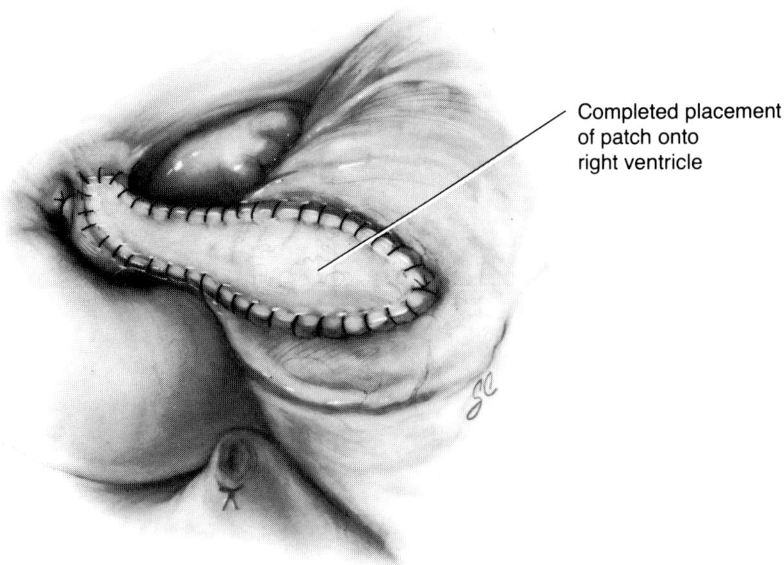

FIGURE 56–7. Once the outflow patch has been completed, the crossclamp can be removed and the patient can be weaned from cardiopulmonary bypass.

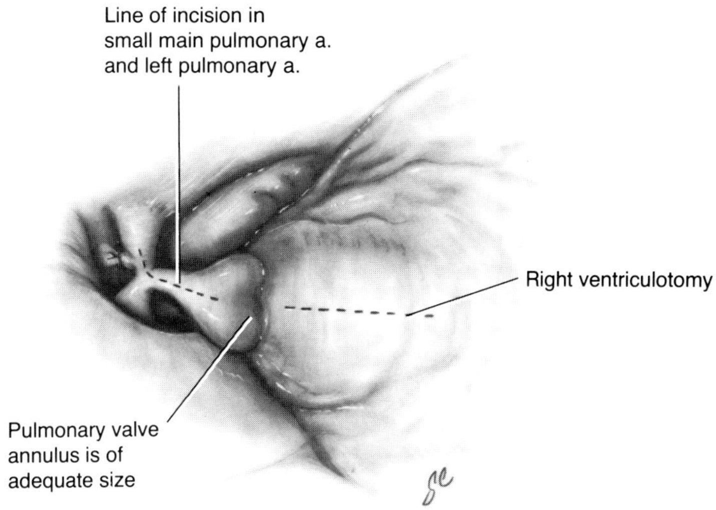

FIGURE 56–8. In many circumstances, the pulmonary valve is of sufficient size that every effort should be made to preserve it. In these instances, the main pulmonary artery above the valve may need to be enlarged with a separate supra-annular incision. A limited ventriculotomy can be performed below the valve for resection of the infundibular muscle and closure of the ventricular septal defect. Alternatively, the VSD can be closed and the obstructing muscle can be resected through a right atrial incision, thus avoiding the need for any incision on the right ventricle.

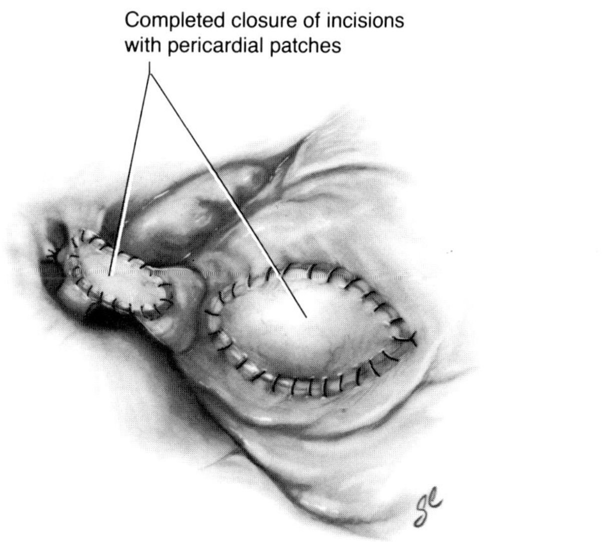

FIGURE 56–9. Both of these incisions can be closed with a patch. If the pulmonary valve is stenotic, a valvotomy along the areas of commissural fusion can be performed through the supra-annular incision. Whenever a transatrial muscle resection and VSD closure is performed, this incision in the main pulmonary artery is necessary to facilitate relief of the RV outflow obstruction, and a supra-annular patch, as described, is necessary.

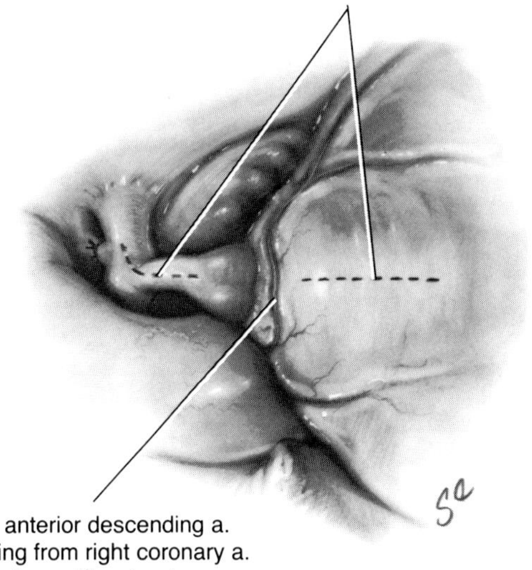

FIGURE 56–10. In patients with an anomalous left anterior descending coronary artery arising from the right coronary artery, a transannular incision should not be performed. In these patients, repair can be accomplished through a transatrial approach or through separate incisions in the infundibular portion of the right ventricle and in the main pulmonary artery (PA), which can be patched separately if the pulmonary valve annulus is adequate (as shown in Fig. 56–9).

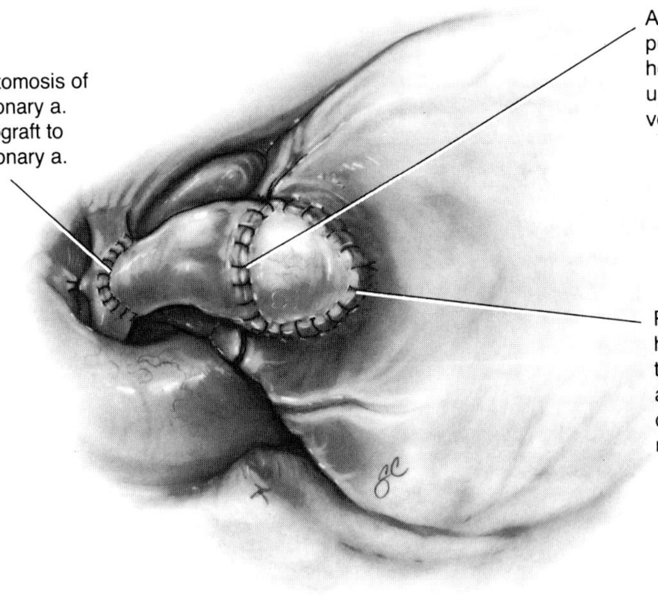

FIGURE 56–11. A pulmonary homograft also can be used to establish RV-to-PA continuity. When a homograft is used to establish RV-to-PA continuity, the anomalous coronary artery courses below the homograft, and its location near the superior aspect of the ventricular incision must be appreciated at the time of eventual conduit replacement.

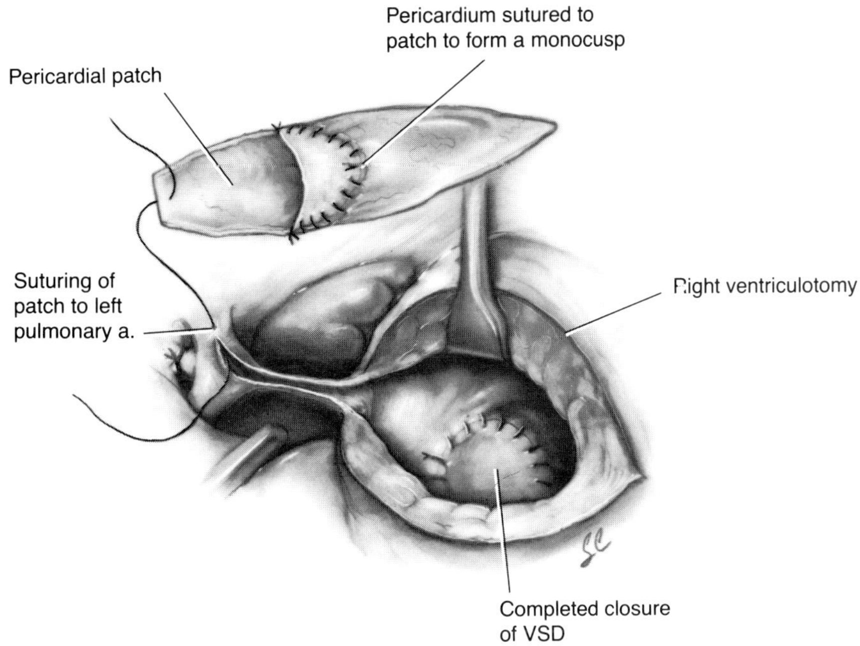

FIGURE 56–12. In patients with extremely hypoplastic main pulmonary arteries, RV outflow reconstruction can be performed with a pericardial patch, and in some instances it is helpful to construct a monocusp valve in this patch using a small piece of autologous pericardium. This technique is especially useful when performing total correction of pulmonary atresia with VSD ("Tet atresia") in infancy.

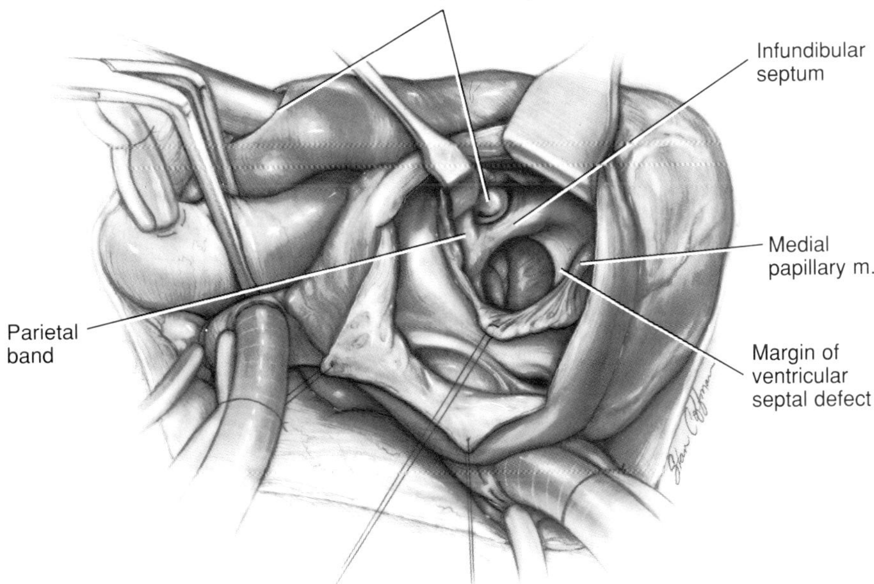

FIGURE 56–13. Another option for patients with tetralogy who have a normal pulmonary valve annulus or for those with an anomalous coronary artery crossing the RV outflow tract is to perform the resection of ventricular muscle by a transatrial approach. This requires bicaval cannulation for venous return (unless circulatory arrest is to be used, in which case single atrial cannulation with removal of the atrial cannula during the arrest period is an alternative). The aorta is crossclamped, and the heart is protected with cardioplegia. A right atriotomy is performed, and the leaflets of the tricuspid valve are retracted to expose the ventricular septal defect. A dilator is placed through the pulmonary valve via an incision in the main pulmonary artery. This dilator helps the surgeon identify the RV outflow tract in relation to the infundibular septum, as viewed through the tricuspid valve. This also allows the surgeon to identify the parietal muscle band, which lies just behind the anterior leaflet of the tricuspid valve.

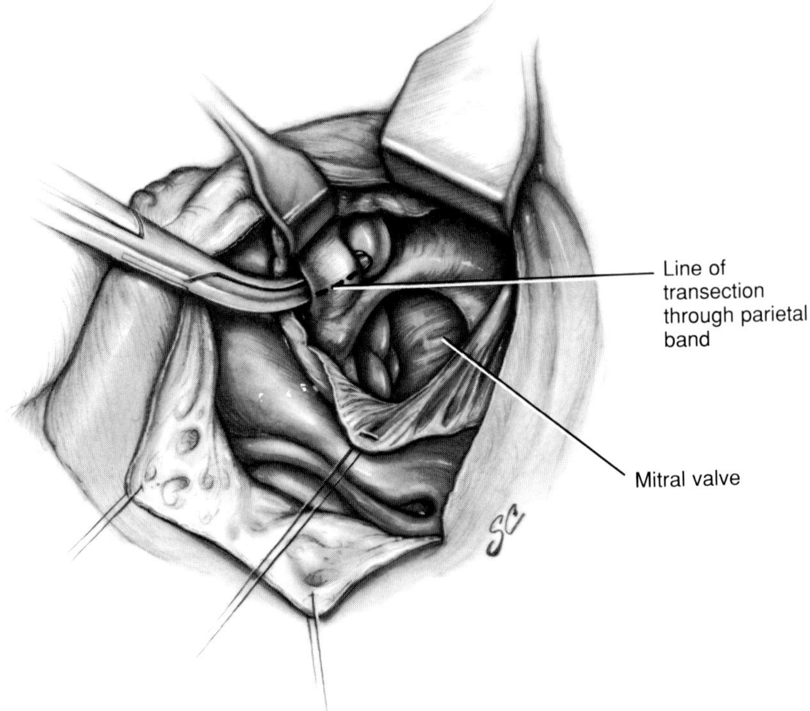

FIGURE 56–14. A clamp is placed behind the parietal band so that it can be divided.

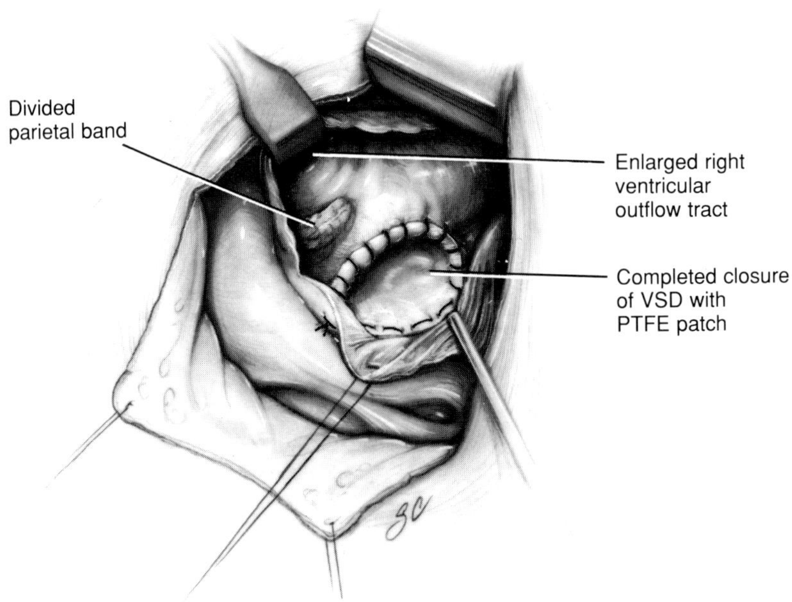

FIGURE 56–15. When the parietal band is divided, the infundibular septum will move posteriorly and enlarge the RV outflow tract. The ventricular septal defect can then be closed with a prosthetic patch using the usual transatrial technique.

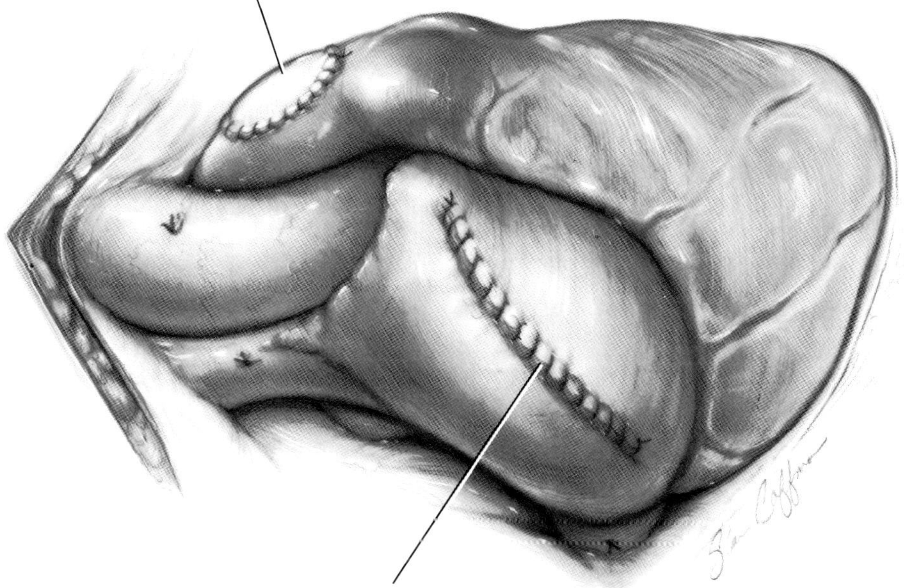

FIGURE 56–16. The completed transatrial repair demonstrates a patch on the main pulmonary artery (which is recommended to repair the site used to insert the dilator) as well as the closed atriotomy. In many instances, no ventricular incision is necessary. Occasionally, the incision in the main pulmonary artery can be extended across the pulmonary valve annulus and then patched if it is necessary to enlarge this area. After the surgeon has obtained experience with this method, it is possible to perform this repair without insertion of a Hegar dilator through the outflow tract, and in properly selected patients this can prevent the need for a patch on the main pulmonary artery.

ROSS M. UNGERLEIDER, M.D.

57 Truncus Arteriosus

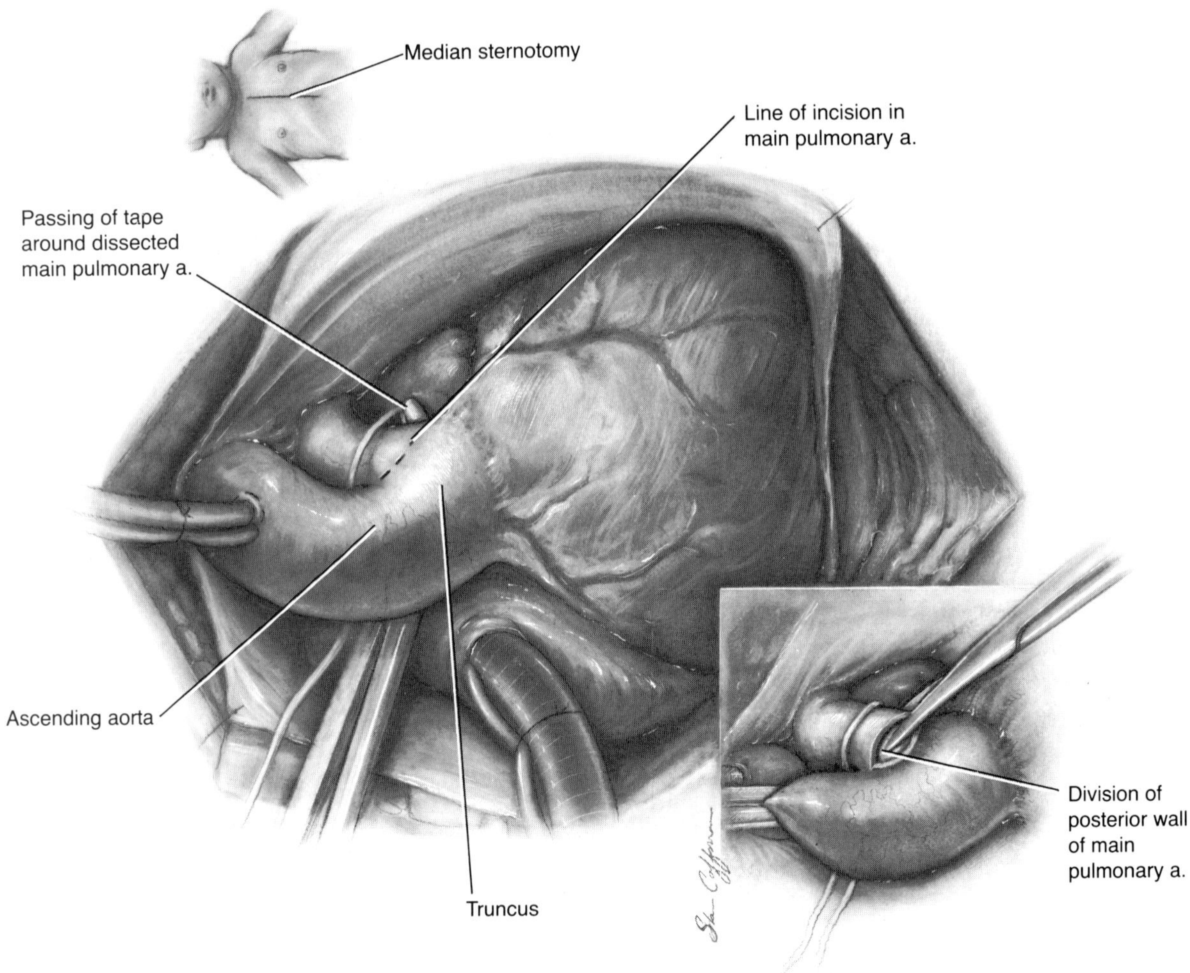

FIGURE 57–1. The heart is exposed through a median sternotomy. Care is taken to avoid excessive manipulation. The physiology of truncus arteriosus can cause excessive diastolic "runoff" into the pulmonary vasculature, with resulting coronary ischemia such that these patients have a high risk for ventricular fibrillation. The main pulmonary artery is encircled with a ligature by placing it between the aorta and pulmonary artery and then pulling it through the transverse sinus. This tie is placed on a snare, which can be occluded as soon as the patient is placed on cardiopulmonary bypass. This prevents excessive perfusion of the pulmonary vasculature during bypass. A cannula with an arterial inflow is placed in the ascending aorta, and a single venous cannula in the right atrium. Immediately after placing the patient on bypass, the main pulmonary artery is occluded. The aorta is then crossclamped *(inset),* and the heart is arrested with cardioplegic solution. The snare is released from around the main pulmonary artery, and the pulmonary artery is excised from the side of the aorta. Care must be taken to avoid injury to the branch pulmonary arteries as well as to the ostium of the left coronary artery, which can arise adjacent to the main pulmonary artery takeoff. The defect in the aorta can then be repaired primarily.

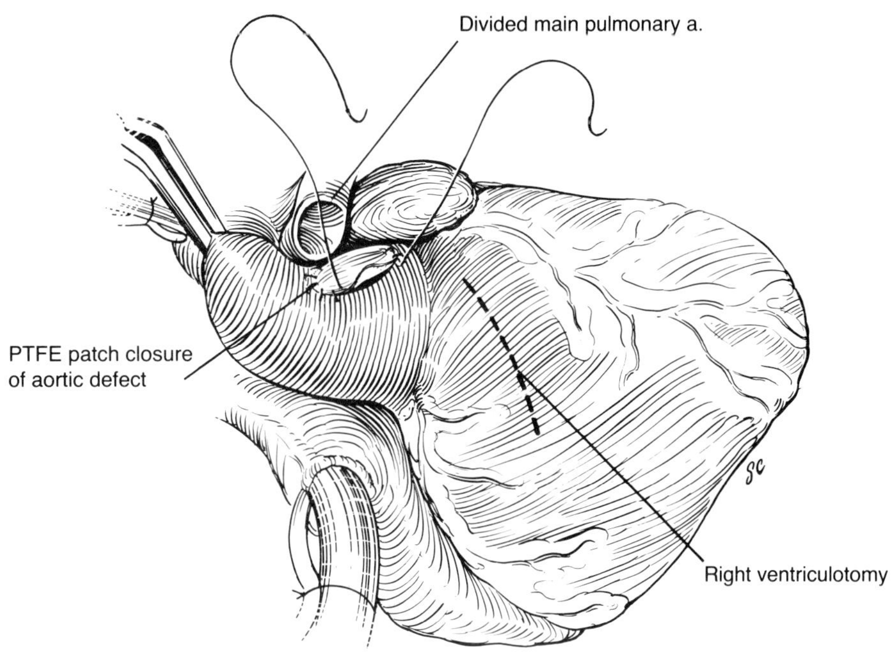

FIGURE 57–2. A ventriculotomy is made on the anterior surface of the right ventricle, as indicated by the dashed line. The defect in the aorta can also be repaired with a patch of homograft or pericardium.

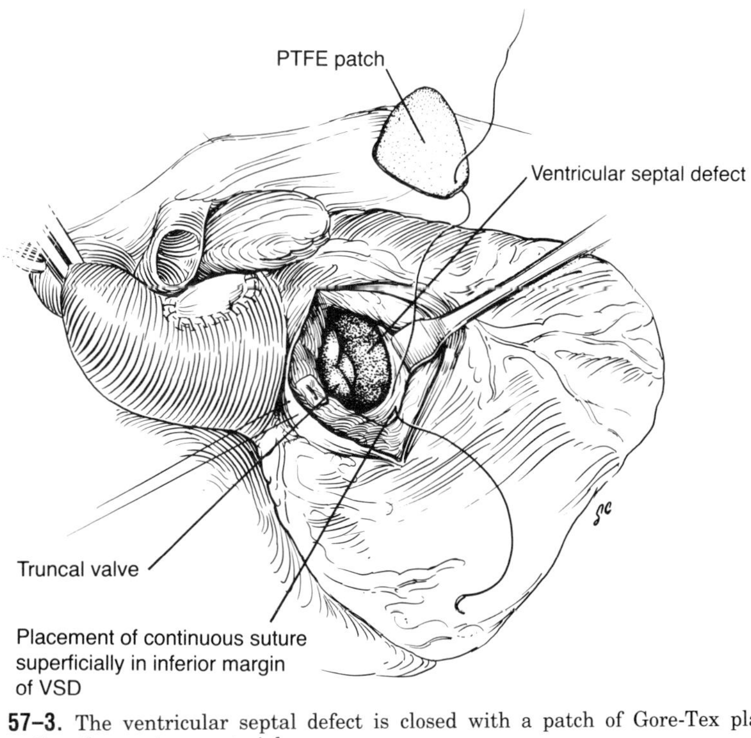

FIGURE 57–3. The ventricular septal defect is closed with a patch of Gore-Tex placed with continuous Surgilene suture material.

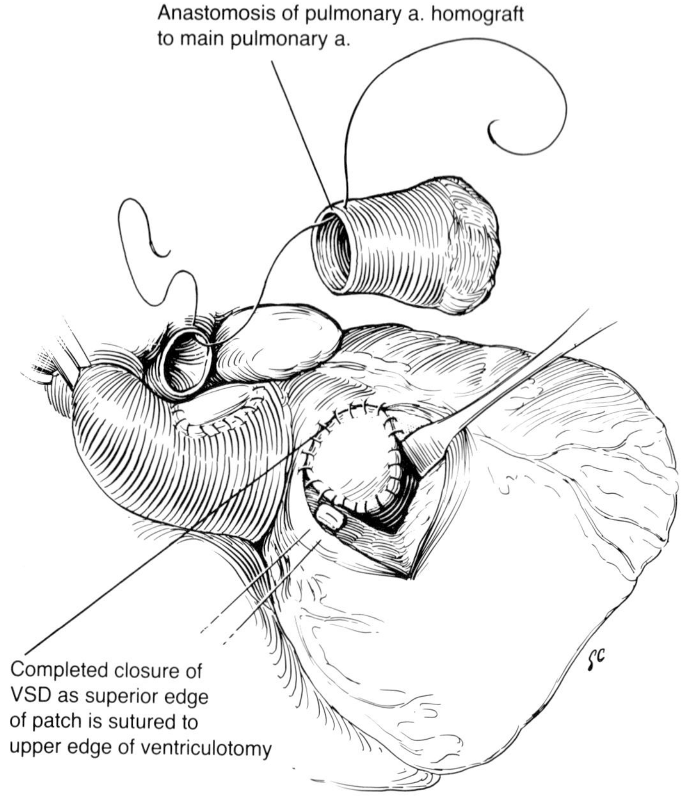

FIGURE 57–4. The uppermost part of this patch is attached to the anterior surface of the right ventricle. A pulmonary homograft is then trimmed and sewn to the distal pulmonary arteries using continuous suture material.

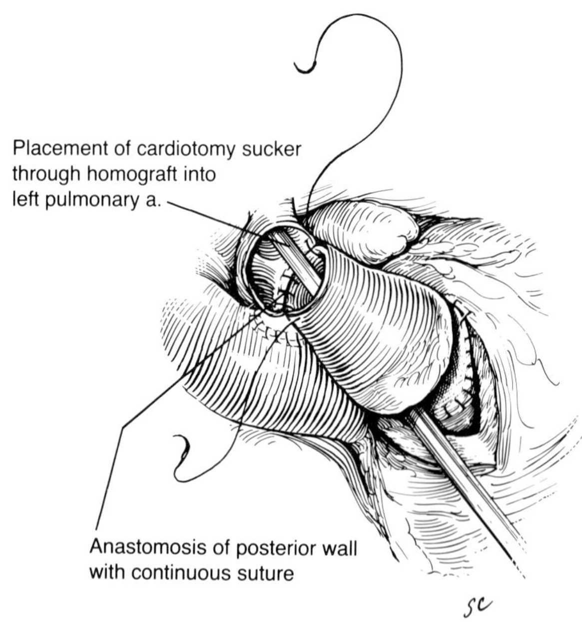

FIGURE 57–5. During the anastomosis of the homograft to the distal pulmonary artery, it is sometimes helpful to place a cardiotomy sucker through the homograft and into the pulmonary arteries to enhance visualization.

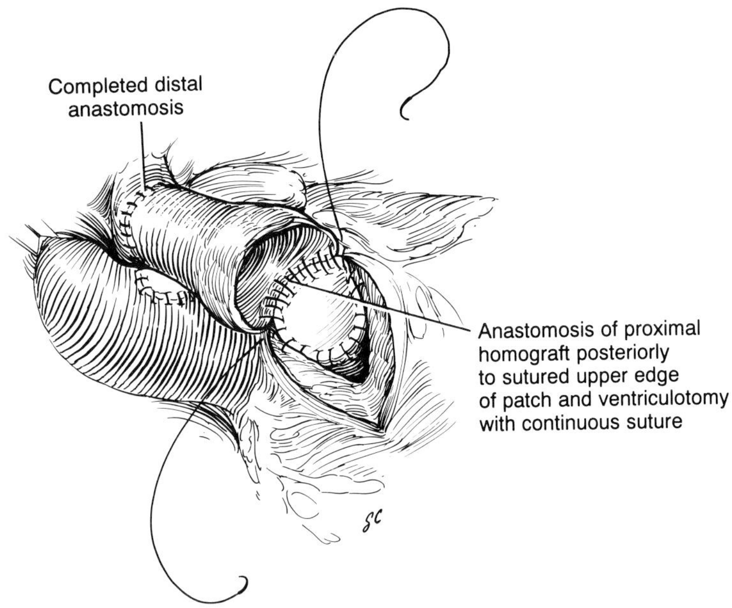

FIGURE 57–6. The proximal homograft is secured to the superior aspect of the ventriculotomy incision with a continuous suture line along the posterior border.

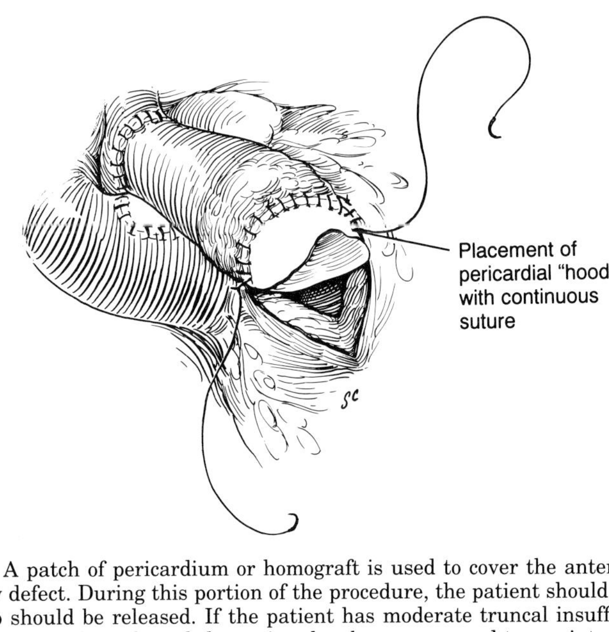

FIGURE 57–7. A patch of pericardium or homograft is used to cover the anterior portion of the ventriculotomy defect. During this portion of the procedure, the patient should be rewarmed and the crossclamp should be released. If the patient has moderate truncal insufficiency, the crossclamp should not be released until the patient has been rewarmed to a point at which the heart begins contracting, so that the patient will be able to eject the regurgitant volume.

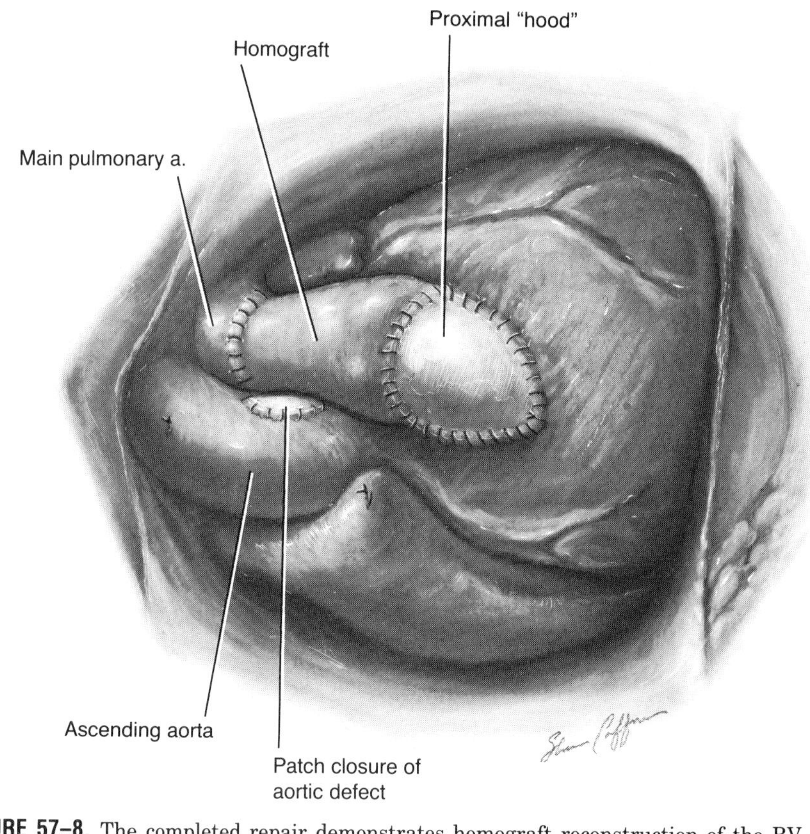

FIGURE 57–8. The completed repair demonstrates homograft reconstruction of the RV outflow tract and patch closure of the defect in the medial aspect of the aorta from where the main pulmonary artery was removed.

ROSS M. UNGERLEIDER, M.D.

58
Congenital Aortic Stenosis

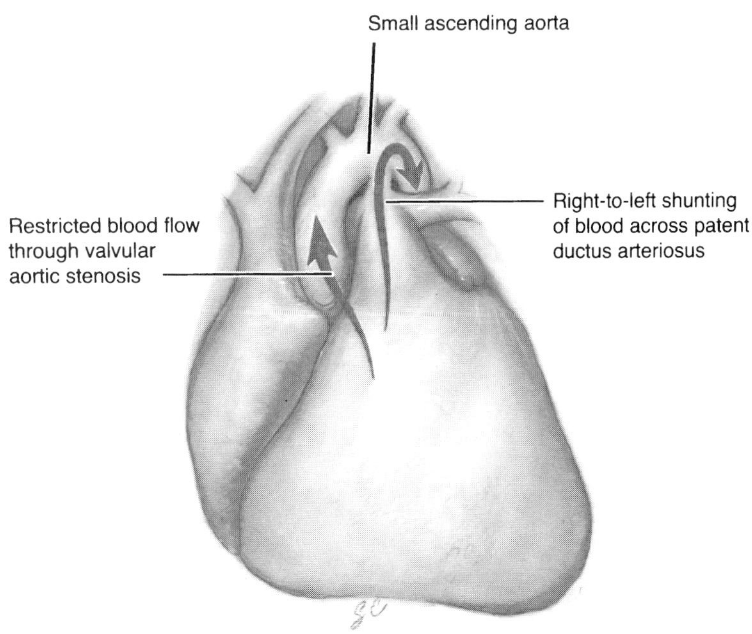

FIGURE 58–1. The physiology of critical aortic stenosis in infancy is benefited by patency of the ductus arteriosus. This allows right ventricular outflow to assist with perfusion of the aorta and provides a method for decompressing the pulmonary hypertension that is often associated with this defect. It is for this reason that these patients often require infusion of prostaglandin E_1 (PGE_1) until more definitive therapy is available.

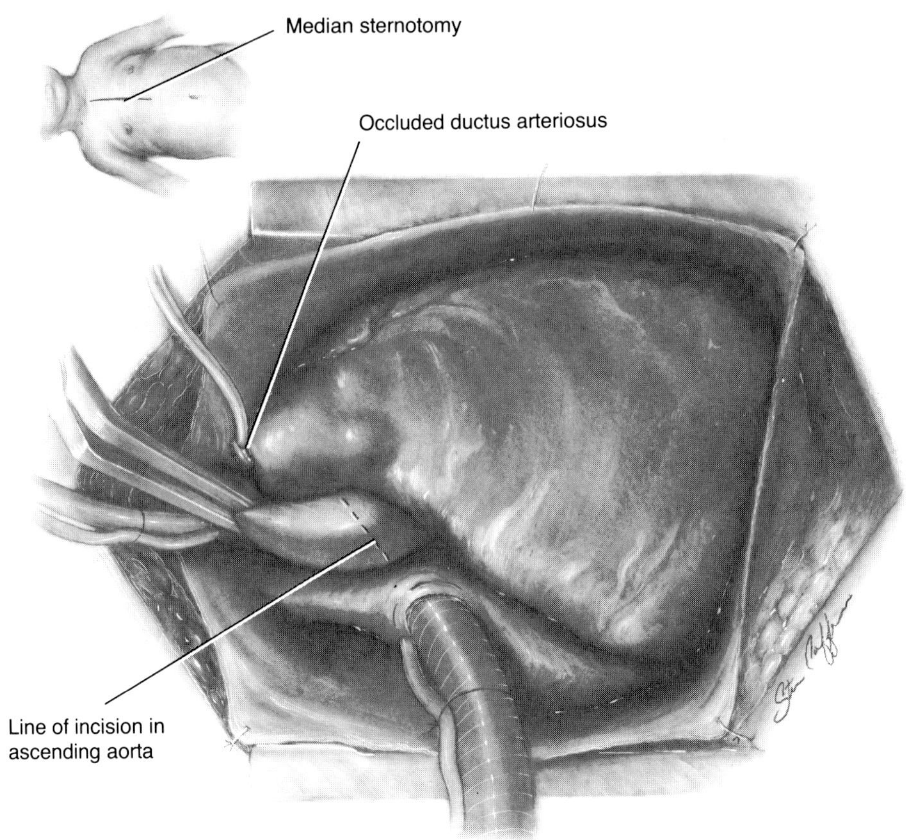

FIGURE 58–2. In neonates with critical aortic stenosis who require valvotomy, the heart is approached through a median sternotomy, and the patient is cannulated for cardiopulmonary bypass using a single atrial cannula. Bypass is begun with a cold (7°C) prime, and immediately after inception of cardiopulmonary bypass, the ductus arteriosus is occluded with a snare. An aortic crossclamp is placed, and the transverse incision is made in the ascending aorta. It is not necessary to provide cardioplegic solution in infants. Rewarming on bypass is begun immediately after the aorta is crossclamped.

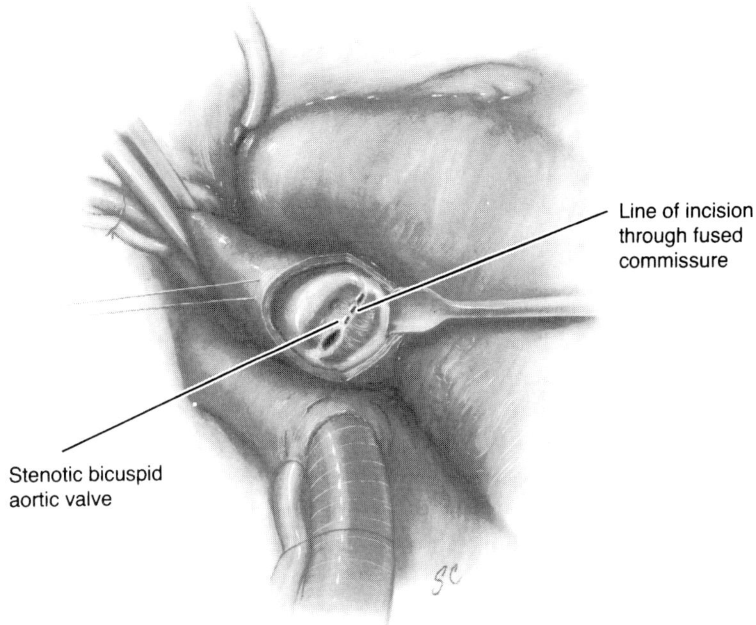

FIGURE 58–3. The stenotic aortic valve is inspected through the aortotomy incision, and the areas of commissural fusion are identified.

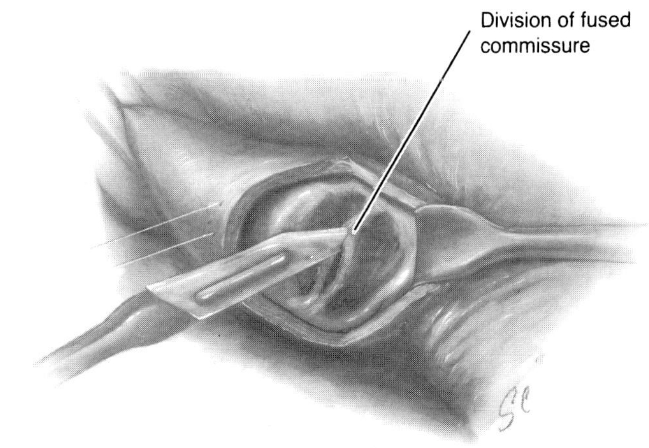

FIGURE 58–4. The fused commissures are usually opened using a knife blade, and the incision should be extended toward the annulus at either extreme. It is important, however, to keep the incision from extending into the annulus, so that postvalvotomy aortic insufficiency is minimized.

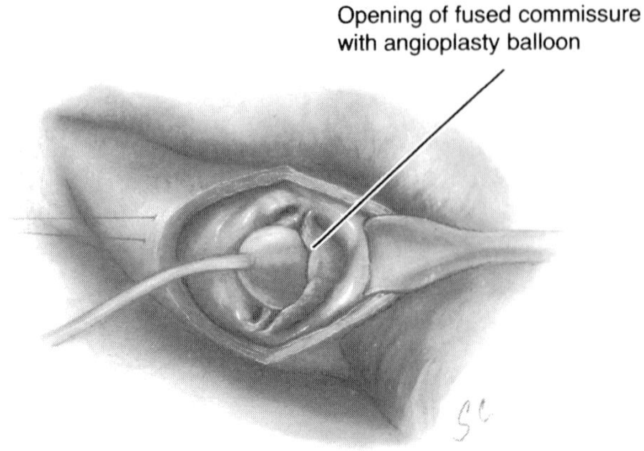

FIGURE 58–5. It is possible to perform the valvotomy with a balloon angioplasty catheter, if one is available.

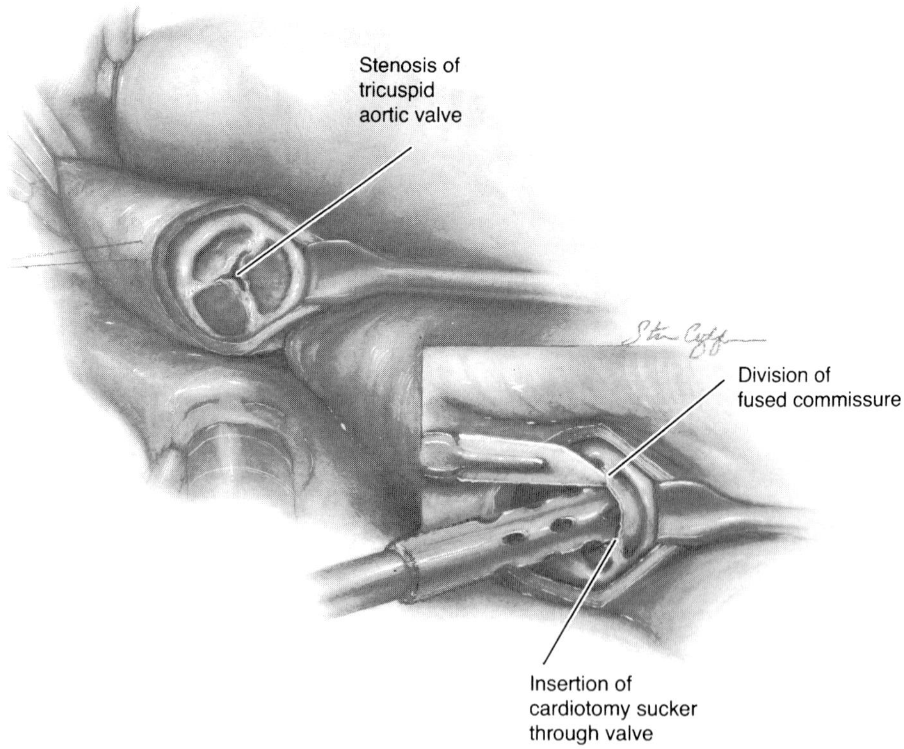

FIGURE 58–6. In some patients with dysplastic but tricommissural aortic valves, it is helpful to insert a cardiotomy sucker through the valve to enable careful incision of all fused commissures.

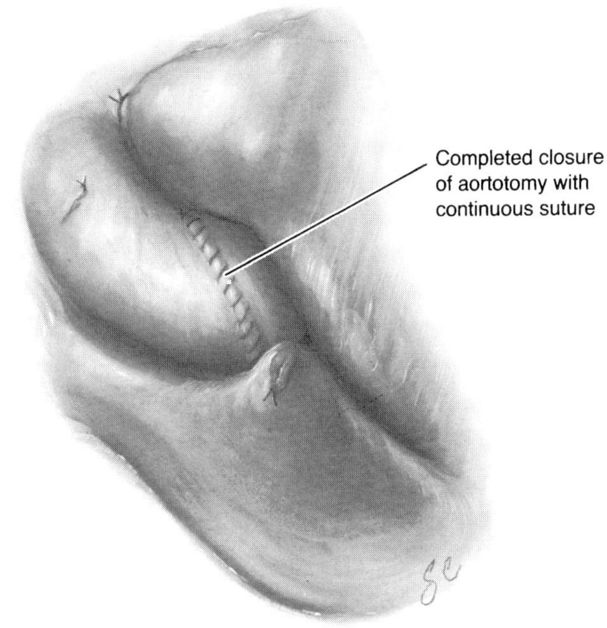

FIGURE 58–7. The aortotomy is repaired with a double line of continuous suture, and the patient is weaned from cardiopulmonary bypass. The ductus arteriosus should be ligated if the patient is stable; but if the patient has persistent pulmonary hypertension and low cardiac output, the ductus can be left open and the patient maintained on prostaglandin infusion during the initial postoperative course, until left ventricular compliance and forward cardiac output through the left ventricle improve.

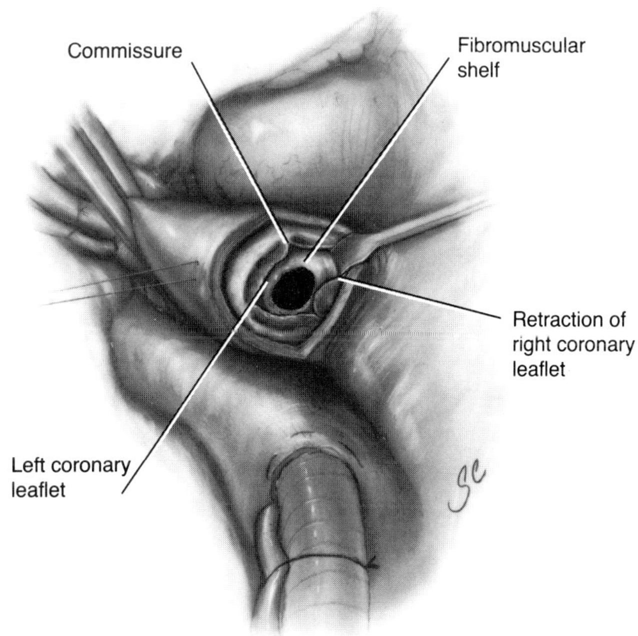

FIGURE 58–8. Subaortic stenosis that is discrete is approached through an aortotomy after the aorta is clamped. Since these patients are usually older and well beyond the neonatal period, it is convenient and helpful to protect the heart with cardioplegic solution. The aortic valve leaflets are carefully retracted, and the fibromuscular shelf can usually be identified below the right and left coronary leaflets.

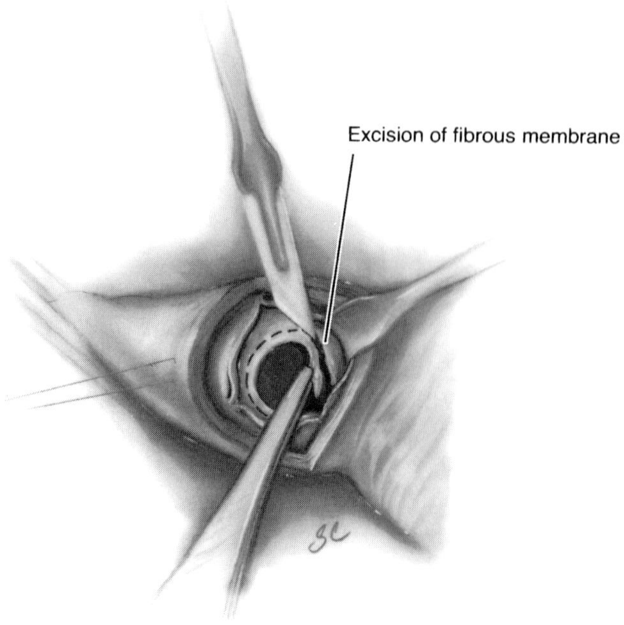

FIGURE 58–9. This membrane is carefully excised with a combination of sharp and blunt dissection. It is important to appreciate the location of the conduction tissue between the noncoronary and right coronary cusps and to avoid deep incision into the interventricular septum in this region.

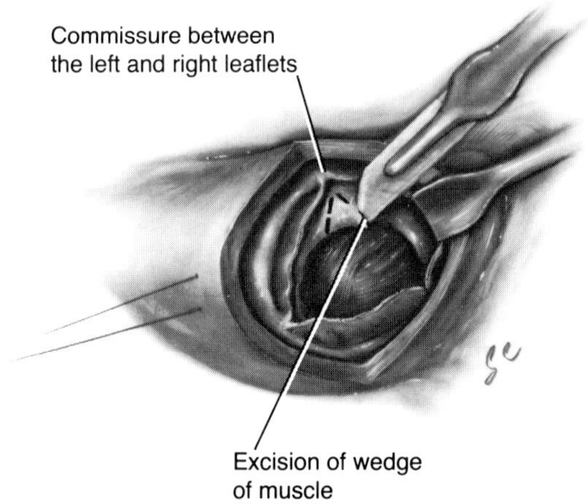

FIGURE 58–10. After the membrane has been completely excised, it is beneficial to remove a wedge of muscle from the interventricular septum below the right and left coronary leaflets. This is a safe region for muscle excision, which does not risk the conduction tissue and which produces further disruption of the fibromuscular ridge.

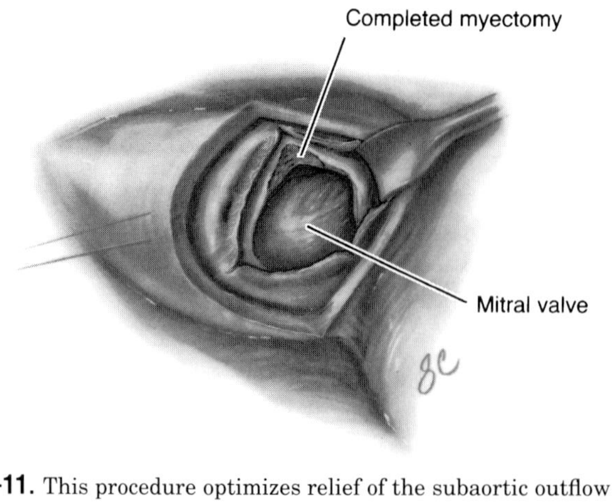

FIGURE 58–11. This procedure optimizes relief of the subaortic outflow obstruction.

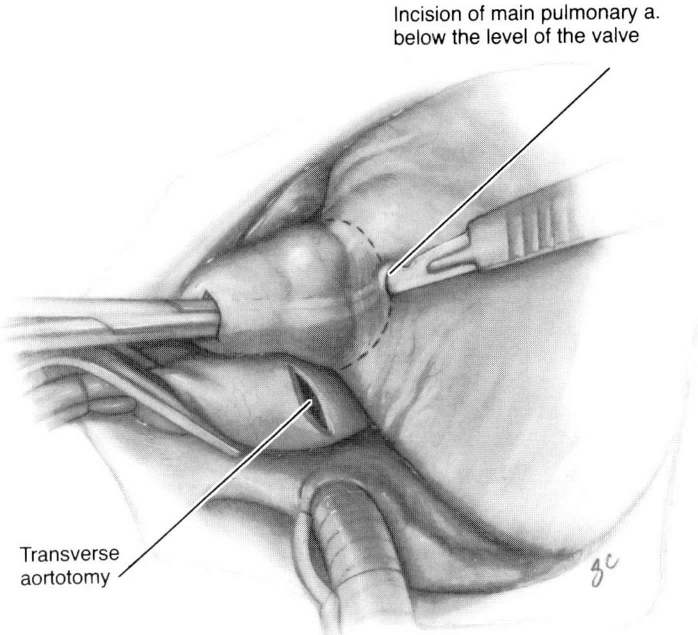

FIGURE 58–12. In patients with severe aortic valve disease who require aortic valve replacement, a pulmonary autograft procedure can be selected in appropriate circumstances. It is currently our preference to use this procedure in young infants in whom the only other alternative for aortic valve replacement would be an extensive annulus-enlarging procedure. After the patient is placed on cardiopulmonary bypass, the aorta is crossclamped and the heart is protected with cardioplegic solution. The aortic valve is inspected through a transverse aortotomy to ensure that it is nonrepairable and that it must be replaced. An incision is then made in the anterior surface of the main pulmonary artery near its junction with the right pulmonary artery. A right-angle clamp is then placed across the pulmonary valve and used to dimple the surface of the right ventricular (RV) outflow tract proximal to the valve leaflets. Incision is made in the RV outflow tract at this point with a knife blade.

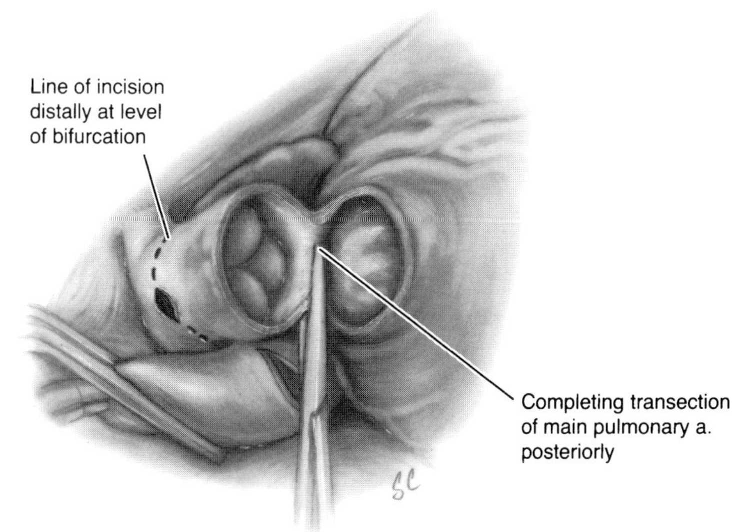

FIGURE 58–13. The proximal portion of the pulmonary valve is excised, with care taken not to damage the pulmonary valve leaflets. The incision along the posterior aspect of the valve should be more horizontal than vertical, to avoid extending deeply into the interventricular septum and risking damage to the first septal perforating branch of the left anterior descending coronary artery.

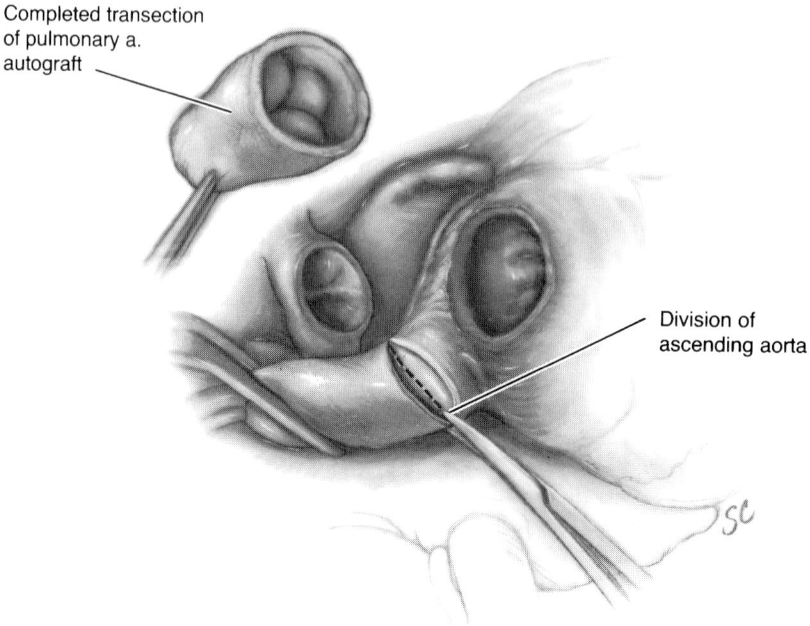

FIGURE 58–14. After the proximal portion of the pulmonary valve has been removed, the distal pulmonary artery is transected at the level of the bifurcation. The transverse aortotomy is then extended so that the aorta is completely divided above the aortic valve.

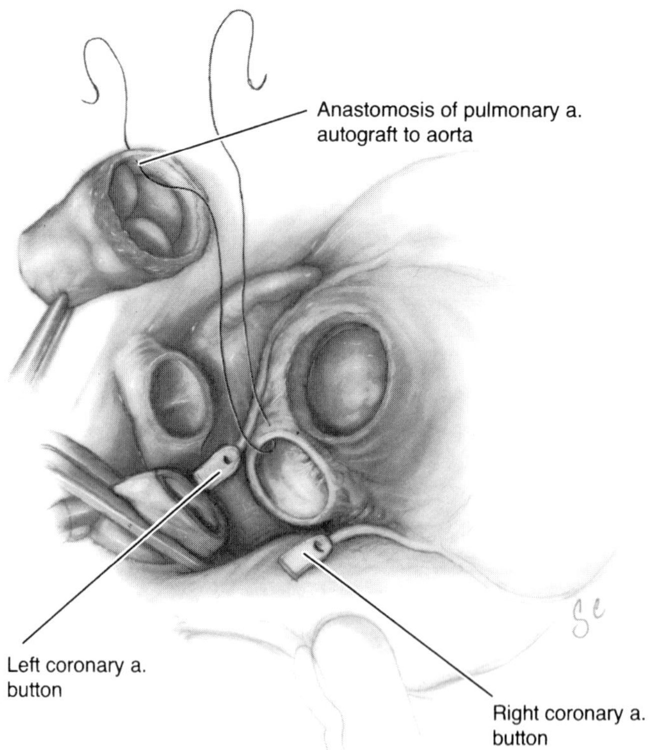

FIGURE 58–15. The coronary arteries are removed as buttons with large amounts of adjacent sinus material. They are gently retracted out of the operative field using fine suture material. The aortic valve and the excess aortic wall tissue are removed from the base of the heart. The pulmonary autograft is then sutured to the base of the heart with continuous suture or interrupted sutures, depending upon the surgeon's preference.

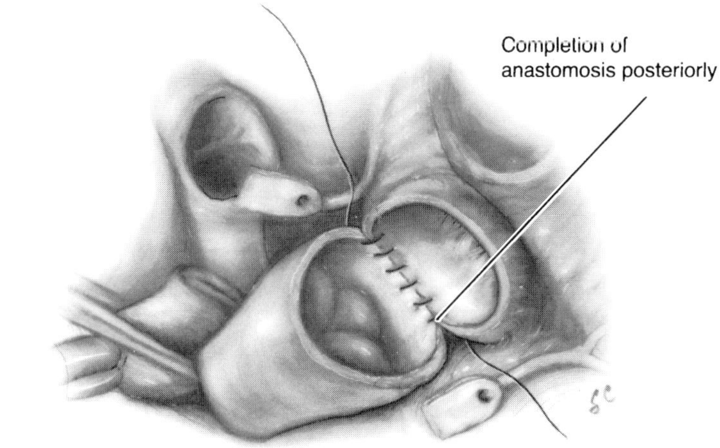

FIGURE 58–16. When a continuous suture line is used, it is best to place the posterior suture line first and to continue the sutures anteriorly along the base of the heart.

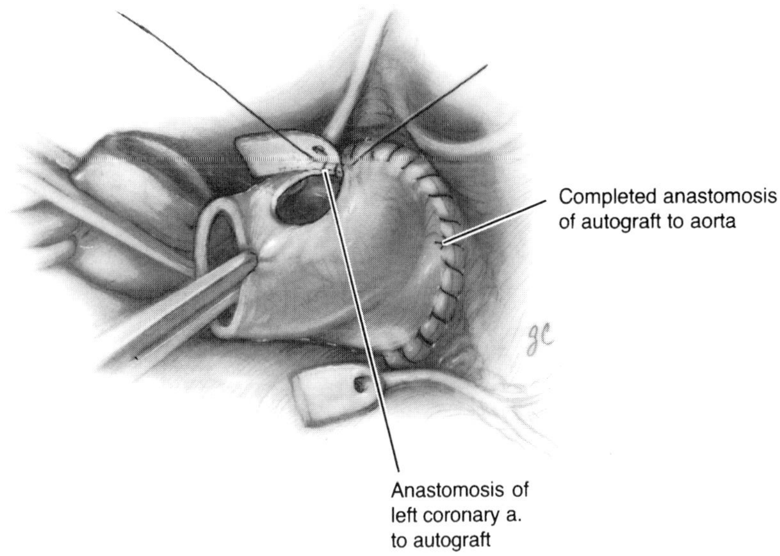

FIGURE 58–17. After the suture line is completed, the left coronary artery is anastomosed to an appropriate portion along the posterior wall of the autograft.

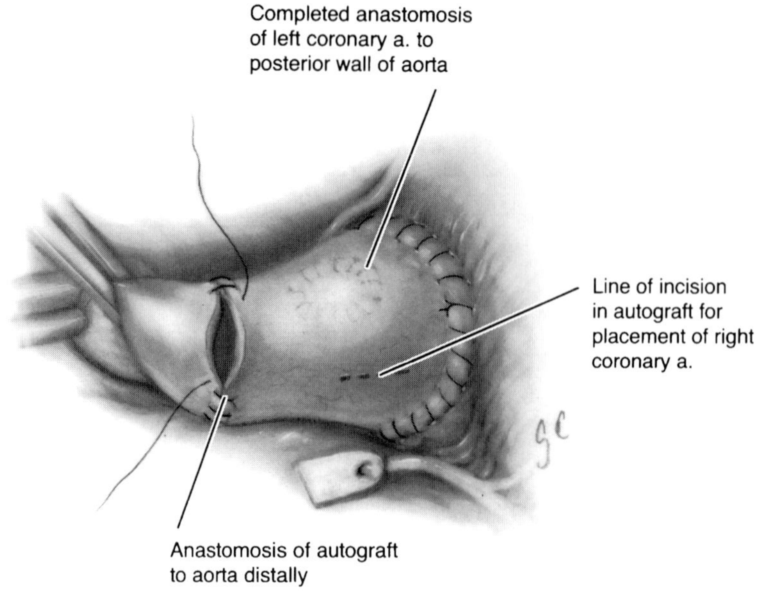

FIGURE 58–18. The autograft is anastomosed to the distal aorta. After this suture line is completed, the neo-aortic root can be distended with a dose of cardioplegic solution, and this will allow determination of the most appropriate spot for placement of the right coronary artery in the expanded autograft. The right coronary anastomosis is then performed before the crossclamp is removed.

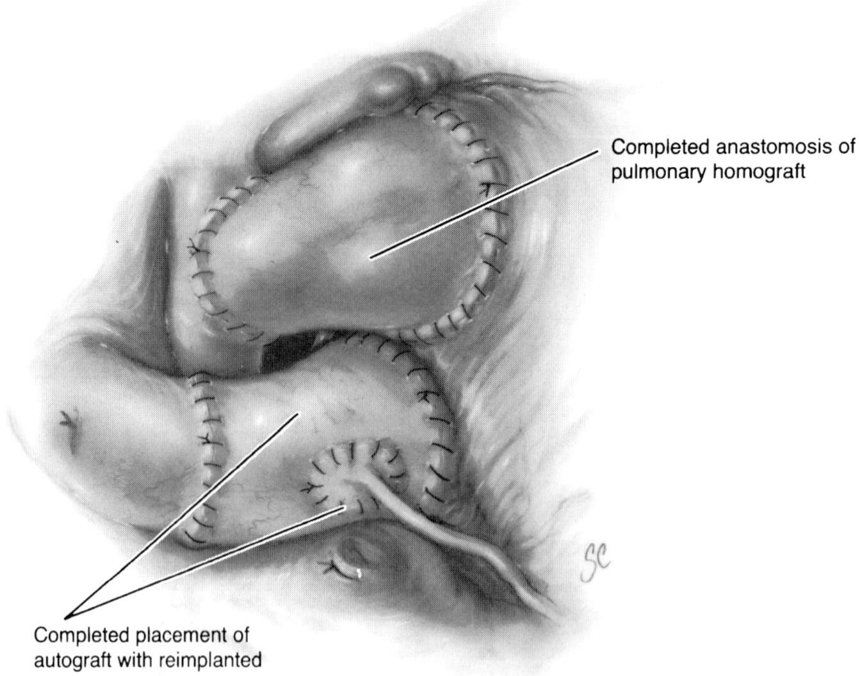

FIGURE 58–19. Continuity between the right ventricle and the pulmonary artery is performed with a cryopreserved homograft (preferably pulmonary), and it is usually easiest to perform the proximal anastomosis first. It is important when performing this anastomosis that the posterior muscle of the right ventricular outflow tract, which was denuded by harvest of the autograft, be carefully inspected for potential bleeding points. In some instances it is useful to place a piece of Teflon felt along this portion of the anastomosis to enhance hemostasis. After completion of all anastomoses, the aortic crossclamp can be removed and the patient can be weaned from cardiopulmonary bypass.

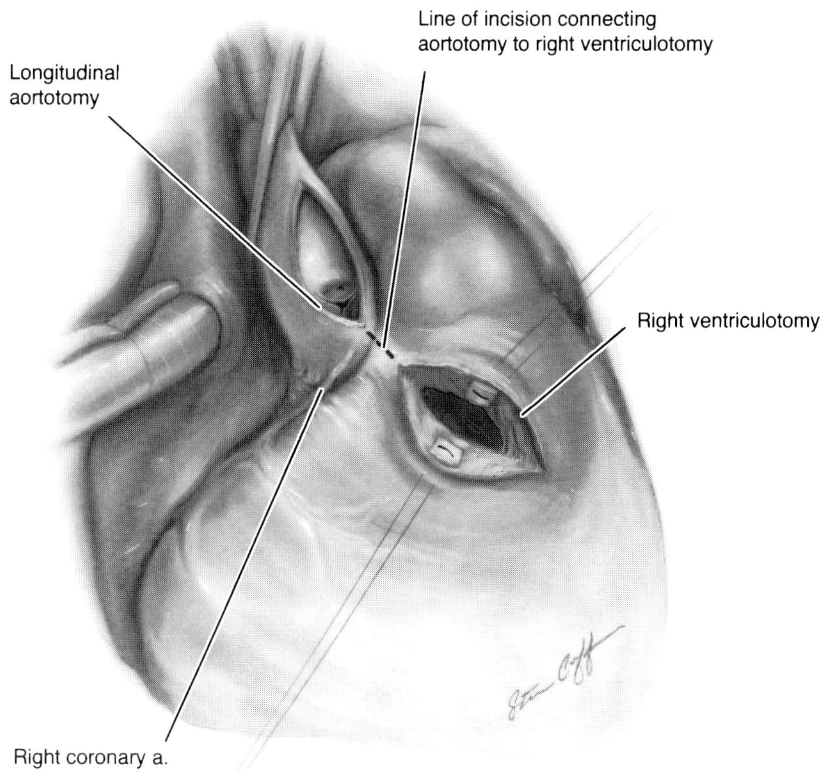

FIGURE 58–20. In patients with significant narrowing of the subvalvular left ventricular outflow tract, a more extensive aortic reconstruction is necessary. This can be performed by protecting the heart with cardioplegia infused proximal to a crossclamp and then joining an aortic incision, which is vertical and aimed to the left of the right coronary artery, with a right ventricular incision, which is performed proximal to the pulmonary valve and also aimed to the left of the right coronary artery.

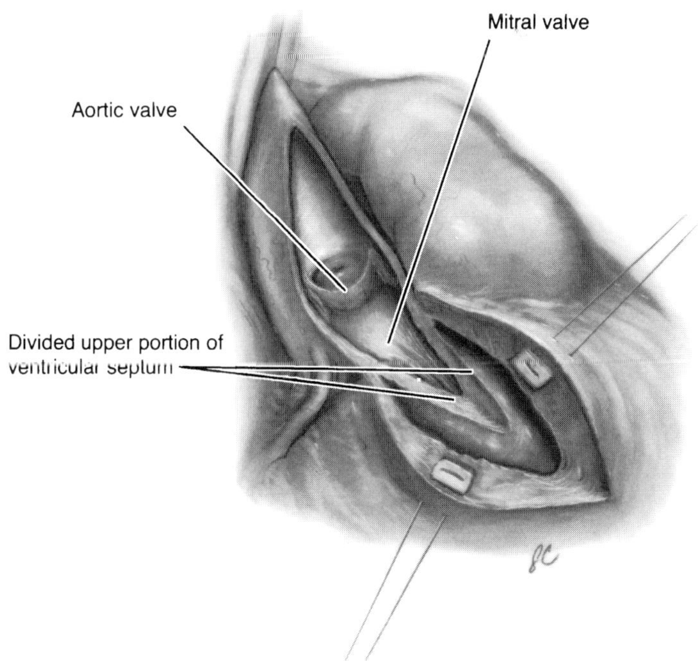

FIGURE 58–21. When these incisions are joined, it is possible to extend an incision across the aortic valve annulus and into the interventricular septum so that the obstruction below the valve can be relieved.

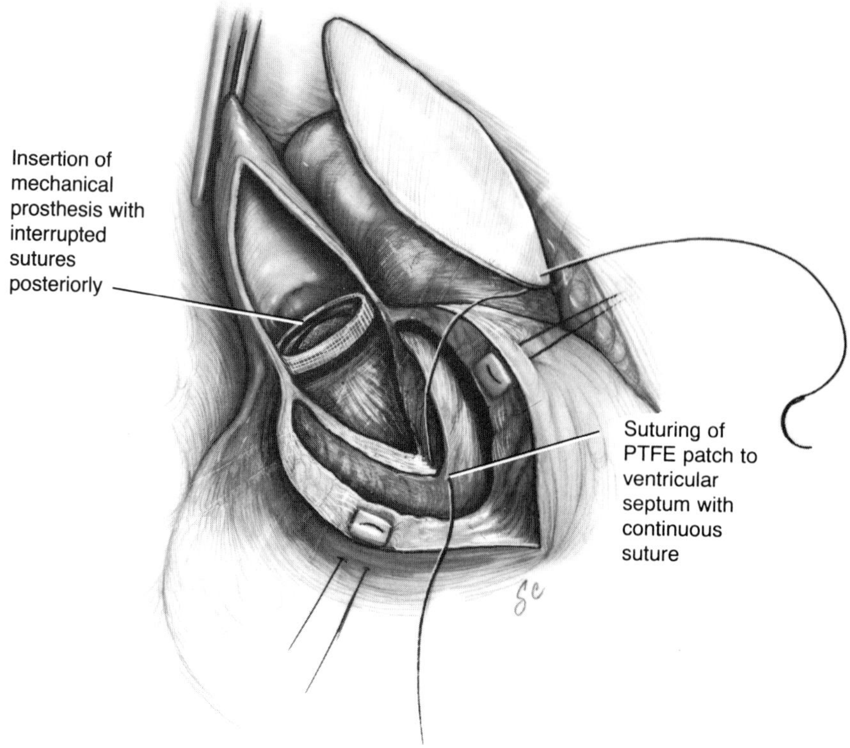

FIGURE 58–22. Reconstruction of the left ventricular outflow tract is performed with a patch of Gore-Tex placed with continuous suture along the edges of the incision in the ventricular septum. The aortic valve is replaced with a prosthetic valve secured posteriorly to its normal location in the annulus.

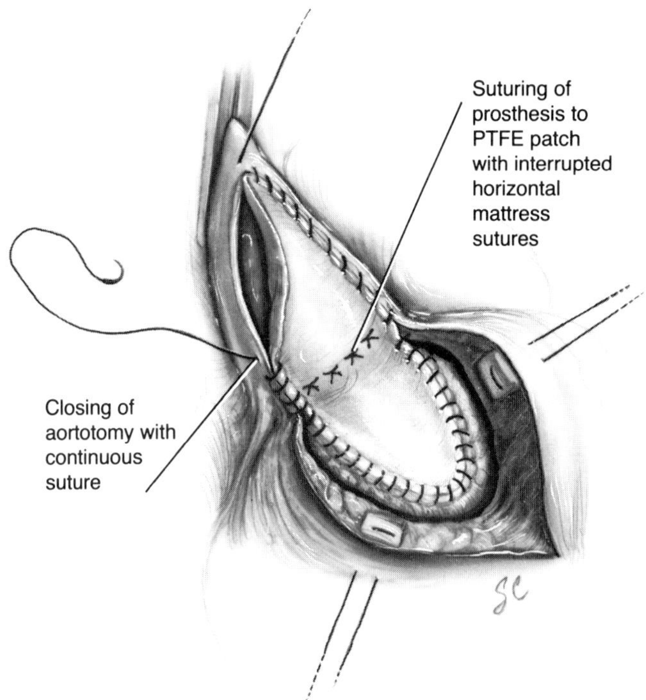

FIGURE 58–23. The Gore-Tex patch is brought over the anterior portion of the prosthetic valve and secured to the valve ring with interrupted sutures. The sutures used to secure the patch to the interventricular septum are then continued along the aorta to complete the left ventricular (LV) outflow reconstruction.

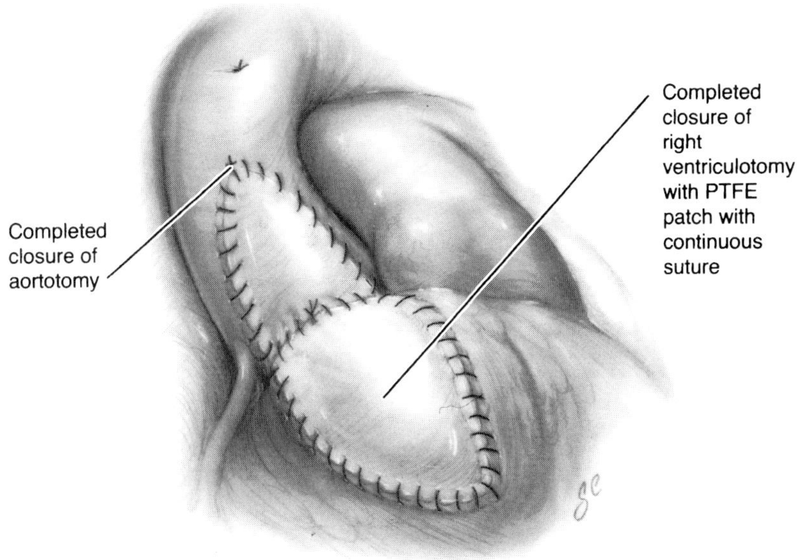

FIGURE 58–24. Reconstruction of the RV outflow tract should be performed with a patch of Gore-Tex or pericardium to provide adequate RV outflow over the enlarged LV outflow tract. The crossclamp can then be removed and the patient weaned from bypass.

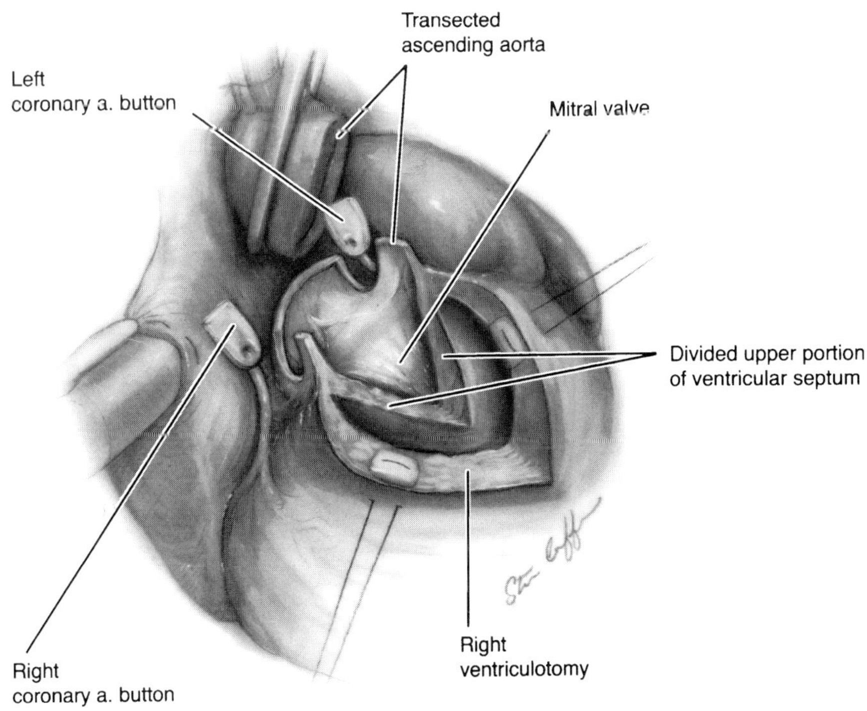

FIGURE 58–25. An aortoventriculoplasty can be performed, using aortic homograft material, by dividing the aorta after the heart has been arrested with cardioplegic solution. The incision into the interventricular septum described in Figure 58–21 is then performed, and the coronary arteries are removed as buttons with a large amount of adjacent sinus material.

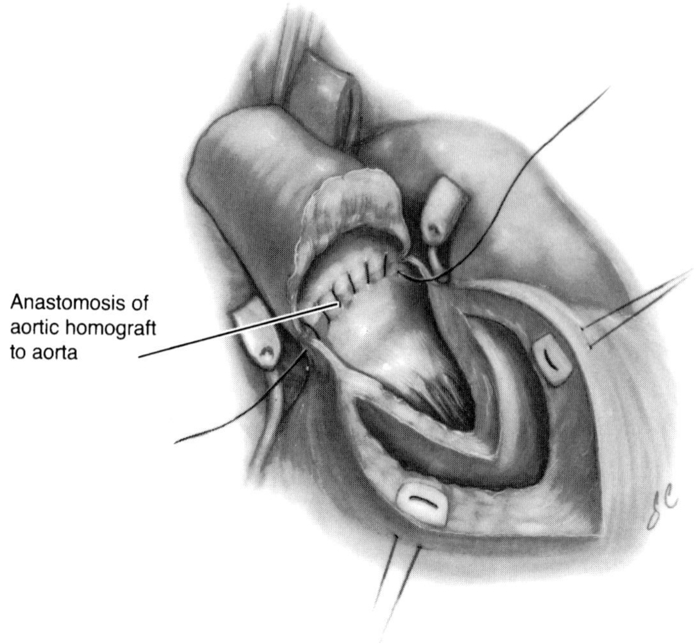

FIGURE 58–26. An aortic homograft is selected, and the posterior portion of the homograft is secured to the base of the heart.

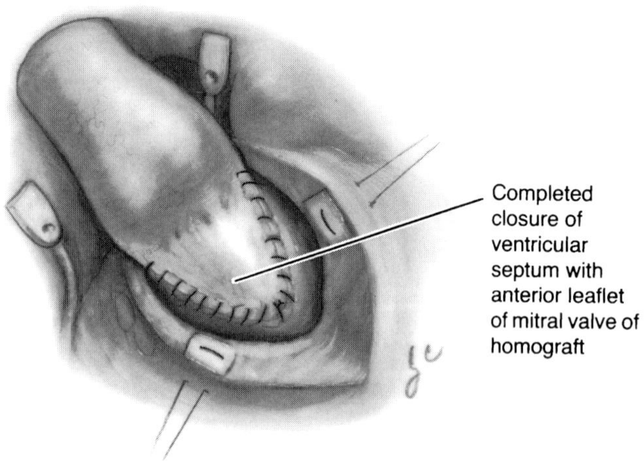

FIGURE 58–27. The mitral valve leaflet that is attached to the aortic homograft is placed anteriorly over the ventricular septal defect, and the suture line is continued along this mitral valve leaflet to secure it to the interventricular septum and to provide LV outflow reconstruction.

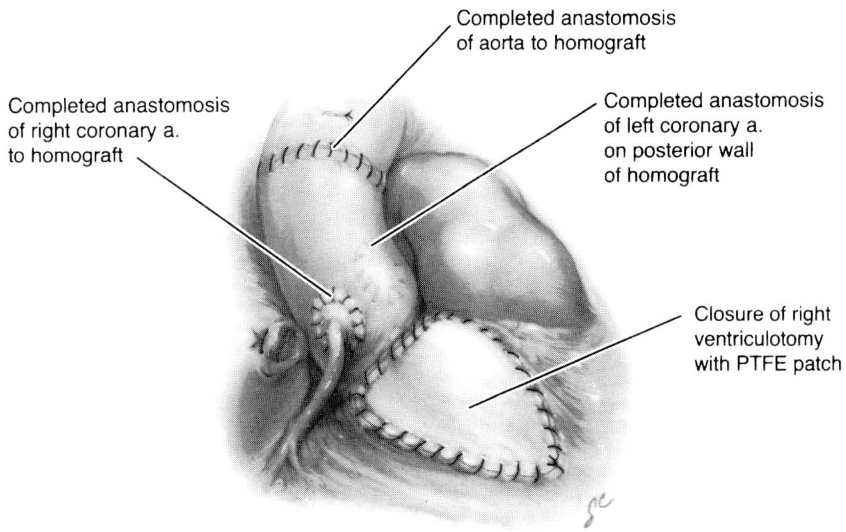

FIGURE 58–28. The coronary artery and distal homograft–to–distal aorta anastomoses are performed in a manner similar to that described in Figure 58–18. Finally, the right ventricular incision is repaired with a patch of Gore-Tex, or with extra homograft material if available.

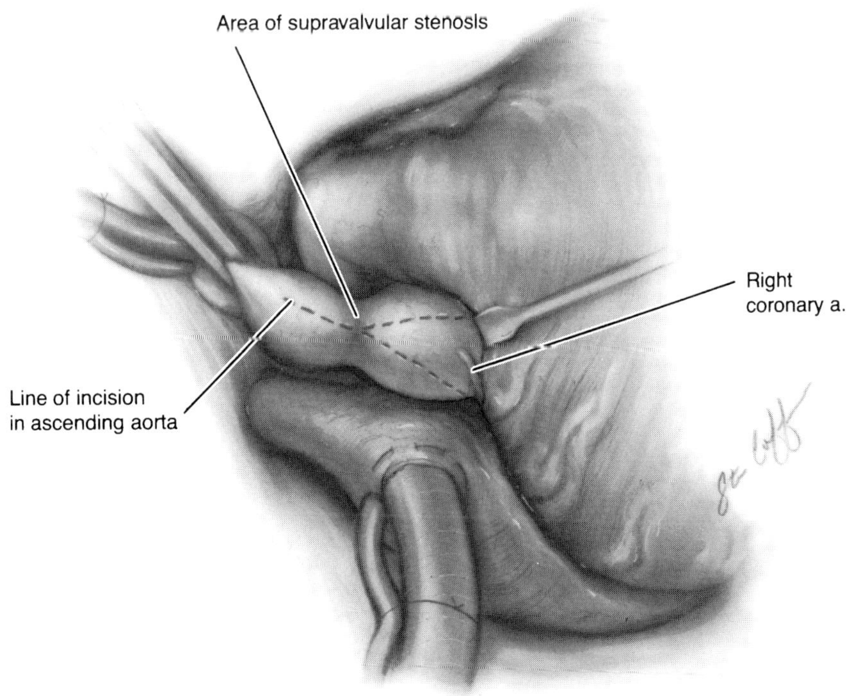

FIGURE 58–29. In patients with discrete supravalvular aortic stenosis, repair can be accomplished after the aorta is crossclamped and the heart is arrested with cardioplegic solution. An incision is made across the area of stenosis and into the sinuses on either side of the right coronary artery.

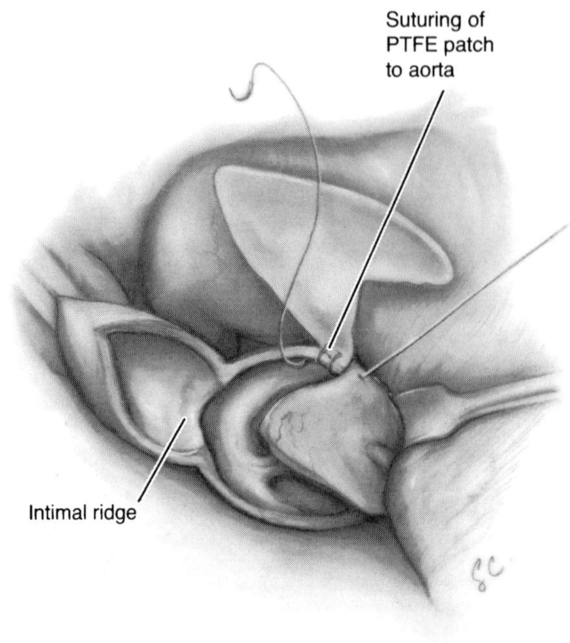

FIGURE 58–30. This incision is repaired with a generous patch of Gore-Tex, which is constructed in a Y shape to fill both sinuses and to enlarge the area of proximal aortic coarctation.

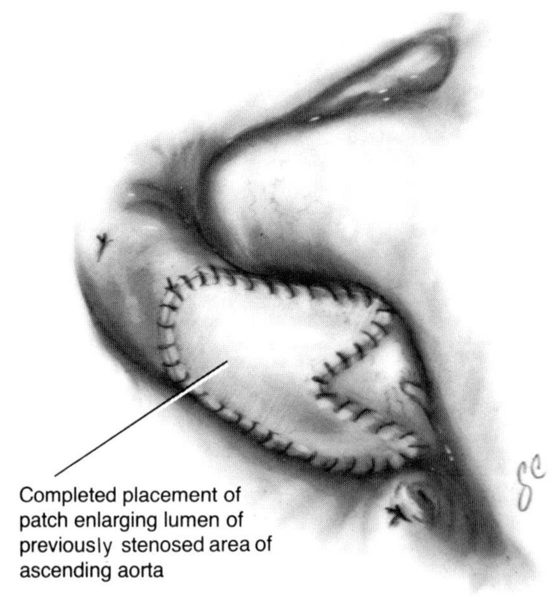

FIGURE 58–31. After the suture line is completed, the ascending aorta is "de-aired" and the crossclamp is removed. The patient is then weaned from cardiopulmonary bypass.

ROSS M. UNGERLEIDER, M.D.

59

Interruption of Aortic Arch

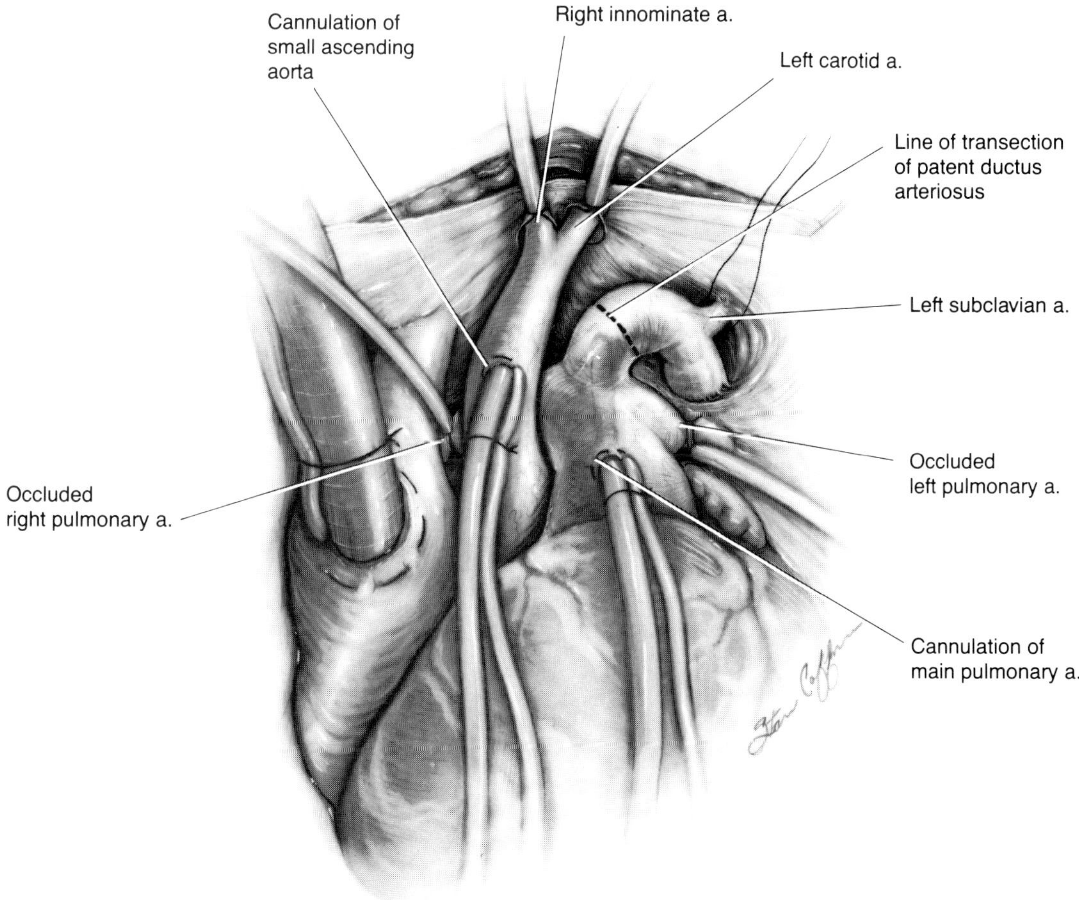

FIGURE 59–1. After the anatomy has been exposed through a median sternotomy, the patient is cannulated for cardiopulmonary bypass. The small ascending aorta and the main pulmonary artery are cannulated for arterial infusion, and snares are placed around the right and left pulmonary artery. After cardiopulmonary bypass is initiated, the snares are occluded to enable perfusion of the descending aorta across the ductus arteriosus to protect the pulmonary vascular bed. Venous return is accomplished easily by a single venous cannula. Some cannulae are configured so that they can be advanced across the ductus arteriosus into the descending aorta for distal perfusion. In these patients, a snare around the ductus allows perfusion of the lower body and enables the surgeon to remove the snares on the pulmonary arteries to facilitate dissection of the descending aorta. Loops are placed around the head vessels as well as the left subclavian artery, and the patient is cooled to 18°C.

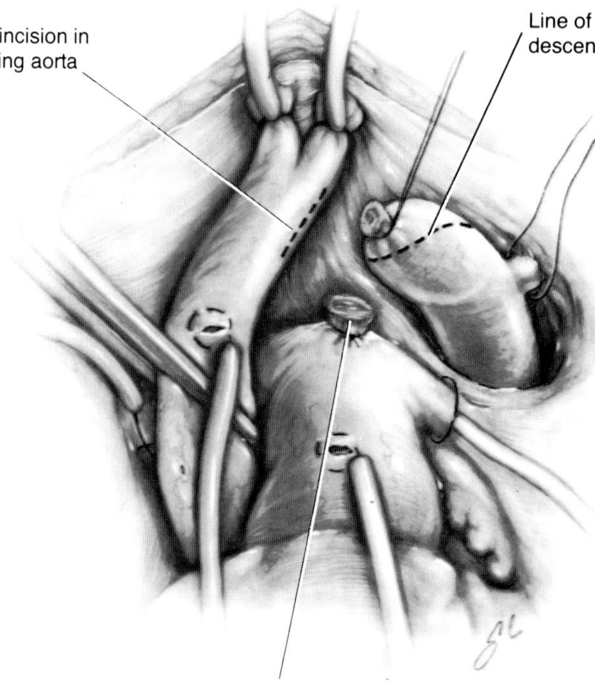

FIGURE 59–2. After adequate cooling, the patient's head is packed in ice, and the heart is arrested with cardioplegic solution infused proximal to the crossclamp. Cardiopulmonary bypass is then discontinued and the cannulae are removed. Snares around the head vessels are occluded, and the ductus arteriosus is divided between ligatures. It is useful to provide gentle traction on the ligature placed on the descending aorta. This gently elevates it and facilitates dissection distally. An incision is then made on the posterior and medial surface of the ascending aorta that extends onto the left common carotid artery. Ductal tissue is removed from the descending aorta, and a large opening in the descending aorta is established.

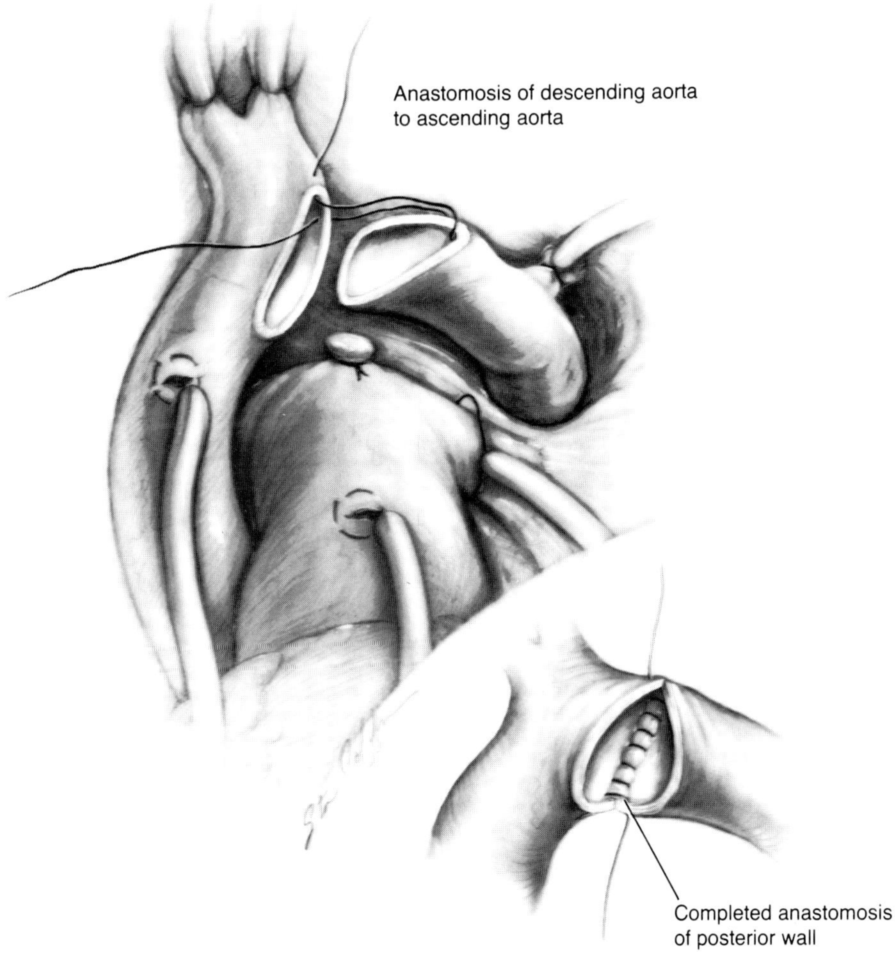

FIGURE 59–3. An anastomosis is performed between the descending aorta and the ascending aorta. This is usually accomplished with a continuous fine monofilament suture.

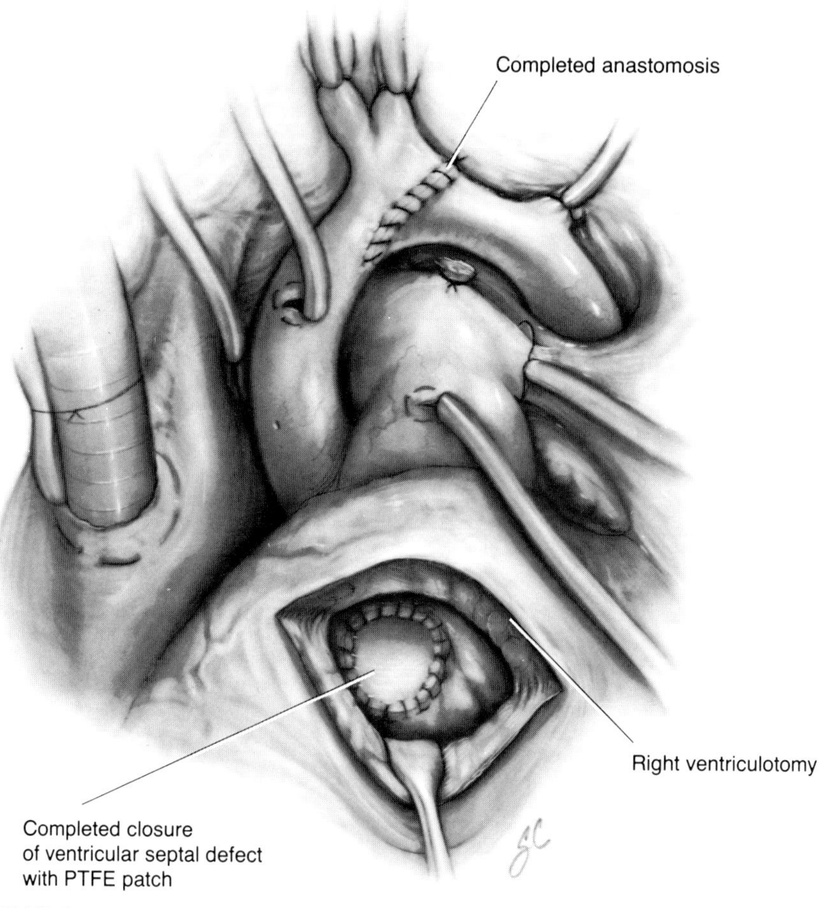

FIGURE 59–4. After the anastomosis is completed, the patient is replaced on bypass at low flow. A ventriculotomy is then performed, and the ventricular septal defect is closed easily with a patch. Alternatively, the ventricular septal defect can be closed through the ventriculotomy (as shown) or by a right atrial approach under a more prolonged period of circulatory arrest.

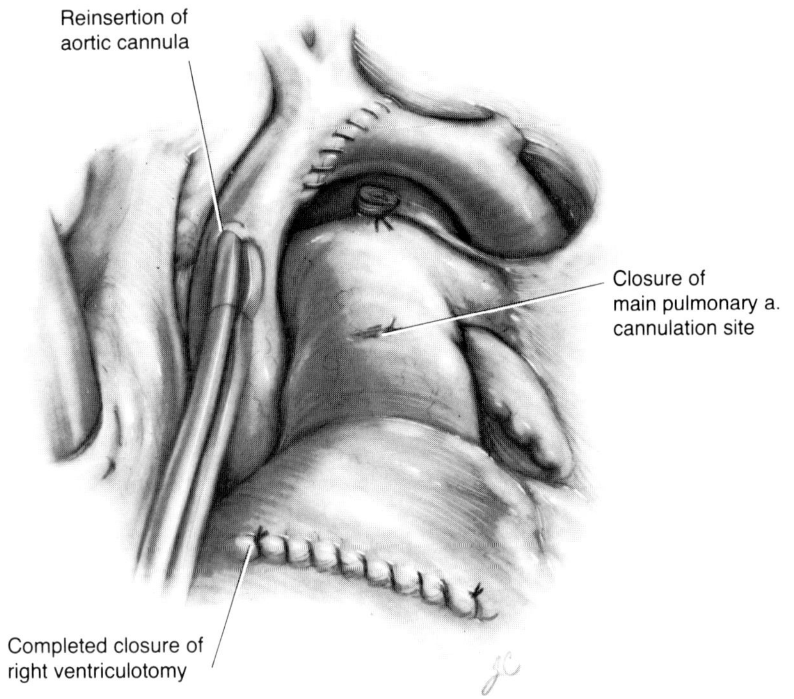

FIGURE 59–5. The ventricular incision is closed primarily, and if the patient has not yet been replaced on cardiopulmonary bypass, that can be accomplished at this time. Arterial infusion is accomplished through a single aortic cannula, and the cannulation site in the main pulmonary artery is securely closed. The patient is rewarmed and removed from cardiopulmonary bypass.

ROSS M. UNGERLEIDER, M.D.

60

Transposition of the Great Arteries

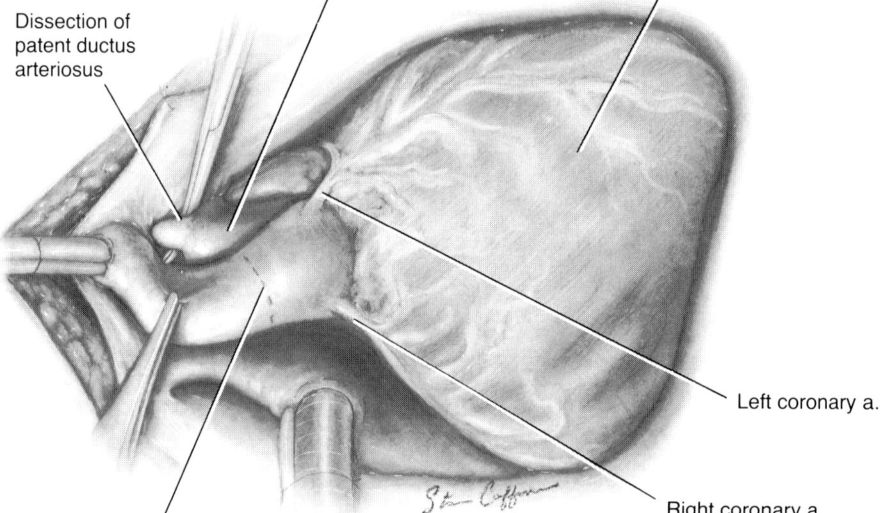

FIGURE 60–1. Prior to administration of heparin and cannulation for cardiopulmonary bypass, the pulmonary arteries are dissected free from the aorta, and the ductus arteriosus is identified. In addition, the coronary arteries are inspected to ensure that no problem is encountered with their transfer. Heparin is then administered to the patient, and cannulae are placed for cardiopulmonary bypass. The arterial cannula should be placed high on the ascending aorta. Venous return is accomplished by a single cannula in the right atrium or by separate caval cannulae placed into the superior vena cava (SVC) and inferior vena cava (IVC). In patients who have transposition with a ventricular septal defect, dual cannulation of the cavae is necessary for venous return unless the ventricular septal defect (VSD) is to be closed using an extended period of circulatory arrest. After the patient is placed on cardiopulmonary bypass, the ductus arteriosus is divided between ligatures; it is occasionally helpful to place an additional mattress suture at the aortic end of the divided ductus to provide security of this ductal closure. During the remaining cooling time on cardiopulmonary bypass, the pulmonary arteries are dissected free of adventitial tissue as far as their hilar branches. In addition, the aorta is dissected away from the main pulmonary artery so that the two structures are completely free from one another.

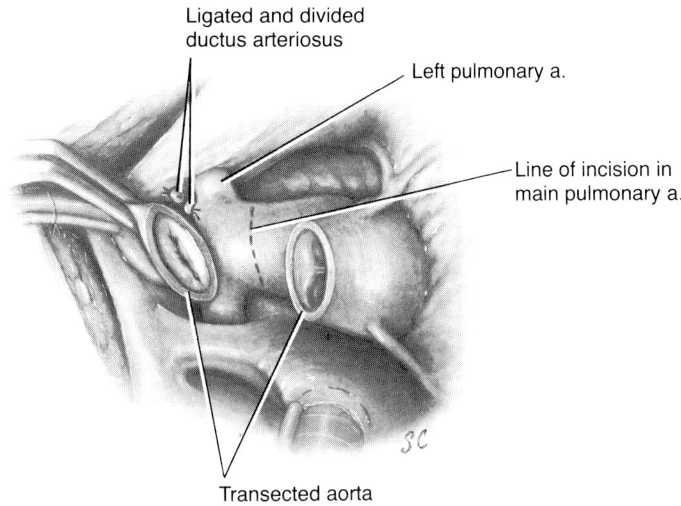

FIGURE 60–2. The aorta is crossclamped, and the heart is arrested with cardioplegic solution. The aorta is then transected above the coronary arteries, and the orifices of the coronary arteries are inspected. The main pulmonary artery is divided at the level of the bifurcation, after which a tape passed around the distal segment can be used to pull the pulmonary arteries anteriorly and to facilitate completion of the distal dissection of the pulmonary arteries so that they are well freed from adventitial connections out to the hilar branches.

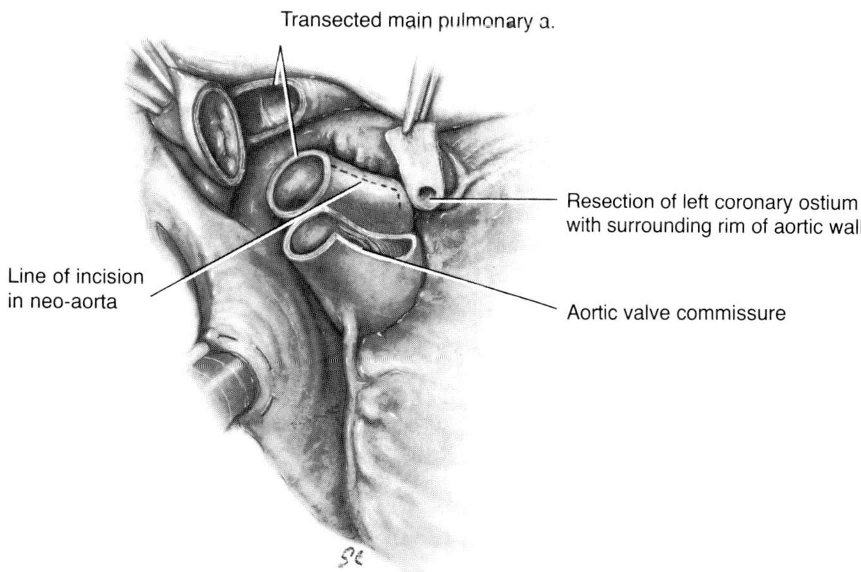

FIGURE 60–3. The coronary artery from sinus 1 (which usually contains the left anterior descending and circumflex coronary arteries) is removed with essentially the entirety of the sinus tissue extending from commissure to commissure. Although the coronary orifice is removed with a large button of tissue, very limited dissection should be performed on the left main coronary artery. An incision can then be made in the posterior pulmonary artery for placement of this translocated coronary artery. It is helpful to curve this incision medially near the base of the great vessel (medial-based flap) to limit torsion on the transferred coronary artery. The coronary artery harvested from sinus 1 should be placed low into the sinus of the neo-aorta.

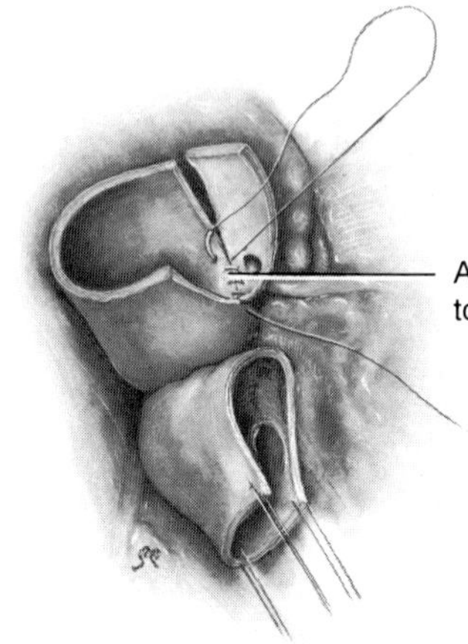

FIGURE 60–4. The coronary artery is sutured in place with a continuous fine monofilament suture. Attention to the orientation of this coronary artery is essential to prevent twisting or kinking.

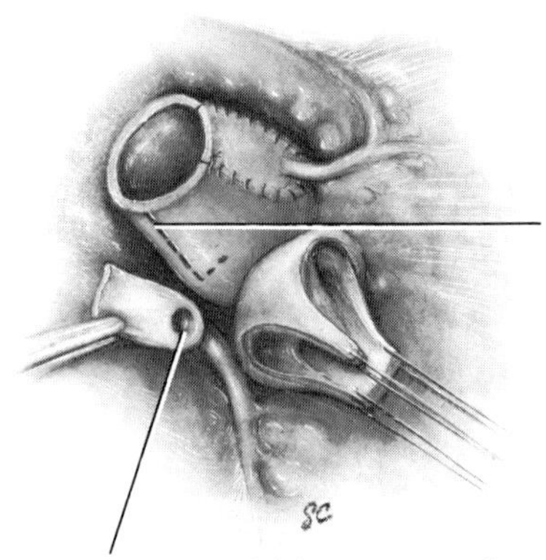

FIGURE 60–5. The coronary artery arising from sinus 2 of the aorta (usually the right coronary artery; however, the circumflex coronary artery may arise from this region as well) is removed with as much of its sinus tissue as possible. It is sometimes helpful to pull the aorta (from which the coronaries have been removed) forward with fine monofilament sutures. This coronary is then placed into a similar incision on the old pulmonary artery (neo-aorta). Again, it is helpful to use a medial-based flap, and it is not necessary to place this coronary as low in the sinus as it was for the left. In fact, when the circumflex coronary artery arises from sinus 2, it is helpful to place the anastomosis somewhat higher on the neo-aorta than usual.

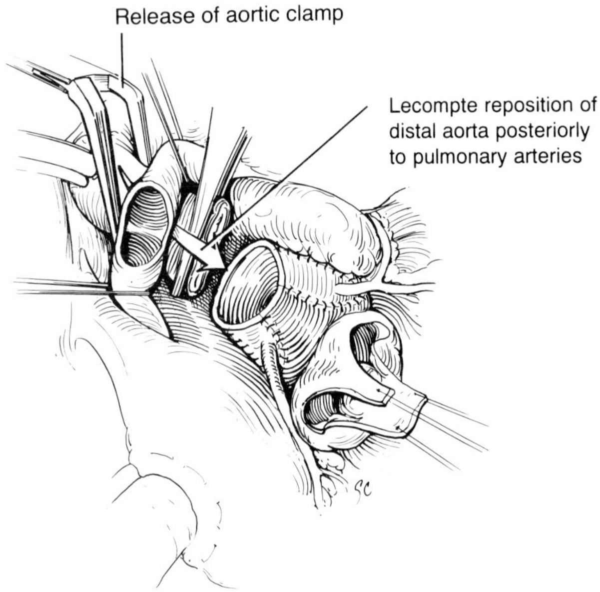

FIGURE 60–6. The pulmonary artery bifurcation is brought anterior to the distal aorta, and the crossclamp is replaced keeping the pulmonary bifurcation above the aorta (Lecompte maneuver).

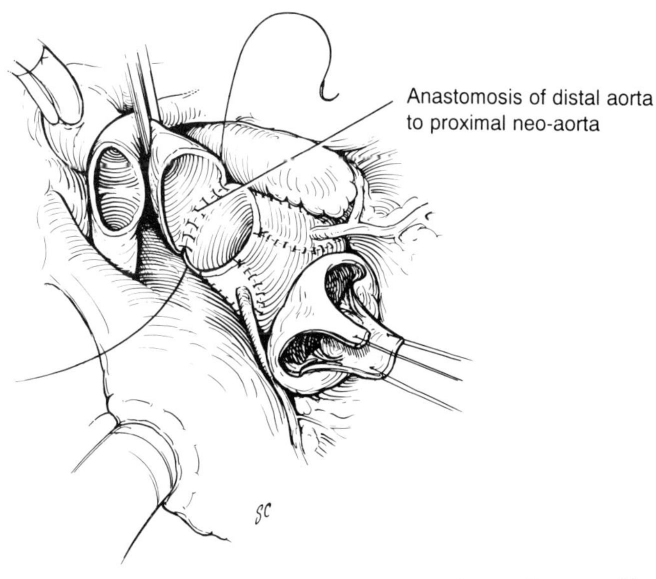

FIGURE 60–7. The neo-aorta can be reconstructed using continuous fine monofilament suture.

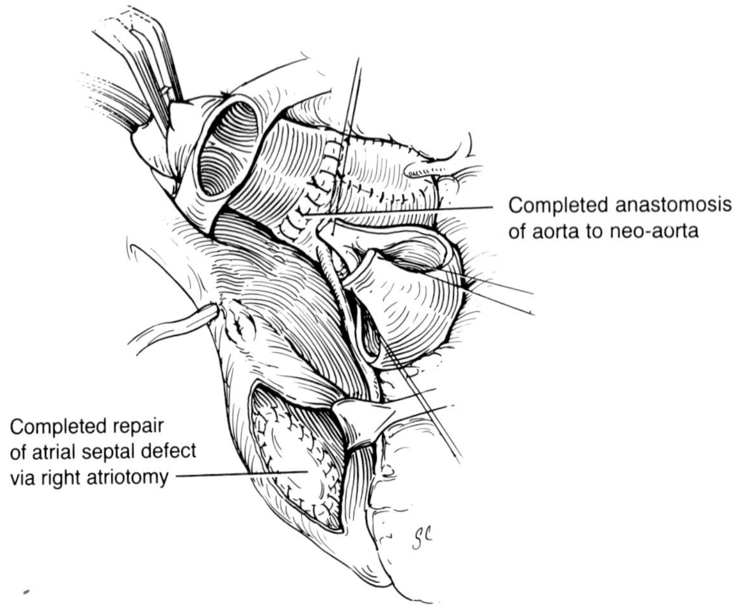

FIGURE 60–8. The right atrium is opened, and the atrial septostomy is repaired during a brief period of circulatory arrest (if one atrial venous return cannula is used) or during continuous flow (if bicaval cannulation has been used). The repair can be performed with a small patch of prosthetic material or primarily using continuous suture, depending on the condition and anatomy of the atrial septum. If bicaval cannulation is to be used, it is helpful to open the right atrium at the beginning of the procedure so that the return to the left atrium can be easily vented (using a sucker) across the atrial septal defect to prevent it from obscuring the operative field. If a ventricular septal defect is present, it can now be closed using appropriate techniques.

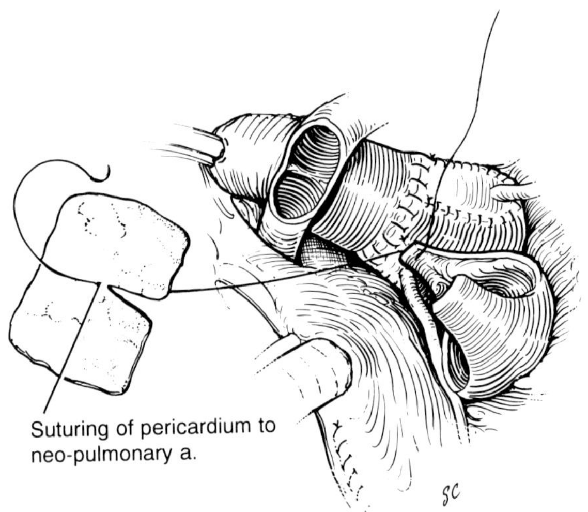

FIGURE 60–9. The aortic crossclamp should be removed, and the neo-aortic suture line including the suture line of the coronary artery transfer should be carefully inspected for bleeding. In addition, the perfusion of the myocardium should be inspected. Even at hypothermia, the heart should be well perfused and should begin to contract readily after removal of the crossclamp. Bleeding on the suture line should be carefully repaired, and any problem with coronary transfer that affects myocardial perfusion should be identified and rectified at this time. The crossclamp can then be replaced if desired during reconstruction of the neopulmonary artery. Alternatively, the crossclamp can be left off while the myocardium is perfused, and the neopulmonary artery can be reconstructed during rewarming. If this latter option is chosen, it is helpful to maintain profound hypothermia until the sinuses of the pulmonary artery have been repaired, because during warming, the heart quickly resumes vigorous contraction, making this portion of the procedure more arduous. The sinuses are repaired with a patch of pericardium using fine monofilament suture material.

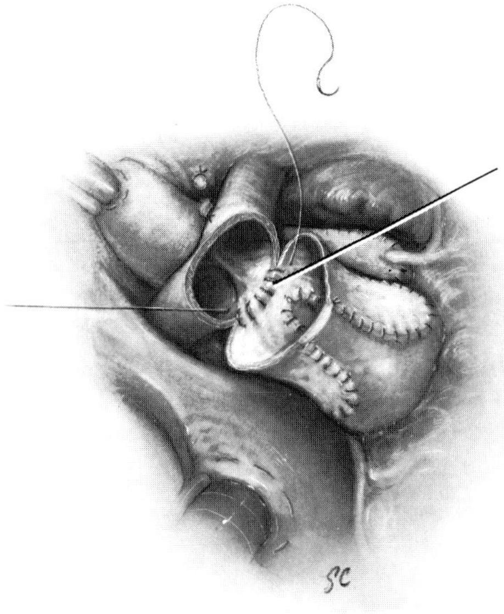

FIGURE 60–10. During completion of warming, the final suture line connecting the reconstructed proximal pulmonary artery to the pulmonary artery bifurcation is performed using a continuous monofilament suture. At the completion of this anastomosis, the heart should be contracting vigorously, and the distal pulmonary arteries should be relatively "loose" over the top of the aorta. By use of a large patch of pericardium, posterior compression on the transferred coronary arteries is limited.

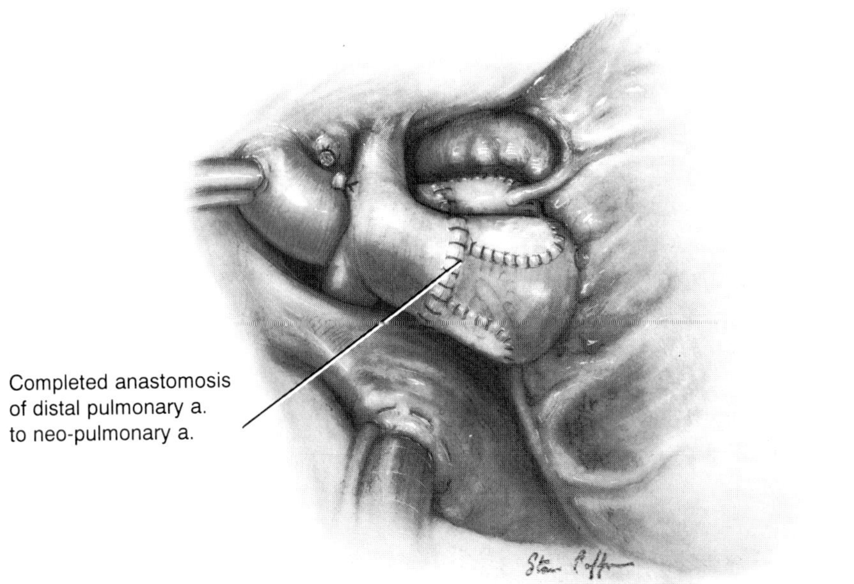

FIGURE 60–11. The completed arterial switch demonstrates the divided ductus arteriosus with the aorta now repositioned below the pulmonary bifurcation. The coronary arteries have been translocated to the posterior great vessel, and the sinuses from which they were removed have been repaired with pericardium. Minimal dissection of the coronary arteries helps prevent twisting and kinking of their proximal portion. Failure of the heart to contract strongly suggests a problem with coronary transfer, as patients usually have no problem tolerating this operation.

ROSS M. UNGERLEIDER, M.D.

61

Pulmonary Atresia with Intact Ventricular Septum

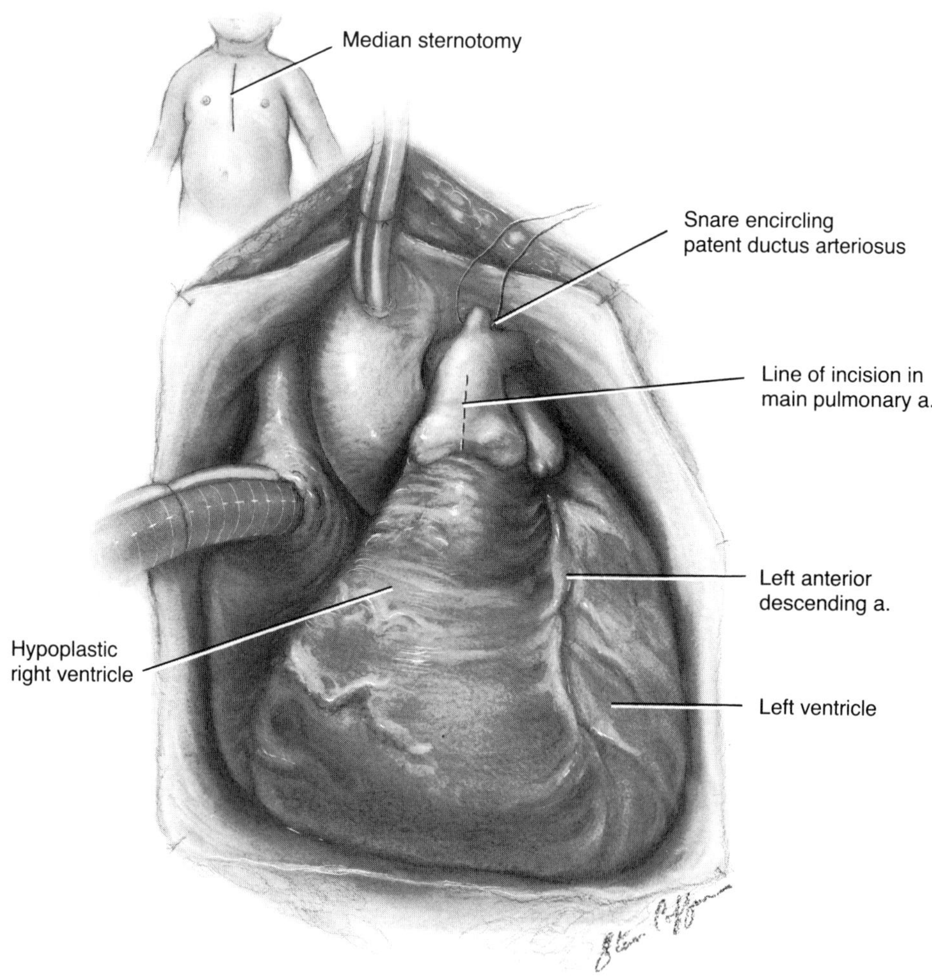

FIGURE 61–1. Patients with an adequate tricuspid valve and right ventricular chamber size are candidates for a procedure that reconstructs communication between the right ventricle and pulmonary artery. This procedure can be accomplished through a median sternotomy and with the patient on cardiopulmonary bypass with venous return provided by a single right atrial cannula. The ductus arteriosus is encircled with a snare that can be occluded immediately after institution of bypass. The sinuses of the pulmonary valve area are usually prominent against the background of the hypoplastic right ventricular infundibulum. The right ventricular chamber size may appear smaller than usual as evidenced by a narrow distance between the right and left anterior descending coronary arteries.

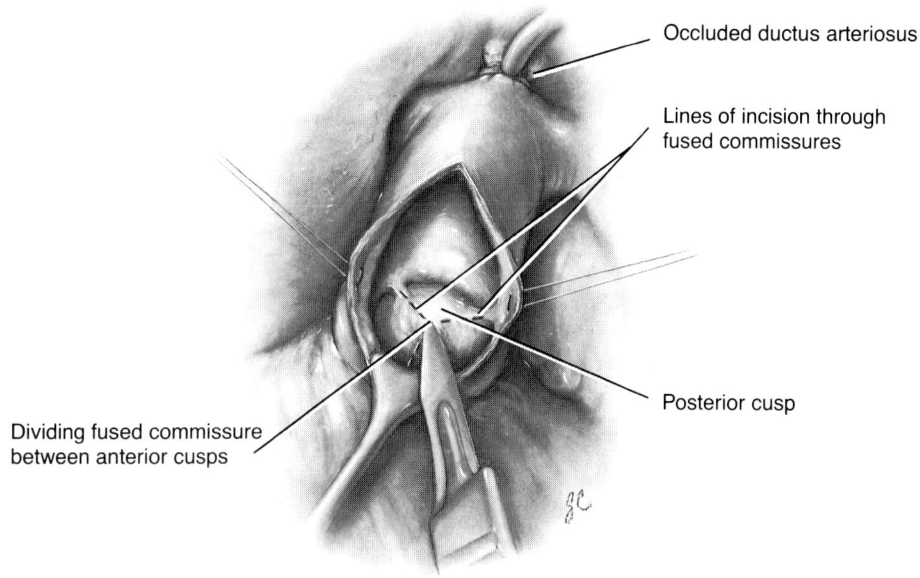

FIGURE 61–2. After the patient is placed on bypass, the ductus arteriosus is occluded with a snare. An incision is made in the main pulmonary artery above the valve annulus, and the pulmonary valve is inspected. If the valve leaflets are fused at their commissures, they may be opened by sharp incision with a scalpel, after which the subvalvular right ventricular outflow tract should be inspected. Any prominent muscle bands can be resected through the valvotomy, and it may not be necessary to enlarge the infundibular portion of the right ventricle.

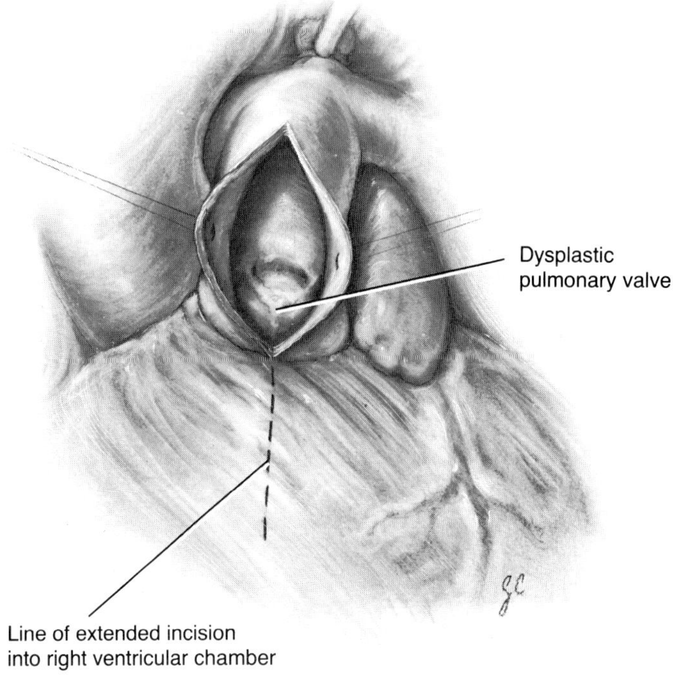

FIGURE 61–3. If the right ventricular outflow tract is hypoplastic, a transannular incision may be necessary, in which case the incision in the main pulmonary artery is extended onto the right ventricular outflow tract. During this time, the heart can be maintained electrically fibrillating, mechanically arrested with cardioplegic solution infused proximal to an aortic crossclamp, or even empty and beating.

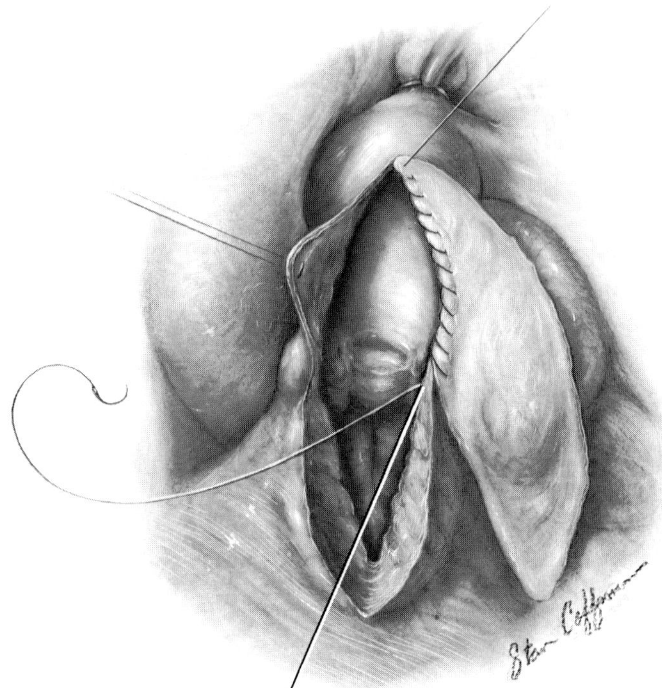

FIGURE 61–4. After an adequate transannular incision has provided unobstructed outflow from the right ventricle to the main pulmonary artery, a patch covering for this incision is created. Usually, this patch is best made of autologous pericardium (which can be stiffened by a short period of preservation in glutaraldehyde), although a piece of bovine pericardium or PTFE (polytetrafluoroethylene) can also be used.

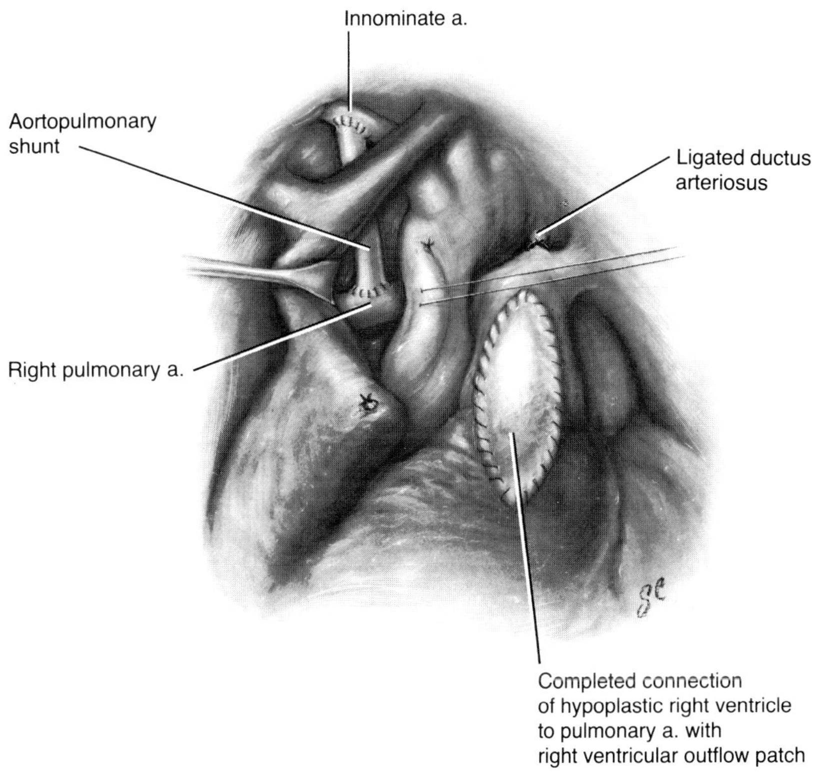

FIGURE 61–5. After completion of a transannular patch or pulmonary valvotomy, it is likely that the patient's right ventricular compliance is such that there continues to be inadequate antegrade flow from the right atrium into the right ventricle and out the newly enlarged right ventricular outflow tract. For this reason, the patient may be dependent on an aortopulmonary connection for several days. In some cases, this can be easily provided by loosening the snare around the ductus arteriosus and maintaining ductal patency on prostaglandin E_1 infusion in the intensive care unit. Alternatively, an aortopulmonary shunt may be placed so that the patient can be removed from mechanical ventilation and sent to the ward with security that adequate pulmonary blood flow will continue until right ventricular compliance improves. These shunts can usually be created between the innominate or subclavian artery and the right pulmonary artery and can be easily closed by interventional catheterization techniques or by relatively simple repeat sternotomy at a future time.

ROSS M. UNGERLEIDER, M.D.

62
Hypoplastic Left Heart Syndrome

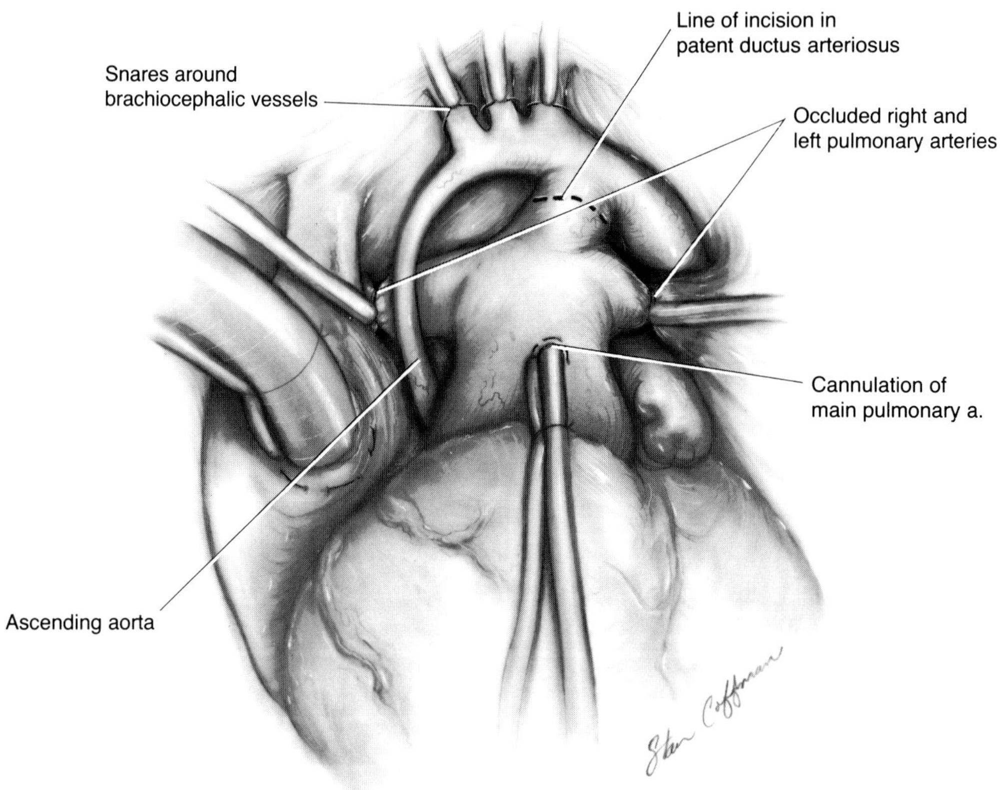

FIGURE 62–1. The anatomy is exposed through a median sternotomy. Arterial inflow is provided by a cannula in the main pulmonary artery, although a cannula that can be advanced across the ductus into the descending artery may be used. Snares are placed around the right and left pulmonary arteries that can be occluded after bypass is initiated. Snares are also placed around the head vessels for later occlusion, and the patient is cooled to 18°C.

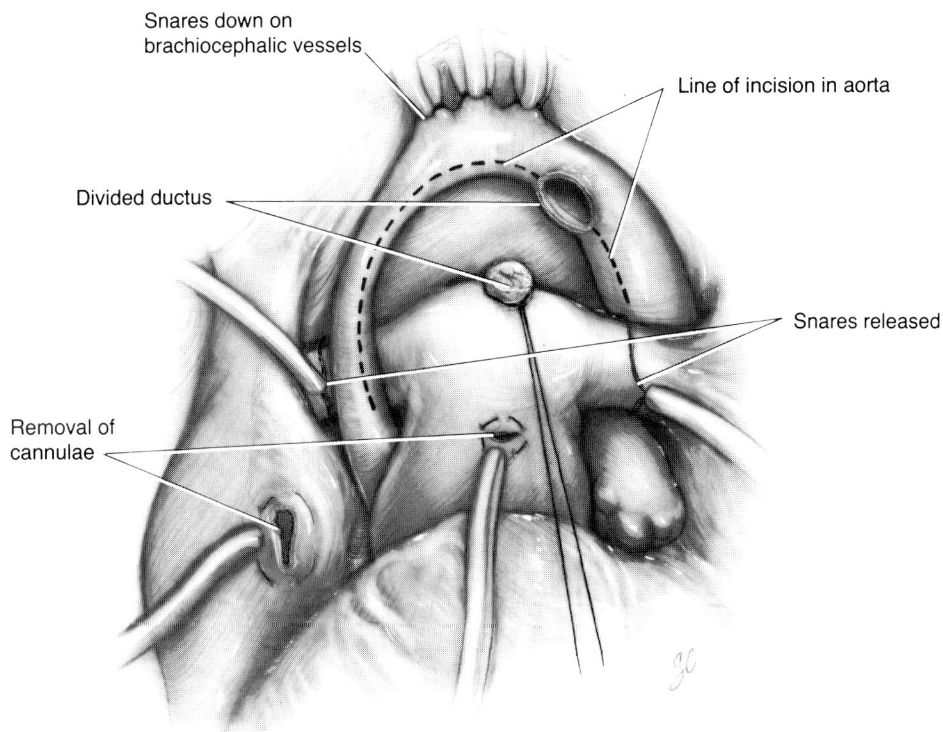

FIGURE 62–2. Cardiopulmonary bypass is discontinued, and the head is packed in ice. Although it is possible to give cardioplegia, it may not be essential and is technically difficult because it requires occlusion of the descending aorta and both branch pulmonary arteries and then infusuion of cardioplegia through the main pulmonary artery. The arterial and venous cannulae are removed. The head vessels are snared. The ductus arteriosus is divided between ligatures, and the ligature on the proximal ductus is left intact. Ductal material distally is removed, enabling a long incision on the hypoplastic aorta extending beyond the area of ductal insertion and onto the descending aorta.

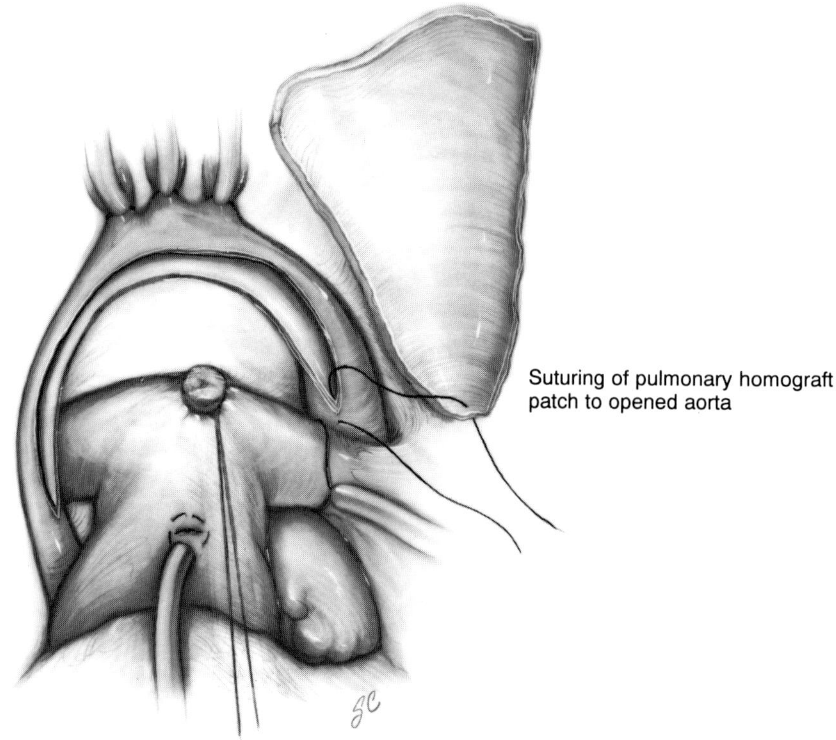

FIGURE 62–3. Once the incision has been made, it is repaired with a patch of pulmonary homograft using a continuous suture. It is convenient to retract the main pulmonary artery segment with the ductal ligature.

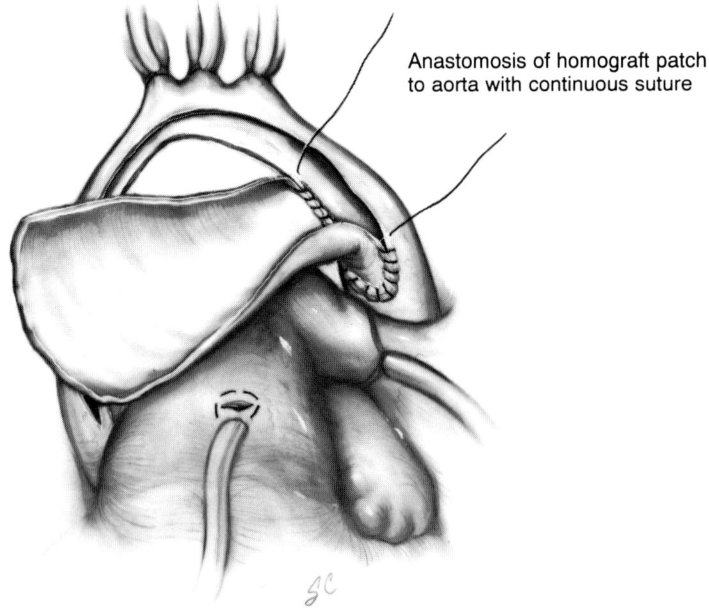

FIGURE 62–4. A large patch of pulmonary homograft should be used, and it should be applied loosely to the underside of the aortic arch so that it does not constrict this area of the aorta.

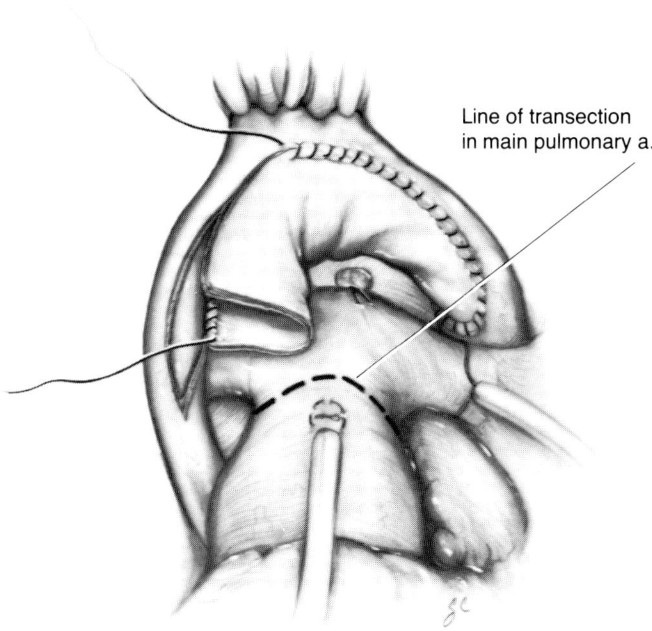

FIGURE 62–5. This patch reconstruction of the aorta is extended to the proximal portion of the aortic incision. At this time, the main pulmonary artery is divided from the branch pulmonary arteries.

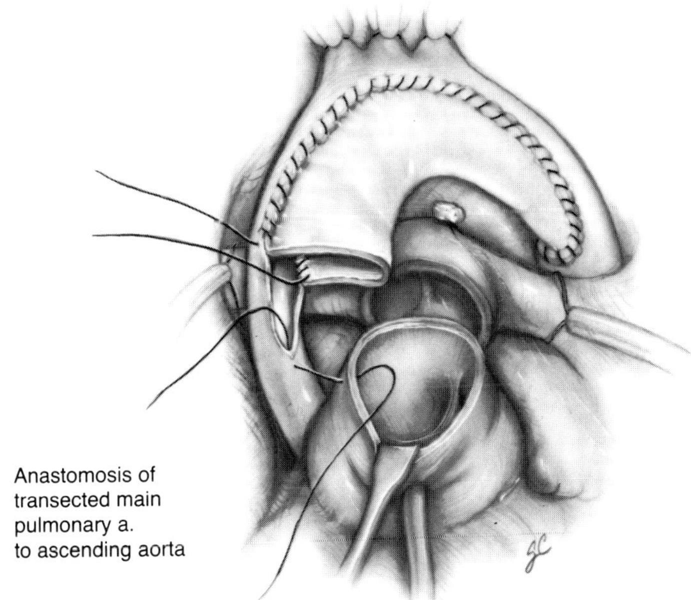

FIGURE 62–6. The main pulmonary artery is incorporated into the aortic arch reconstruction.

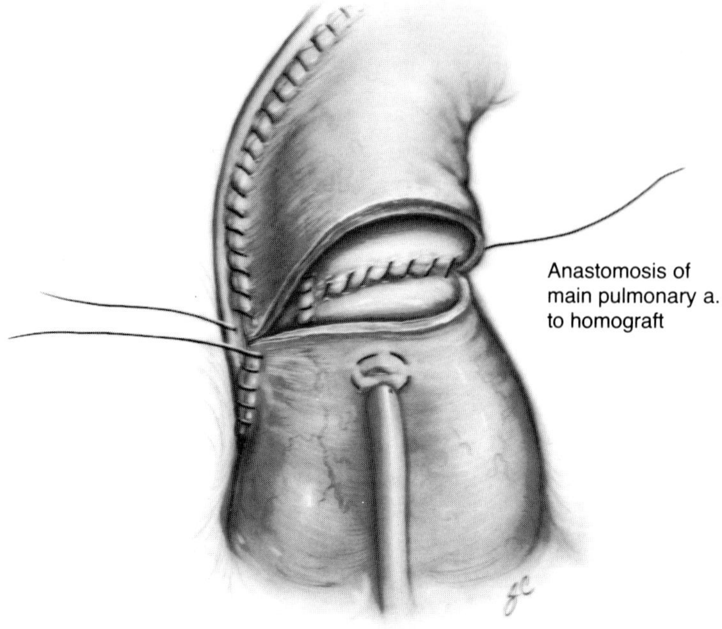

FIGURE 62–7. The main pulmonary artery is connected to the large patch of pulmonary homograft so that the "neo-aorta" reconstruction is complete.

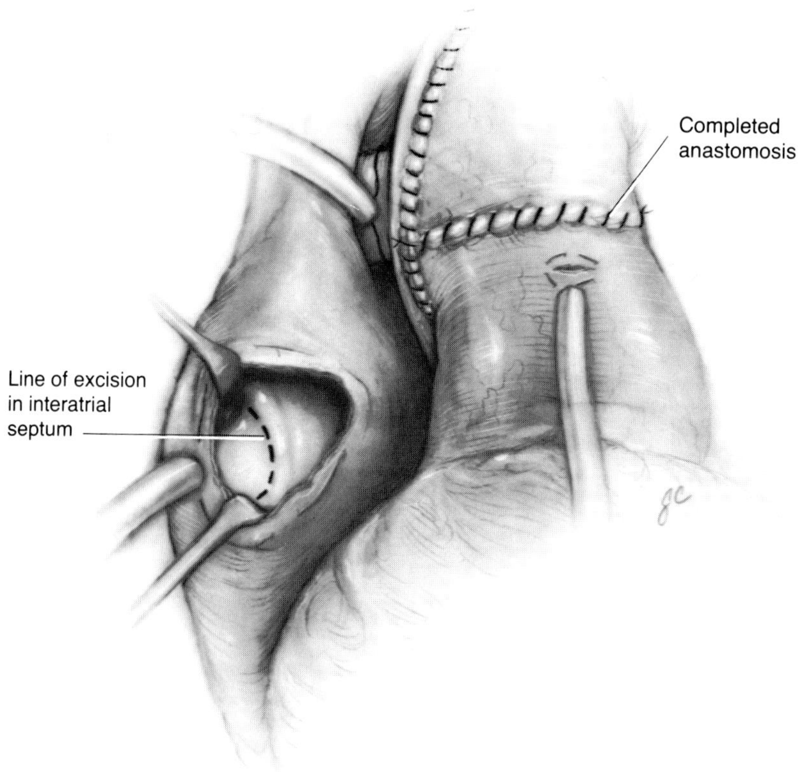

FIGURE 62–8. The atrial septum must be excised, and this can often be done through the venous cannulation site through the atrial pursestring suture, as shown. Alternatively, an incision can be made in the right atrium.

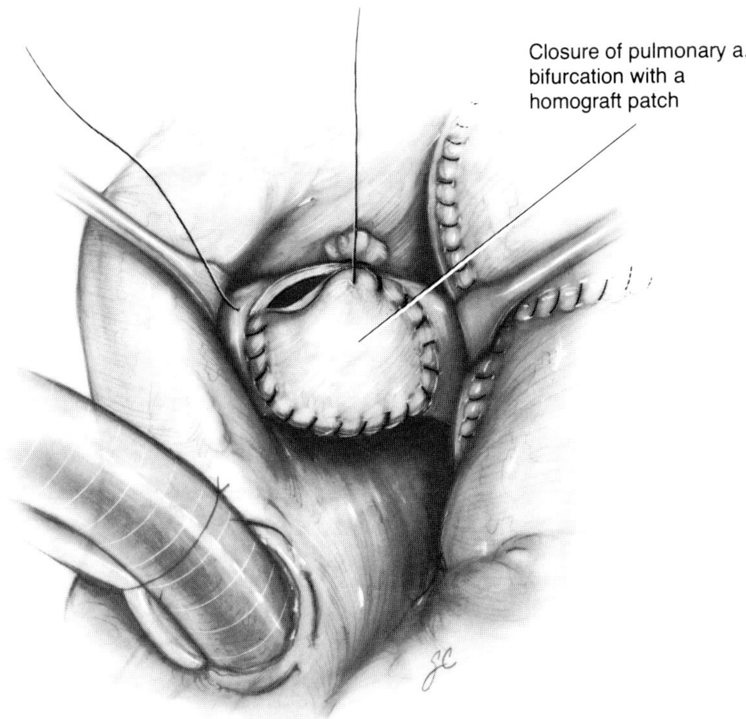

FIGURE 62–9. The patient is replaced on bypass, and during warming the bifurcation of the pulmonary arteries is repaired with a patch of homograft. This usually can be done by bringing the pulmonary arteries below the aorta and performing this reconstruction between the aorta and the superior vena cava.

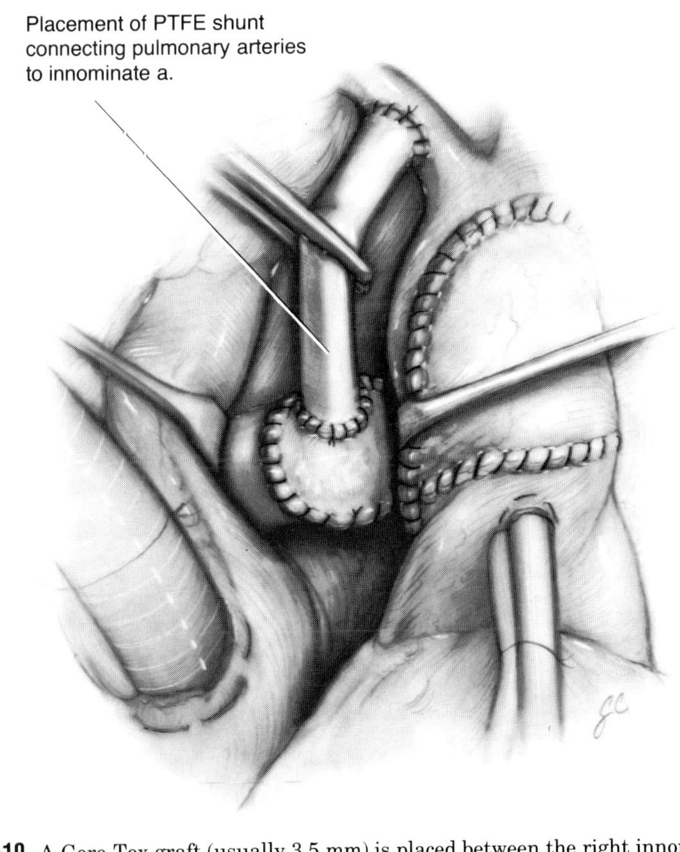

FIGURE 62–10. A Gore-Tex graft (usually 3.5 mm) is placed between the right innominate artery and the top of the pulmonary bifurcation. This graft should be kept occluded until the patient is removed from bypass.

ROSS M. UNGERLEIDER, M.D.

63

Tricuspid Atresia

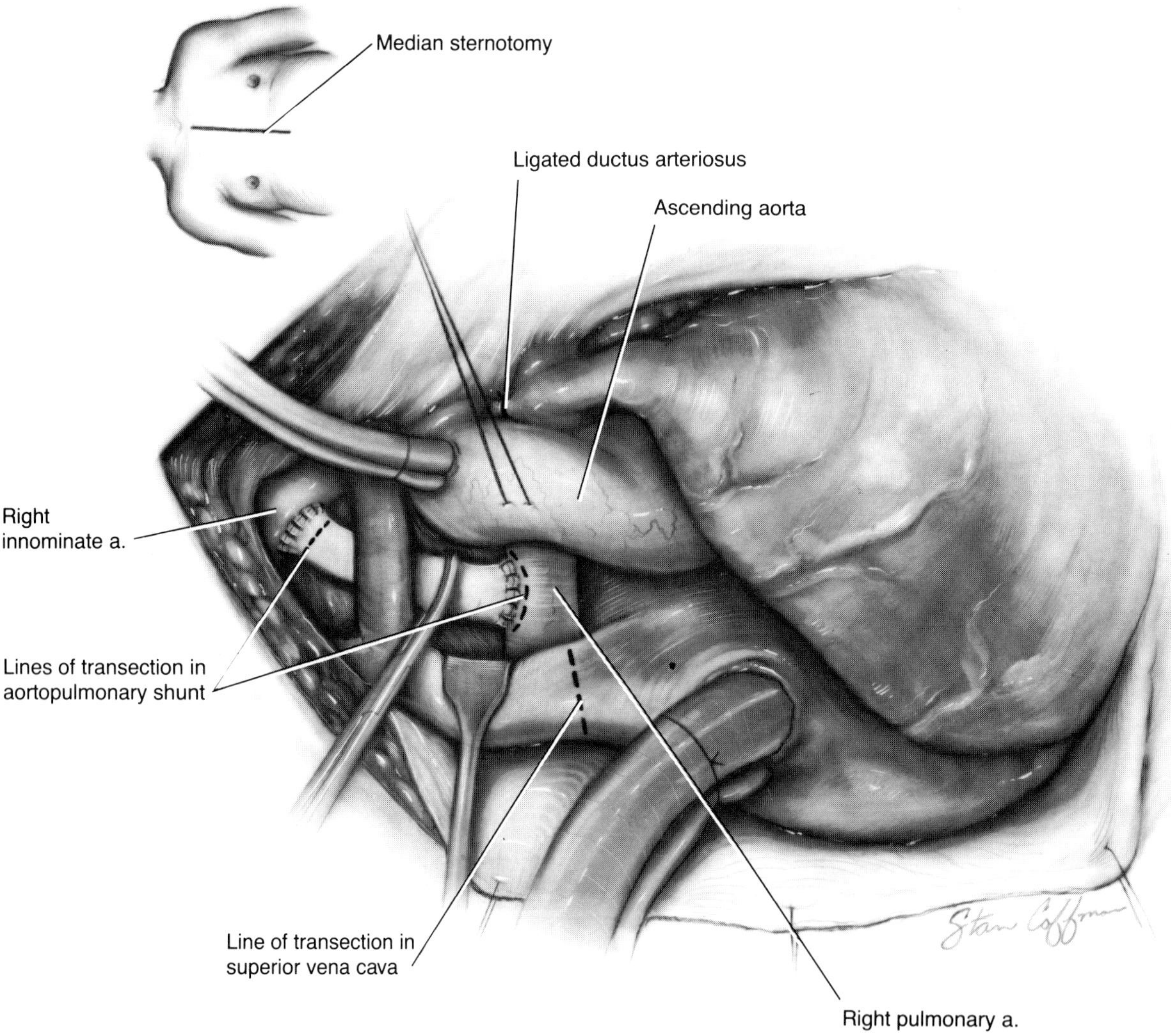

FIGURE 63–1. The anatomy is exposed through a median sternotomy. Patients with tricuspid atresia usually have undergone an aortopulmonary shunt in infancy. This illustration depicts a Gore-Tex shunt between the innominate artery and the right pulmonary artery. The patient is placed on cardiopulmonary bypass using a single venous cannula. Once bypass is established, the shunt is clamped and divided. The proximal end is oversewn, and the distal end is removed from the pulmonary artery. The superior vena cava (SVC) is then divided at its site of connection with the right atrium.

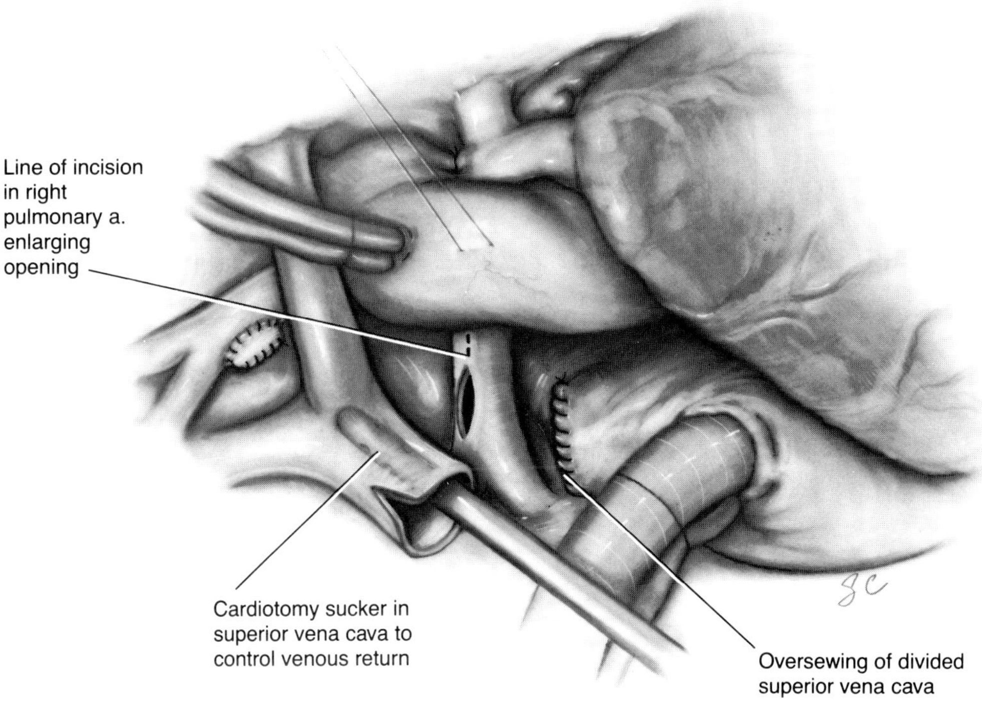

FIGURE 63–2. The atrial end of the superior vena cava is oversewn with a continuous suture. The heart is maintained empty and beating throughout the procedure because the cardiac chambers are not entered. The opening in the right pulmonary artery is incised to enlarge the pulmonary arteriotomy. A cardiotomy sucker is used to control blood returning from the superior vena cava. Alternatively, the superior vena cava can be cannulated with a separate cannula placed near the junction of the jugular and innominate veins.

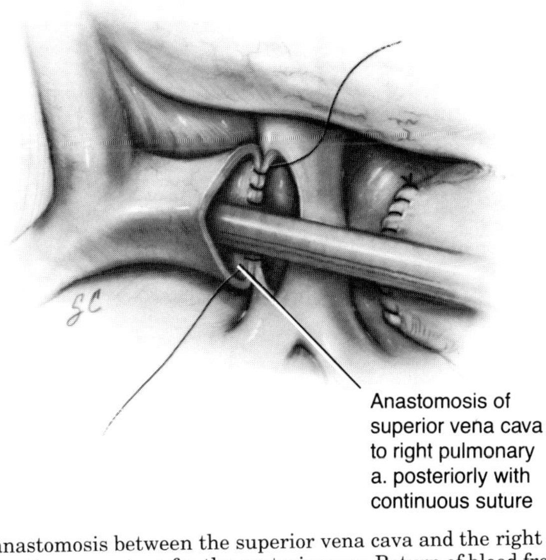

FIGURE 63–3. An anastomosis between the superior vena cava and the right pulmonary artery is performed using a continuous suture for the posterior row. Return of blood from the superior vena cava is controlled with a cardiotomy sucker.

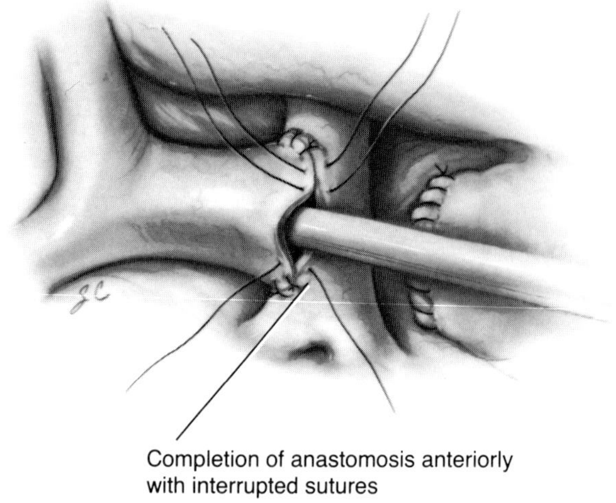

FIGURE 63–4. The anterior anastomosis of the Glenn shunt usually is performed with interrupted sutures to prevent pursestringing. At the completion of the anastomosis, the patient is removed from cardiopulmonary bypass, and pulmonary blood flow is provided by the SVC-pulmonary anastomosis.

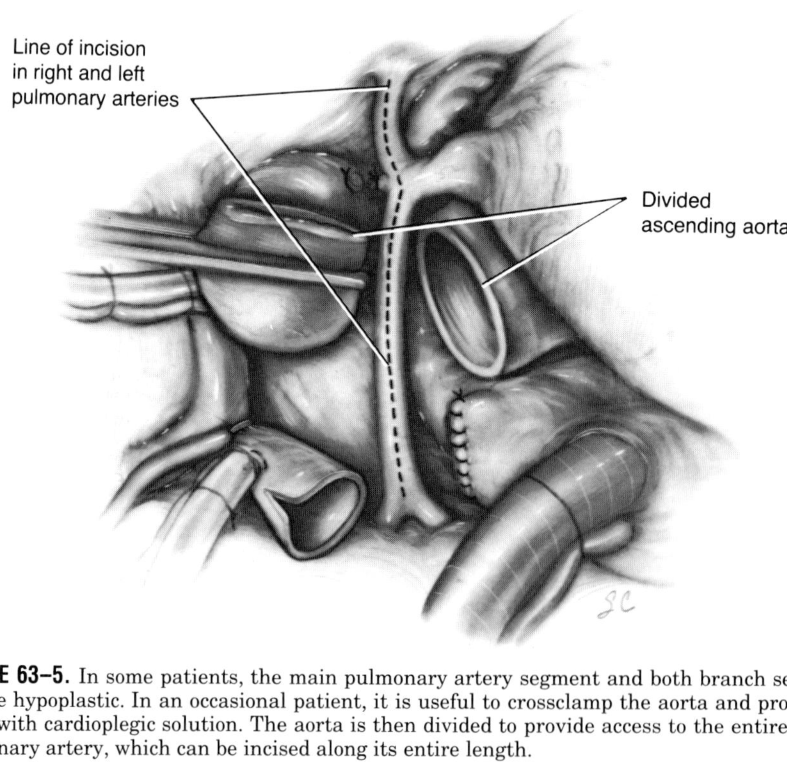

FIGURE 63–5. In some patients, the main pulmonary artery segment and both branch segments may be hypoplastic. In an occasional patient, it is useful to crossclamp the aorta and protect the heart with cardioplegic solution. The aorta is then divided to provide access to the entire central pulmonary artery, which can be incised along its entire length.

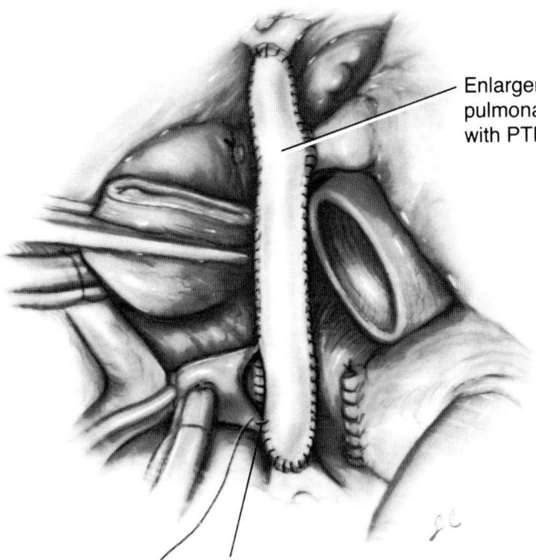

FIGURE 63–6. The pulmonary artery is enlarged with a patch of Gore-Tex or homograft. A Glenn anastomosis is incorporated into this patch reconstruction. In these patients, it is useful to perform separate cannulation of the superior vena cava (as shown), because the reconstruction is a bit more complicated than the standard bidirectional Glenn procedure. The aorta is then repaired. Occasionally it is useful to interpose a short section of graft material to prevent the aorta from compressing the newly enlarged pulmonary artery.

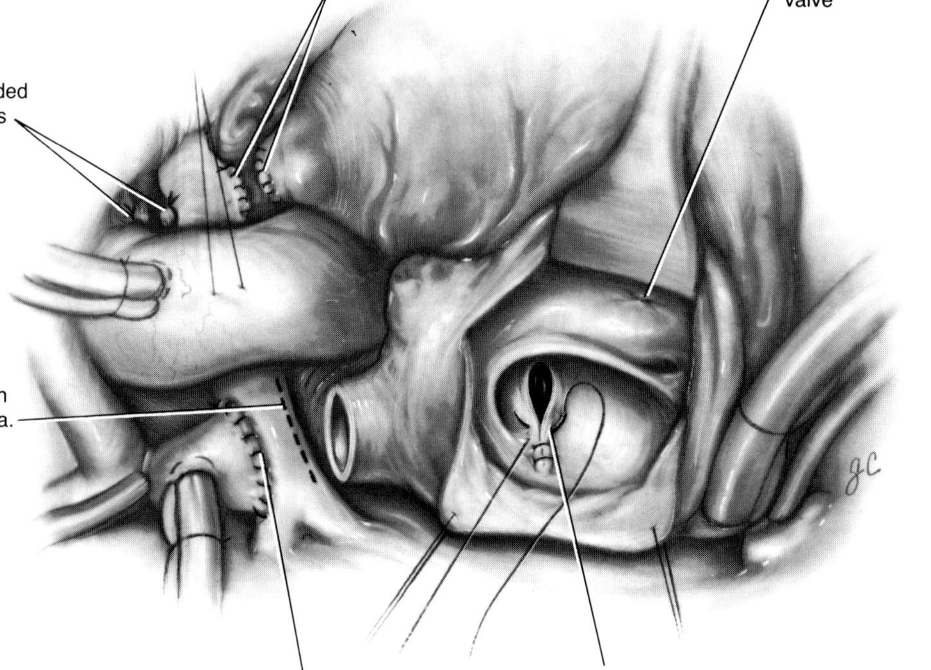

FIGURE 63–7. A Fontan procedure is performed for many patients with tricuspid atresia as part of the initial conversion from an aortopulmonary shunt. In these patients, the Glenn anastomosis is performed to the right pulmonary artery (at the site of the previous shunt insertion), as previously described. The main pulmonary artery is divided and oversewn if desired. Likewise, the ductus arteriosus is divided, which, along with division of the main pulmonary artery, enables mobilization of the central pulmonary artery behind the aorta to reduce any tension on the anastomoses. The inferior vena caval return is collected through a separate cannula. With the heart arrested with cardioplegic solution or electrical fibrillation, a right atriotomy is performed, and the atrial septal defect is repaired directly or with a patch (not shown). The atrial end of the superior vena cava is prepared for anastomosis with the inferior border of the right pulmonary artery.

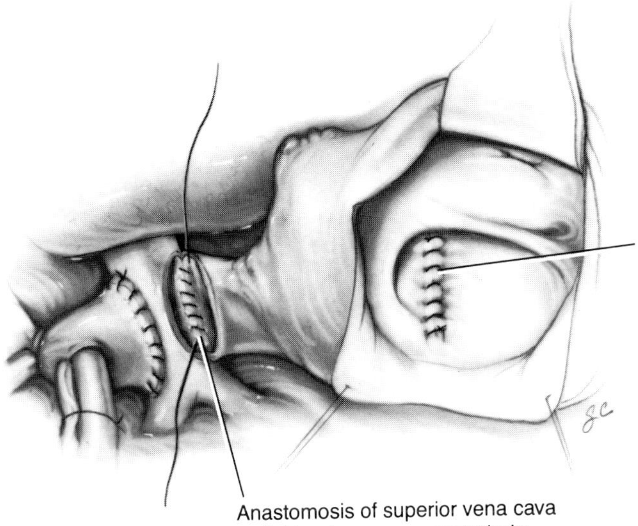

FIGURE 63–8. This anastomosis is made as large as possible and, like the anastomosis of the superior vena cava, is performed with a continuous suture posteriorly but with interrupted sutures anteriorly.

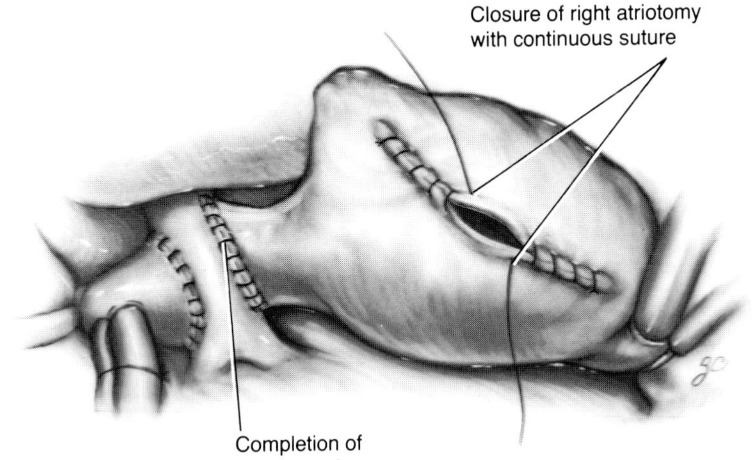

FIGURE 63–9. The right atriotomy is closed such that all systemic venous return is directed into the pulmonary artery.

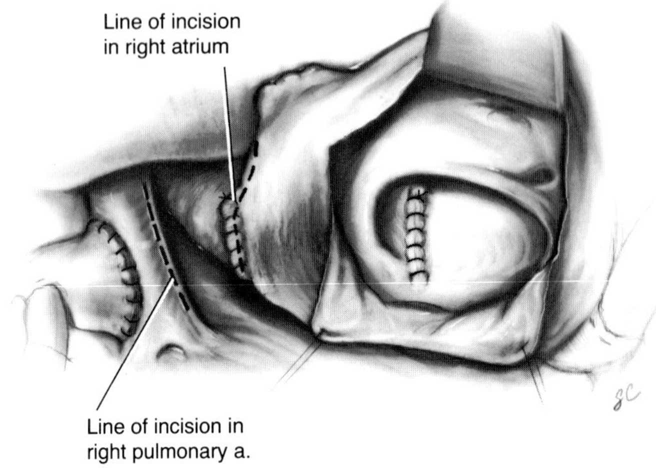

FIGURE 63–10. Occasionally a patient returns for completion of a Fontan procedure after having undergone a previous bidirectional Glenn procedure. In these patients, cardiopulmonary bypass is initiated with separate caval cannulation. With the heart electrically fibrillating or arrested with cardioplegic solution, a right atriotomy is performed and the atrial septal defect is closed. The previously oversewn atrial end of the superior vena cava is incised, with the incision extending medially onto the roof of the right atrium.

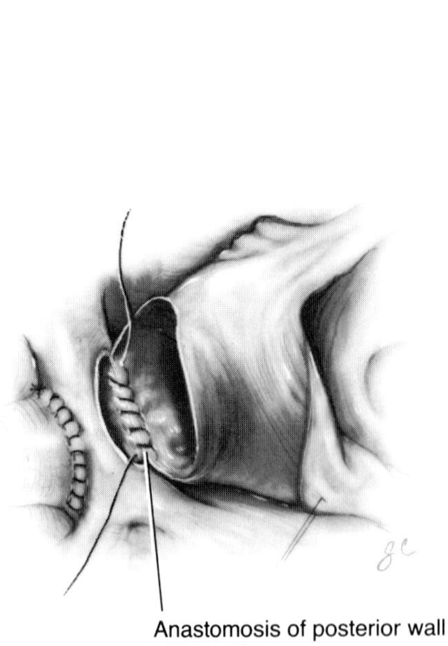

FIGURE 63–11. A large anastomosis is performed between the enlarged SVC opening and the inferior aspect of the right pulmonary artery. Usually it is best to perform this with continuous posterior suture.

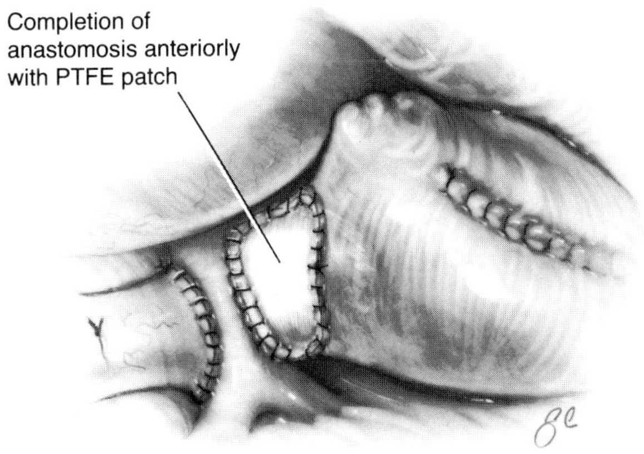

FIGURE 63–12. For these patients, a tension-free anastomosis is usually best accomplished with a patch of Gore-Tex or homograft for the roof of this connection.

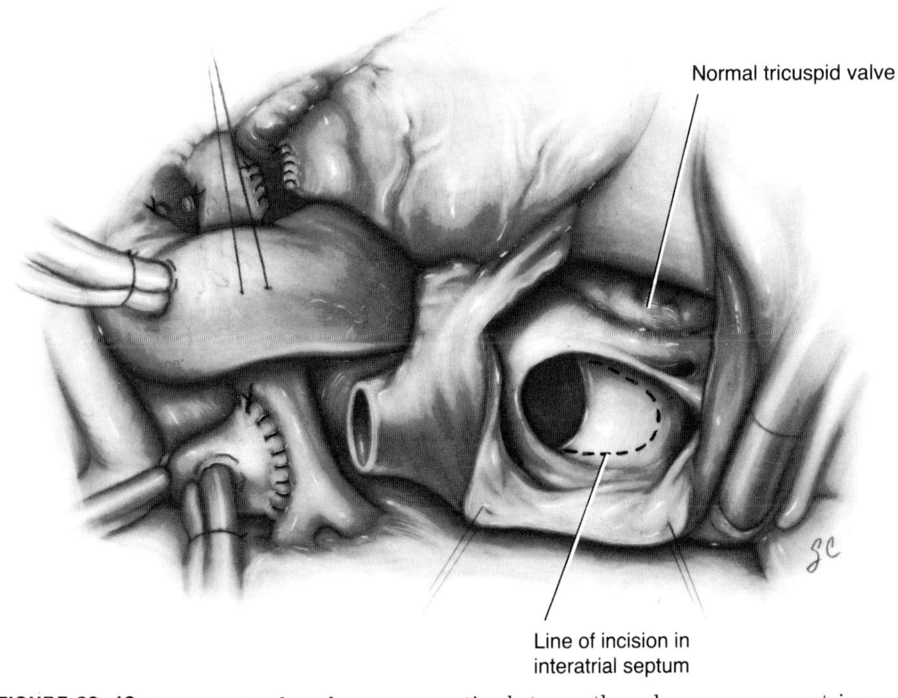

FIGURE 63–13. In patients who rely on a connection between the pulmonary venous atrium and the tricuspid valve (e.g., those with hypoplastic left heart syndrome), the Fontan procedure is best accomplished by excising the atrial septum to reduce the likelihood of obstruction to pulmonary venous return.

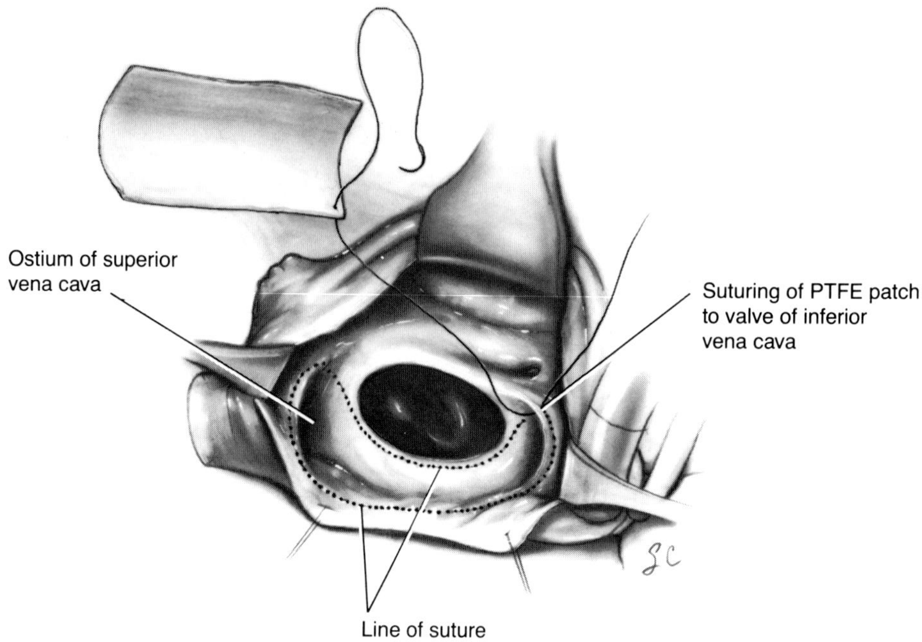

FIGURE 63–14. A Gore-Tex graft is opened longitudinally to provide a convex patch that can be placed (as shown by dashed lines) such that it creates a "tunnel" for the blood of the inferior vena cava (IVC) to be directed toward the SVC.

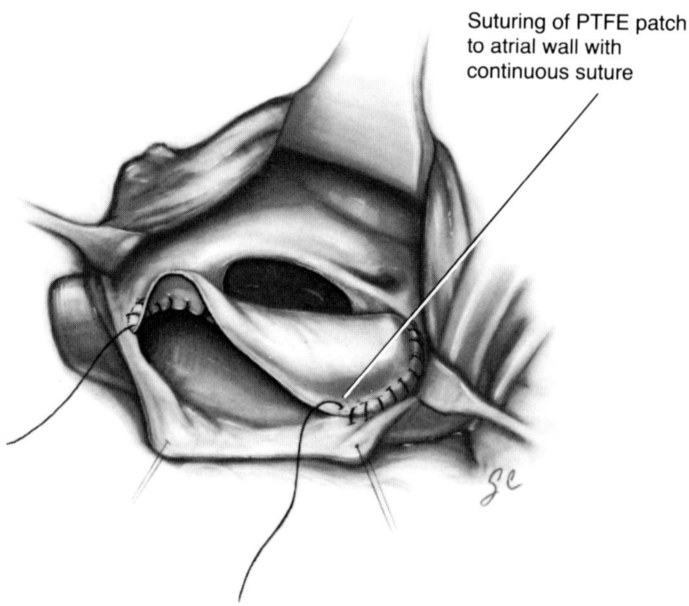

FIGURE 63–15. This baffle is sewn in place with a continuous suture so that the inferior vena caval return is directed toward the pulmonary arteries without interfering with pulmonary venous return across the atrial septal defect into the tricuspid valve. It is easiest to begin this suture line at the eustachian valve by the IVC and continue along the medial border of the patch all the way up to the SVC. The suture is then brought around the IVC and along the lateral border of the atrium (as shown).

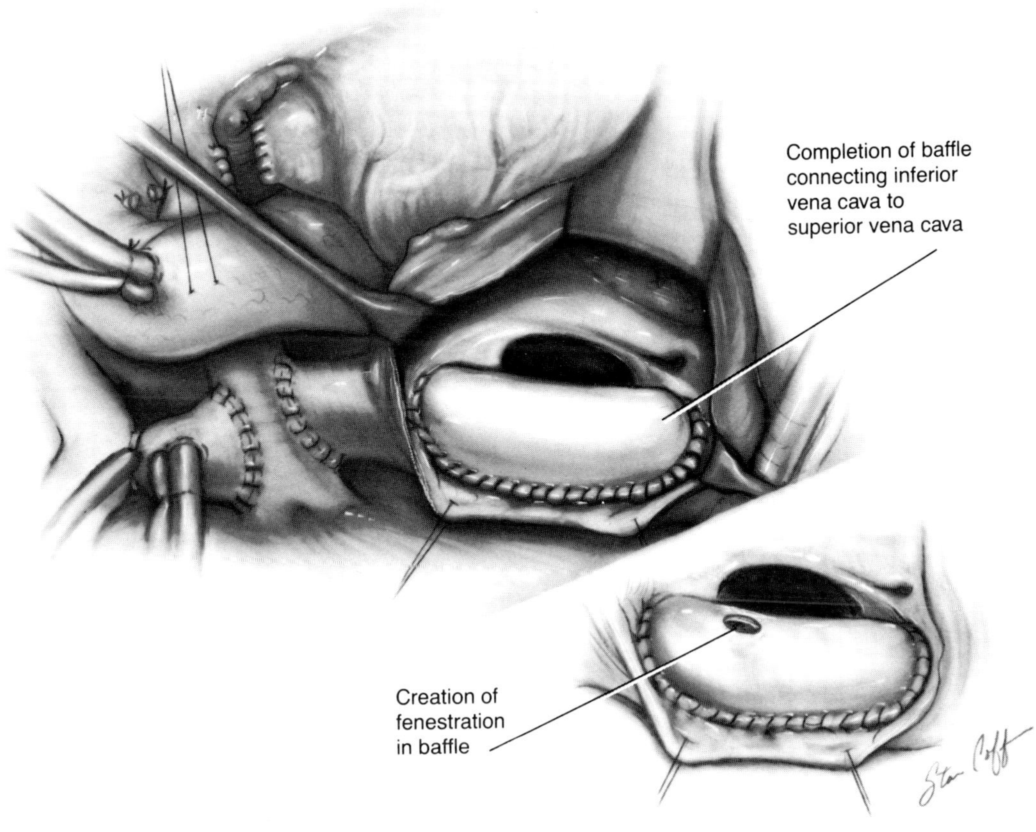

FIGURE 63–16. When this "lateral tunnel Fontan" is complete, the right atrium is closed. In some patients it is useful to place a small hole (fenestration) in this baffle to help the patient adapt to the physiology of a Fontan procedure. This lateral tunnel Fontan is now becoming the procedure of choice for all Fontan patients, including those with tricuspid atresia.

ROSS M. UNGERLEIDER, M.D.

64

Ebstein's Anomaly

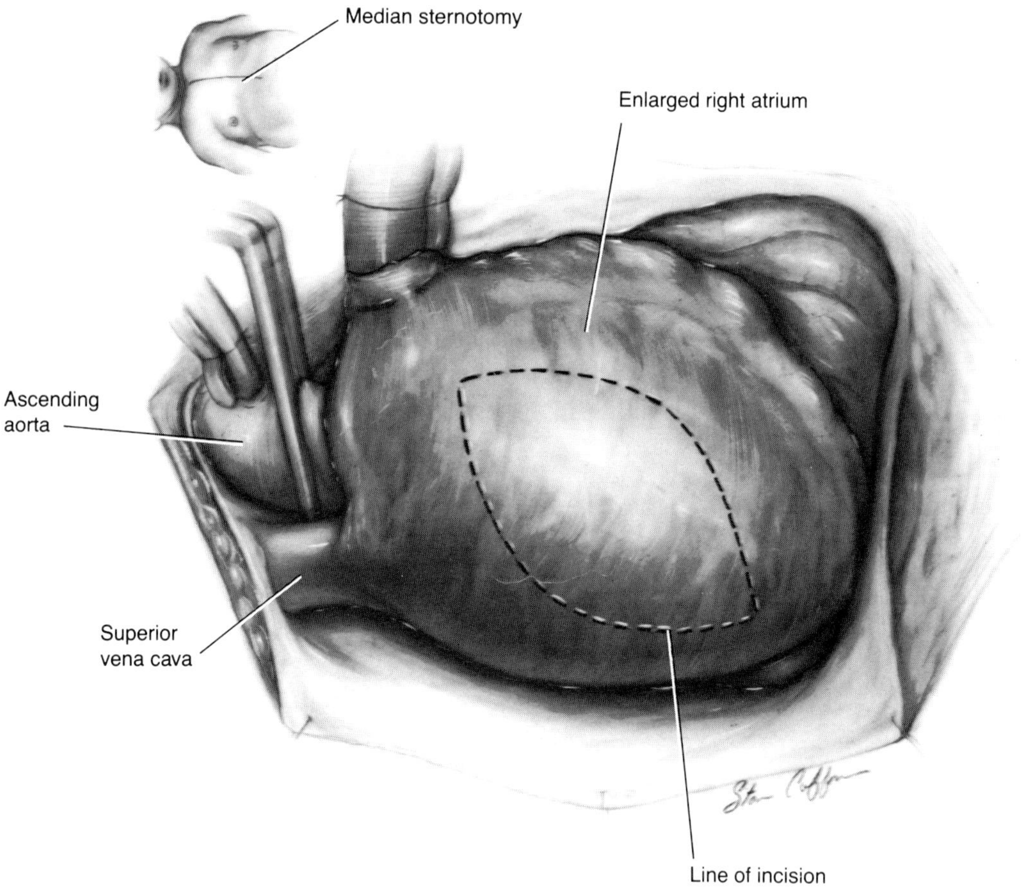

FIGURE 64–1. Infants who present with Ebstein's anomaly may require prostaglandin infusion to support pulmonary blood flow. In many cases, these infants slowly recover as the pulmonary vascular resistance falls and the heart is able to provide pulmonary blood flow. The occasional infant with Ebstein's anomaly (and the resulting tricuspid insufficiency with concomitant pulmonary stenosis) may present with marked cardiomegaly and inability to be weaned from prostaglandins. Such a patient should have a surgical procedure, and the heart is approached through a median sternotomy. After the pericardium is opened, the extremely enlarged right atrium must be retracted inferiorly to expose the aorta for cannulation. The patient can be placed on cardiopulmonary bypass with a single venous cannula through the right atrial appendage. Once on bypass, the patient is cooled to 18°C. The aorta is then crossclamped, and the heart is arrested with cardioplegic solution. Alternatively, with the patient on bypass, the right atrium can be retracted medially, exposing the superior vena cava (SVC) and inferior vena cava (IVC) for dual cannulation. If dual cannulation is preferred, it is easier to perform this once the patient is on bypass and the enormous right atrium is decompressed. When the patient is prepared for the intracardiac portion of the operation, a large elliptic portion of right atrial wall is excised, as shown by the dashed lines.

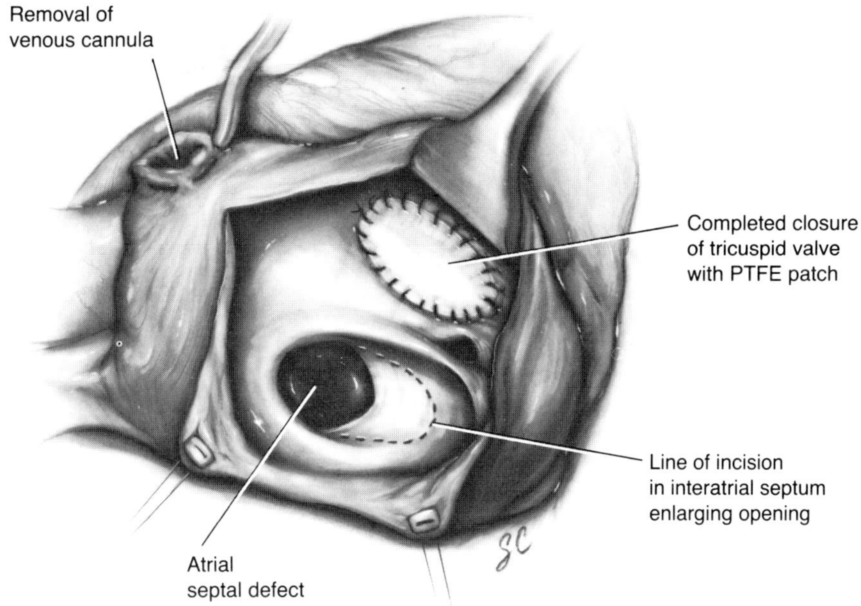

FIGURE 64–2. The internal anatomy of the right atrium is examined. There is commonly a large atrial septal defect of the secundum variety, and this is enlarged by excising the remaining septum primum to produce a totally unrestrictive intra-atrial communication. The tricuspid valve is closed with a patch of Gore-Tex placed through the leaflet material along the septal region to limit the risk of damage to the conduction tissue.

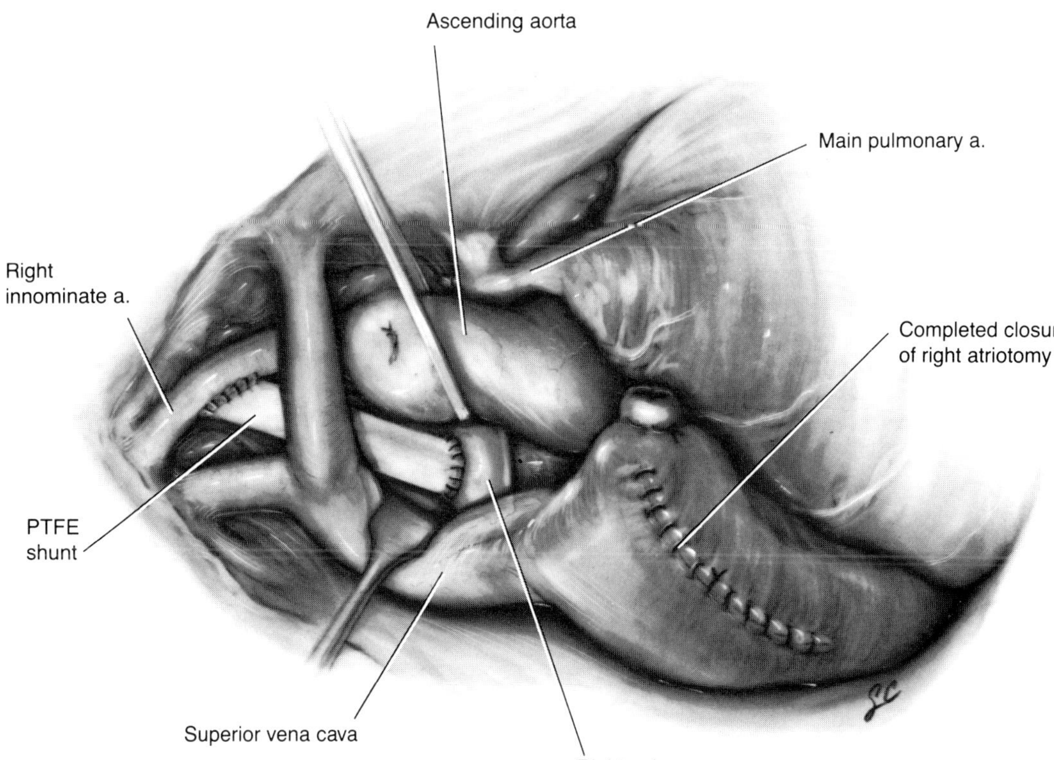

FIGURE 64–3. The right atriotomy is closed primarily, and the size of the right atrium should be dramatically reduced by the excision of part of the right atrial wall. The patient is replaced on bypass (if total circulatory arrest has been used), and the crossclamp can be removed. During the remainder of the rewarming period, a Gore-Tex shunt (usually 4.0 mm) is placed between the right innominate artery and the right pulmonary artery. This procedure effectively creates the physiology of tricuspid atresia and provides the first stage toward a Fontan procedure. Infants who present with Ebstein's anomaly in the neonatal period may have the best chance of survival as well as the best long-term outcome if staged toward a Fontan procedure in this manner.

SECTION XIII

Acquired Cardiac Valvular Disease

PETER VAN TRIGT, III, M.D.

65

Closure of Wounds of the Heart

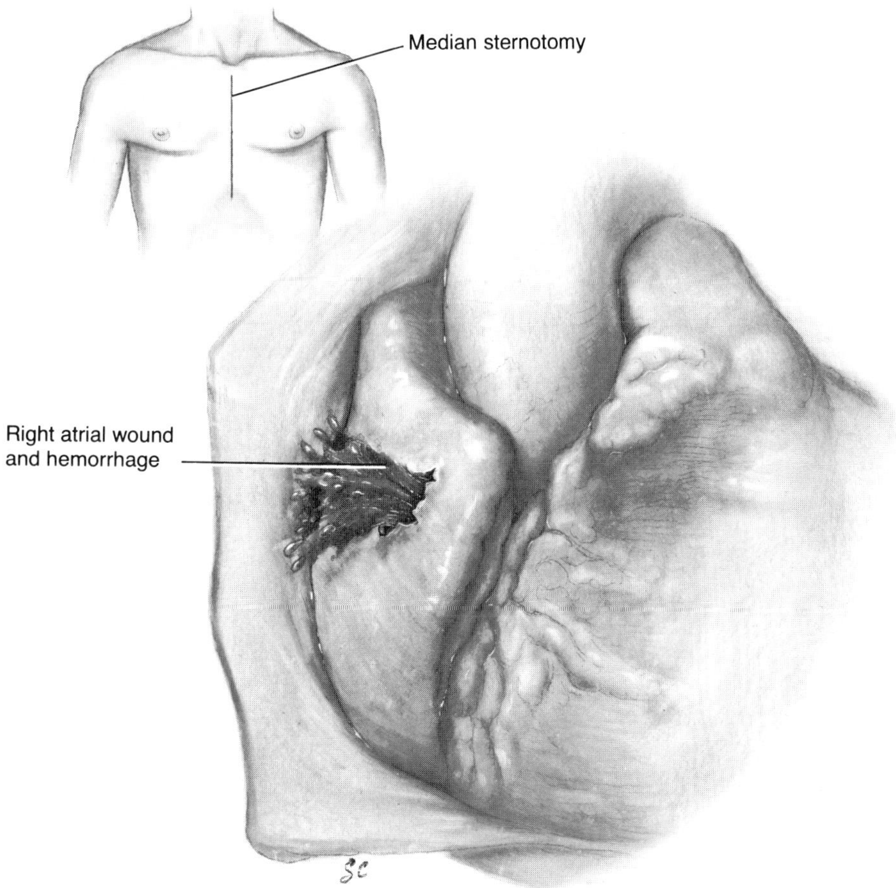

FIGURE 65–1. Penetrating wounds of the heart are best approached through a median sternotomy with standby cardiopulmonary bypass. The pericardium is widely opened, and the site of bleeding must be identified quickly. Atrial injuries generally produce significant tamponade, as the thin-walled structure freely bleeds into the pericardial space.

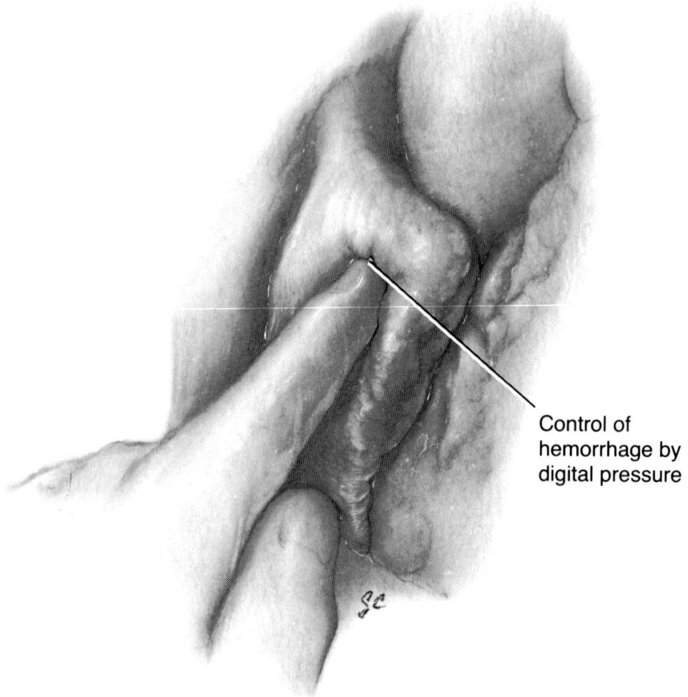

FIGURE 65–2. The site of hemorrhage is quickly controlled with digital pressure.

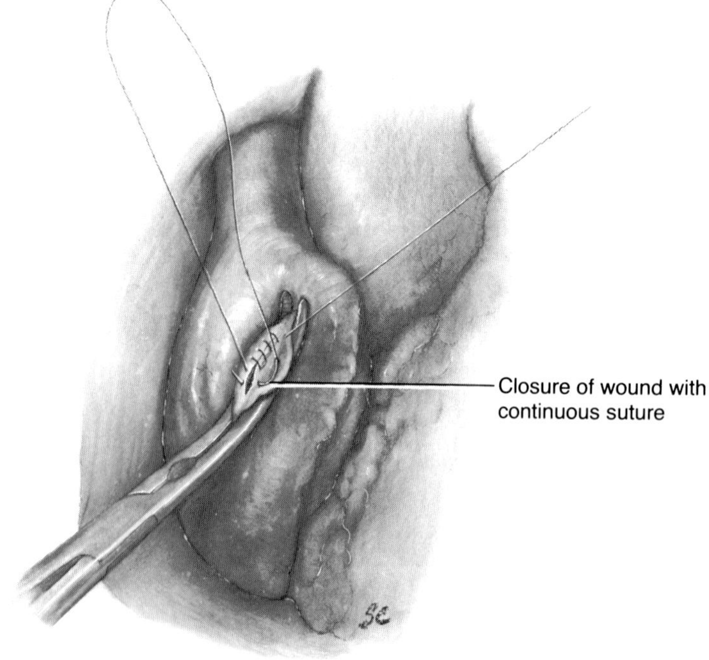

FIGURE 65–3. A vascular clamp is placed below the site of the right atrial injury, and the defect is closed with a continuous suture.

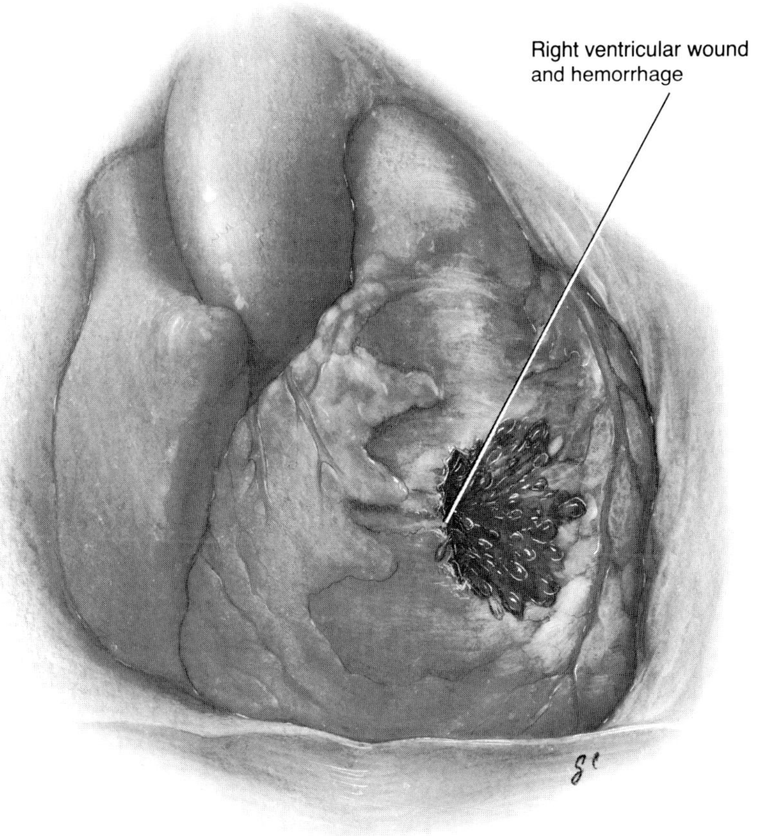

FIGURE 65–4. When the defect is in the anterior surface of the heart in the right ventricle, the site of bleeding is immediately controlled with a sponge stick or direct digital pressure.

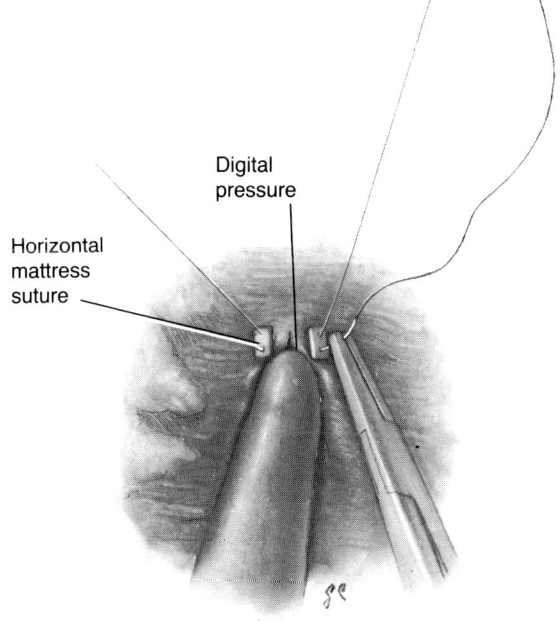

FIGURE 65–5. Interrupted horizontal mattress sutures are placed through pledgets to initially close the defect and control hemorrhage while digital pressure is being applied.

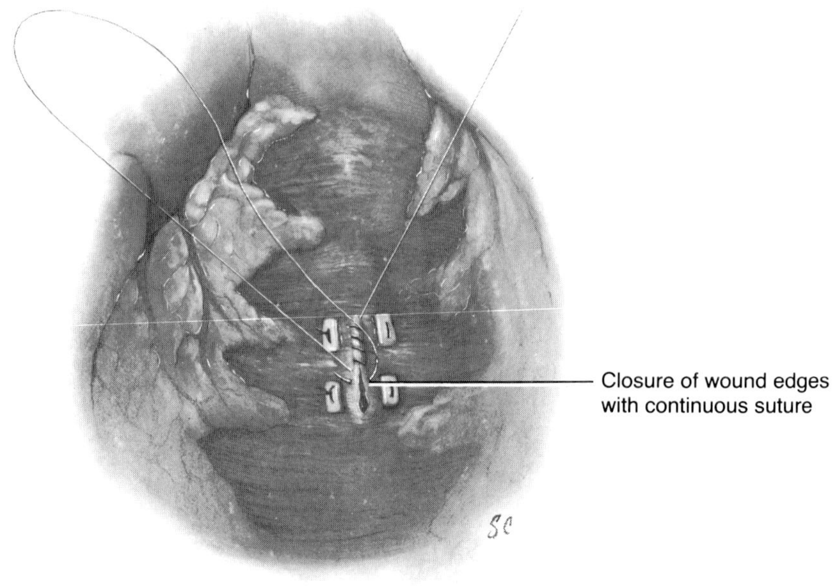

FIGURE 65–6. After placement of the interrupted mattress sutures, a continuous suture is used to obtain complete hemostasis by approximating the edges of the wound.

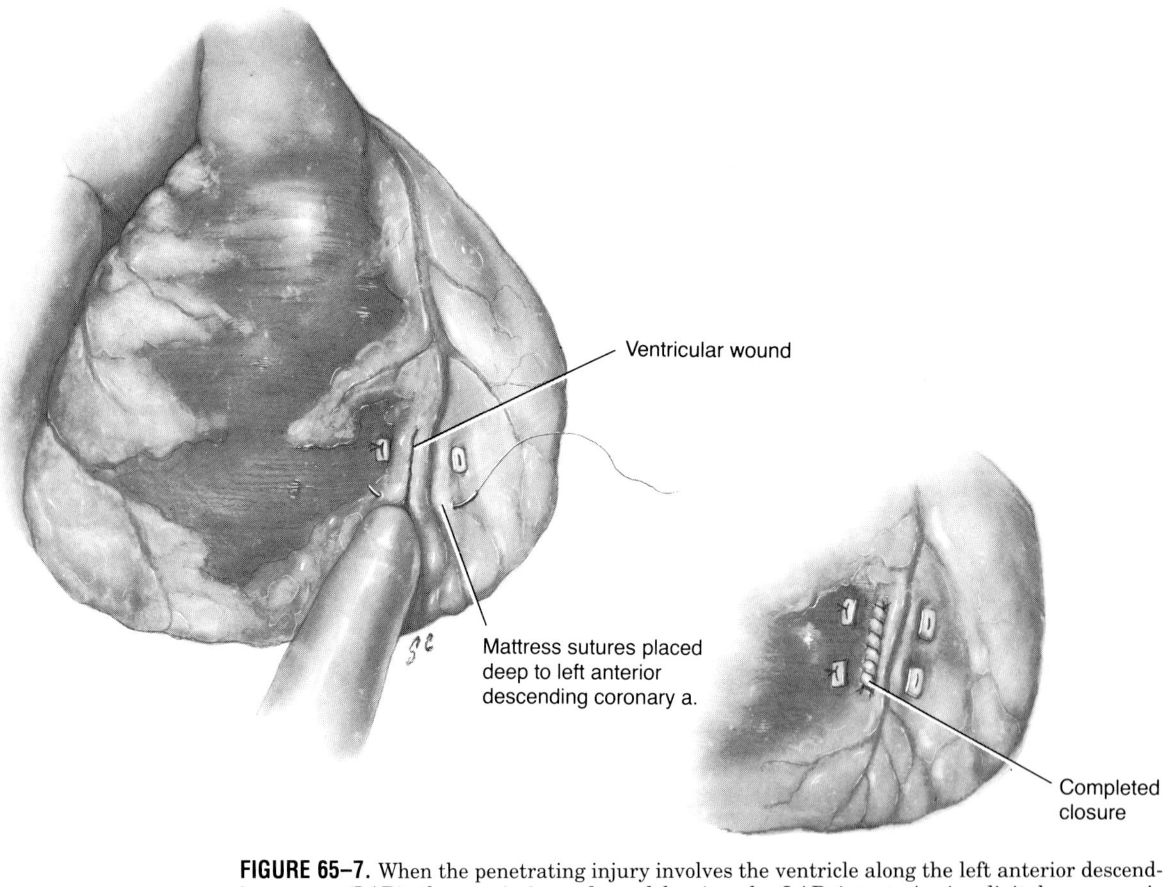

FIGURE 65–7. When the penetrating injury involves the ventricle along the left anterior descending artery (LAD), the repair is performed leaving the LAD intact. Again, digital pressure is applied while opposing pledgeted mattress sutures are used to gain control of the bleeding. They are carefully passed deep to the left anterior descending artery without compromising the myocardium of the ventricular apex. A continuous suture is again used to obtain complete hemostasis.

PETER VAN TRIGT, III, M.D.

66

Tricuspid Valve Replacement for Tricuspid Stenosis

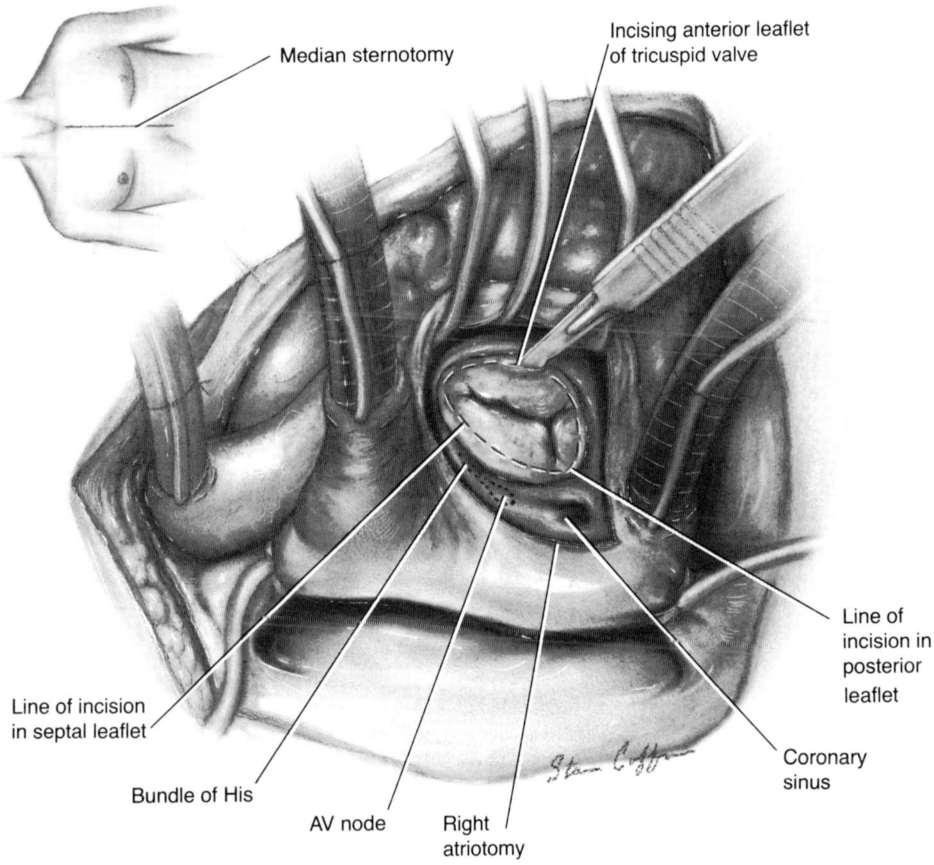

FIGURE 66–1. Tricuspid valve replacement is performed with the patient on cardiopulmonary bypass and the heart beating, usually after the crossclamp has been removed following mitral (and sometimes also aortic) valve replacement. The tricuspid valve is exposed by a transverse right atrial incision. Systemic venous return is diverted through individual venous cannulae placed into the superior and inferior venae cavae and snared by tapes. The anterior and posterior leaflets are excised at their junction to the annulus. The septal leaflet is excised so as to leave a margin along the inferior aspect of the annulus, along which the conduction system is located.

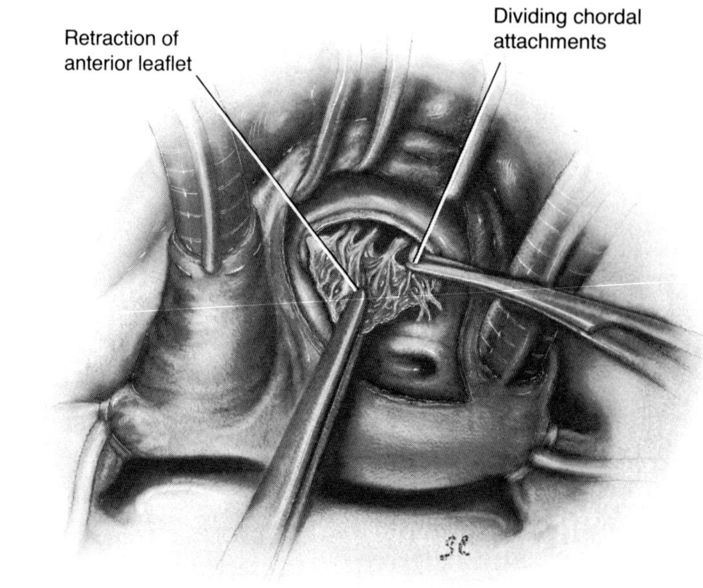

FIGURE 66–2. The chordal attachments to the leaflets are divided at their junction with the papillary muscles.

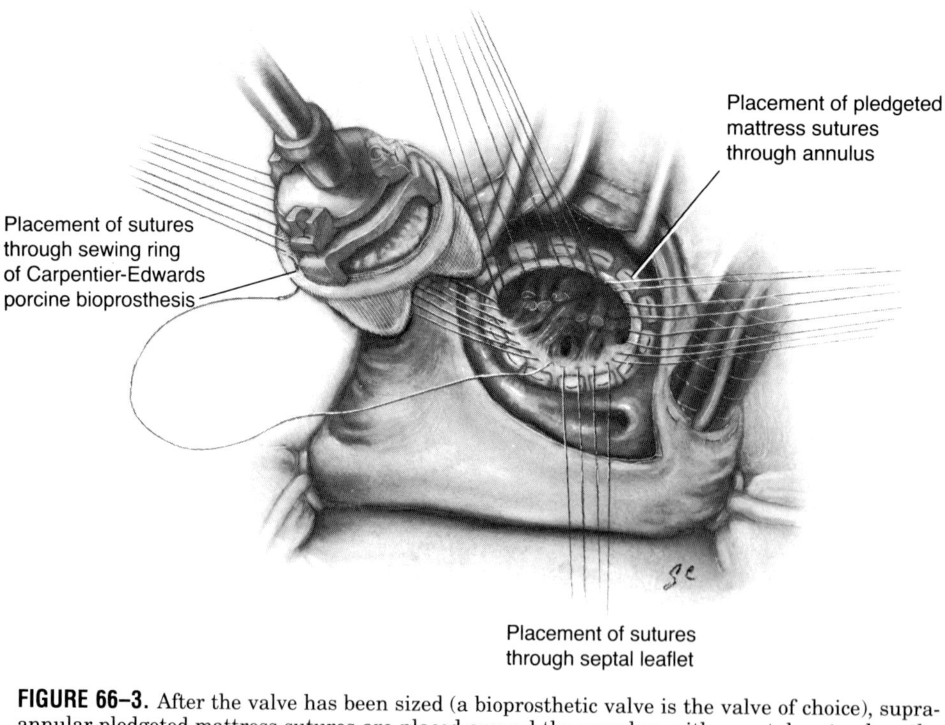

FIGURE 66–3. After the valve has been sized (a bioprosthetic valve is the valve of choice), supra-annular pledgeted mattress sutures are placed around the annulus, with care taken to place the sutures through the remnant of the septal leaflet to avoid injury to the conduction system. The sutures are then passed sequentially through the Dacron sewing ring of the bioprosthetic valve.

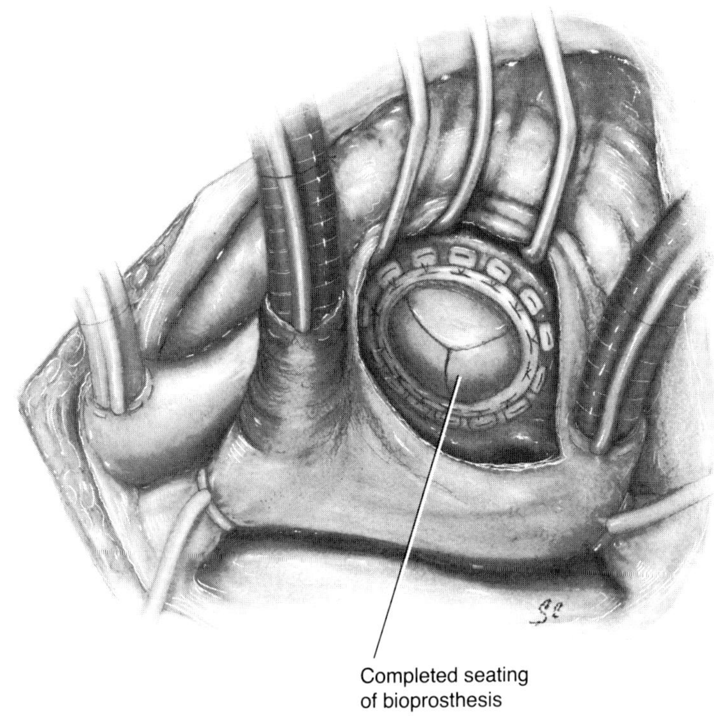

FIGURE 66–4. The valve is carefully seated with the struts passing into the right ventricle, and the sutures are individually tied. Air is vented from the right side of the heart, and the atriotomy is closed with a continuous mattress suture.

JAMES M. DOUGLAS, JR., M.D.

67
Tricuspid Valve Repair

The tricuspid valve is frequently rendered insufficient as a consequence of diseases of the left side of the heart or pulmonary circulation, including mitral valve disease and aortic valve disease. Dilatation of the tricuspid annulus occurs as a result of volume overload or excessive right ventricular pressures. The decision to restore competence to the tricuspid valve can be quite complicated. However, when the surgeon determines that restoration of tricuspid valve competence is advisable, and the native leaflets of the tricuspid valve are normal, tricuspid valve annuloplasty is clearly the treatment of choice. Tricuspid valve replacement should rarely, if ever, be considered when the tricuspid valve leaflets and chordal attachments are normal. Numerous techniques exist for performing a satisfactory tricuspid annuloplasty. This chapter describes the insertion of a Carpentier tricuspid annuloplasty ring.

PROCEDURE

The patient is placed on cardiopulmonary bypass with bicaval cannulation. If the tricuspid operation is performed in association with other cardiac procedures, the annuloplasty is generally performed last. The annuloplasty may be performed under cardioplegic arrest or during hypothermic ventricular fibrillation.

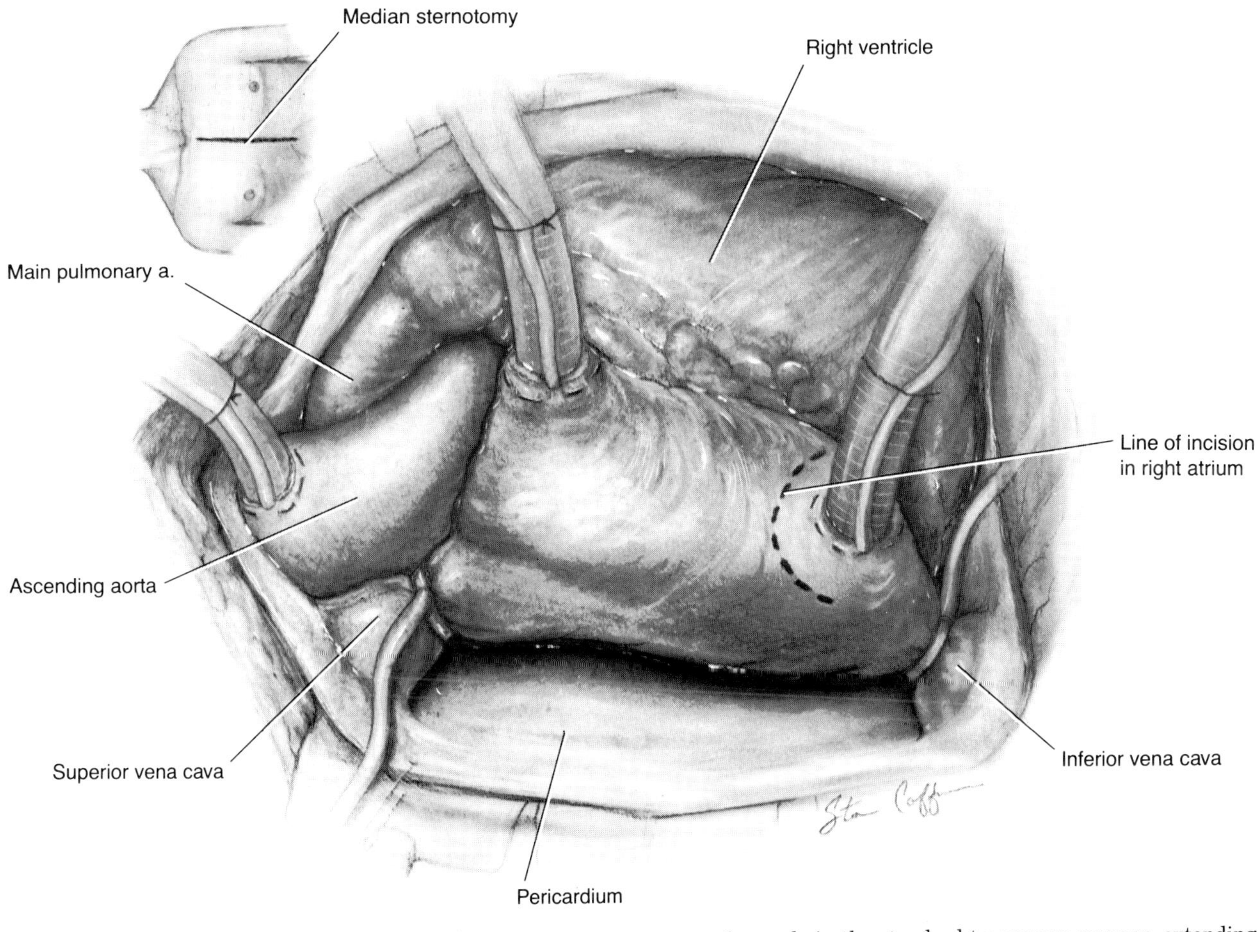

FIGURE 67–1. The initial atriotomy can be made in the standard transverse manner, extending from the right atrial appendage down toward the inferior vena caval cannulation site. Alternatively, a preferable incision is a semicircular one performed low in the atrium, approximately 1.5 to 2 cm away from the insertion site of the inferior vena caval cannula. This allows excellent exposure of the tricuspid valve and easy subsequent closure.

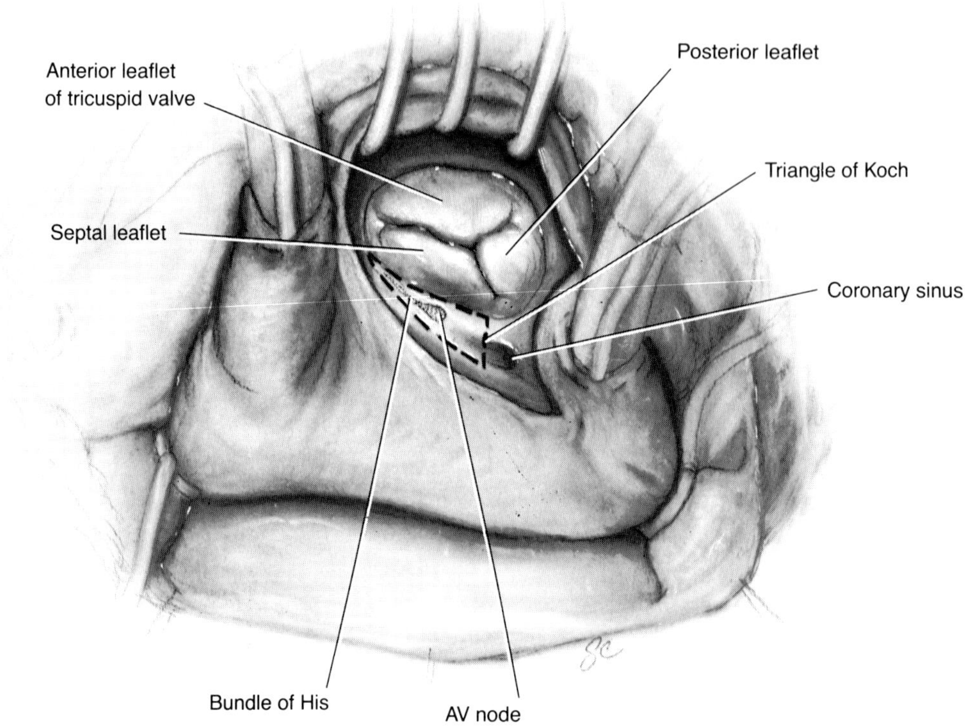

FIGURE 67–2. The primary considerations in performing a tricuspid annuloplasty are choosing the appropriate-size ring and proper orientation of the ring so that its placement does not interfere with the cardiac conduction system—the bundle of His and the atrioventricular node. The annuloplasty ring is oriented so that the open end corresponds to the region of the conduction tissue. This area is defined by the apex of the triangle of Koch.

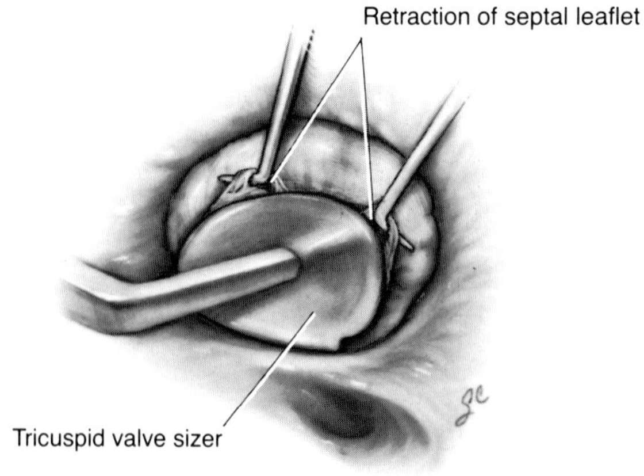

FIGURE 67–3. The annuloplasty ring chosen should be one that matches the area of the unfurled septal leaflet. The size is measured using an annuloplasty ring obturator. Typically, the normal-size adult female patient requires a #31 ring, and the normal-size adult male requires a #33 ring.

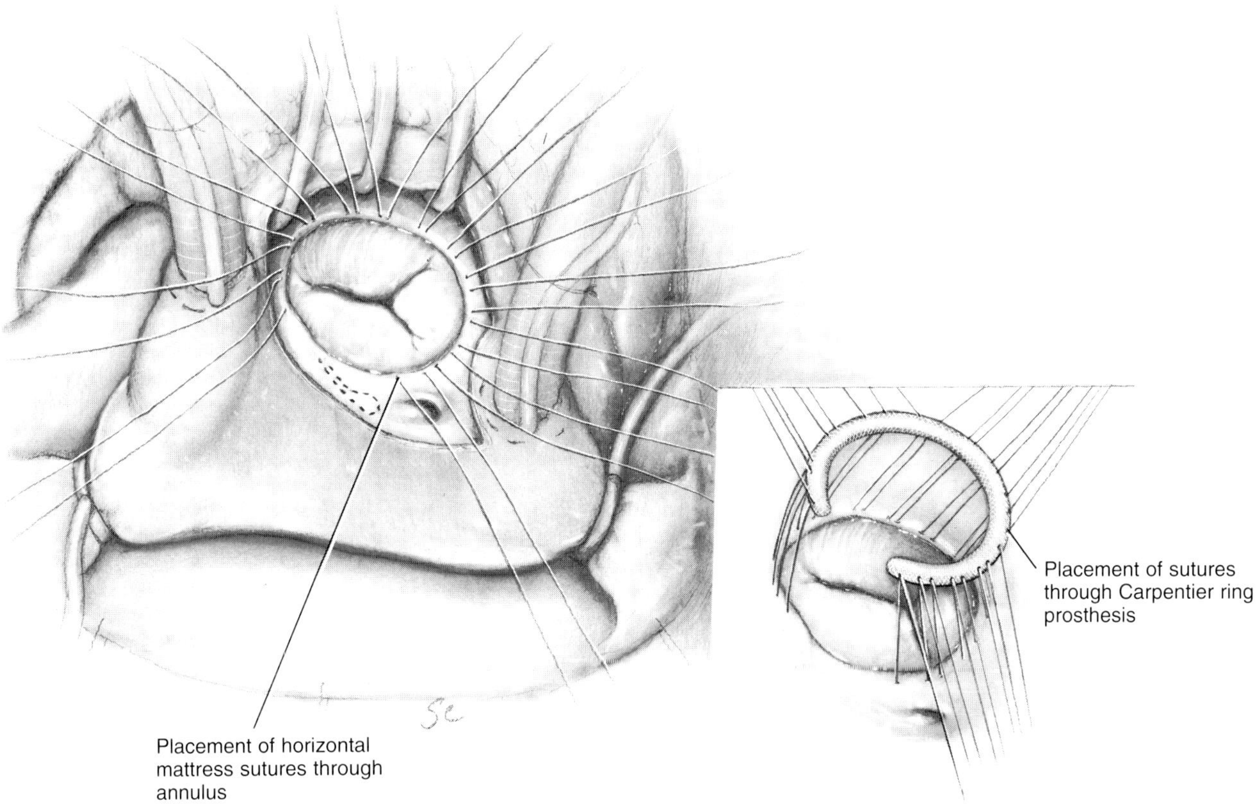

FIGURE 67–4. The annuloplasty sutures are placed in horizontal mattress form through the tricuspid annulus. This area lies approximately 1 mm away from the junction of the tricuspid leaflet with the muscular tissue. The sutures should be spaced so that the commissural areas, not the leaflet areas, are plicated for annular narrowing. This is performed by placing equal bites through the heart tissue and the ring in the areas at the base of the leaflets, but narrower bites are placed on the ring than on the heart tissue in the regions corresponding to the commissures.

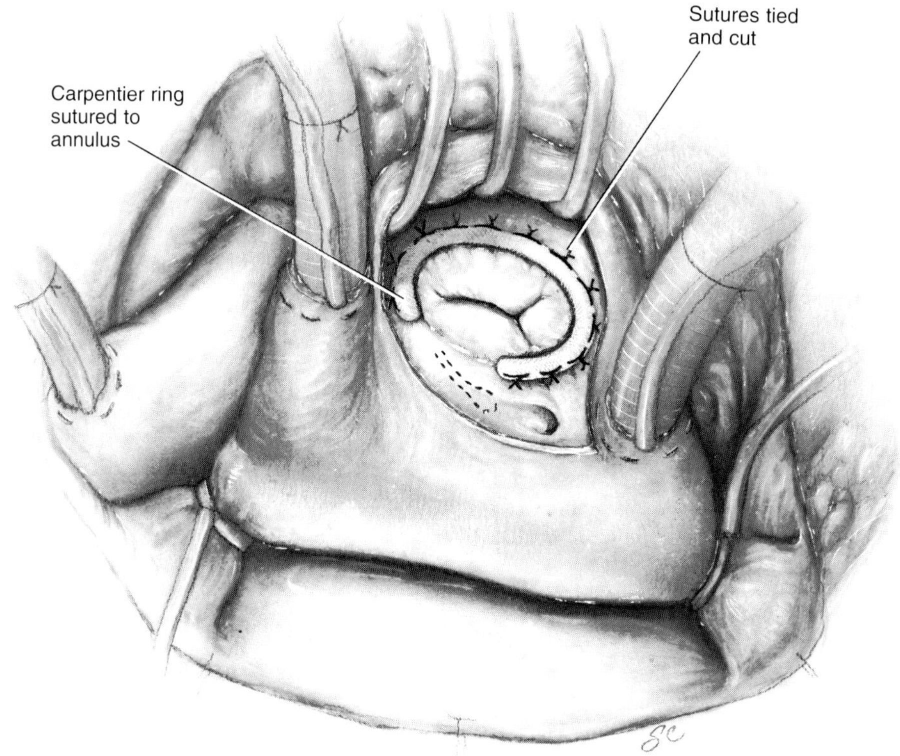

FIGURE 67–5. The sutures are tied securely for completion of the annuloplasty. Reliable testing of the competence of the valve is not possible in the tricuspid position before cardiac function is restored. However, if the appropriate-size ring has been chosen and the valve leaflets and underlying chords are normal, valve competence can be ensured.

JAMES M. DOUGLAS, JR., M.D.

68

Mitral Valve Replacement

Mitral valve replacement is indicated whenever disease of the valve leaflet is so severe or the valve pathology so complex that a lasting and functional mitral valve repair is not likely. Additionally, mitral valve replacement is indicated in patients for whom the surgeon feels the ultimate long-term outcome or immediate postoperative course would be jeopardized by attempted mitral valve repair.

Adequate exposure of the mitral valve is the most important step in ensuring a safe and effective operation. The valve is most commonly approached by a median sternotomy. This approach allows the best general access to the great vessels and cardiac chambers. In selected circumstances, a right anterolateral thoracotomy through the fourth intercostal space can be employed. This can provide good visualization of the mitral valve, but access to the aorta is limited, and cannulation of the femoral artery is required for arterial inflow. It is not an acceptable approach in the setting of aortic insufficiency, and removal of cardiac air can be problematic. Very rarely, the valve can be approached through a left posterolateral thoracotomy.

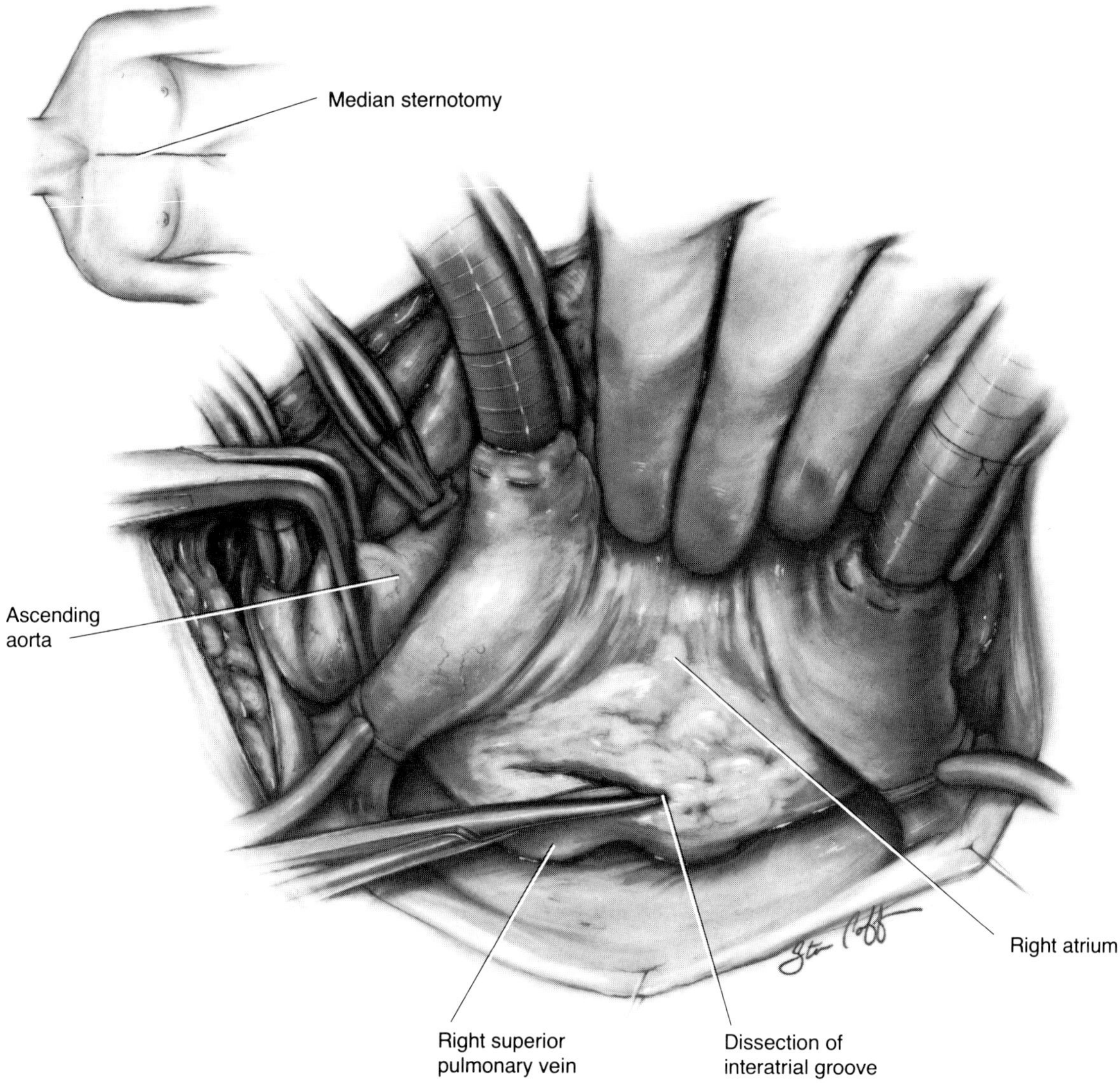

FIGURE 68–1. After sternotomy and opening of the pericardium, the heart is cannulated for cardiopulmonary bypass. Double venous cannulation of the venae cavae by way of the right atrium is generally employed. This author prefers straight venous cannulae. In most adult patients, a size 32 French cannula in the superior vena cava and a size 38 French cannula in the inferior vena cava provide excellent venous drainage and an easy fit. Encircling of the venae cavae and their generous mobilization aid in the subsequent exposure of the mitral valve. Umbilical tapes secured with Rumel tourniquets can be used for subsequent upward retraction on the cavae. They may be tightened following cardioplegic arrest in order to minimize blood return into the right atrium and its subsequent delivery through the right heart and pulmonary circuit into the left atrium. The interatrial groove is dissected just anterior to the right superior pulmonary vein. This dissection is carried all the way to the level of the atrial septum. During the course of the aforementioned dissections, the core temperature of the body is reduced to 28°C. After the dissection is completed, the aorta is crossclamped and cardioplegic solution delivered through the aortic root. In operations that may be lengthy or in patients with associated coronary disease, the author has found it useful to additionally use the coronary sinus route for retrograde delivery of cardioplegia. This improves myocardial protection and reduces the need to change exposure of the valve during the course of the operation to deliver cardioplegic solution.

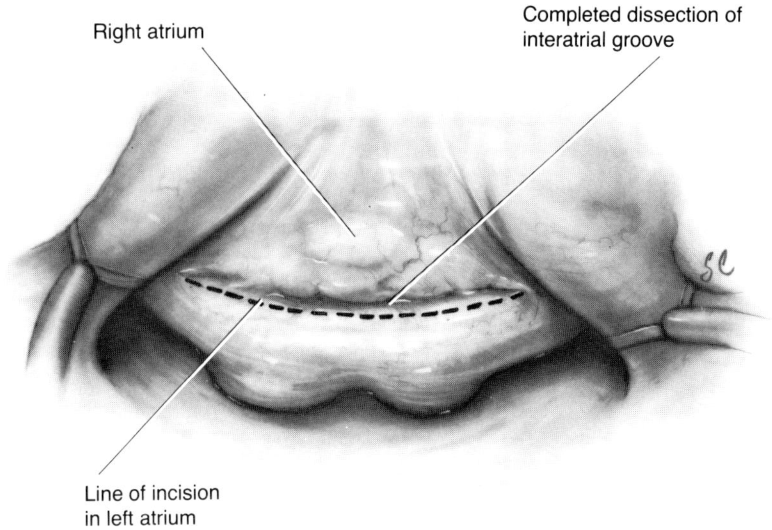

FIGURE 68–2. After the cardioplegic solution is delivered, the Rumel tourniquets encircling the cavae are tightened and retracted upward. A transverse left atriotomy is performed and extended superiorly and inferiorly beneath the venae cavae. The mitral valve is then exposed by superior traction using a hand-held atrial retractor. In more lengthy cases, self-retaining retracting systems such as the Carpentier or Cosgrove retractors may be preferable.

Valve replacement is frequently preceded by excision of some part of the native valve tissue. However, preservation of the posterior leaflet with its chordal attachments is strongly recommended. Preserving these attachments is a strong deterrent against the risk of potentially fatal atrioventricular separation. Furthermore, preservation of chordal attachments helps maintain left ventricular geometry, thereby improving ventricular function. Preservation of both the anterior and posterior leaflets should be strongly considered in the setting of ventricular impairment.

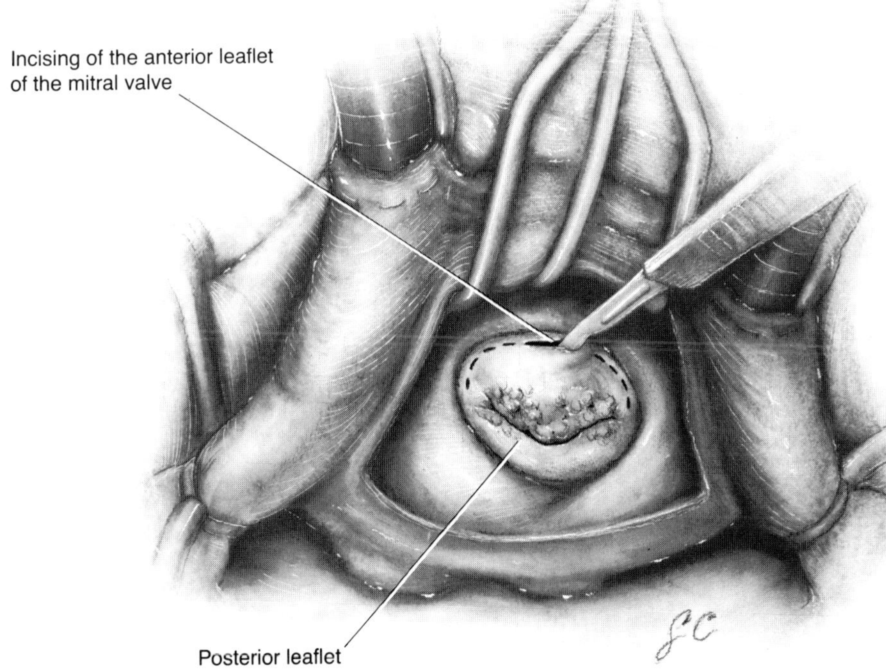

FIGURE 68–3. The anterior leaflet usually is excised, particularly if the valve leaflets are thickened or calcified. The line of incision is performed leaving approximately 1 to 2 mm of leaflet tissue along the circumference.

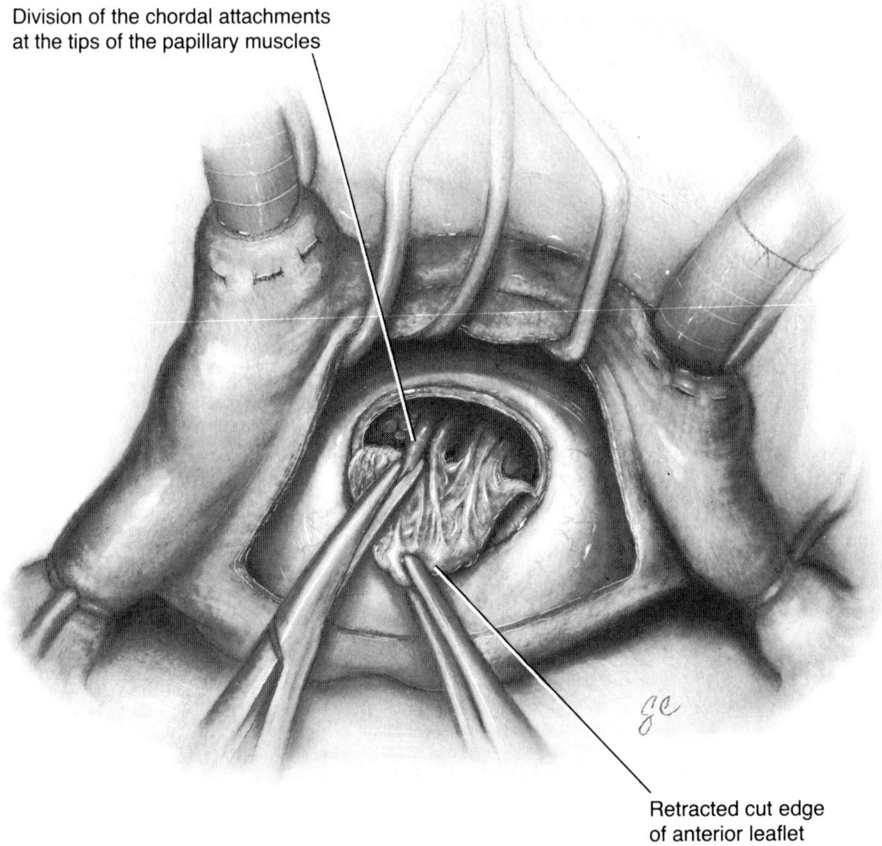

FIGURE 68–4. The chordal attachments are divided at the tips of the papillary muscles without division of the muscles themselves.

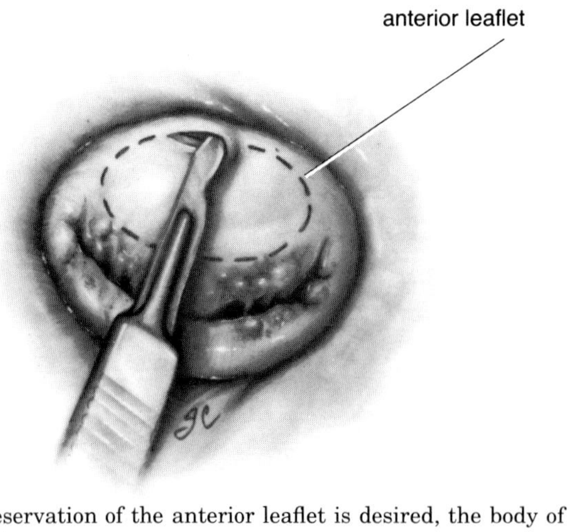

FIGURE 68–5. If preservation of the anterior leaflet is desired, the body of the leaflet is excised from its central portion.

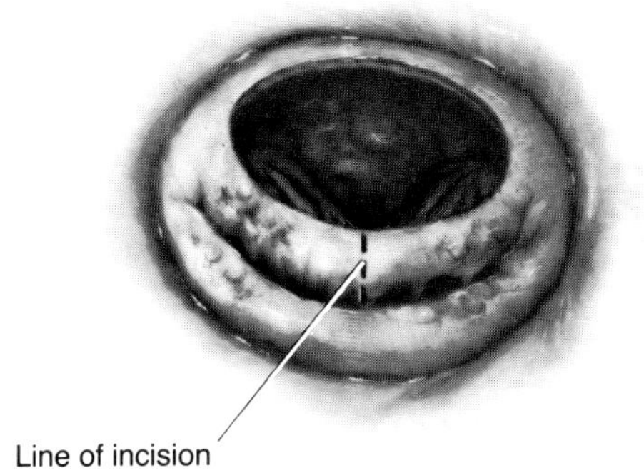

FIGURE 68–6. The leaflet is divided in the midportion between the chordal attachments and the free edge of the leaflet, and its associated chords are maintained in continuity.

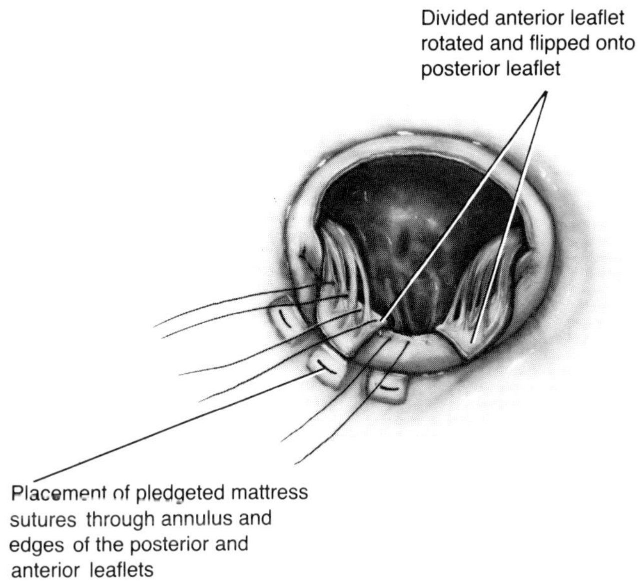

FIGURE 68–7. These leaflet edges are folded backward along the rim of the posterior leaflet and incorporated into the subsequent valve sutures.

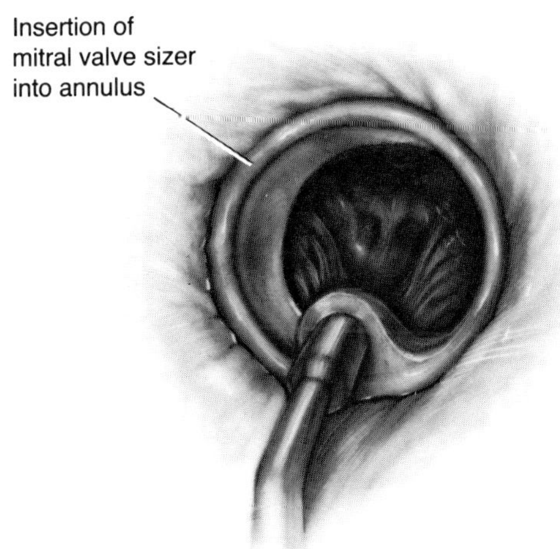

FIGURE 68–8. The valve orifice is sized by passing the largest valve obturator that goes easily through the orifice into the ventricle. The appropriate valve is then selected.

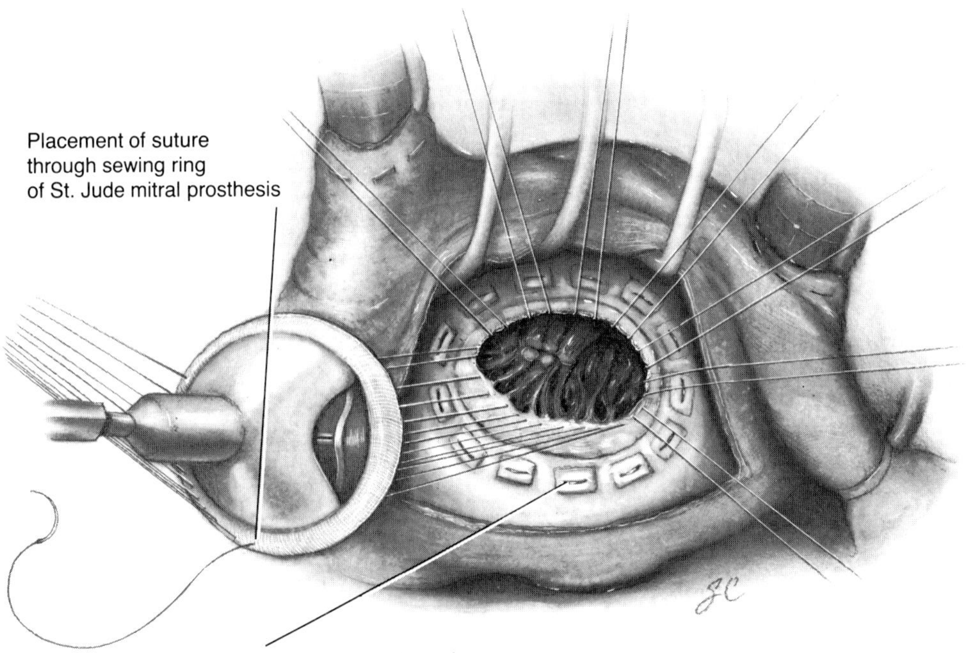

FIGURE 68–9. The valve is sutured into place using 2–0 braided, polyester, horizontal mattress, pledgeted, supra-annular stitches. Stitch placement within the horizontal mattress suture is at a width of approximately 3 to 4 mm. Each suture is placed 1 to 2 mm apart. Sutures are brought out through the valve tissue at the free edge.

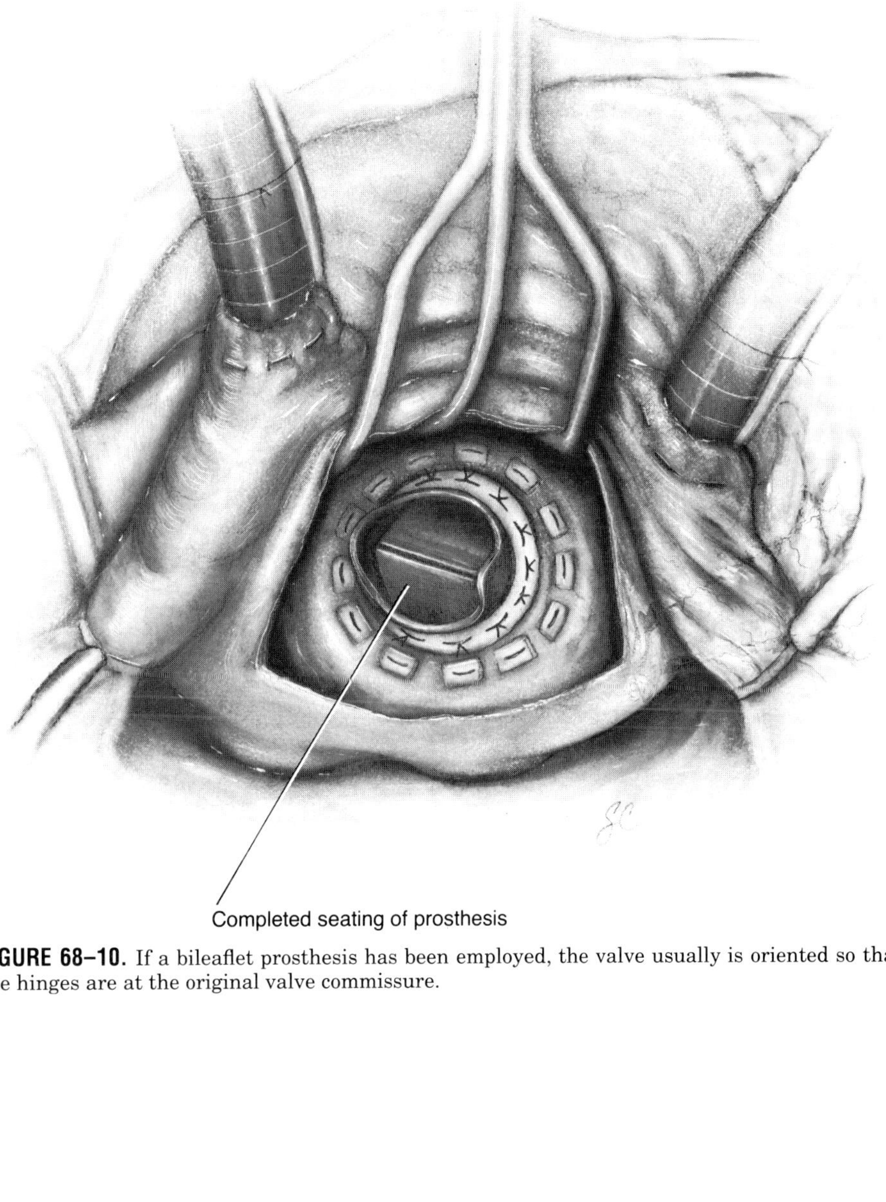

FIGURE 68–10. If a bileaflet prosthesis has been employed, the valve usually is oriented so that the hinges are at the original valve commissure.

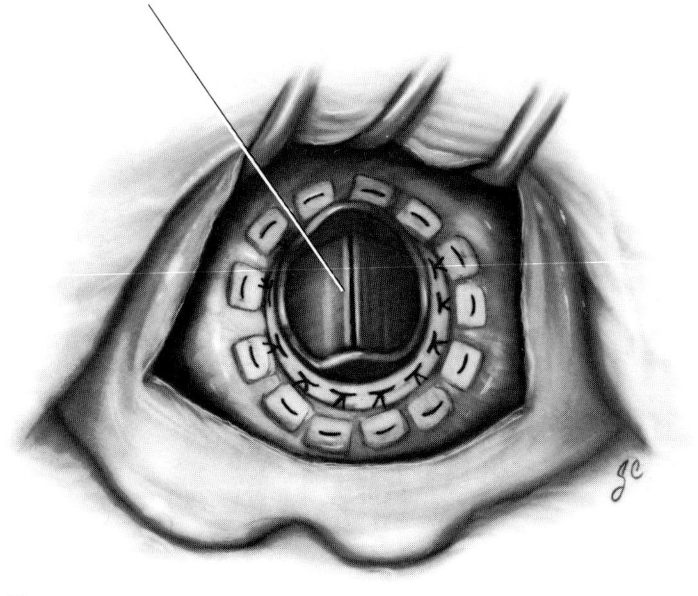

FIGURE 68–11. However, if chordal attachments to both anterior and posterior leaflets have been preserved, it is preferable to orient the valve at a 90-degree angle so that the hinges are in the anteroposterior orientation. This helps prevent slack chords from interfering with the valve mechanism.

Valve orientation is not critical when ball-in-cage valves are employed. Strutted porcine valves are oriented so that the strut does not lie in the left ventricular outflow tract, beneath the aortic valve.

REWARMING, REMOVAL OF CARDIAC AIR, ATRIAL CLOSURE, AND SEPARATION FROM CARDIOPULMONARY BYPASS

Rewarming of the patient typically is begun while the valve sutures are being tied down. In obese patients, in whom rewarming may be prolonged, this process may have to start somewhat earlier. In that case, additional cardioplegia is given if necessary to ensure good myocardial protection.

Removal of air from the heart is accomplished primarily through the opened left atrium. However, supplementary de-airing is also performed through the aorta. In preparation for de-airing, the prosthetic valve is kept incompetent by means of a Foley catheter or ventricular vent passed through the orifice of the valve. The vena caval tapes are loosened, and the perfusionist is instructed to restrict venous return to the pump so that the right heart fills with blood. The patient is rotated on the table away from the surgeon, and the head is declined so that air tends to rise toward the left atrial opening and aortic root at the level of the cardioplegic cannula. Any retrograde cardioplegic cannula that was placed is removed. The anesthesiologist then forces air out of the pulmonary veins into the left atrium by slow hyperexpansion of the lungs. Simultaneously, the surgeon gently massages the left ventricle and disturbs the left atrial appendage so that entrapped air evacuates through the left atrium.

Overvigorous massage of the heart when a strutted valve is in place may puncture the ventricular wall. Additionally, the elevation of the apex of the heart is to be avoided once the mitral prosthesis is in place. Elevating the heart with this rigid structure in place risks causing iatrogenic atrioventricular separation. While cardiac filling and massage is ongoing, suction is placed on the aortic vent to evacuate air through the aorta.

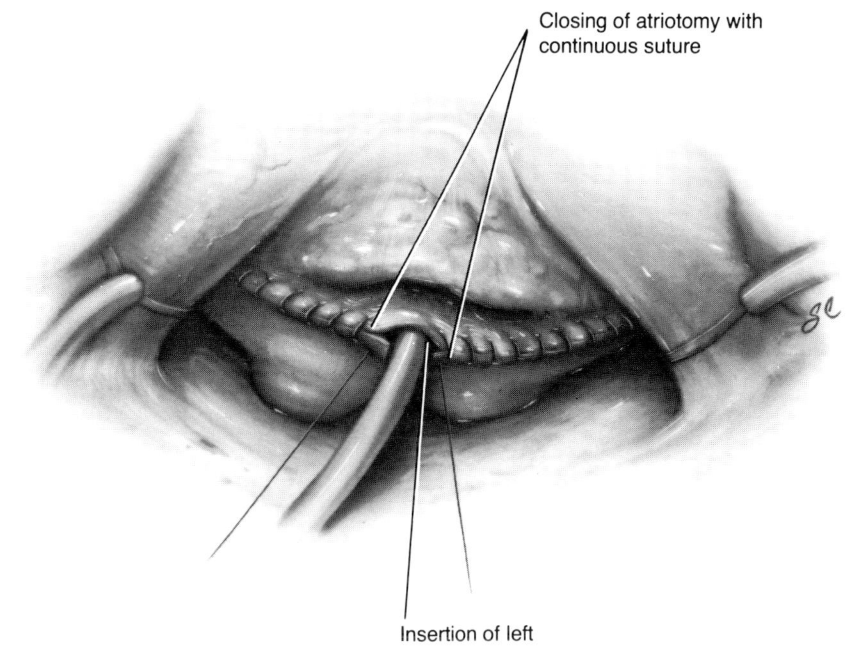

FIGURE 68–12. After this process, which should not be hurried, the atriotomy is closed and the aortic crossclamp is removed. Full venous return is then allowed to drain into the cardiopulmonary bypass circuit, and the heart is collapsed. When cardiac contractions resume, the heart is allowed to fill while suction is maintained on the aortic root. When the patient is fully warmed and cardiac function is restored, cardiopulmonary bypass is discontinued. Removal of air continues even after the heart resumes its function. Initially this is performed with direct suction via the aortic vent. After bypass is discontinued, this can be accomplished by allowing the aorta to bleed through the puncture site in the aortic root until the surgeon believes that adequate removal of air has been accomplished.

JAMES M. DOUGLAS, JR., M.D

69
Mitral Valve Repair

Techniques for mitral valve repair continue to evolve. This chapter adapts the principles advocated by Alain Carpentier. Any discrepancies are due to the author's interpretation and practice.

REPAIR OF MITRAL STENOSIS

Mitral stenosis is almost always caused by rheumatic heart disease. Valve repair is preferred in cases with moderate pathologic changes characterized by commissural fusion and minimal or moderate chordal shortening and fusion. Although extensive leaflet calcification and/or annular calcification may be repaired by advanced techniques, the overall results may be unsatisfactory except in the most experienced hands. Consequently, under these circumstances, valve replacement is recommended.

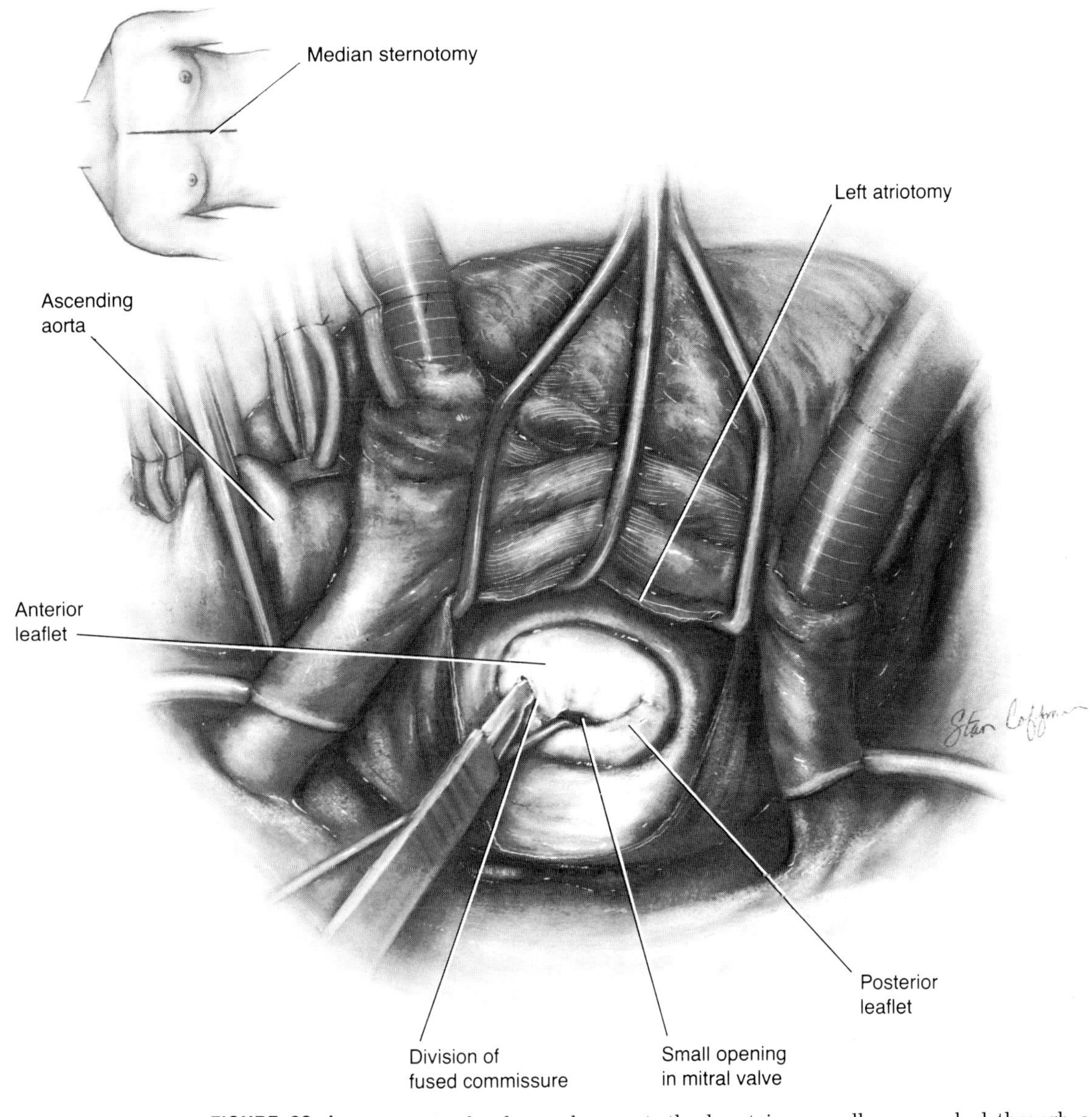

FIGURE 69–1. As in mitral valve replacement, the heart is generally approached through a median sternotomy. Cannulation for cardiopulmonary bypass is performed as described under mitral valve replacement. Full mobilization of the venae cavae and extensive dissection of the interatrial groove are recommended for all mitral valve repairs. Adequate exposure of the mitral valve is paramount for a satisfactory mitral valve repair.

Commissural fusion is treated by open commissurotomy. The actual commissurotomy is performed using a #15 blade scalpel beginning 3 to 4 mm from the valve annulus and extending in the direction of the valve orifice. If the commissural area is difficult to identify, recognition may be enhanced by grasping both the anterior and posterior leaflets of the mitral valve and bringing them together so that a natural fold in the commissure region may be induced. Observing the underlying chordal attachments sometimes reveals the symmetry of chordal attachments, which generally should be distributed equally in the commissural areas.

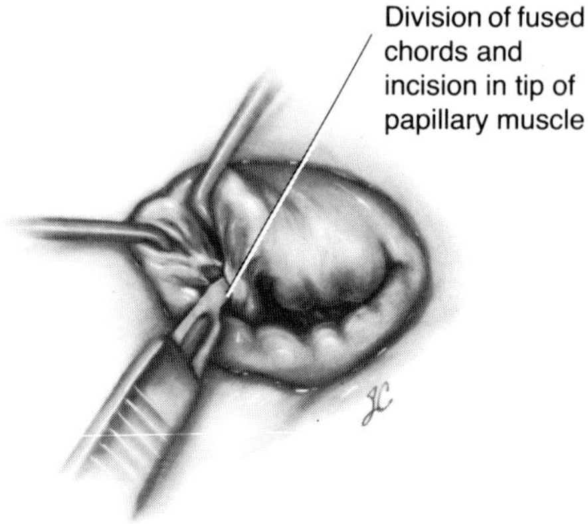

FIGURE 69–2. The incision is extended to the subvalvular apparatus to separate underlying fused chords or fused papillary muscles.

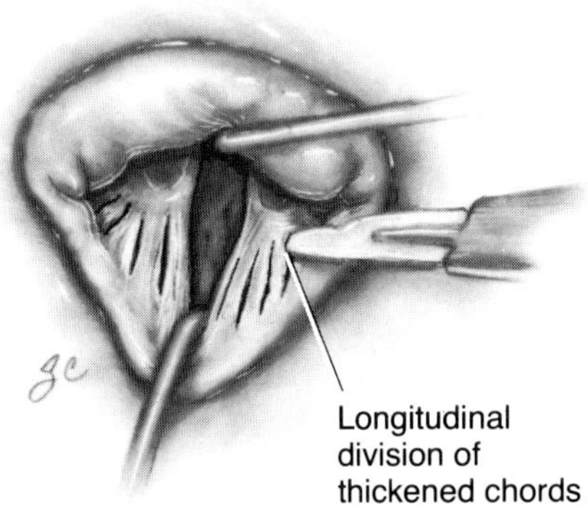

FIGURE 69–3. The posterior leaflet is typically restricted in its motion by the underlying thickened and fused chords. A degree of mobility may be restored by division of basilar chords to the posterior leaflet, which extend directly from the ventricular muscle to the body of the posterior leaflet. Additionally, separation of these chords can be accomplished by longitudinal division using a #11 blade.

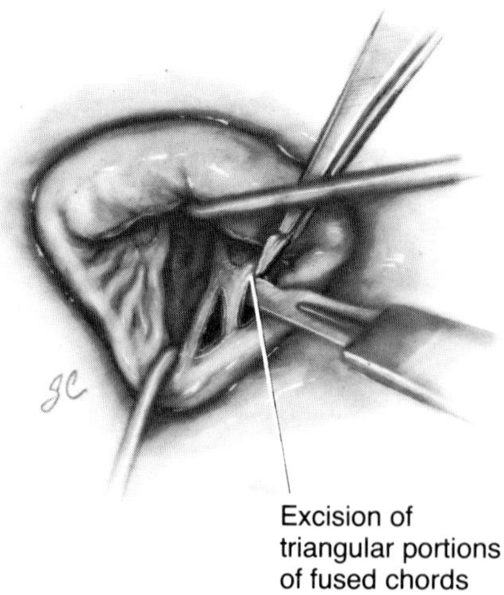

FIGURE 69–4. Very thickened chords can be mobilized more freely by actual excision of a core of the fibrosed structure (fenestration). Similar fenestration may be accomplished on the chords to the anterior leaflet. However, if extensive intervention with the anterior leaflet is required to accomplish a more normal valve, strong consideration should be given to valve replacement.

If there is associated valvular insufficiency as a result of leaflet prolapse or annular dilatation, this pathology is repaired as described under "Repair of Mitral Insufficiency."

REPAIR OF MITRAL INSUFFICIENCY

Mitral insufficiency is generally caused by leaflet prolapse, leaflet restriction, leaflet perforation, or annular dilatation.

The most important step in valve repair is proper analysis of the valve pathology. Valve prolapse is best assessed while tone remains in the cardiac muscles. Consequently, in regurgitant valves, it is preferable to analyze the cause of valvular regurgitation with the heart under cool fibrillatory arrest. During core cooling, ventricular arrest usually occurs at temperatures less than 30°C. If the aortic valve is competent, the left atrium may be opened widely and the valve examined without fear of air embolism, as long as perfusion pressure is maintained. The presence of aortic insufficiency necessitates crossclamping of the aorta while ventricular fibrillation is ongoing. With the heart cooled to 28°C or lower, several minutes of aortic occlusion can be tolerated without myocardial damage, as long as intermittent coronary perfusion is allowed. Two minutes of aortic occlusion may be induced safely in almost all circumstances at these temperatures. For the purpose of analyzing valve prolapse, it should rarely be necessary to extend the clamping beyond this time period. It should be remembered that after aortic crossclamping, air may accumulate within the aortic root. Consequently, aortic suction should be performed and the operating table leveled to allow evacuation of air through the aortic root by way of the aortic vent once the clamp is removed.

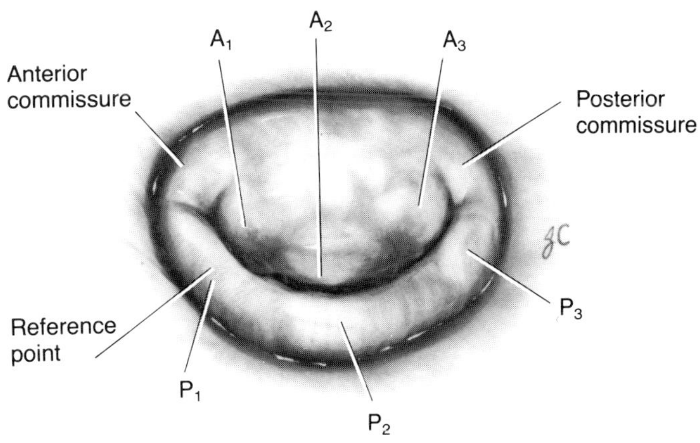

FIGURE 69–5. Carpentier has established a reproducible approach to analysis of prolapse and has divided each leaflet into definable regions.

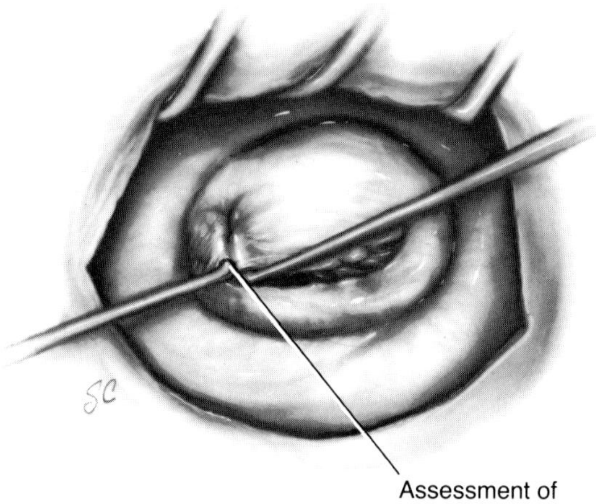

FIGURE 69–6. The area of the posterior leaflet closest to the anterolateral commissure (P_1) is rarely prolapsed and should be used as a reference point (RP) for evaluating prolapse in the remainder of the posterior leaflet and along the anterior leaflet. To do this, a nerve hook is employed to unfurl the free edge of the leaflet in this region and place the leaflet and the underlying chords under tension. A second nerve hook is then used to sequentially evaluate the midportion of the posterior leaflet (P_2), posteromedial portion of the posterior leaflet (P_3), anterolateral portion of the anterior leaflet (A_1), midpoint of the anterior leaflet (A_2), posteromedial portion of the anterior leaflet (A_3), and the anterior and medial commissural areas. In a sequential manner, these points are approximated toward the reference area, and the relative height above the normal leaflet coaptation level is identified. Areas of valve prolapse may be marked by placing stay sutures on either side around normal, intact chords.

After valve prolapse is assessed, preparations are made for cardioplegic arrest. If aortic crossclamping with ventricular fibrillation has been performed, reperfusion is allowed to proceed for 1 or 2 minutes. The aorta is then formally crossclamped and cardioplegic solution administered. The left atrium is then carefully retracted to ensure maximal exposure of the mitral valve apparatus. Careful note is made of the pathologic processes present.

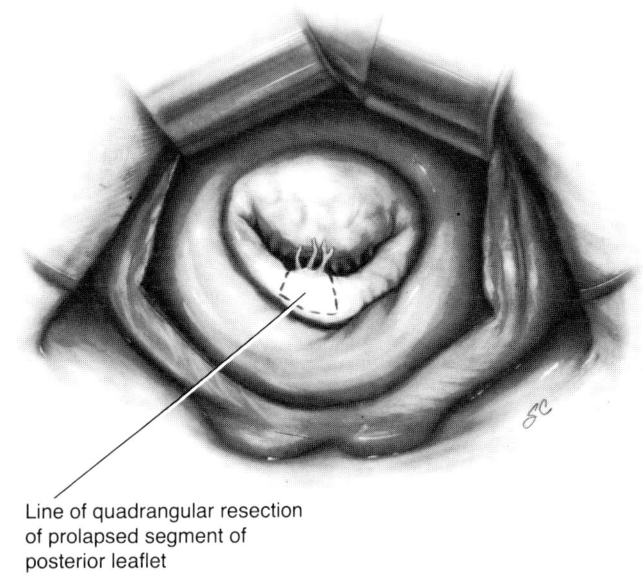

FIGURE 69–7. Posterior leaflet prolapse may be easily treated with quadrangular resection of the involved leaflet tissue. This approach is acceptable whenever 40% or less of the posterior leaflet is involved. Additionally, for best results, resection should be limited to the areas of the posterior leaflet away from the commissures. After the leaflet tissue is resected, it is convenient to place any sutures for an associated annuloplasty while this gap exists in the leaflet tissue, to improve visualization and assist proper placement of the annuloplasty sutures.

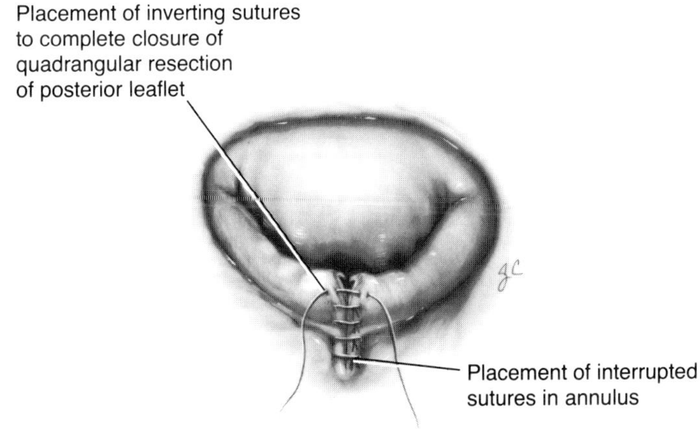

FIGURE 69–8. The leaflet is repaired with interrupted 5–0 sutures. When the leaflet resection is extensive, the annulus should be shortened by placement of one or two figure-of-eight sutures through the annulus to allow a tension-free repair of the leaflet tissue. Tension may also be reduced by incising the junction of the posterior leaflet with the annulus over several millimeters and reattaching the leaflet to the annulus in a sliding manner toward the center of the repair. Interrupted 4–0 braided polyester suture works well for this reattachment.

Treatment of Chordal Elongation

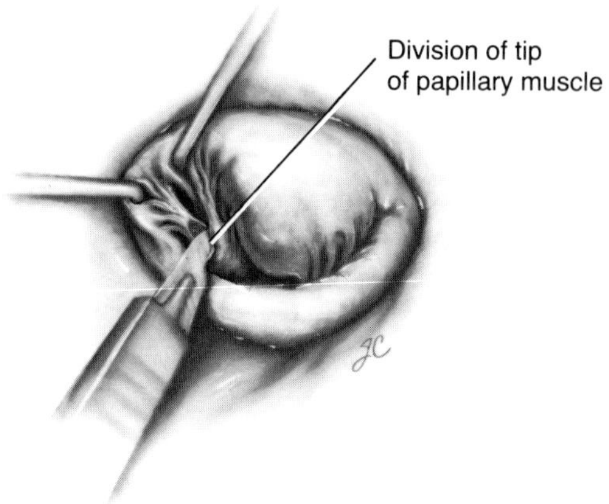

FIGURE 69–9. Elongated chords have been reproducibly treated successfully with shortening techniques designed to adjust the point of origin to a point beneath the tip of the papillary muscle.

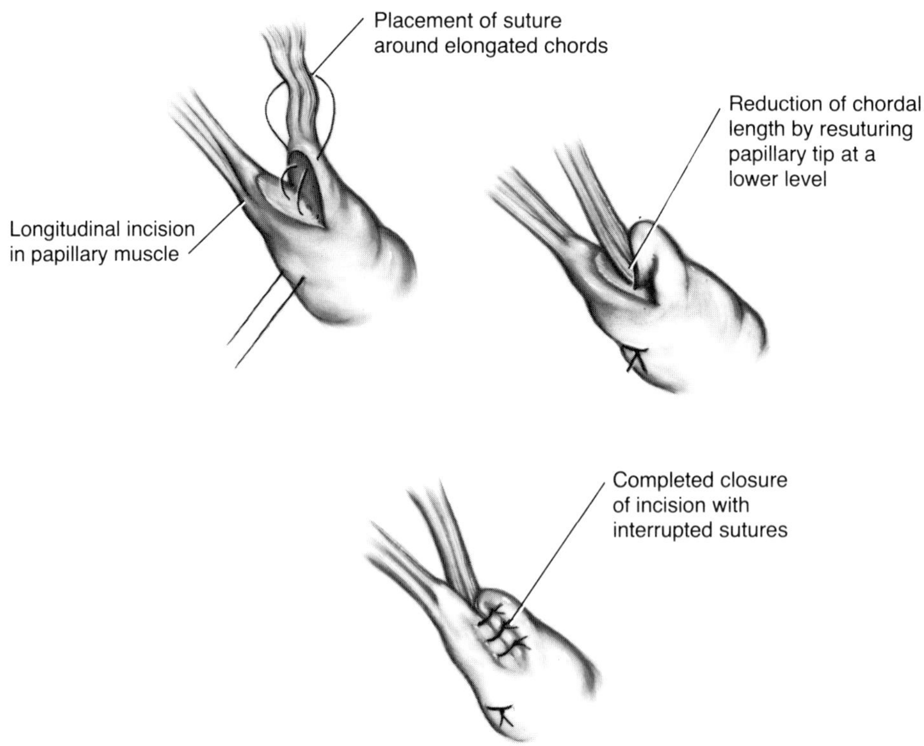

FIGURE 69–10. Areas requiring minimal shortening may be treated with a so-called papillary muscle sliding plasty.

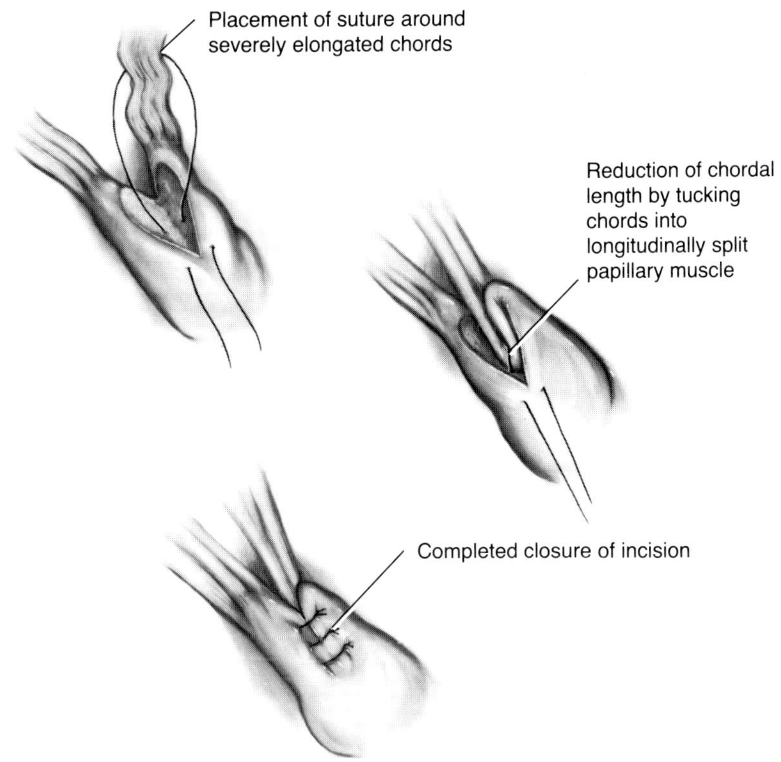

FIGURE 69–11. Greater degrees of chordal elongation are treated with chordal shortening. In this case, the surgeon should recognize that the looped chord will be repositioned at the base of a small trench placed in the head of the papillary muscle. The length of chordal shortening will be twice the depth of the trench. The amount of required chordal shortening is estimated by the initial assessment of prolapse. The trench is closed with 4–0 interrupted braided polyester suture. Care is taken to avoid abrasion of the shortened chord by sutures employed to close the trench.

Treatment of Chordal Rupture

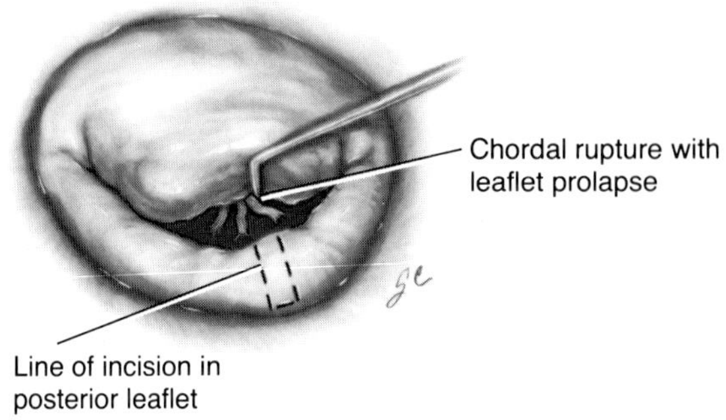

FIGURE 69–12. Ruptured chords to the anterior leaflet may be treated in one of several ways. If the opposing posterior leaflet is at the normal level, without prolapse, a segment of this leaflet with its accompanying chords may be transferred and attached to the anterior leaflet. This may be done by using a small rectangular resection of the entire area of the opposing posterior leaflet or simply the free edge of the leaflet with the attached chords.

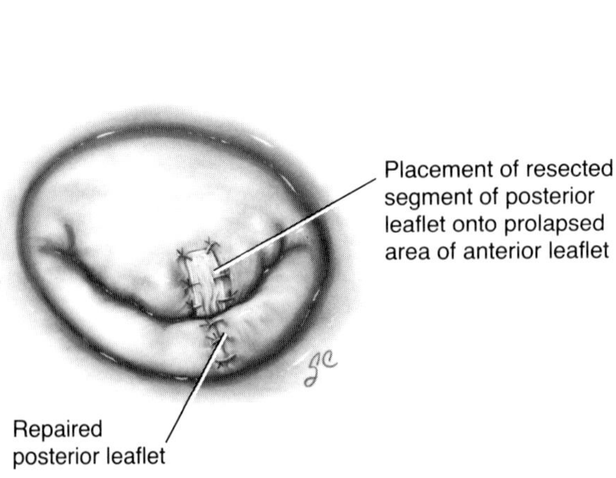

FIGURE 69–13. The leaflet is repaired with interrupted 5–0 braided polyester suture, and the attachment is likewise made to the anterior leaflet with the same type of suture.

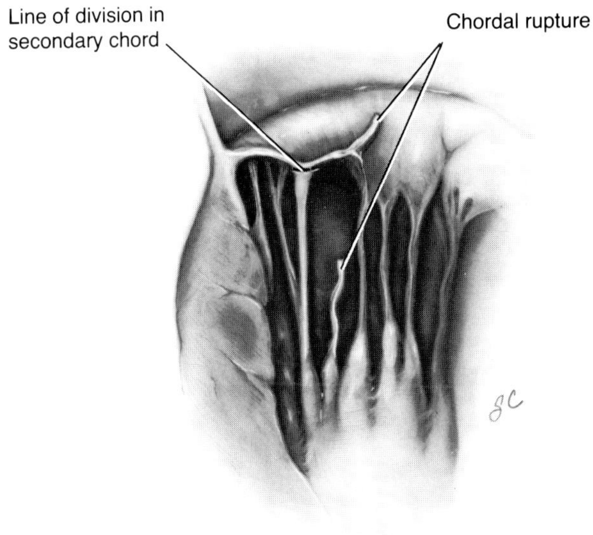

FIGURE 69–14

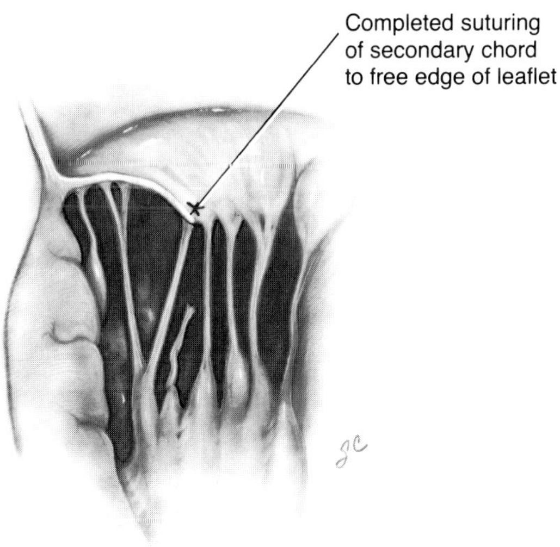

FIGURE 69–15

FIGURES 69–14 and 69–15. Chordal rupture of the anterior leaflet may also be treated by transfer of a healthy secondary chord from the adjacent nonprolapsed portion of the anterior leaflet to the free edge of the prolapsed anterior leaflet.

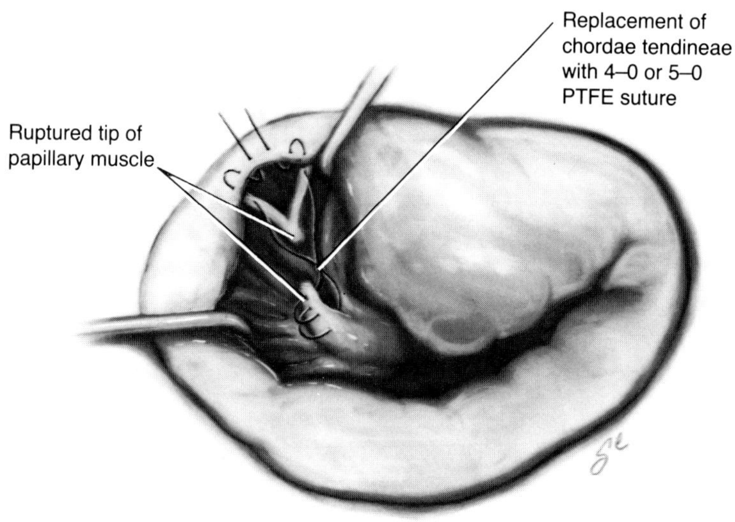

FIGURE 69–16. Early success has been reported using Gore-Tex suture to replace ruptured chords as well as chordal elongation on both the anterior and posterior leaflets. For this purpose, 5–0 Gore-Tex suture appears to work quite well. The suture must be placed through the fibrous tips of the papillary muscle as well as the thickened area of the free edge of the leaflet being repaired. While the suture is being tied, appropriate adjustment of the length of the artificial chord must be carefully gauged by applying traction on the nonprolapsed portions of the leaflet. This can be accomplished by placing a nerve hook along chords on the free edge of adjacent normal leaflet. Additionally, some surgeons have found it helpful to adjust the chordal length by tying the chords at the completion of the remainder of the valve repair while the ventricle is distended with iced saline. The long-term results of this technique have yet to be defined.

Treatment of Commissural Prolapse

Prolapse of the commissural areas of the mitral valve may be treated with chordal shortening, papillary muscle shortening, or Gore-Tex suture chordal replacement.

Ring Annuloplasty for Annular Dilatation

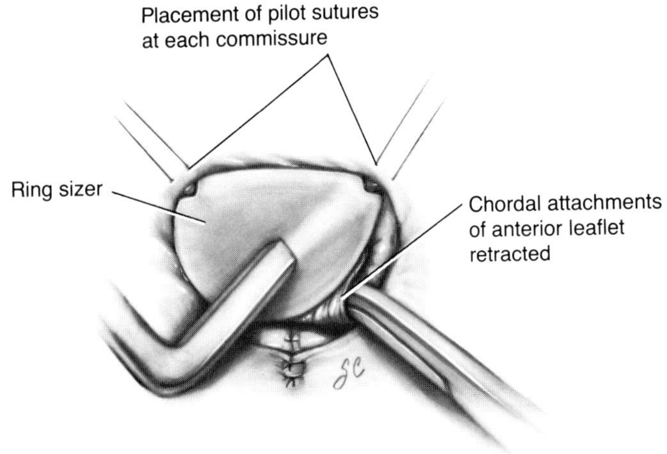

FIGURE 69–17. Valve repair for treatment of all degenerative diseases of the mitral valve should be accompanied by placement of an annuloplasty ring. This ring successfully treats annular dilatation and supports any leaflet repairs. Proper sizing of the annuloplasty ring is of extreme importance. The appropriate ring is one that corresponds to the area of the anterior leaflet of the mitral valve. Stay sutures are placed at each commissural area so that the base measurement of the leaflet can be accurately assessed. The leaflet is then unfurled by placing tension to all primary chords using an angled clamp or nerve hooks. The notches in the ring sizer correspond to the areas of the commissures. The leaflet shape and size should match those of the valve ring sizer.

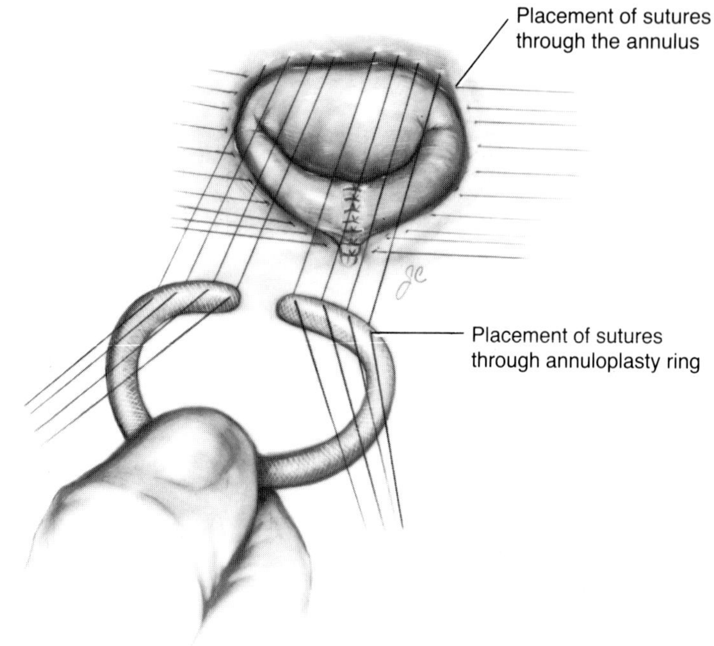

FIGURE 69–18. When the appropriate ring is chosen, it is fixed to the annulus with interrupted horizontal mattress sutures passed through the annulus. Care is taken to ensure that good solid annular tissue is incorporated. Typically, the annulus lies approximately 1.5 mm away from the junction of the valve leaflet with the cardiac muscular tissue. The valve ring may be slightly bent into a more saddle shape if the conformation of the adjoining aortic root and annulus is particularly prominent.

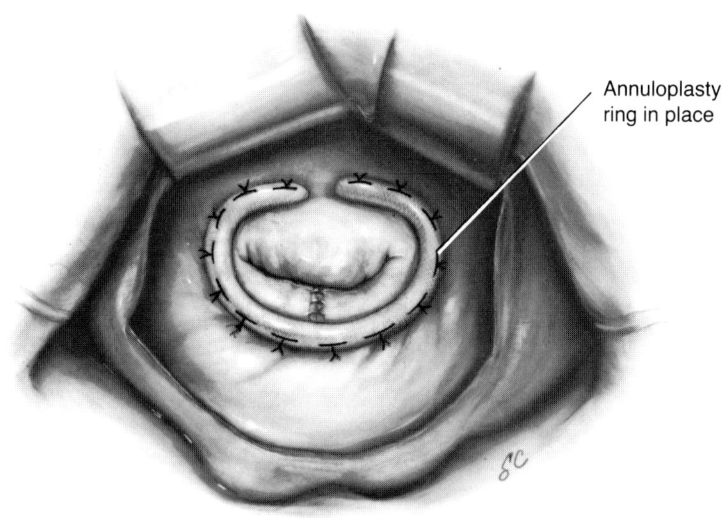

FIGURE 69–19. Following completion of the ring placement, the closure line of the valve should be symmetrical. A "smile" that runs parallel to the circumference of the ring should be evident. Filling the ventricle with iced saline solution will close the valve so that this closure line can be carefully examined. Any asymmetry of this closure indicates residual leaflet prolapse or restriction. A symmetrical closure line guarantees valve competence even if some saline leak is evident. An asymmetrical line of closure is often associated with some incompetence following resumption of cardiac contraction even if the saline solution does not seem to escape with ventricular filling.

Repair of Leaflet Perforations

Occasionally, the leaflets may contain actual perforations. These may be repaired easily with native pericardium tanned at the table for 10 minutes in glutaraldehyde solution. The pericardial tissue is then washed with saline and attached to the leaflet with interrupted 5–0 sutures after freshening of any ragged or diseased leaflet edges.

Repair of Deformities of the Anterior Leaflet

Localized anterior leaflet perforations may be treated with pericardial patches, as previously described. However, severe leaflet retraction and severe anomalies of anterior leaflet shape require treatment by surgeons experienced in valve repair techniques and are beyond the scope of this section.

Prevention of Left Ventricular Outflow Obstruction Secondary to Systolic Anterior Motion of the Mitral Valve

Rarely, mitral valve repair has been associated with the development of marked systolic anterior motion of the mitral valve and subsequent left ventricular outflow tract obstruction. Detailed evaluation of this problem has been performed by Carpentier and others. It is now clear that this complication occurs primarily with redundancy of the posterior leaflet tissue in association with severe myxomatous degeneration, and improper downsizing of the annuloplasty ring used for remodeling of the annulus.

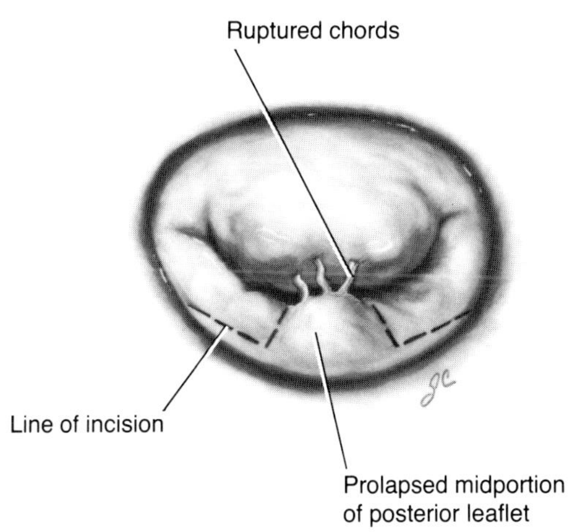

FIGURE 69–20. When excess leaflet tissue is identified, it is important that the height or span of the posterior leaflet be reduced before a ring annuloplasty is performed, particularly when a rigid ring is employed. Most commonly, a very redundant valve leaflet is found in association with prolapse of the posterior leaflet. Quadrangular resection of the appropriate portion of the leaflet should include extension into the attachment of the remaining posterior leaflet to the annulus along the area of suspected redundancy.

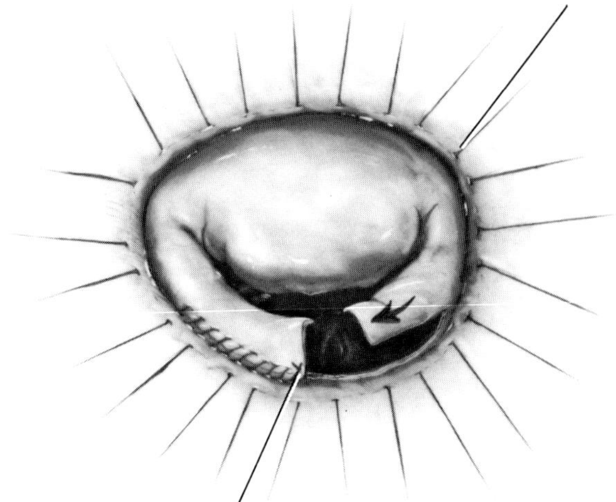

FIGURE 69–21. The leaflet is reattached to the annulus with a continuous 4–0 suture. For convenience, the annuloplasty sutures may be placed before the repair of the posterior leaflet is completed.

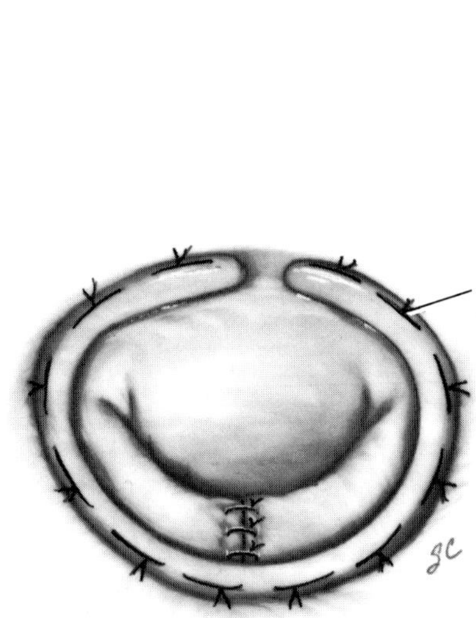

FIGURE 69–22. The annuloplasty ring to be placed is determined by sizing the entire area of the anterior leaflet using a valve ring obturator. Care must be taken not to choose too small a ring. After the appropriate annuloplasty ring is selected, the annuloplasty is performed.

PETER VAN TRIGT, III, M.D.

70
Aortic Valve Replacement for Aortic Stenosis

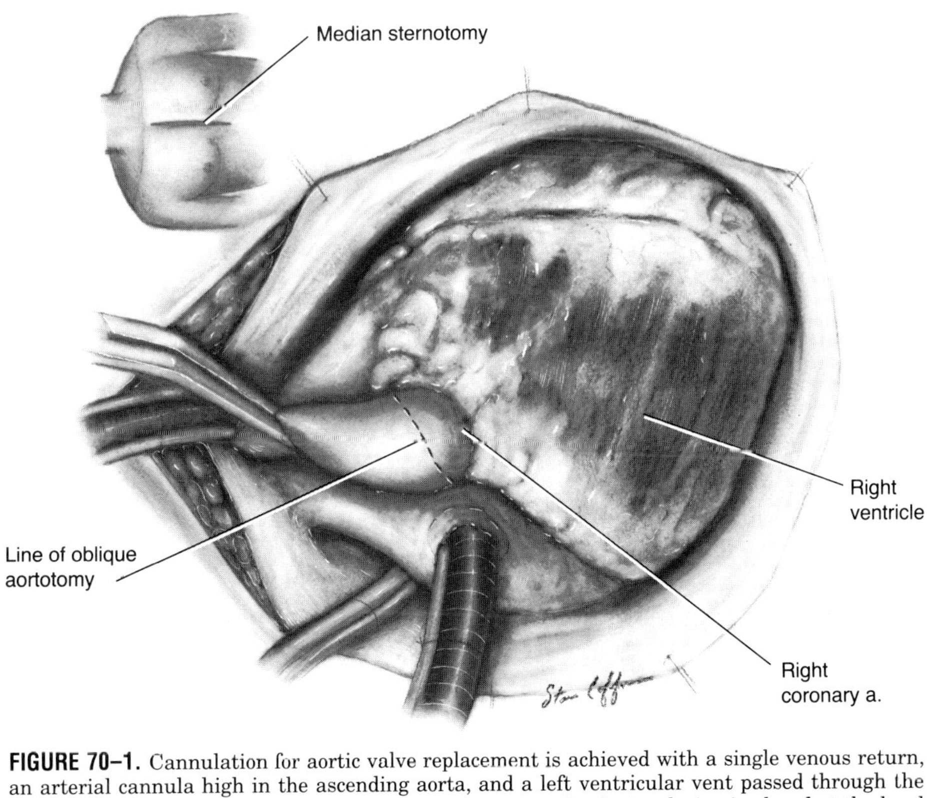

FIGURE 70–1. Cannulation for aortic valve replacement is achieved with a single venous return, an arterial cannula high in the ascending aorta, and a left ventricular vent passed through the right superior pulmonary vein. A needle for delivery of cardioplegic solution is placed at the level of the aortotomy, which is directed obliquely toward the noncoronary cusp of the aortic valve.

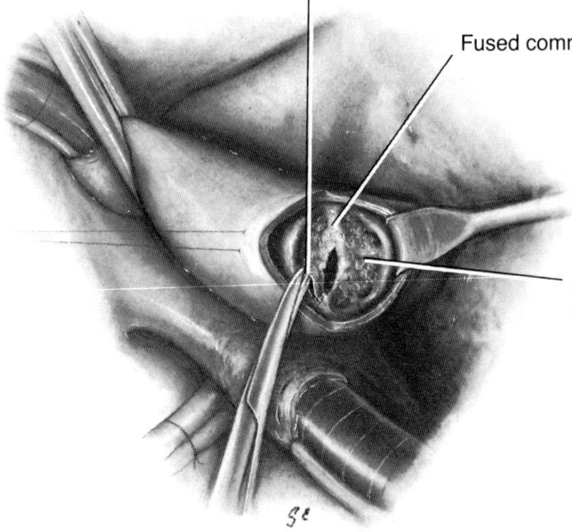

FIGURE 70–2. After delivery of cardioplegic solution, the aortotomy is performed and the anterior wall of the aorta is carefully retracted. The valve leaflets are excised so as to remove the scarred and calcified tissue up to the valvular annulus.

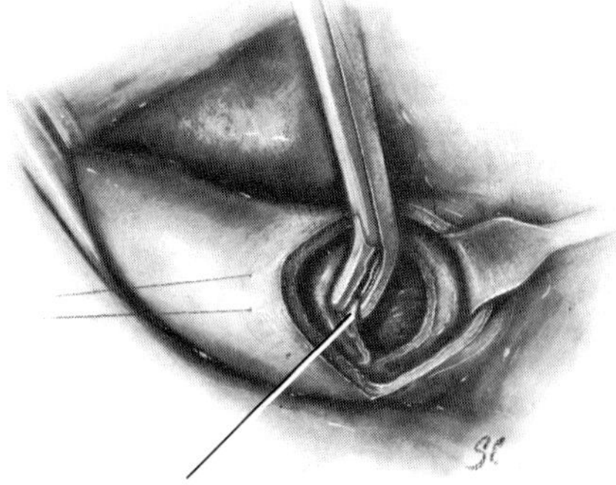

FIGURE 70–3. The remaining annular calcium, which can interfere with proper seating of the prosthetic valve, is removed by crushing the deposits with the pituitary rongeur and sharply removing the calcified tissue with scissors.

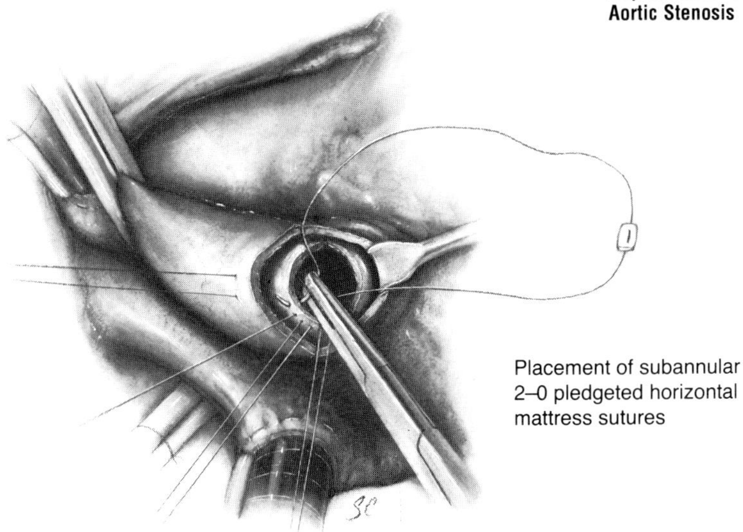

FIGURE 70–4. Subannular pledgeted mattress sutures are placed sequentially around the aortic annulus. They are passed through the fibrous annular tissue and not into ventricular muscle.

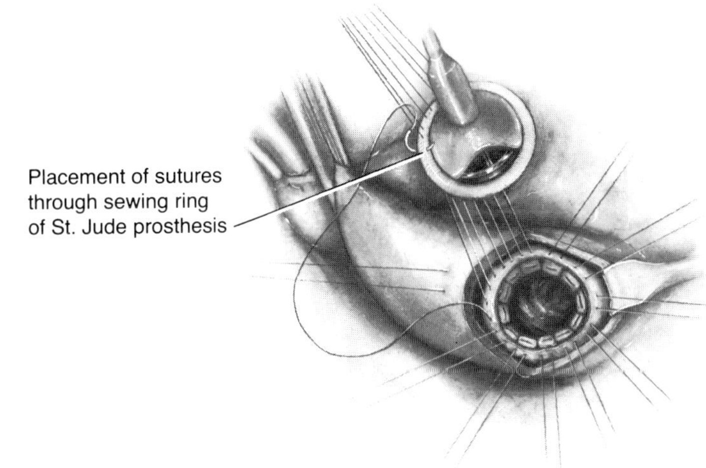

FIGURE 70–5. The valve sutures are passed sequentially through the Dacron sewing ring of the prosthetic valve. The valve is seated and the sutures are tied, first along the area of the left coronary cusp below the left main ostium, with the other sutures to follow.

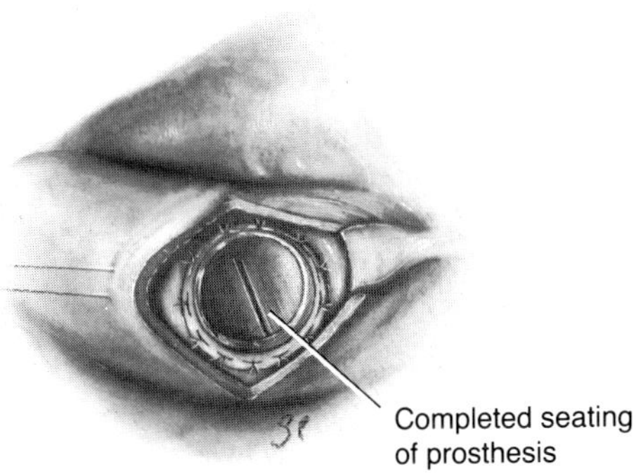

FIGURE 70–6. The valve is inspected after the sutures have been tied, and a cotton-tipped applicator is used to open the leaflets to inspect proper seating of the pledgeted sutures beneath the annulus.

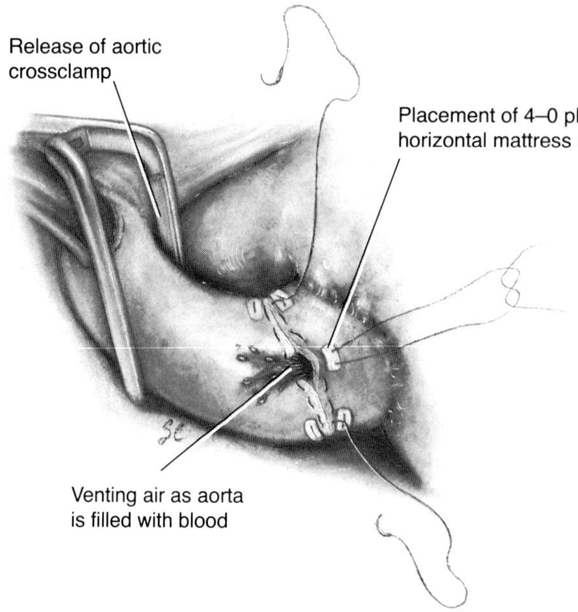

FIGURE 70–7. Air is removed by filling the heart with blood from the cardiopulmonary bypass circuit and briefly releasing the crossclamp prior to tying the continuous horizontal mattress suture.

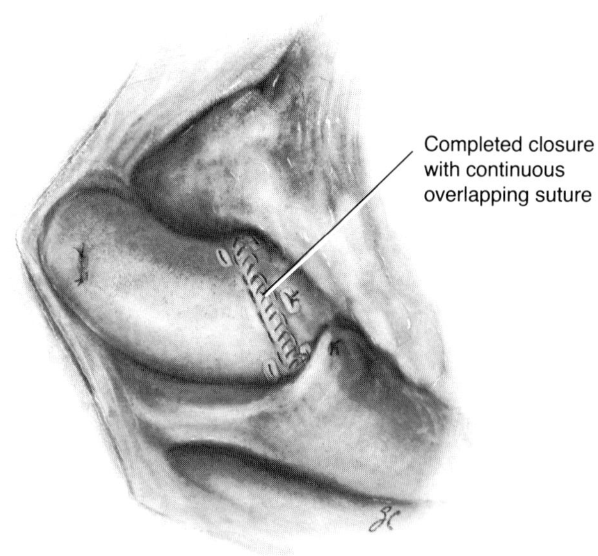

FIGURE 70–8. A second continuous suture is placed above the horizontal mattress suture for complete hemostasis.

PETER VAN TRIGT, III, M.D.

71

Aortic Valve Replacement for Aortic Insufficiency

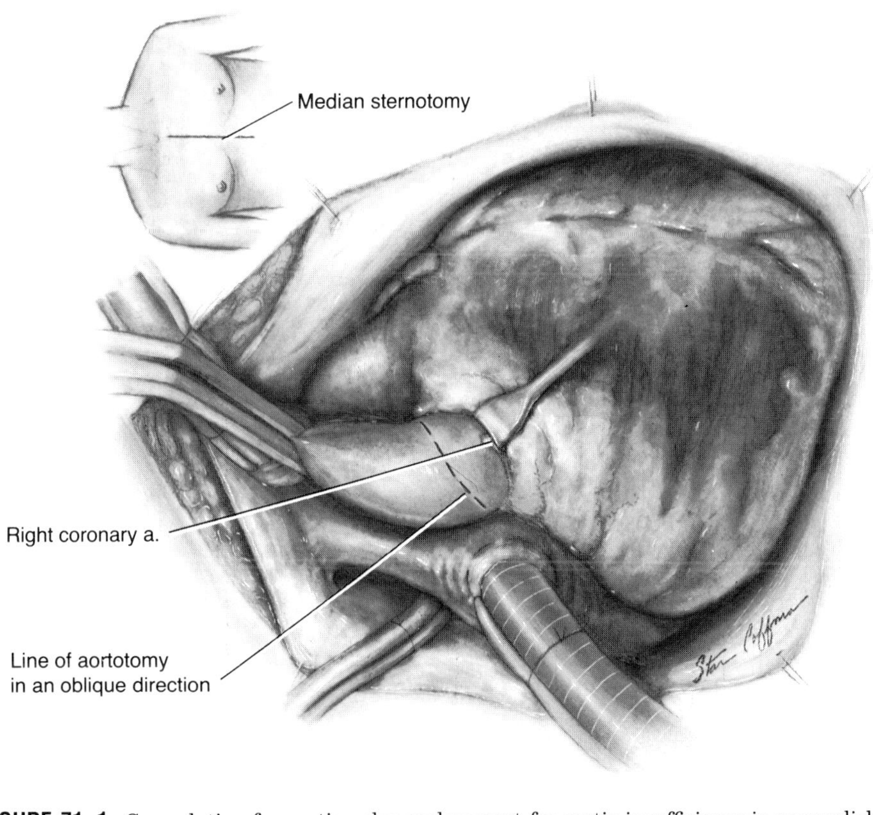

FIGURE 71–1. Cannulation for aortic valve replacement for aortic insufficiency is accomplished with a single cannula for venous return, an arterial cannula high on the ascending aorta, and a left ventricular vent passed through the right superior pulmonary vein. Moderate systemic hypothermia is achieved to 28°C, and the ascending aorta is crossclamped. An oblique aortotomy is performed several millimeters above the ostium of the right coronary artery, directed toward the noncoronary cusp of the aortic valve.

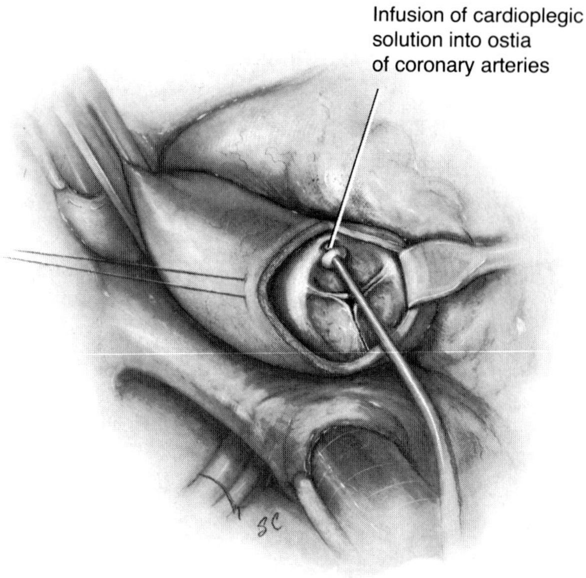

FIGURE 71–2. The anterior wall of the aorta is carefully retracted, and the hand-held cardioplegia cannula is seated in the left main ostium as topical hypothermia is also accomplished with cold saline. Generally, two thirds of the cardioplegic solution is administered to the left main artery, and one third to the ostium of the right coronary artery. The right coronary ostium can be better visualized by gentle cephalad pressure on the right ventricular outflow track.

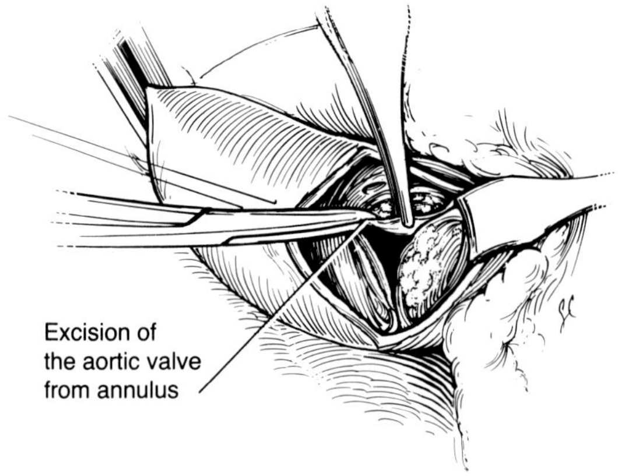

FIGURE 71–3. The leaflets are excised individually, leaving the annular tissue intact.

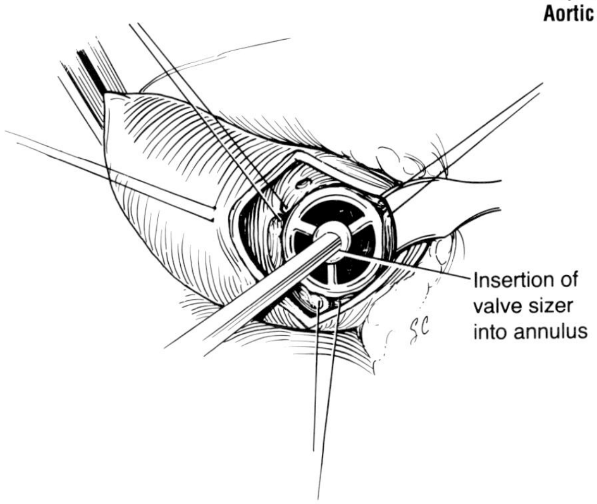

FIGURE 71–4. A valve sizer is used to determine the proper diameter of the prosthetic valve. It is especially important to avoid oversizing the prosthesis.

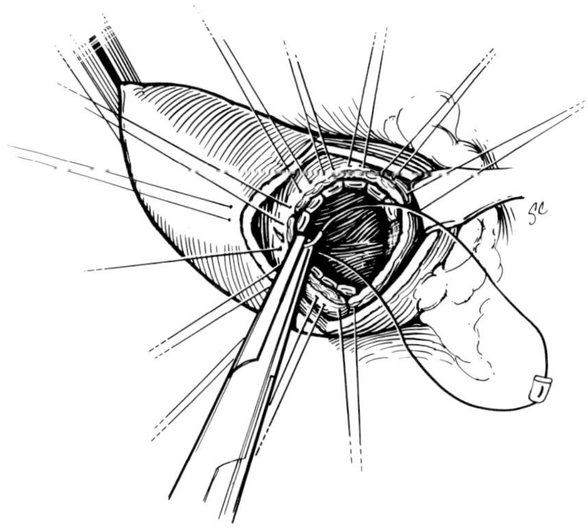

FIGURE 71–5. Subannular mattress pledgeted sutures are placed sequentially around the aortic annulus, passed through the fibrous annular tissue and not the ventricular muscle.

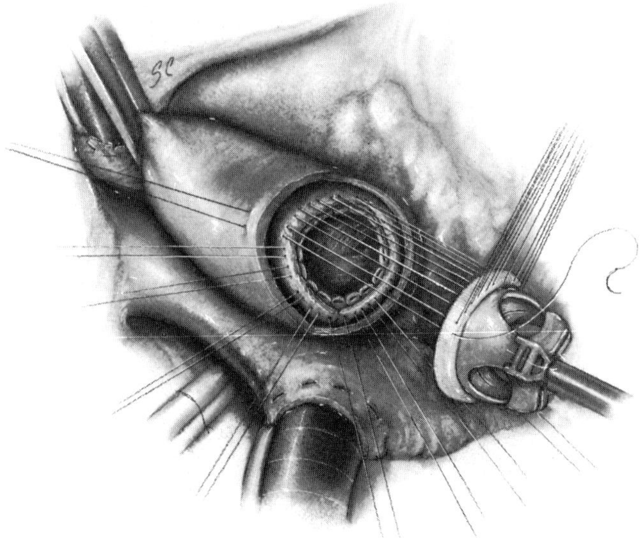

FIGURE 71–6. The valve sutures are passed sequentially through the Dacron sewing ring of the prosthetic valve. The valve is seated and sutures are tied, first along the area of the left coronary cusp below the left main ostium, with the other sutures to follow.

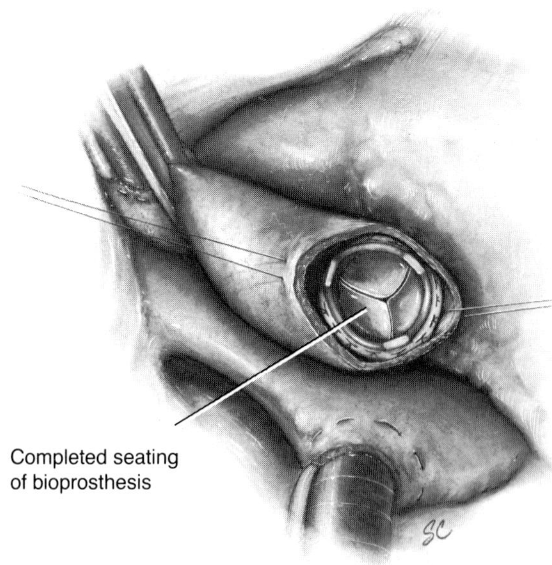

FIGURE 71–7. After the sutures have been tied, the valve leaflets are gently opened to inspect the proper seating of the subannular pledgeted sutures. The aortotomy is closed, and air is vented.

DONALD D. GLOWER, JR., M.D.

72
Closure of Aortic Wounds

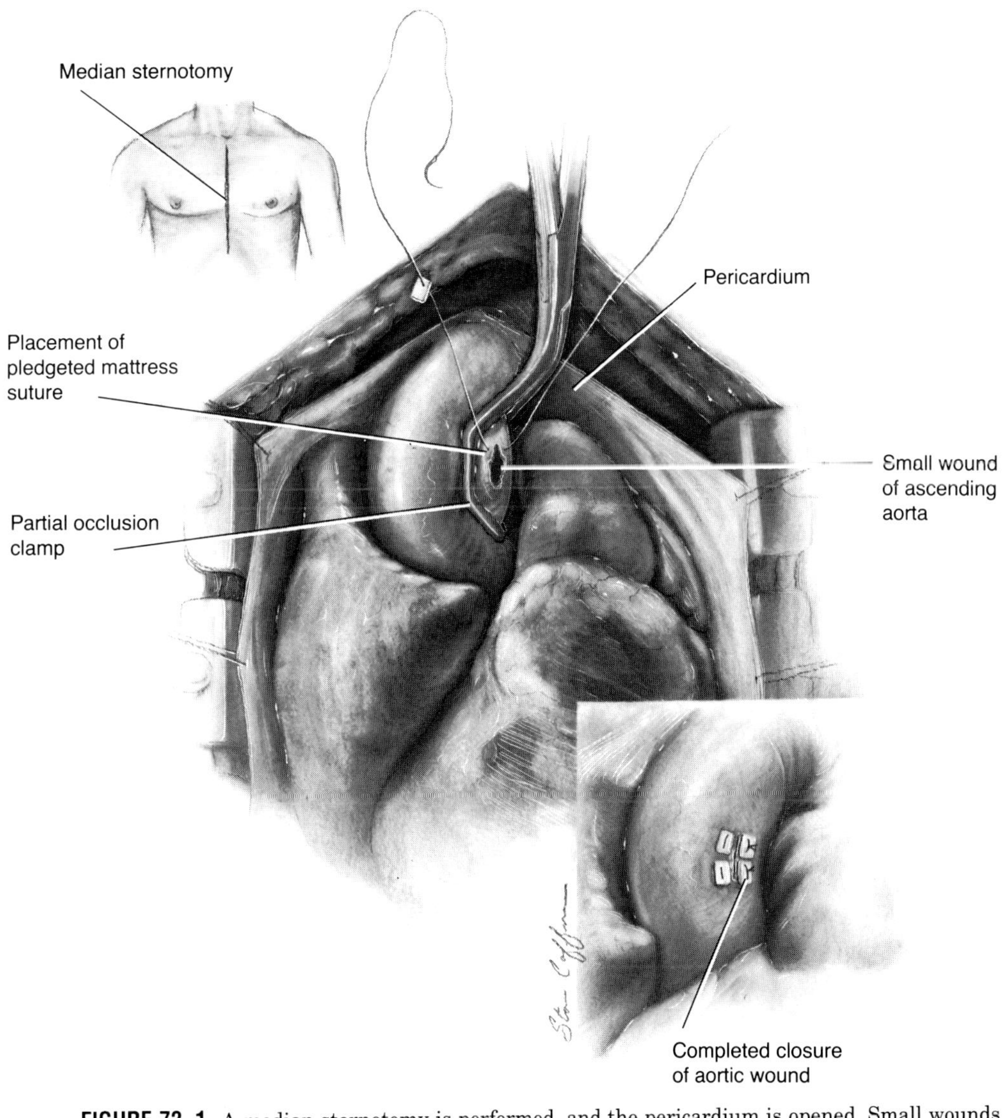

FIGURE 72–1. A median sternotomy is performed, and the pericardium is opened. Small wounds of the ascending aorta may be repaired directly with pledgeted mattress sutures, using a partial occlusion clamp on the aorta.

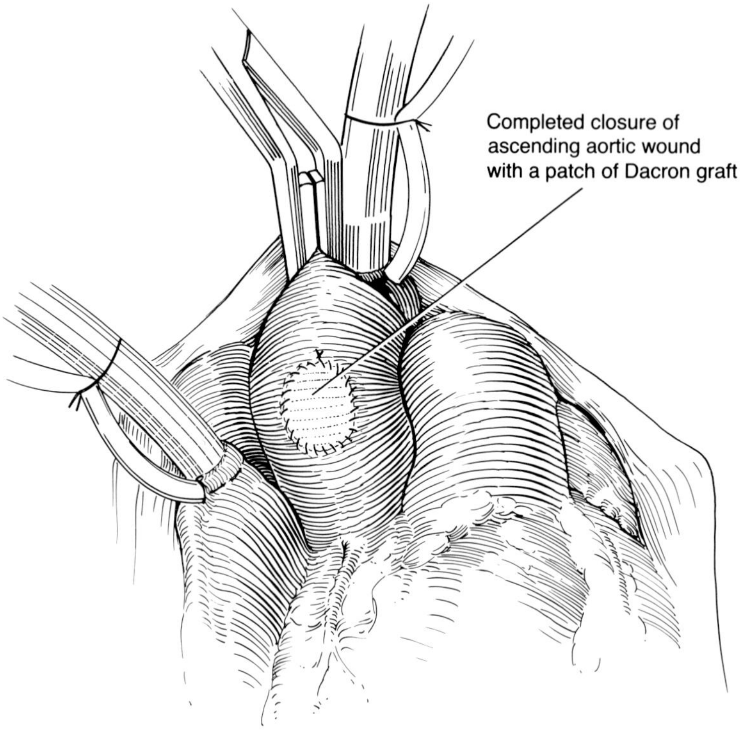

FIGURE 72–2. Larger wounds require cardiopulmonary bypass with cannulation of the right atrium and the aortic arch or femoral artery. The aorta is clamped proximal to the innominate artery, and the heart is arrested with cardioplegia. The aortic defect may be closed with a patch of Dacron.

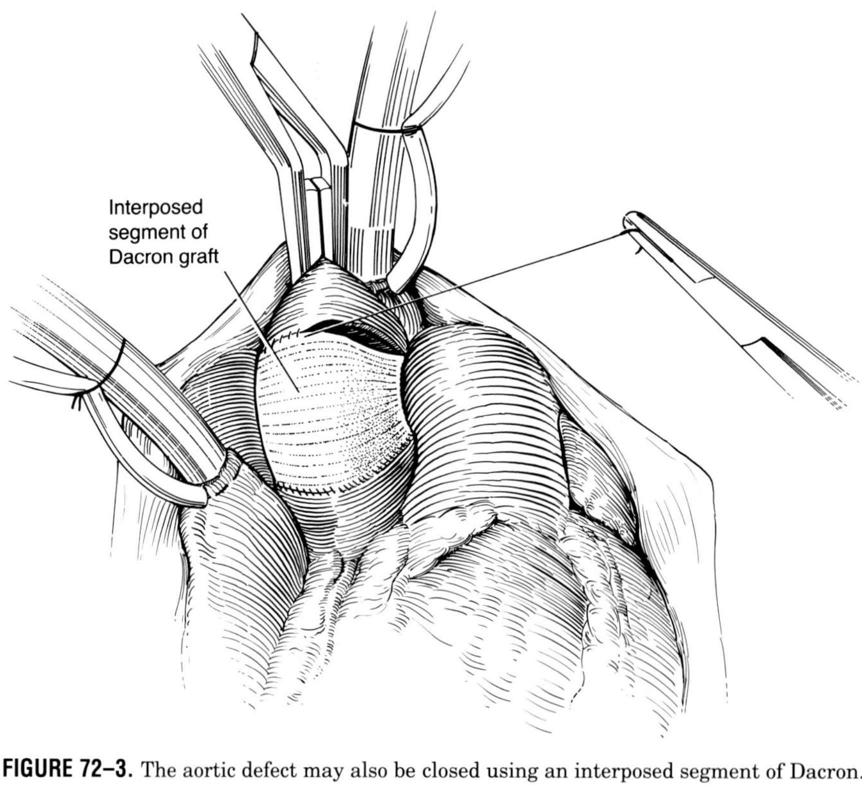

FIGURE 72–3. The aortic defect may also be closed using an interposed segment of Dacron.

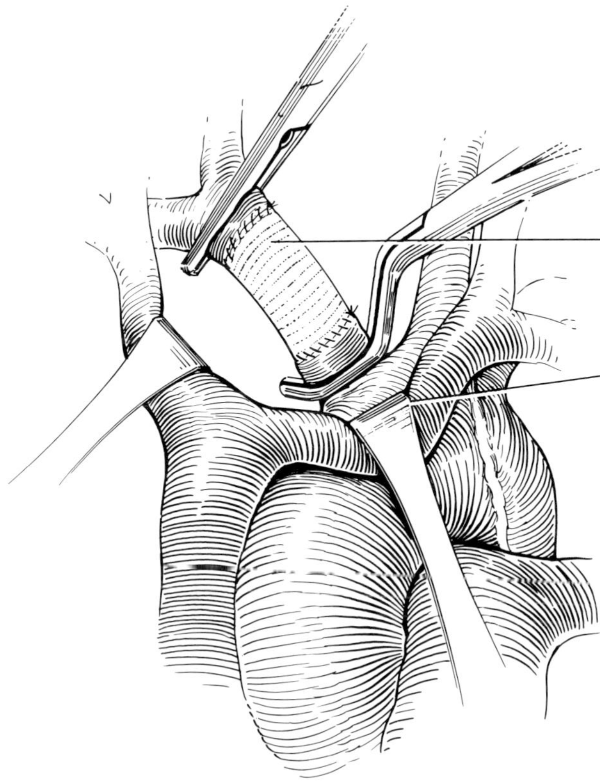

FIGURE 72–4. Injuries of the innominate artery require proximal and distal control obtained by mobilization of the innominate vein. The innominate artery may be repaired primarily or with a prosthetic patch or interposition graft.

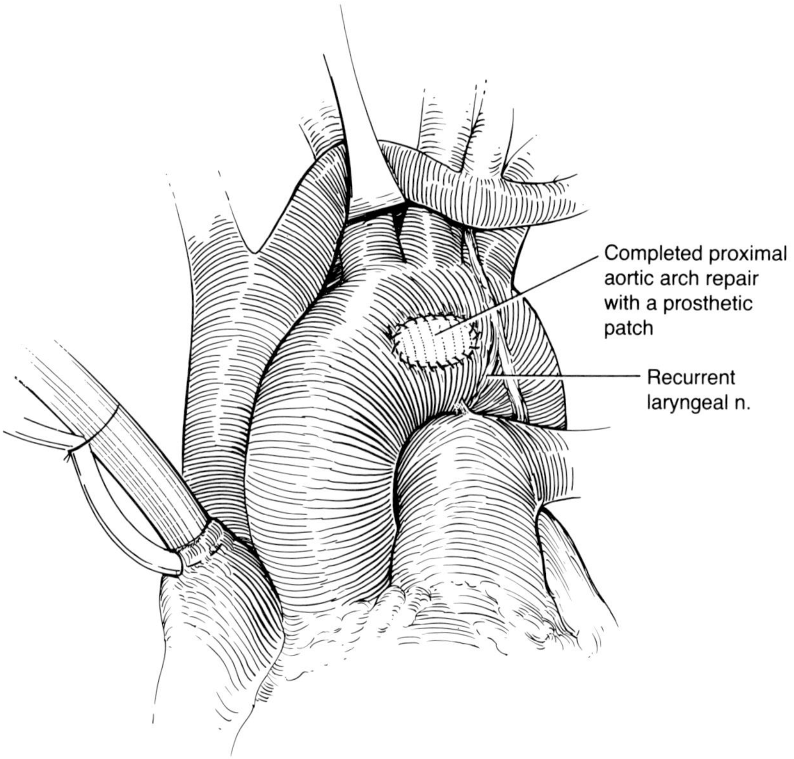

FIGURE 72–5. Injuries of the proximal aortic arch require mobilization of the proximal arch, with care taken to preserve the phrenic and recurrent laryngeal nerves. Small injuries may be repaired primarily with pledgeted mattress sutures. Larger injuries require cardiopulmonary bypass with cannulation of the right atrium and femoral artery, profound systemic hypothermia, and a period of circulatory arrest in Trendelenburg position to avoid air embolism to the cephalic vessels. The aortic wall defect is replaced with prosthetic material.

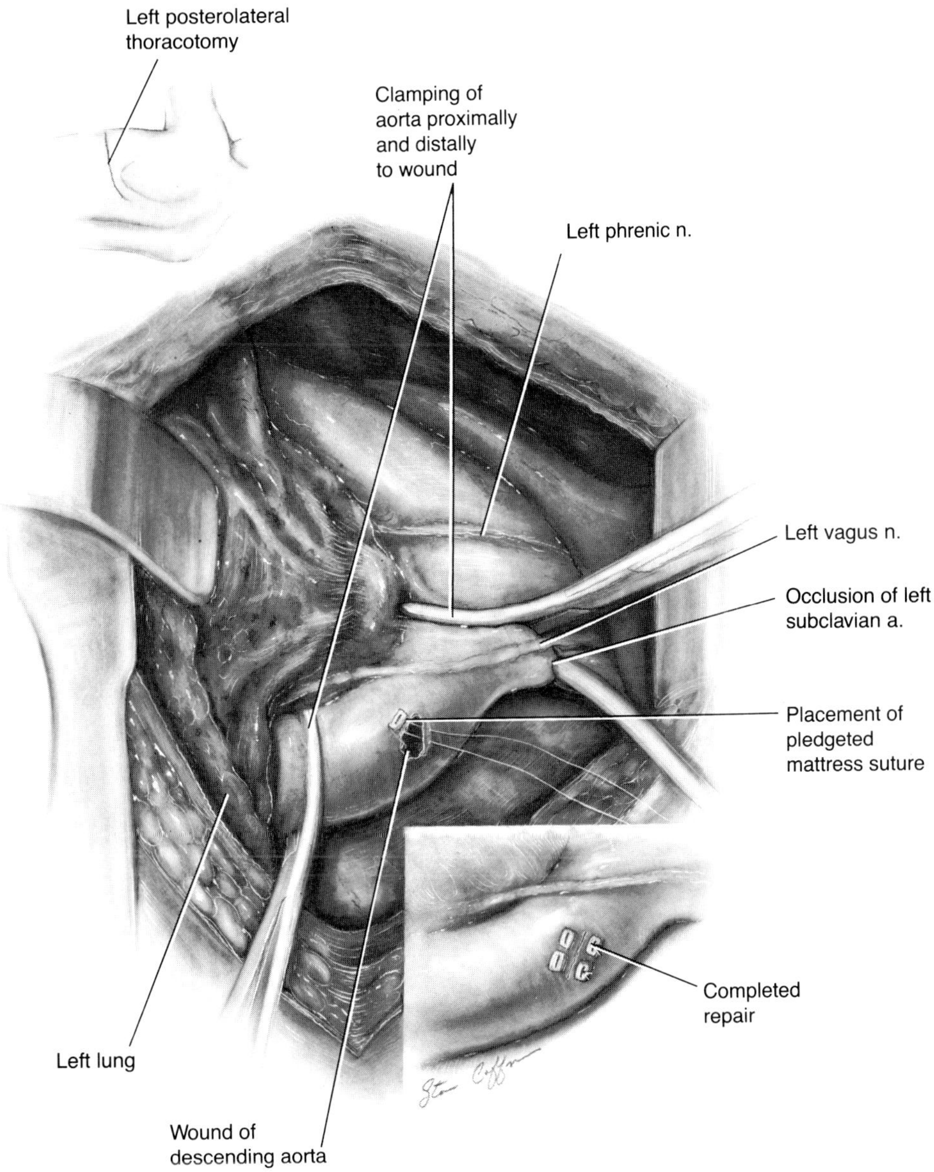

FIGURE 72–6. Wounds of the distal aortic arch and descending thoracic aorta require a left posterolateral thoracotomy in the fourth to seventh interspace, depending on injury location. Small wounds may be repaired primarily using a partial occluding clamp. Larger wounds require clamping of the aorta proximal and distal to the injury. Large aortic wounds may be repaired using pledgeted mattress sutures, patch grafting, or interposition grafting with prosthetic material. Large injuries may require support of the distal circulation with a shunt or circulatory bypass.

WALTER G. WOLFE, M.D.

73

Aneurysms of the Ascending Aorta

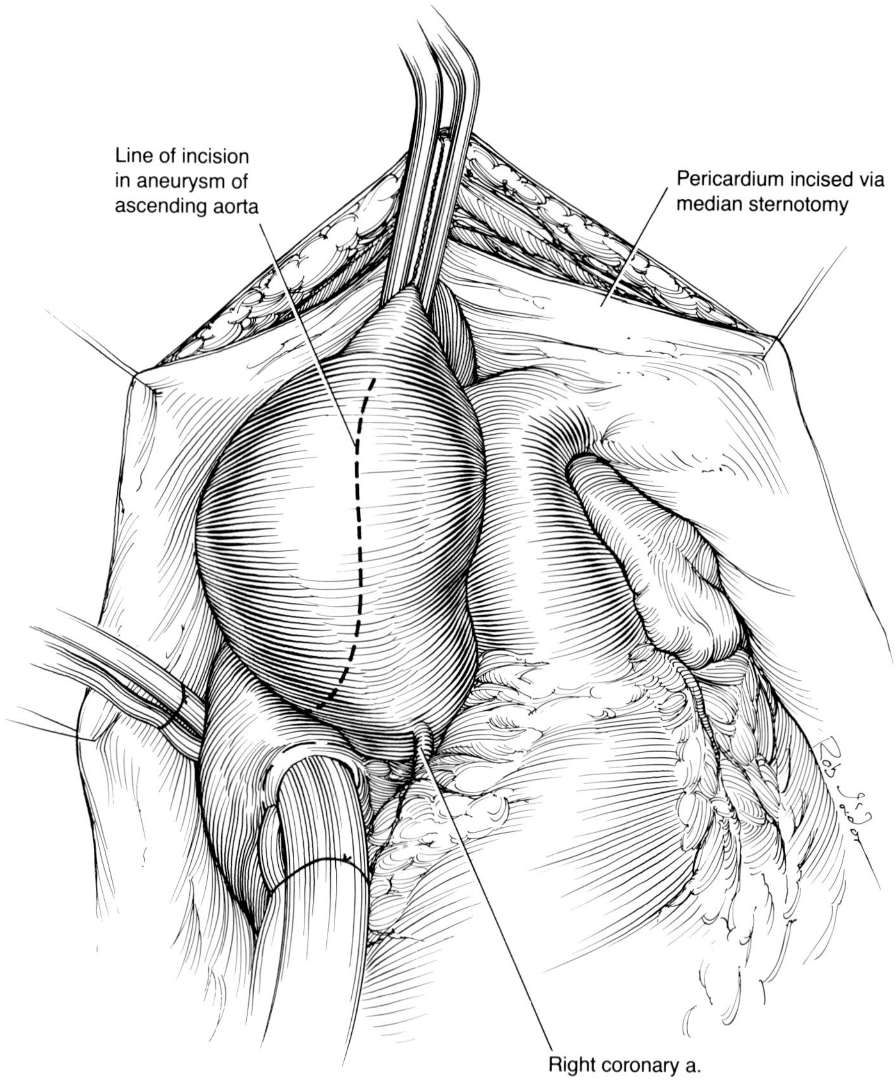

FIGURE 73–1. A median sternotomy is made in the standard manner, and the femoral artery usually is cannulated for aortic inflow. The venous cannula is placed in the right atrium, and the ventricles are vented through the superior vein. Cardiopulmonary bypass is instituted, and the patient is cooled to 32°C. Before the aorta is clamped, a Teflon strip is placed around the neck distally. If there is an adequate neck to clamp the aorta, it is not necessary to use hypothermic circulatory arrest. The aorta is then crossclamped and cardioplegic solution infused directly through the aneurysm if the valve is competent. If the valve is incompetent, retrograde cardioplegia is used along with direct cannulation of the coronary arteries in some cases. The aneurysm is then opened, and thrombus and debris are removed.

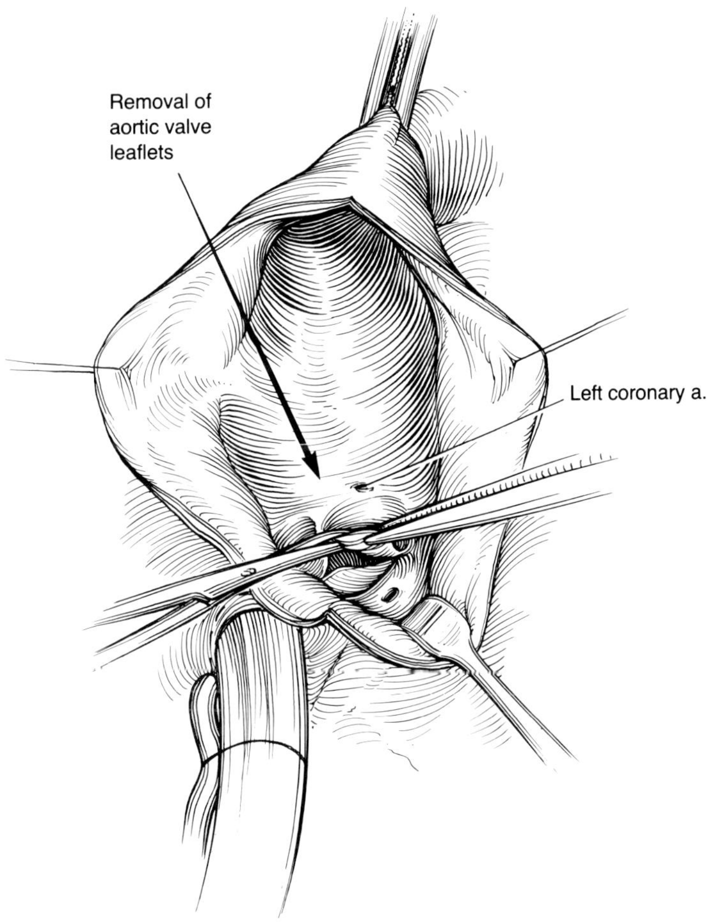

FIGURE 73–2. The valve leaflets are excised.

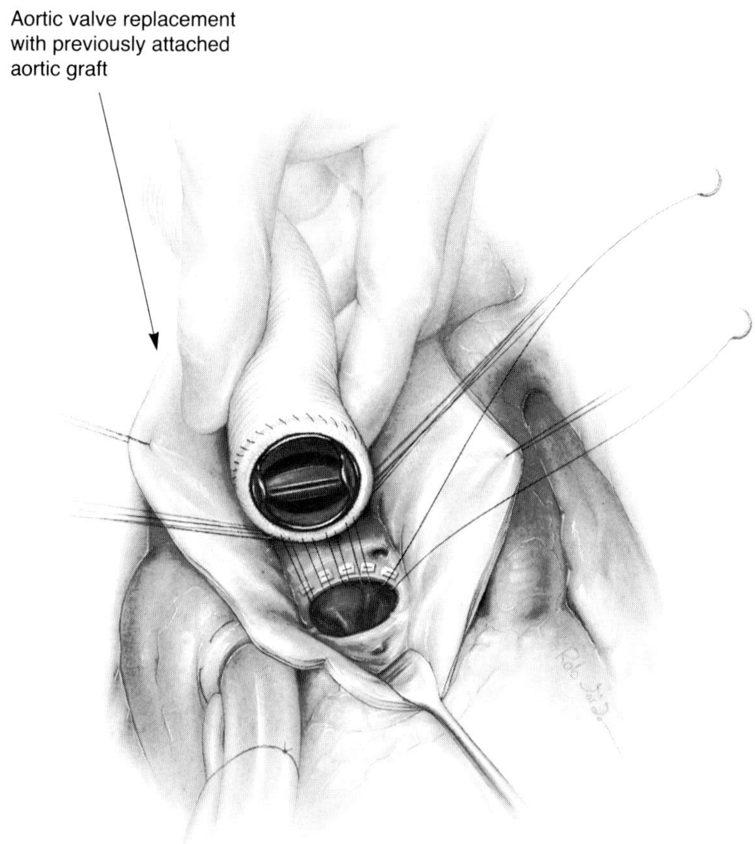

FIGURE 73–3. The valve conduit is selected in the usual manner by sizing the annulus. It is then sutured in place with interrupted pledgeted supra-annular stitches.

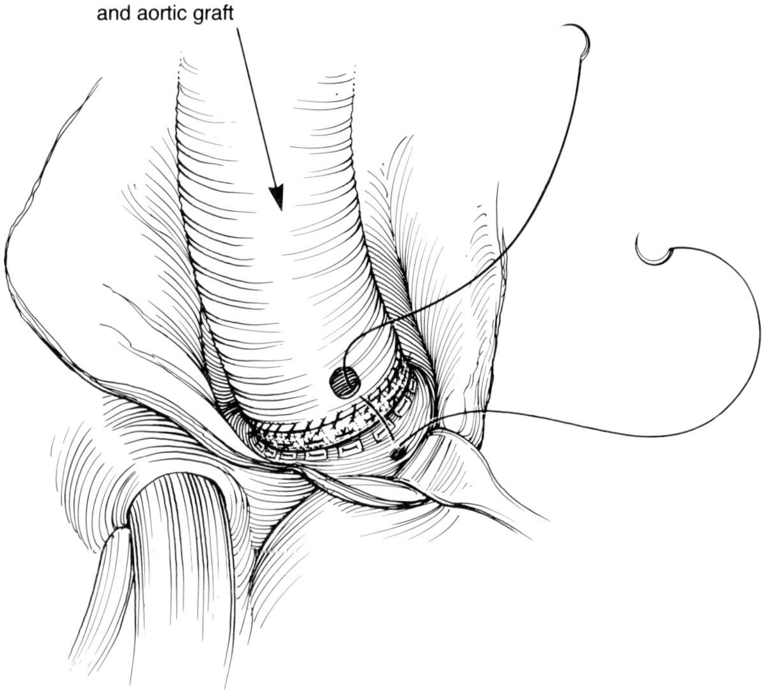

FIGURE 73–4. A button is made in the graft, and the left coronary artery is anastomosed to it with a continuous Prolene suture. A button is then made for the right coronary artery, which is implanted into the graft in a similar manner. The graft is cut to length, and the distal anastomosis is completed with a continuous 3–0 or 4–0 Prolene suture.

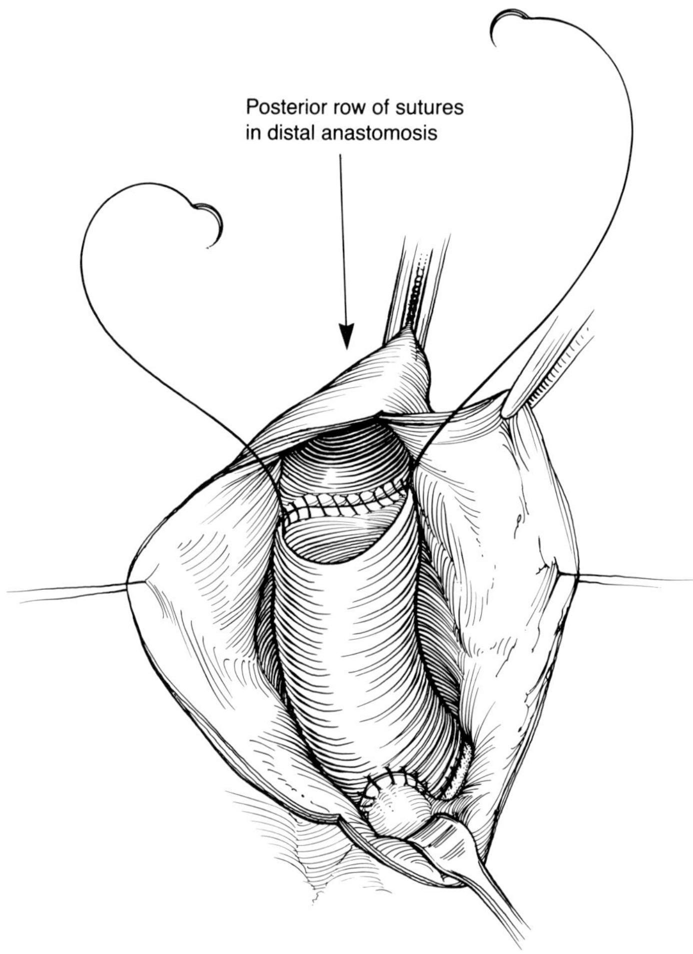

FIGURE 73–5. The distal anastomosis is buttressed with a Teflon strip externally, and the crossclamp is released.

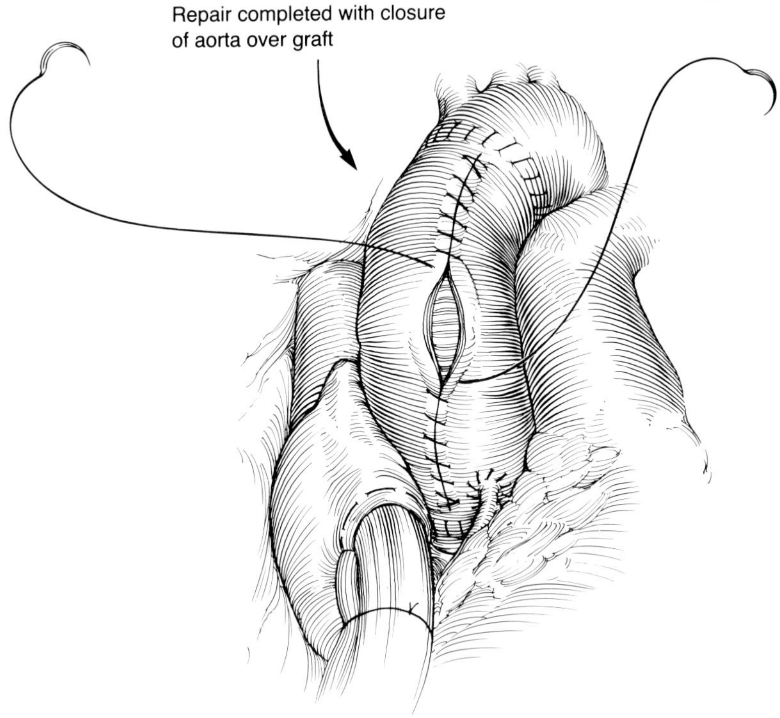

FIGURE 73–6. Once the hemostasis of the suture line is established, any remaining wall of the aneurysm is partially or completely closed over the graft to isolate it from the mediastinal structures. The patient is rewarmed during the distal anastomosis and removed from cardiopulmonary bypass in the usual manner.

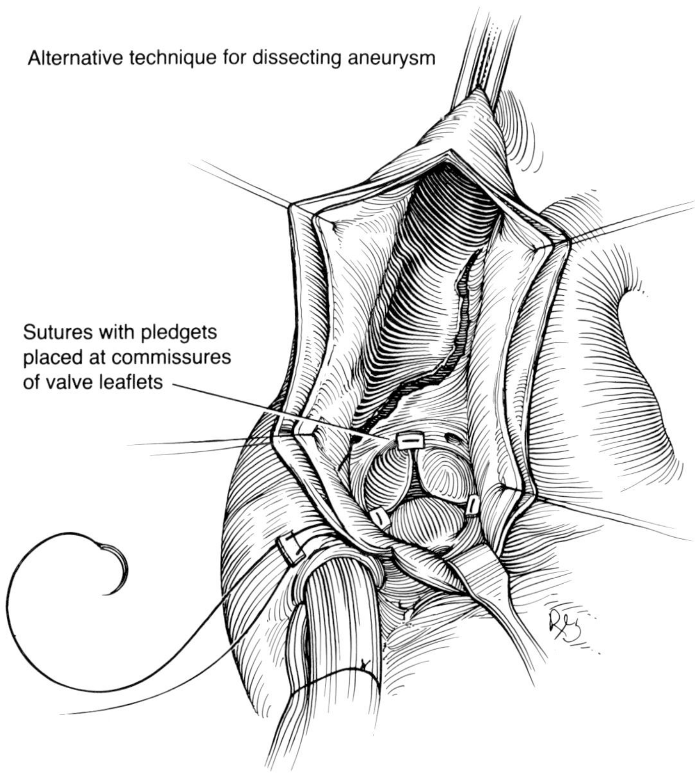

FIGURE 73–7. If the patient does not have an incompetent valve or if the operation is being done for an ascending dissecting aneurysm, the valve is resuspended at the commissures.

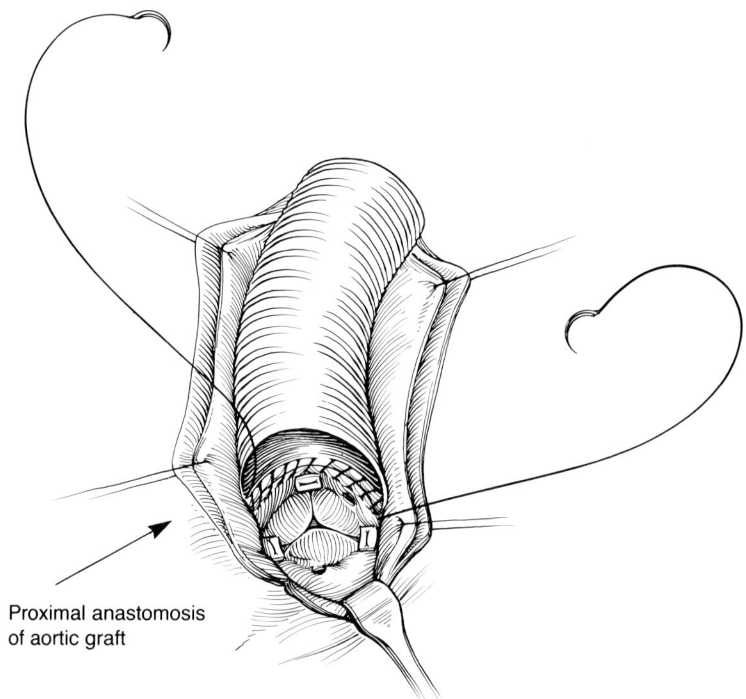

FIGURE 73–8. A woven Dacron graft is sutured in the supracoronary position with a continuous 3–0 Prolene suture. With some ascending dissecting aneurysms, the distal anastomosis is done first (under hypothermic circulatory arrest) using an open method of inserting the graft up into the aortic arch. Once the distal anastomosis is completed, the graft is clamped. The patient is rewarmed, and the proximal anastomosis is done in the supracoronary position.

In general, for dissecting aortic aneurysms, cannulation is through the femoral artery and venous return through the atrium with a left ventricular vent. Once cardiopulmonary bypass is instituted, the patient is immediately cooled to 16°C. The aorta may then be clamped and opened, and the valve resuspended. Myocardial protection is accomplished in most patients by using retrograde coronary perfusion. Occasionally, direct effusion of cardioplegia into the coronary arteries is done when the aorta is opened. Once sufficient cooling is obtained, the aorta is unclamped and the flow is slowed so that the arch can be inspected. If necessary, the distal anastomosis can be done first. If not, the artery is reclamped. Then the patient is rewarmed while the proximal and distal anastomoses are being done. The distal anastomosis is supported with a Teflon strip placed before the aorta is clamped.

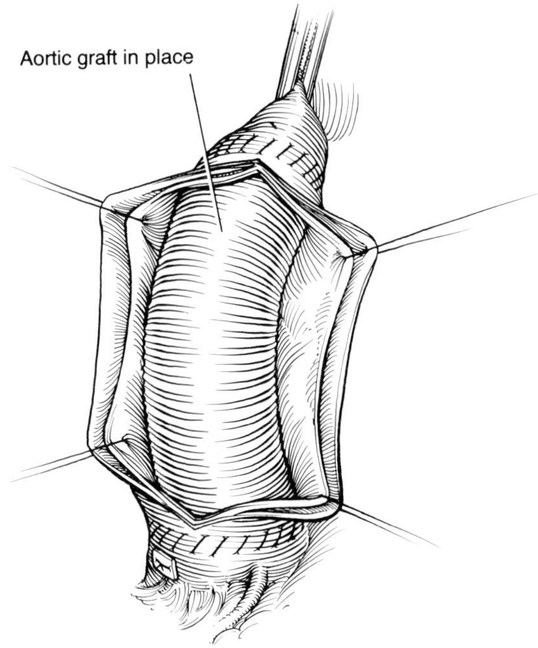

FIGURE 73–9. Once the graft is sutured in place, the clamp is released. When hemostasis is ensured, the remaining tissue, if any, is closed over the graft to protect the mediastinal structures.

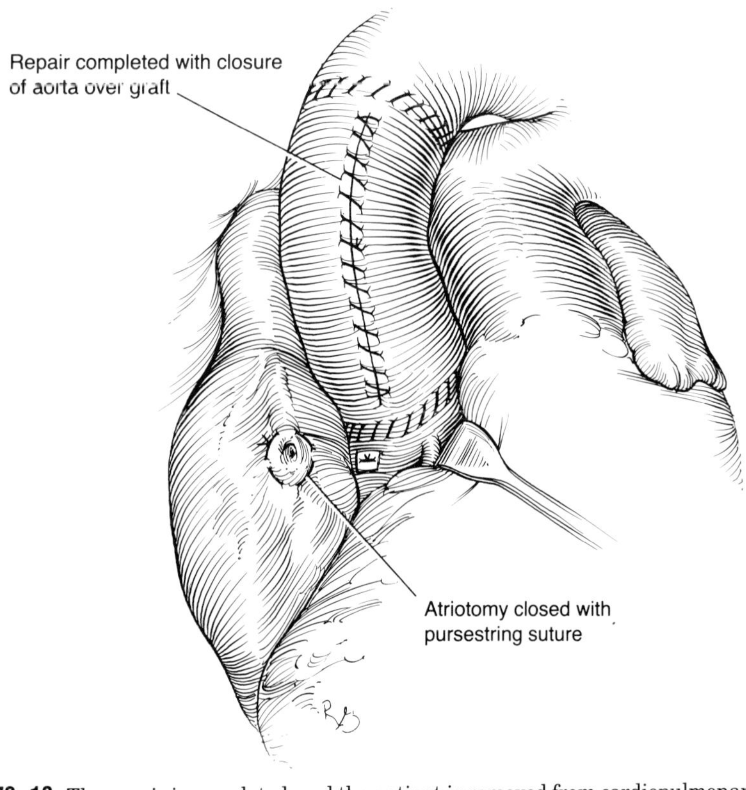

FIGURE 73–10. The repair is completed, and the patient is removed from cardiopulmonary bypass.

WALTER G. WOLFE, M.D.

74

Aneurysms of the Transverse Aortic Arch

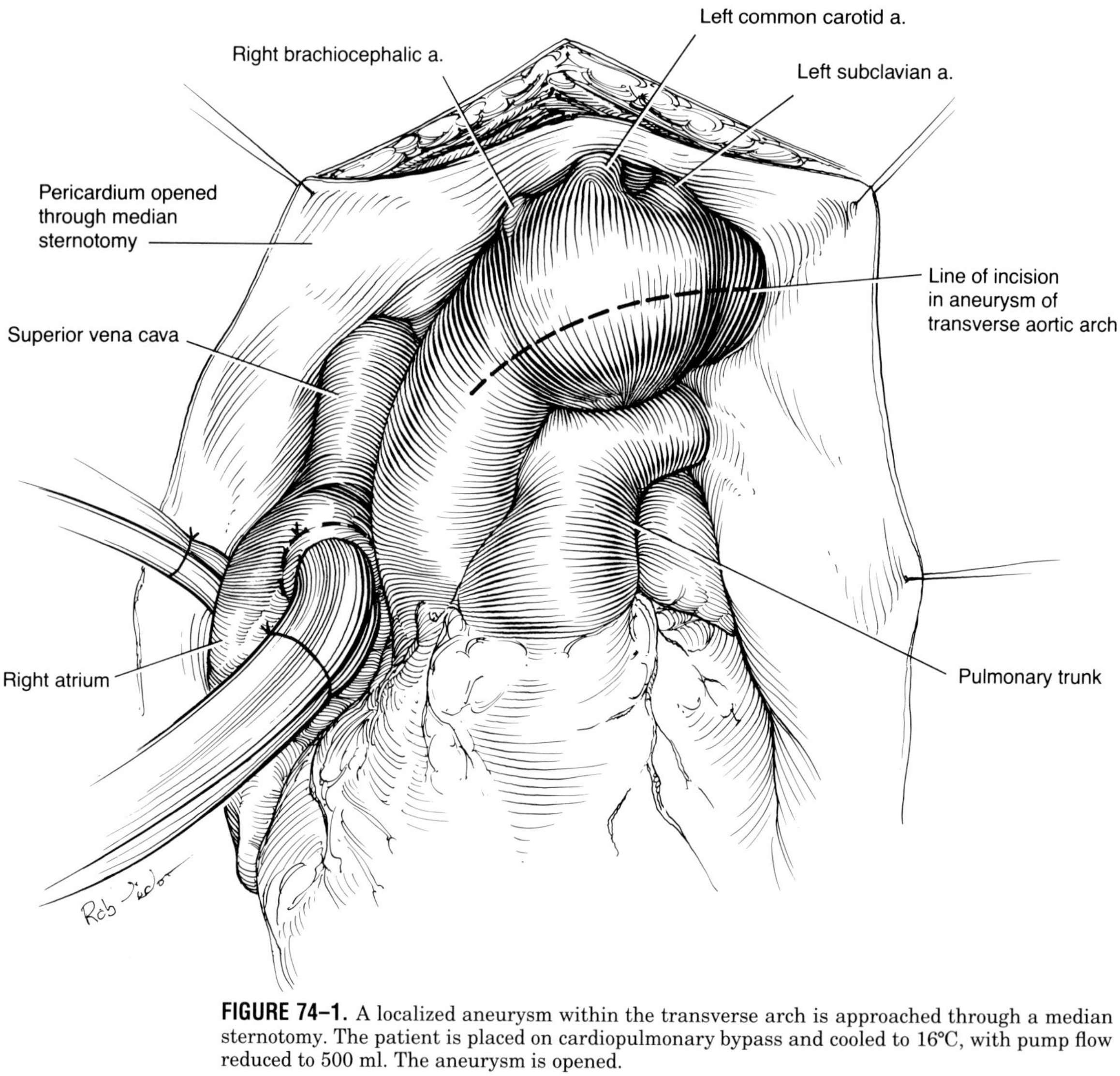

FIGURE 74–1. A localized aneurysm within the transverse arch is approached through a median sternotomy. The patient is placed on cardiopulmonary bypass and cooled to 16°C, with pump flow reduced to 500 ml. The aneurysm is opened.

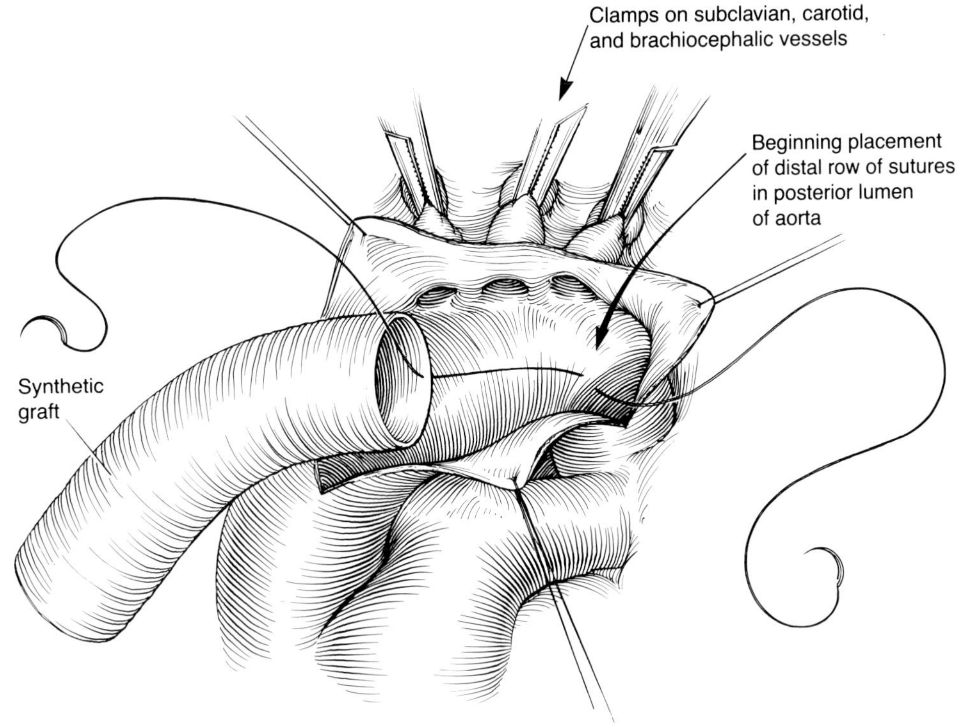

FIGURE 74–2. The distal suture line is usually completed just below or at the area of the subclavian artery.

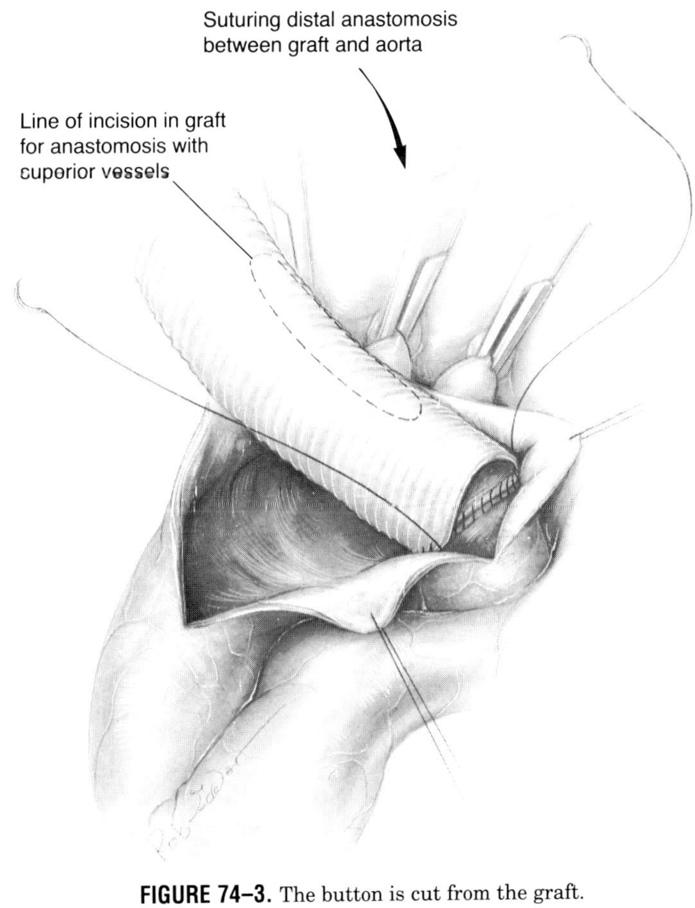

FIGURE 74–3. The button is cut from the graft.

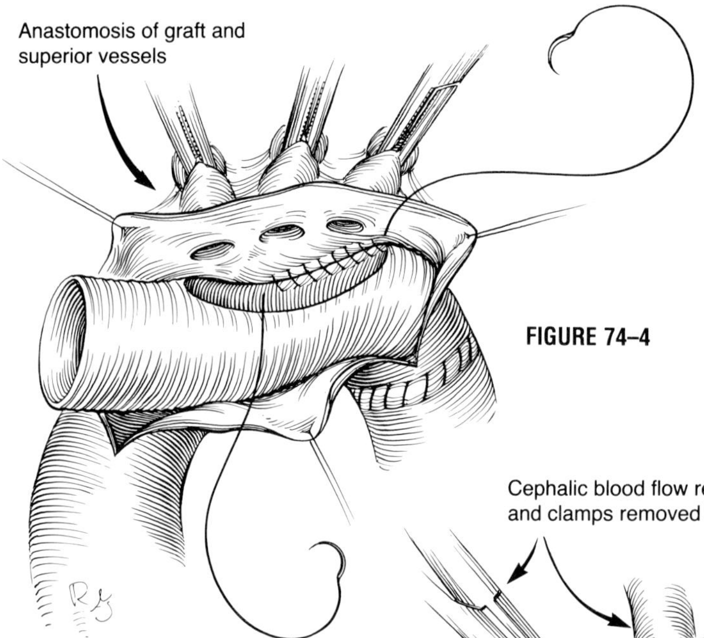

FIGURE 74–4

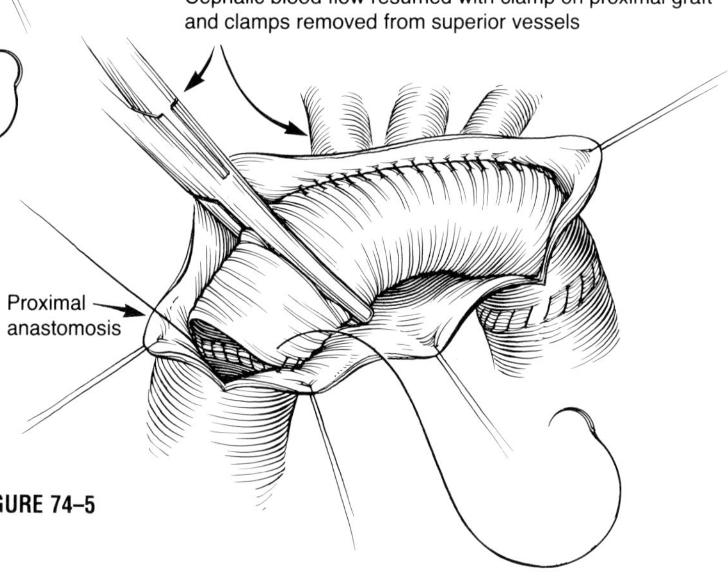

FIGURE 74–5

FIGURE 74–4. The three arch vessels are inserted with a single suture line.

FIGURE 74–5. Once the suture line is completed, the graft is de-aired and clamped, and the pump flow is increased. The patient is then rewarmed, and blood flow to the brain is re-established. A proximal anastomosis is completed, and the graft is opened. When the patient is rewarmed, cardiopulmonary bypass is discontinued.

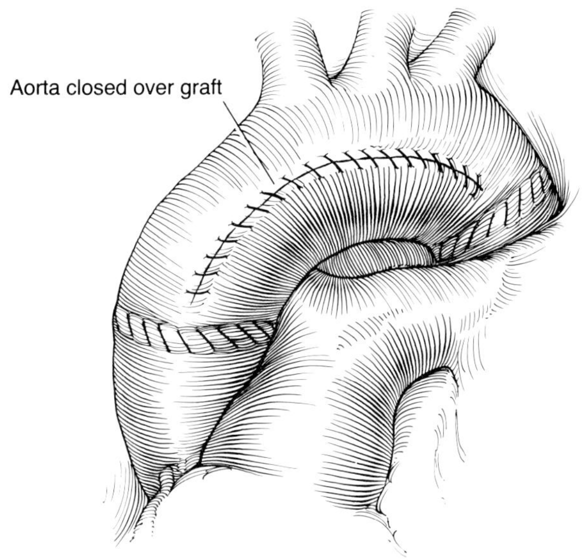

FIGURE 74–6. If enough tissue remains, it is closed over the graft.

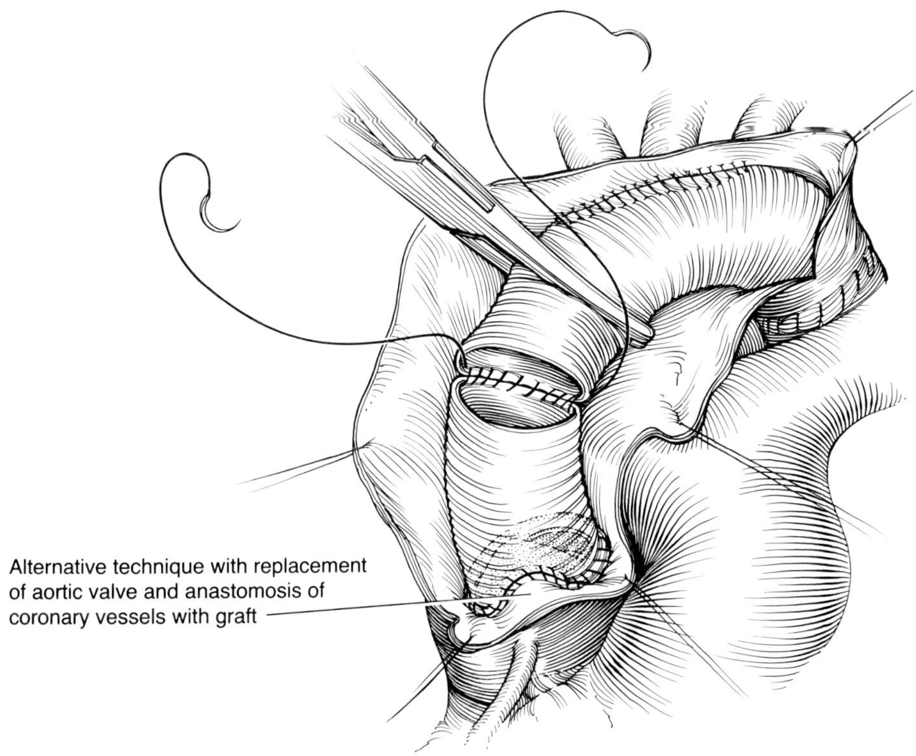

FIGURE 74–7. If an aortic valve replacement or conduit procedure is necessary to replace the entire ascending aorta and arch, the conduit is placed after circulation has been restored to the brain. The conduit is placed in the usual manner, and the coronary arteries are reimplanted. The conduit is sutured to the transverse graft.

WALTER G. WOLFE, M.D.

75
Aneurysms of the Descending Aorta

FIGURE 75–1. The chest is usually entered through a left thoracotomy at the fifth intercostal space. Placement depends on the length and position of the aneurysm and the aorta, and may be made lower or in the fourth intercostal space if there is concern about possible control high into the subclavian artery. Depending on the size of the patient, a second, lower incision may be required to help complete the anastomosis. For an acute or chronic dissection of the aorta with an aneurysm just distal to the subclavian artery, a Bio-Medicus pump is used with insertion of a cannula in the left atrium either through the appendage or vein, with cannulation of the distal thoracic aorta. The pericardium is opened if the appendage is used, but not if the inferior vein is used. For aneurysms involving the entire descending thoracic aorta, if the distal circulation is to be supported with the pump, the cannula is inserted into the femoral artery for inflow. If femoral-femoral bypass is used, both the vein and the femoral artery are cannulated.

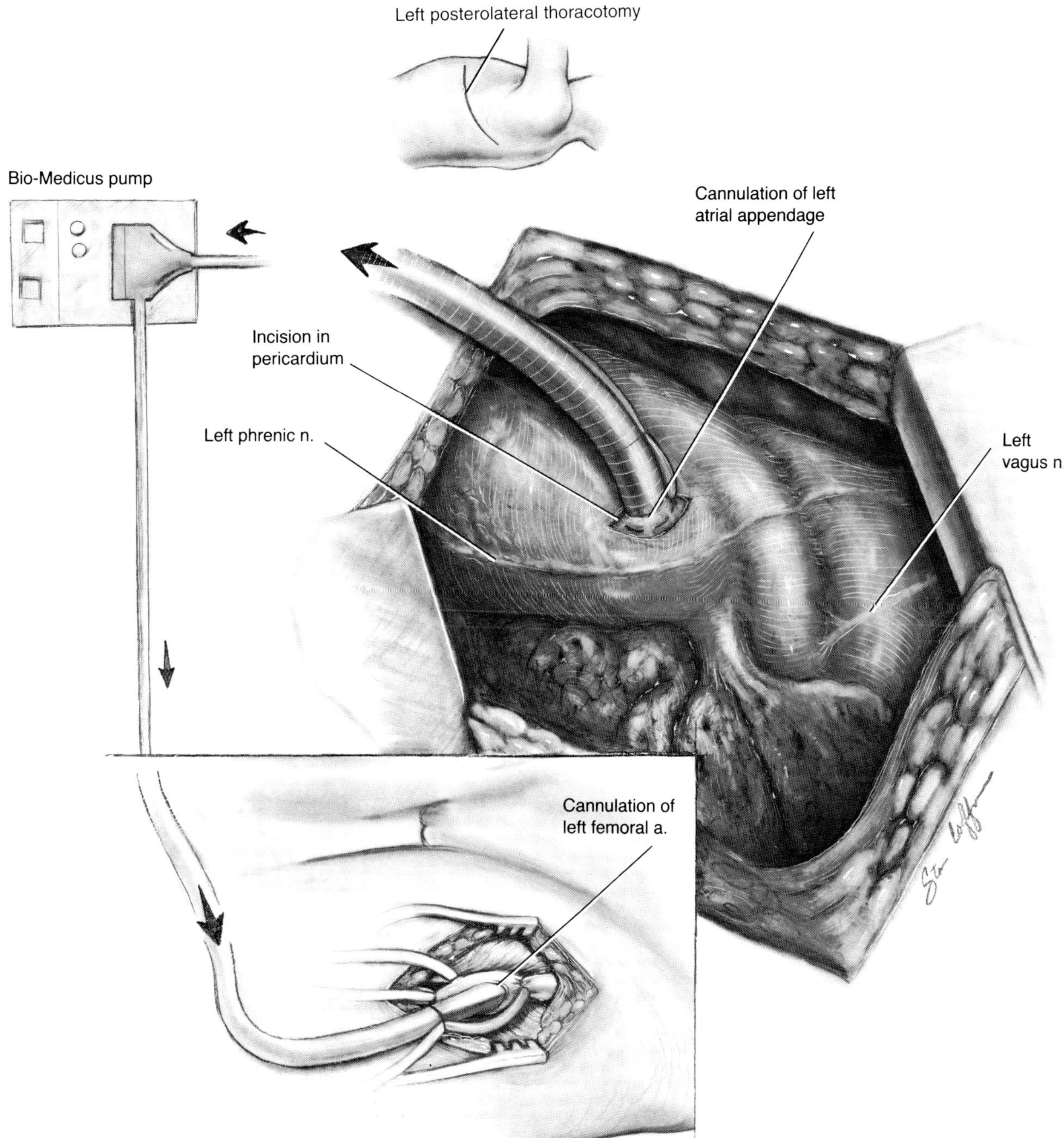

FIGURE 75–1 *See legend on opposite page*

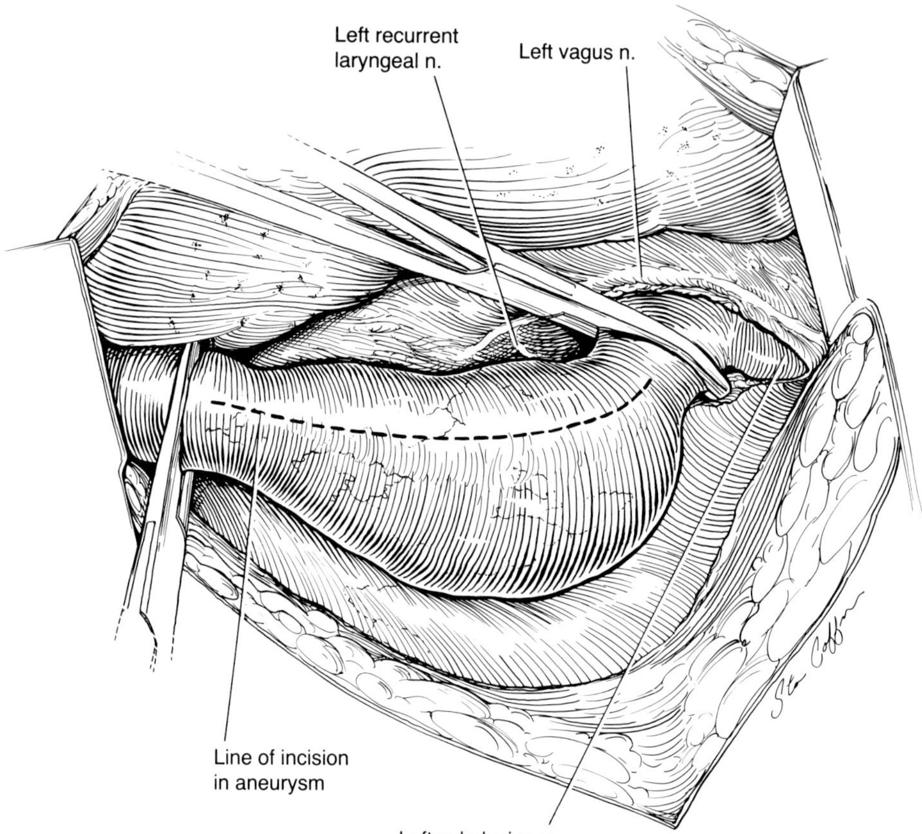

FIGURE 75–2. The aorta is dissected in the area of the left subclavian artery such that, if necessary, the vessel can be clamped between the subclavian and the carotid arteries. Distal control is necessary if bypass is used. During this dissection, care is taken not to injure the pulmonary artery or the esophagus and to preserve the recurrent and phrenic nerves.

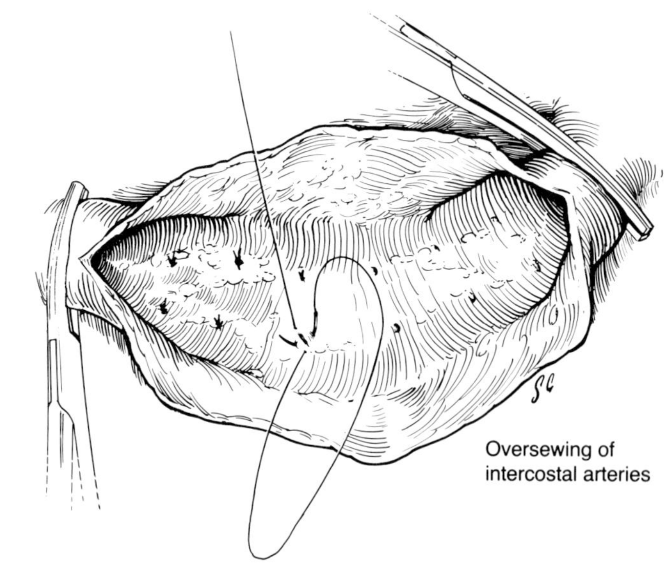

FIGURE 75–3. The aneurysm is opened and a few intercostal arteries may need to be ligated. The intercostal arteries may be implanted in the graft, but this is not generally done by this author.

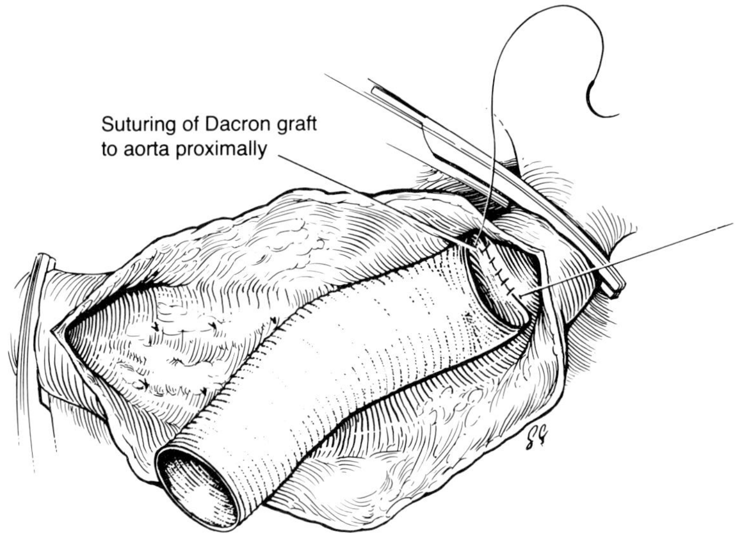

FIGURE 75–4. A proximal anastomosis is done using a continuous 3–0 Prolene suture. If there is concern over the quality of the aorta being sutured, Teflon felt strips are placed around the anastomoses to secure them both distally and proximally.

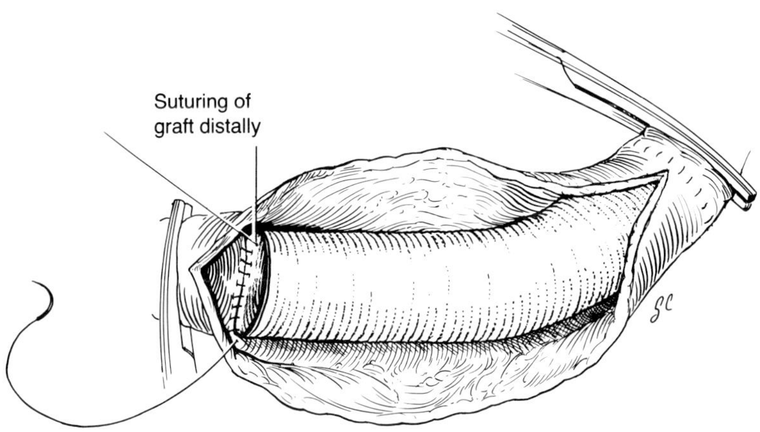

FIGURE 75–5. Once the distal anastomosis is completed, the clamp is opened and air is removed from the graft. The proximal clamp is then released.

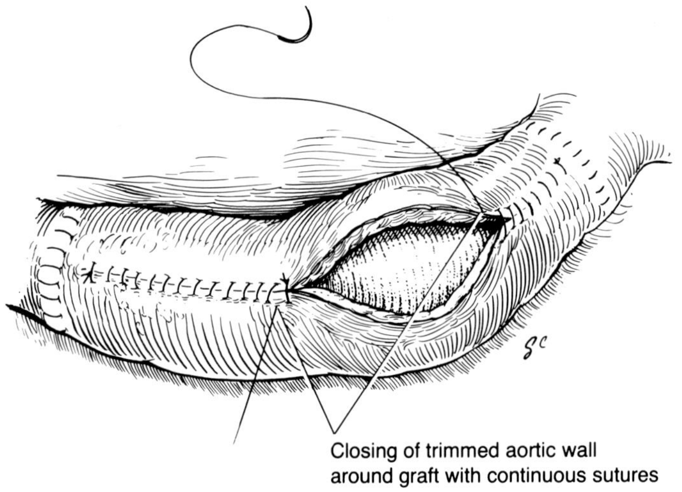

FIGURE 75–6. If enough aneurysm wall remains after the graft is inserted, it is closed over the graft. Two chest tubes are placed to drain the pleural space, and the incision is closed in the usual manner.

SECTION XIV

Cardiac Arrhythmias

JAMES E. LOWE, M.D.

76

Placement of Implantable Cardiac Defibrillator

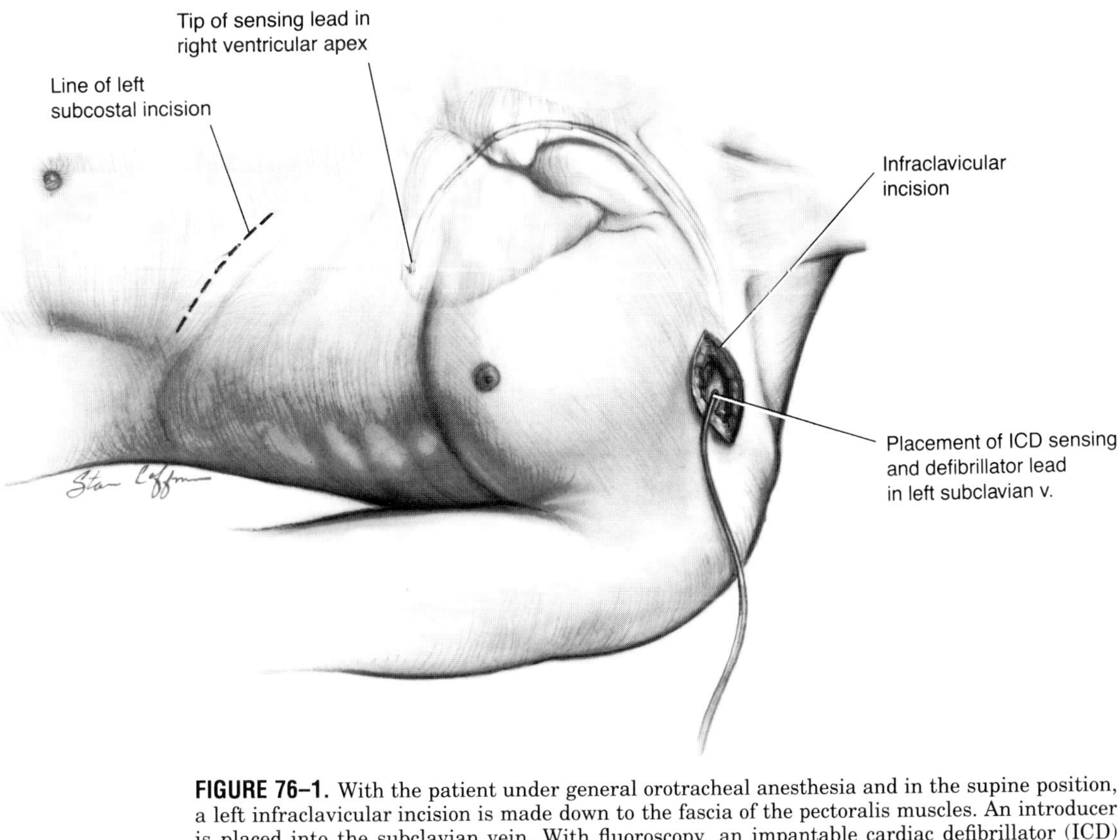

FIGURE 76–1. With the patient under general orotracheal anesthesia and in the supine position, a left infraclavicular incision is made down to the fascia of the pectoralis muscles. An introducer is placed into the subclavian vein. With fluoroscopy, an impantable cardiac defibrillator (ICD) sensing and shocking lead is positioned and secured in the right ventricular apex. The R wave sensed by the sensing lead and the pacing thresholds are determined. After adequate sensing and pacing thresholds are obtained, ventricular fibrillation or ventricular tachycardia is induced, and defibrillation thresholds are determined. After lead testing is completed, a left subcostal incision is made *(dashed line)*.

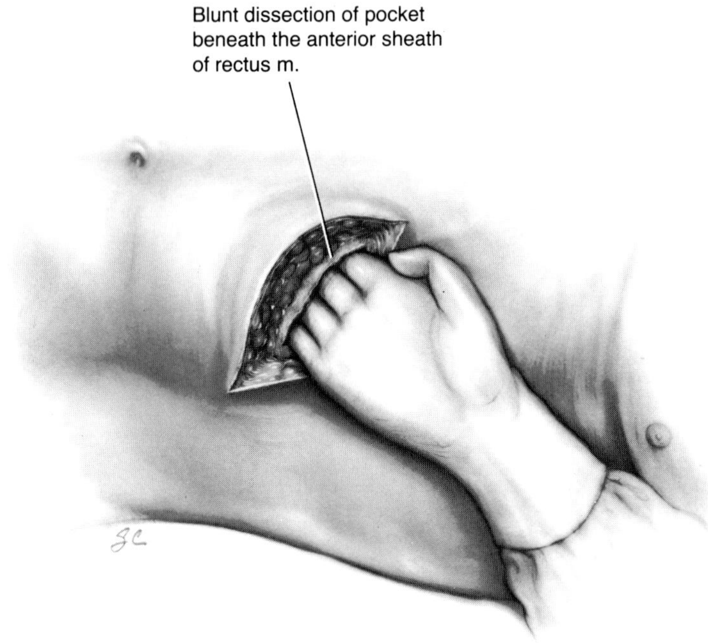

FIGURE 76–2. The anterior rectus sheath is opened, and both blunt and sharp dissection are used to create a pocket large enough to accommodate the implantable cardiac defibrillator generator beneath the anterior rectus sheath.

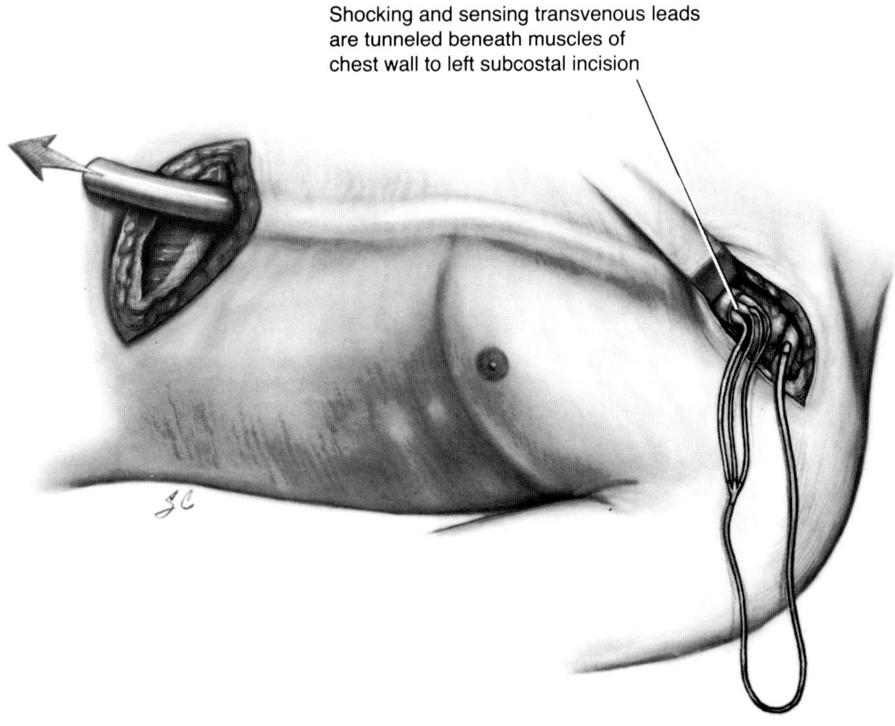

FIGURE 76–3. A tunnel is created from the left upper quadrant beneath the anterior rectus sheath over the anterior chest wall to the left infraclavicular incision. The shocking and sensing transvenous leads are then tunneled beneath the muscles of the anterior chest wall into the left subcostal incision.

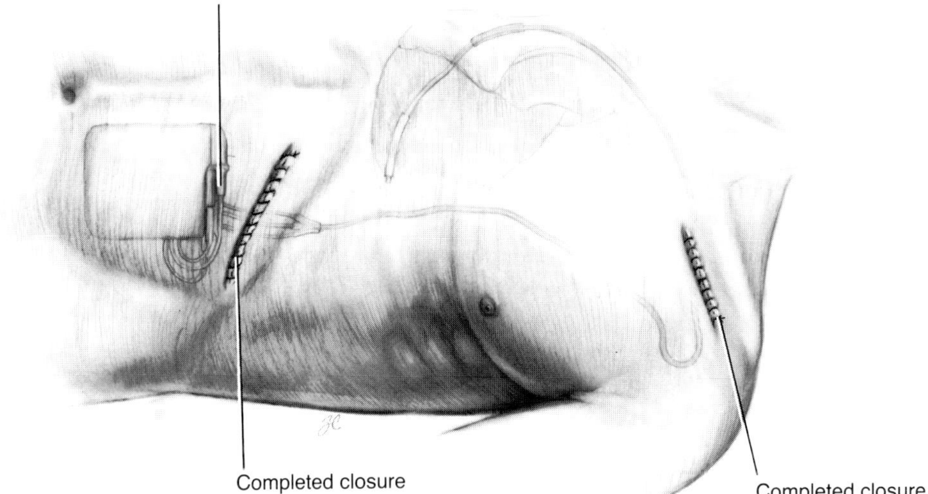

FIGURE 76–4. The shocking and sensing leads are connected to the ICD generator. Ventricular fibrillation or ventricular tachycardia is induced to verify normal function of the entire system. The ICD generator with attached shocking and sensing leads is then placed beneath the anterior rectus sheath. The anterior rectus sheath is closed with a continuous suture of 0 Prolene, and the subcostal and infraclavicular incisions are closed in a routine manner.

JAMES E. LOWE, M.D.

77

Surgical Procedures for Cardiac Arrhythmias

SURGICAL TREATMENT OF THE WOLFF-PARKINSON-WHITE SYNDROME AND CONCEALED ATRIOVENTRICULAR CONNECTIONS

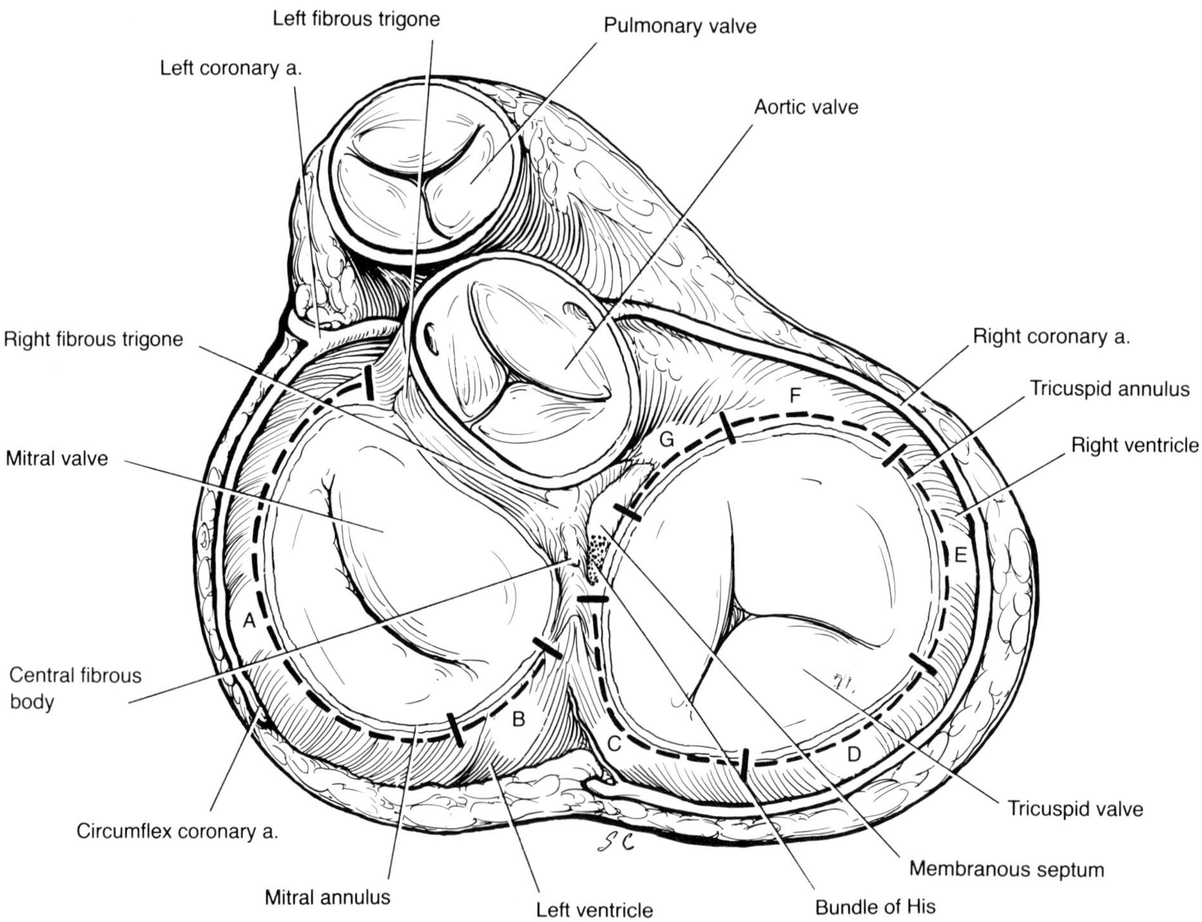

FIGURE 77–1. This superior view of the heart with the atria removed demonstrates the location of various accessory atrioventricular pathways that produce the Wolff-Parkinson-White (WPW) syndrome as well as paroxysmal supraventricular tachycardia due to concealed accessory atrioventricular connections (accessory ventricular connections that conduct in the retrograde direction only). Left free-wall pathways pass beneath the posterior mitral valve annulus in the location indicated by *A*. Left paraseptal pathways are indicated by *B*. Right posteroseptal pathways are closely adjacent to the bundle of His and atrioventricular (AV) node, as indicated in *C*. Right-sided free-wall pathways can be located in the right posterior free wall *(D)*, right lateral free wall *(E)*, anterior free wall *(F)*, and anteroseptal position *(G)*. It is important to note that accessory atrioventricular connections are not located in the region of the fibrous skeleton of the heart between the left fibrous trigone and right fibrous trigone, anterior to the mitral annulus.

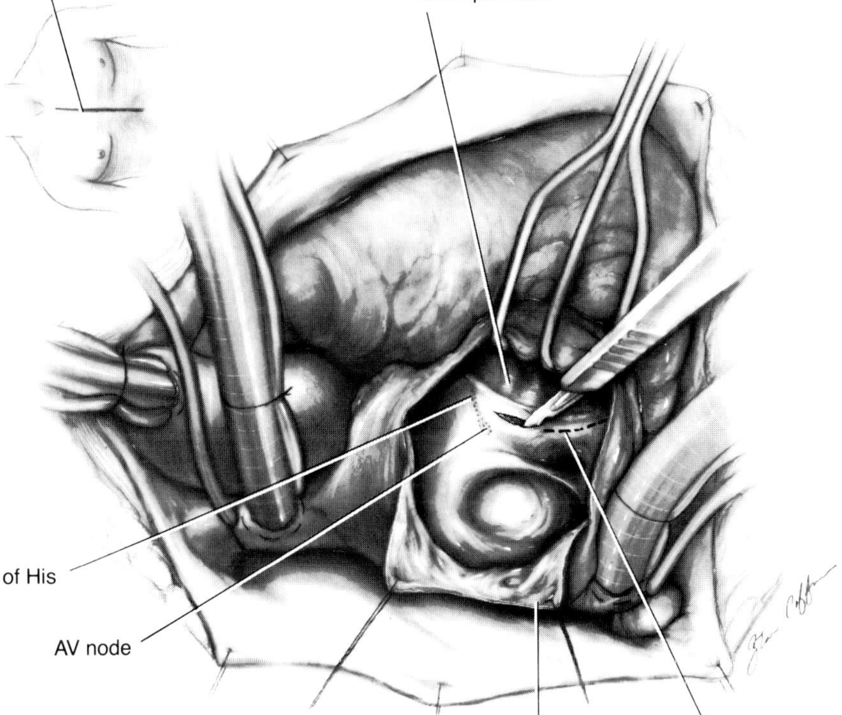

FIGURE 77–2. Cannulation techniques in the operative approach for right-sided WPW pathways are shown. For right-sided accessory connections, the right atrium is opened during normothermic cardiopulmonary bypass after transesophageal echocardiography has confirmed that neither a patent foramen ovale nor an atrial septal defect is present. A right atrial incision is continued superiorly and directed toward the right atrial appendage to avoid injury to the sinoatrial node. With the heart in sinus rhythm, the His bundle electrogram is first identified with a hand-held probe. A supra-annular incision *(dashed line)* is then made just posterior to the identified site of the His bundle electrogram and 2 mm above the posterior tricuspid valve annulus. This incision is extended counterclockwise onto the posterior right atrial free wall from within the atrium.

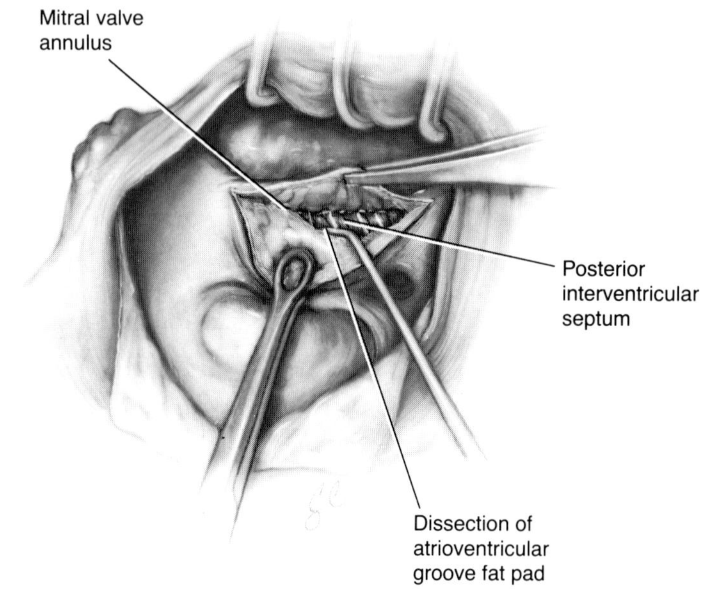

FIGURE 77–3. After the right atrial endocardium is divided, a plane of dissection is established between the fat pad and the top of the posterior interventricular septum with the heart in sinus rhythm. The dissection is extended deep into the posterior pyramidal space overlying the posterior interventricular septum and is extended medially until the annulus of the mitral valve is visualized and posteriorly to the epicardial reflection of the right ventricle at the crux of the heart.

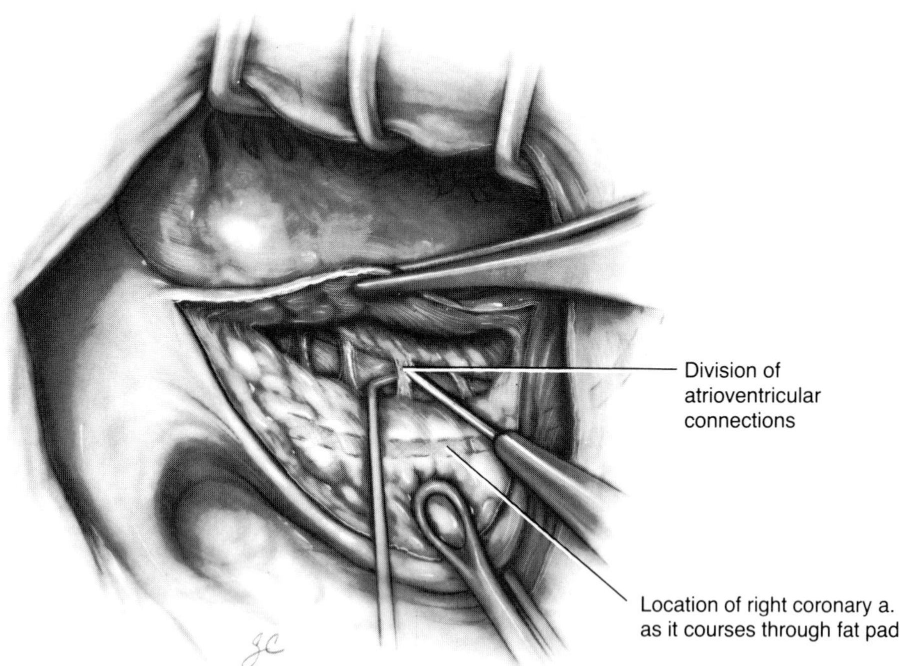

FIGURE 77–4. Several accessory AV connections in the posteroseptal region are depicted. Each of these is divided using a nerve hook and electrocautery.

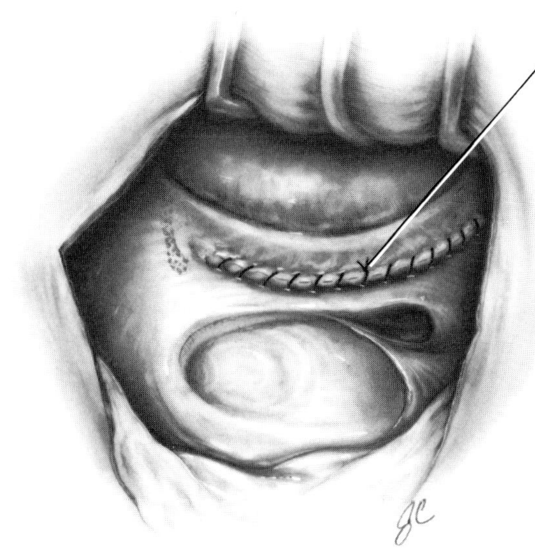

FIGURE 77–5. After the posteroseptal dissection is completed, the supra-annular incision above the tricuspid valve annulus is closed with a continuous suture of 4–0 Prolene.

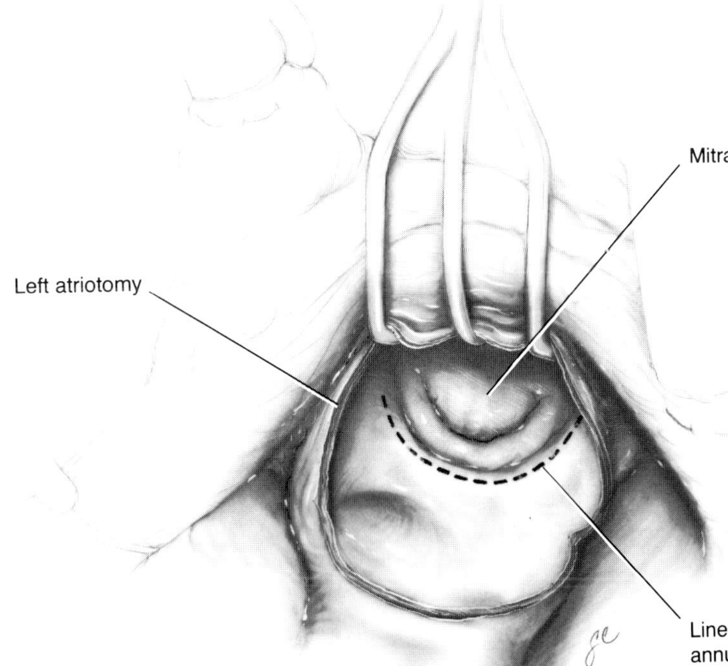

FIGURE 77–6. Left-sided pathways creating the WPW syndrome are surgically divided with the heart arrested by cold potassium cardioplegia. The interatrial groove is dissected, and a standard left atrial incision is made similar to the approach taken for mitral valve replacement or repair. Because the left atrium is of normal size, exposure is facilitated by cannulating the superior vena cava through the right atrial appendage and the inferior vena cava through a separate pursestring suture over the inferior midportion of the right atrium. In addition, the pericardial reflection over the superior and inferior venae cavae is divided to allow rotation of the heart to the left. After the left atrium is opened under cardioplegic arrest, a specially modified hand-held mitral retractor is placed across the mitral valve to expose the posterior mitral valve annulus. A supra-annular incision is then placed 2 mm above the posterior mitral valve annulus, as indicated by the dashed line. This incision begins just below the left fibrous trigone and is extended counterclockwise to the area of the posterior interventricular septum.

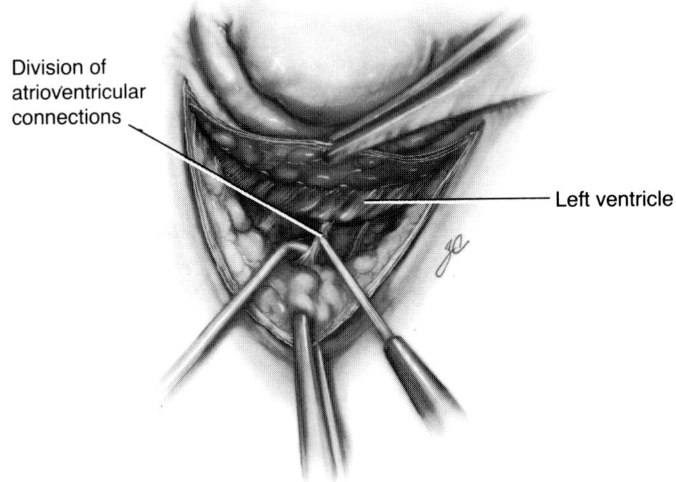

FIGURE 77–7. After the endocardium is divided, the fat pad of the AV groove is entered, and the left atrium is disconnected from the top of the posterior left ventricle throughout the length of the supra-annular incision. The AV groove fat pad is then exposed, and accessory AV connections between the posterior left atrium and posterior left ventricle are divided using a nerve hook and electrocautery. Ring forceps are used to grasp the posterior mitral valve annulus and posterior aspect of the left ventricle for exposure. The dissection is extended to the epicardial reflection of the posterior left ventricle to completely disconnect the left atrium from the left ventricle. A sharp nerve hook is used to transect any remaining fibers connecting the atrium to the ventricle along the posterior mitral valve annulus.

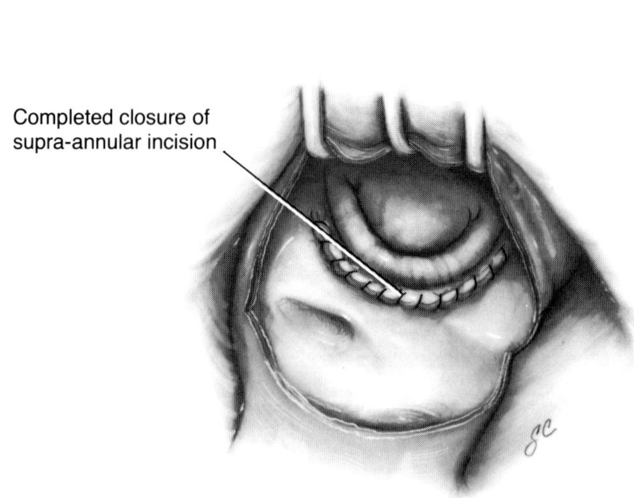

FIGURE 77–8. After the left-sided dissection is completed, the supra-annular incision is closed with a continuous suture of 4–0 Prolene, and the left atrium is closed in a routine manner. The total crossclamp time required to complete the left-sided dissections averages 20 to 30 minutes.

SURGICAL TREATMENT OF AUTOMATIC ATRIAL TACHYCARDIAS

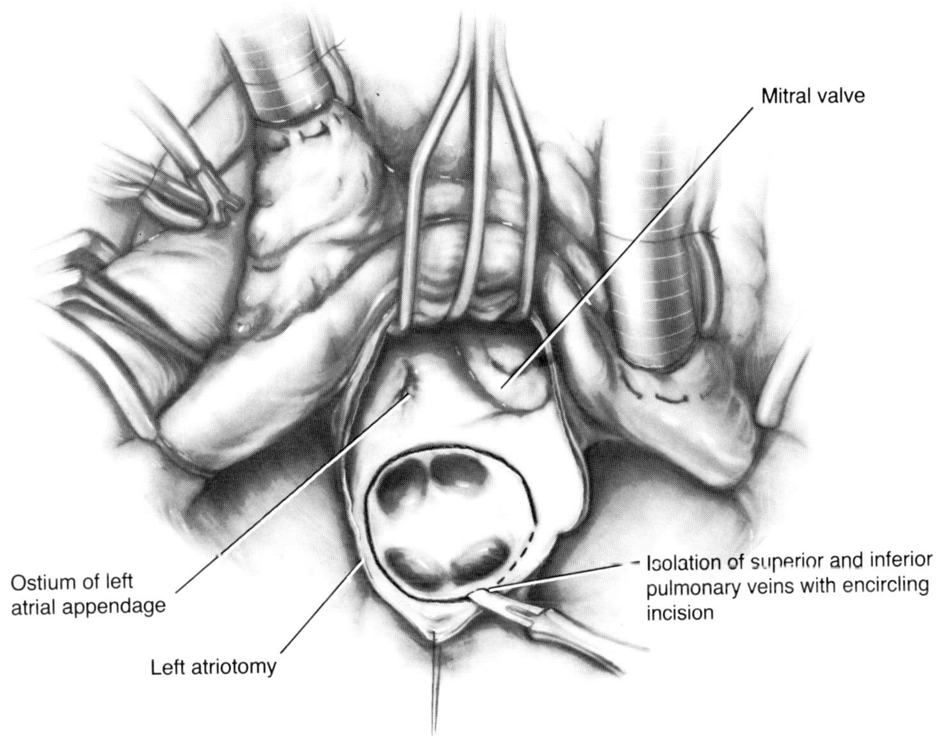

FIGURE 77–9. Automatic atrial tachycardia is an uncommon dysrhythmia caused by a single extranodal automatic focus. Dilated cardiomyopathy and congestive heart failure eventually develop in most patients with sustained supraventricular tachycardia. In these patients, control of the tachycardia by surgical correction usually improves ventricular function. The site of origin of automatic atrial tachycardia can be in either the left or the right atrium and can be either discrete or diffuse. Therefore, a variety of surgical approaches must be considered, depending on the site and size of origin.

In this patient, intraoperative mapping confirms a focus of ectopic atrial tachycardia that originated between the insertion of the pulmonary veins into the posterior left atrium. Because the exact site is unknown, a partial left atrial isolation procedure is performed using cardioplegic arrest.

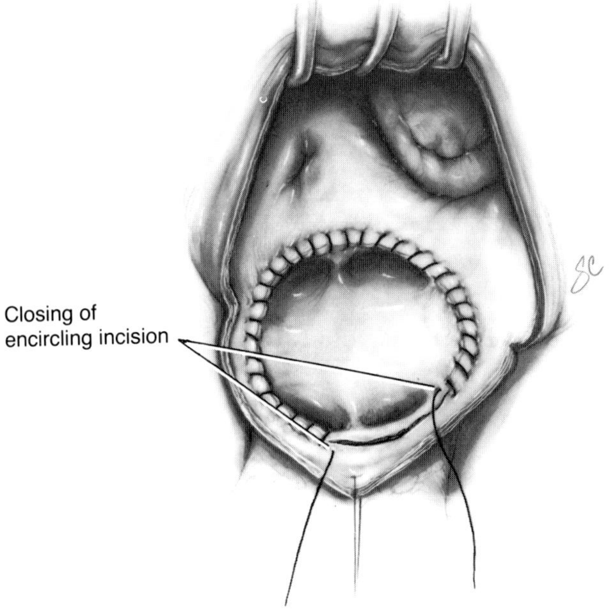

FIGURE 77–10. After complete isolation of all pulmonary veins from the left atrium, the incision is closed with a continuous suture of 4–0 Prolene.

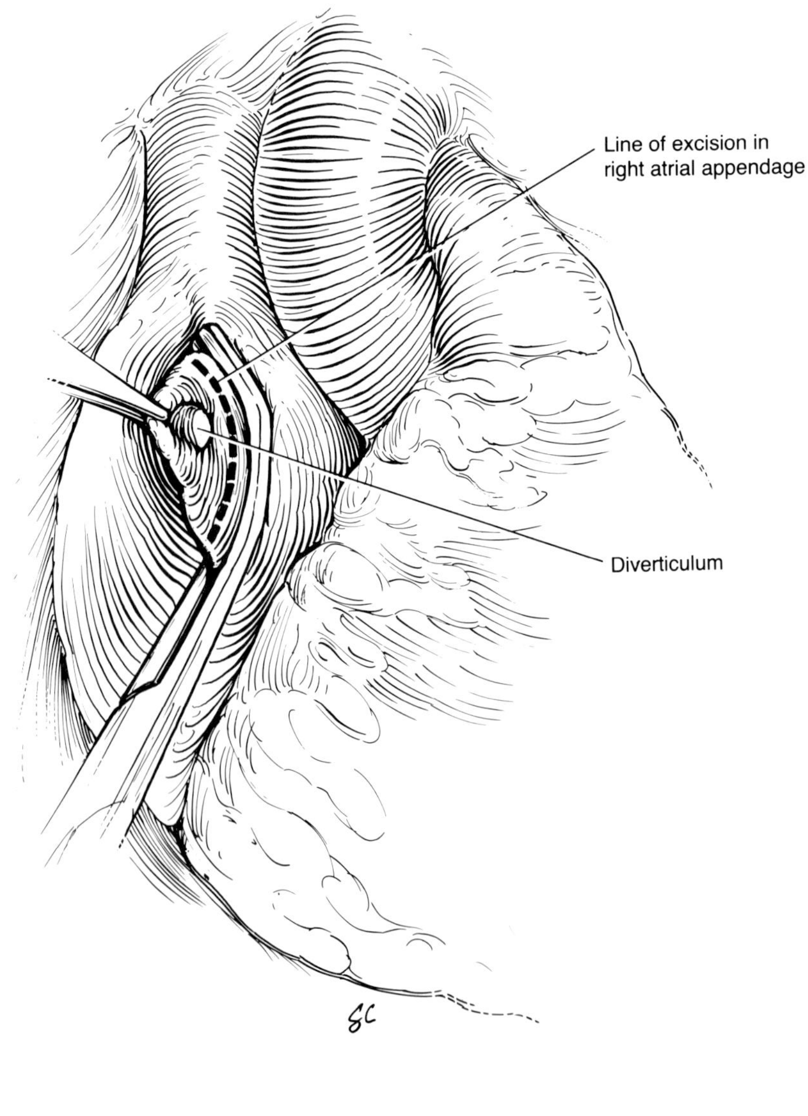

FIGURE 77–11. A focus causing chronic ectopic atrial tachycardia originated in a small right atrial diverticulum. The diverticulum and surrounding right atrium are easily excised and repaired primarily without requiring cardiopulmonary bypass.

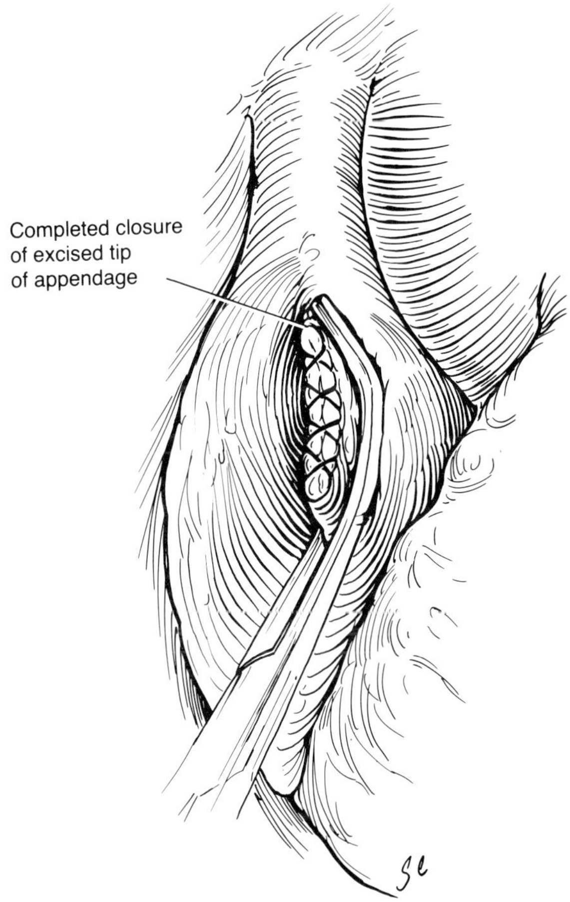

FIGURE 77–12. An occluding clamp is placed at the base of the atrial appendage, and the appendage containing the diverticulum is excised and closed with 4–0 Prolene.

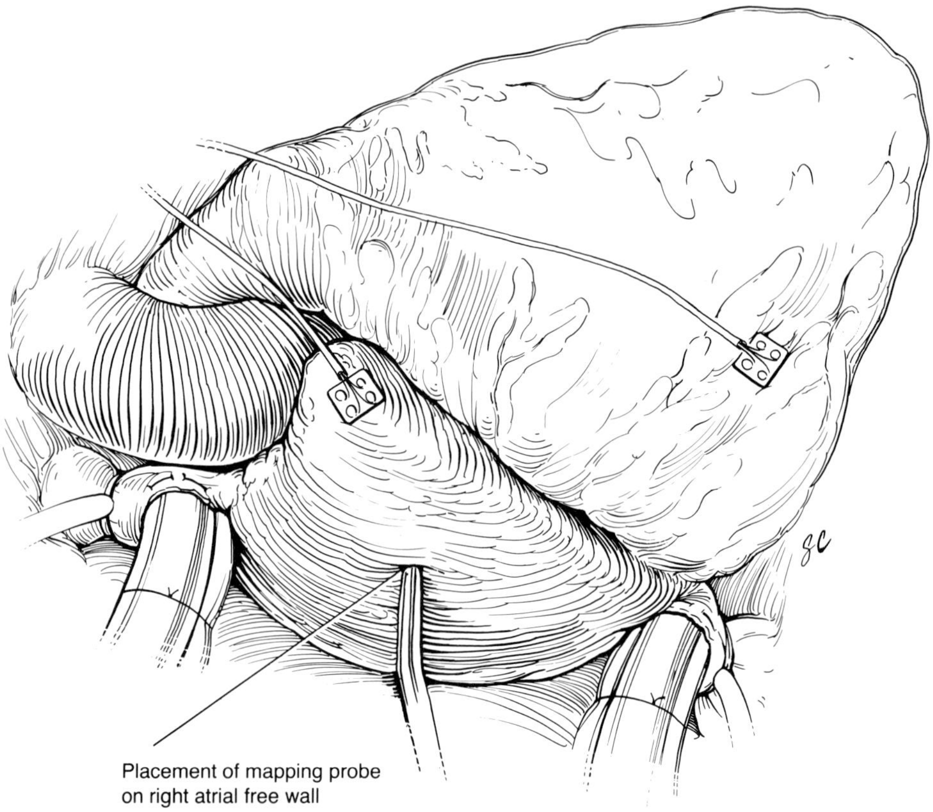

FIGURE 77–13. A focus of ectopic atrial tachycardia is localized to an area over the right atrial free wall using a bipolar mapping probe.

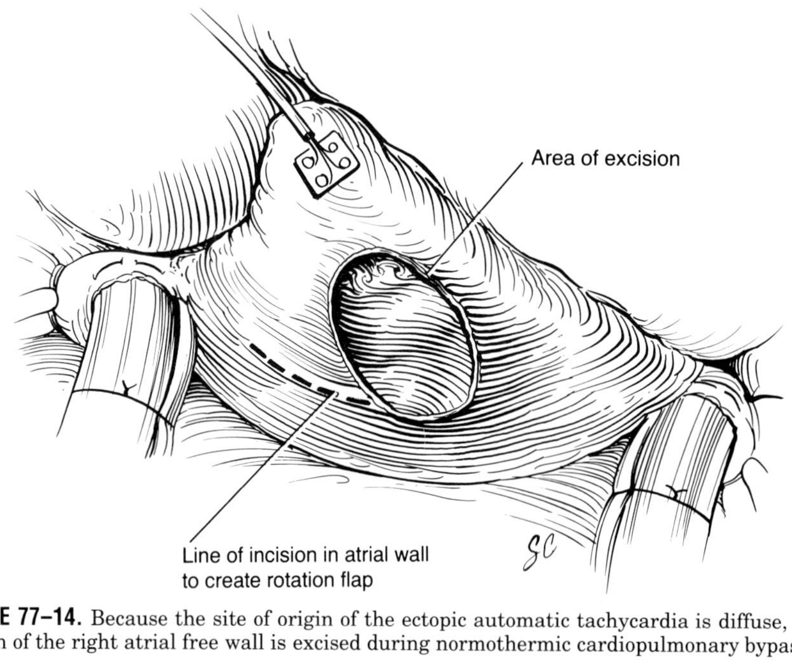

FIGURE 77–14. Because the site of origin of the ectopic automatic tachycardia is diffuse, a large portion of the right atrial free wall is excised during normothermic cardiopulmonary bypass.

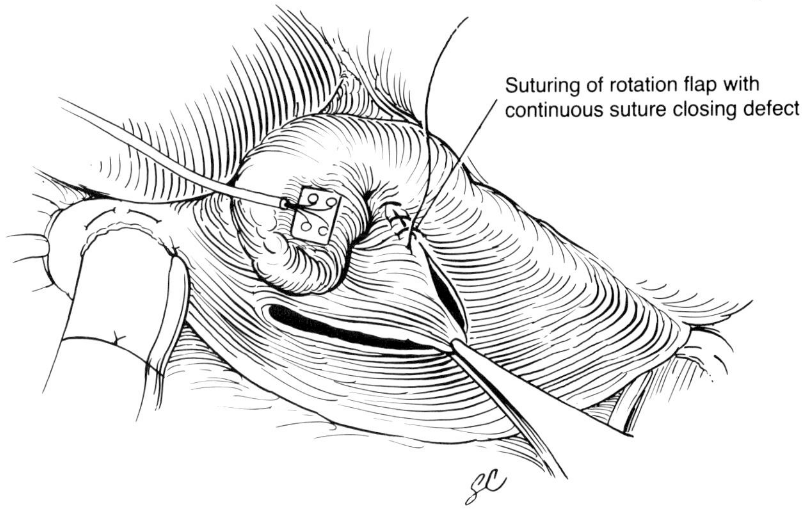

FIGURE 77–15. The large defect in the right atrial free wall is repaired with a rotation flap of the remaining right atrium including the right atrial appendage.

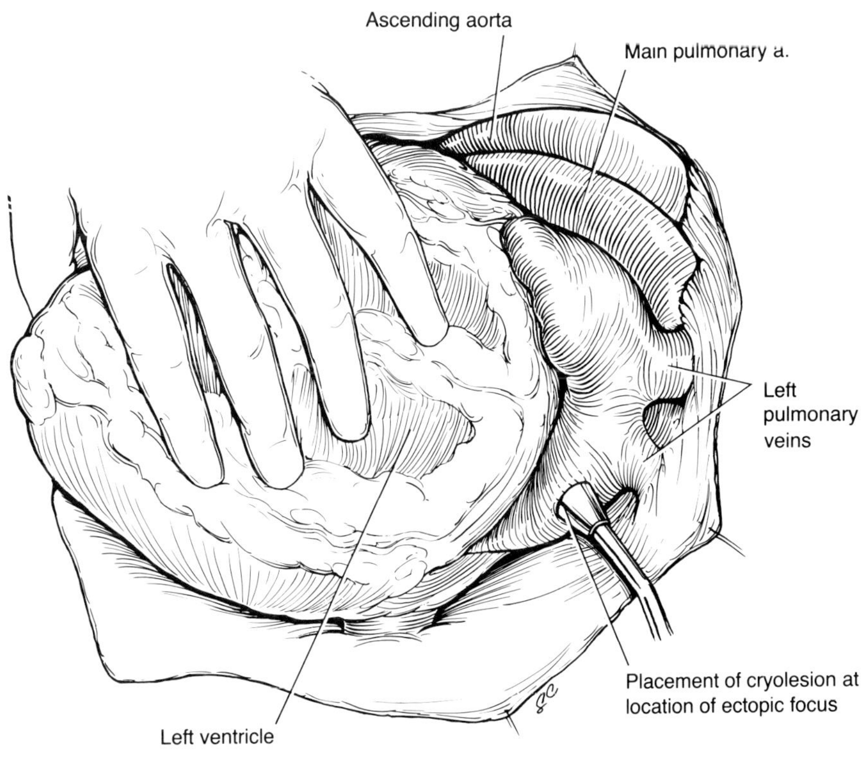

FIGURE 77–16. Cryoablation is used to ablate a small focus of ectopic atrial tachycardia near the left inferior pulmonary vein. This procedure is performed under normothermic cardiopulmonary bypass and does not require cardioplegic arrest.

SURGICAL TREATMENT OF RE-ENTRANT VENTRICULAR TACHYCARDIA

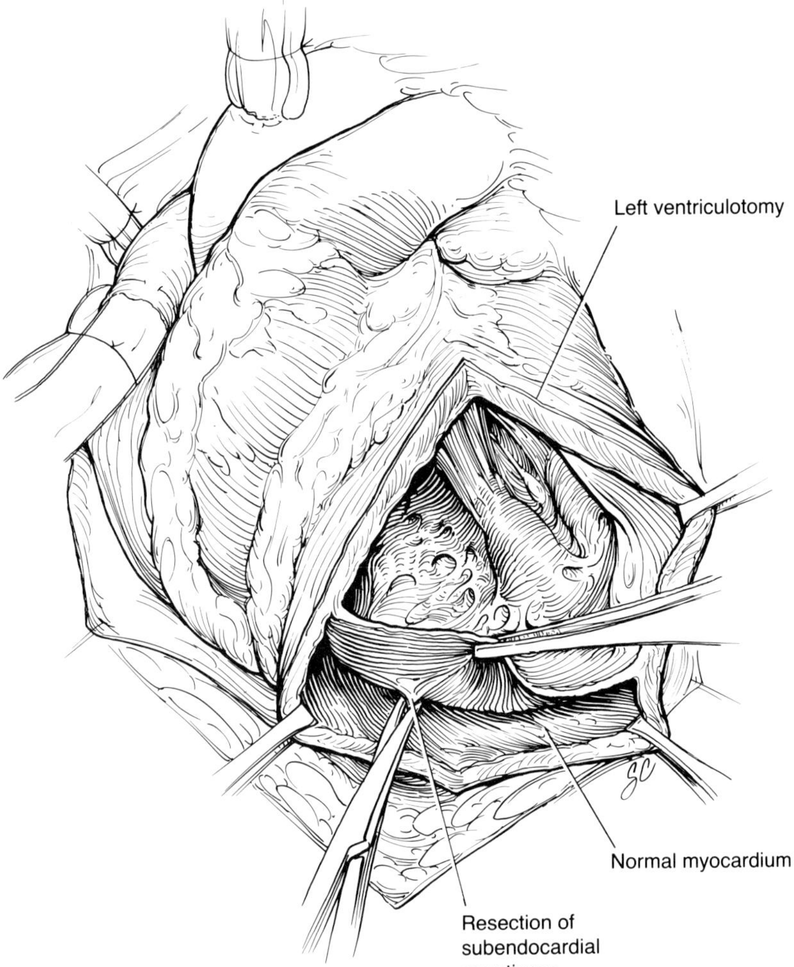

FIGURE 77–17. A subendocardial resection procedure is used to ablate an arrhythmogenic re-entrant region identified by endocardial mapping. The subendocardial scar tissue is excised where it joins normal myocardium at the border of a left ventricular aneurysm. Shown is an anteroapical left ventricular aneurysm that has been opened in its midportion during normothermic cardiopulmonary bypass. After endocardial mapping, all visible scar tissue is removed.

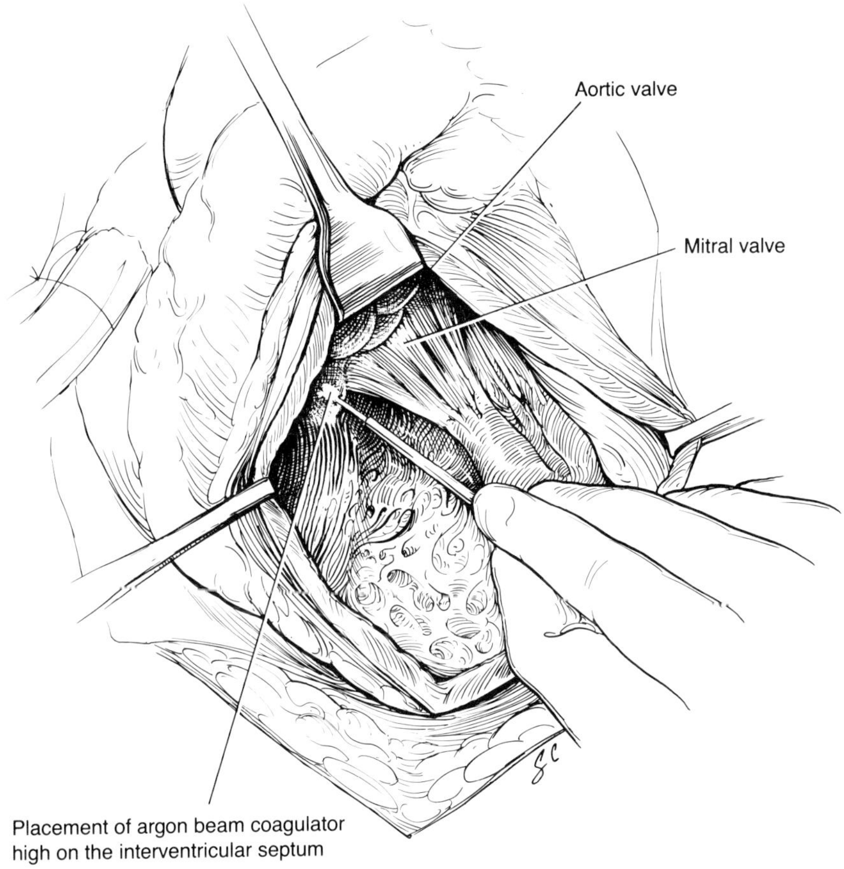

FIGURE 77–18. Often the site of origin of the re-entrant ventricular tachycardia is located high on the interventricular septum. This area can be ablated using a nonlaser argon beam coagulator. This technique is preferred because subendocardial resection in this area may create a ventricular septal defect. In addition, the argon beam coagulator destroys tissue much more rapidly than does placement of multiple cryolesions.

JAMES L. COX, M.D.

78

The Maze III Procedure for Treatment of Atrial Fibrillation

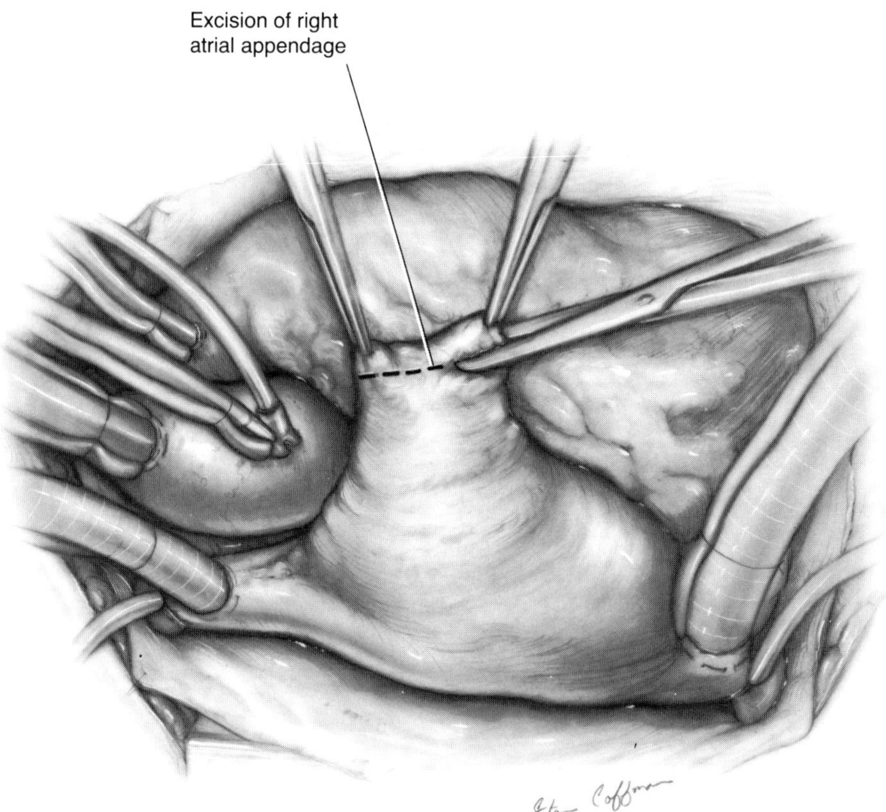

FIGURE 78–1. After total cardiopulmonary bypass is established and the caval tapes are secured, the right atrial appendage is excised. At least 2 cm of visible atrial muscle should be preserved between the superior end of the excised appendage *(dashed line)* and the orifice of the superior vena cava (SVC). Note that the SVC is cannulated directly approximately 2 cm above the right atrium and that the inferior vena cava also is cannulated low. A pulmonary artery vent is shown in position, as is the combined cardioplegia infusion-aortic vent in the ascending aorta.

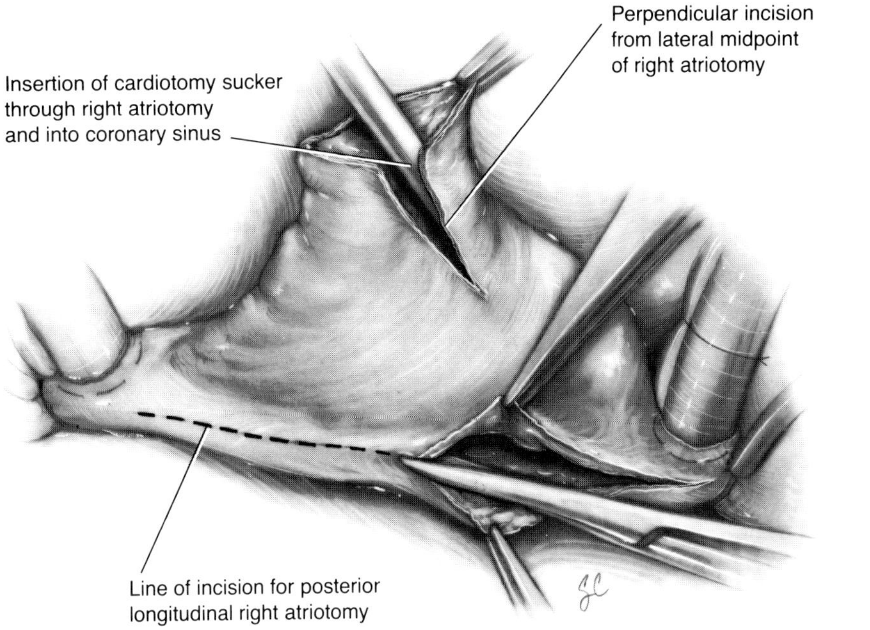

FIGURE 78–2. A lateral incision, parallel to the right atrioventricular groove, is placed from the base of the excised atrial appendage toward the inferior vena cava (IVC), leaving 5 to 6 cm of right atrial free wall between the lower end of the incision and the IVC cannula. A posterior longitudinal incision is then placed from well into the SVC *(dashed line)* to well into the IVC. It is helpful to place a cardiotomy sucker into the opening of the coronary sinus via the atrial appendage during placement of the posterior longitudinal incision.

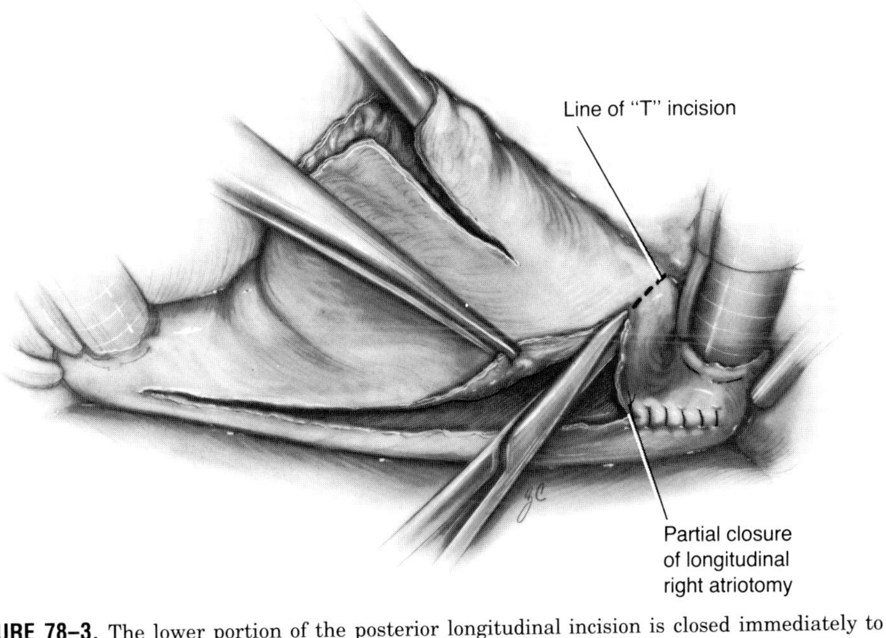

FIGURE 78–3. The lower portion of the posterior longitudinal incision is closed immediately to prevent inadvertent tearing and extension of the incision into the IVC during later retraction. The incision usually is closed to the level of the top of the IVC cannula. A T incision is then made from this point across the lower right atrial free wall approximately 1 cm above the IVC cannula. The T incision is extended to the top of the right atrioventricular groove *(dashed line)*. The remainder of the incision, extending to the tricuspid valve annulus, must be made from inside the right atrium.

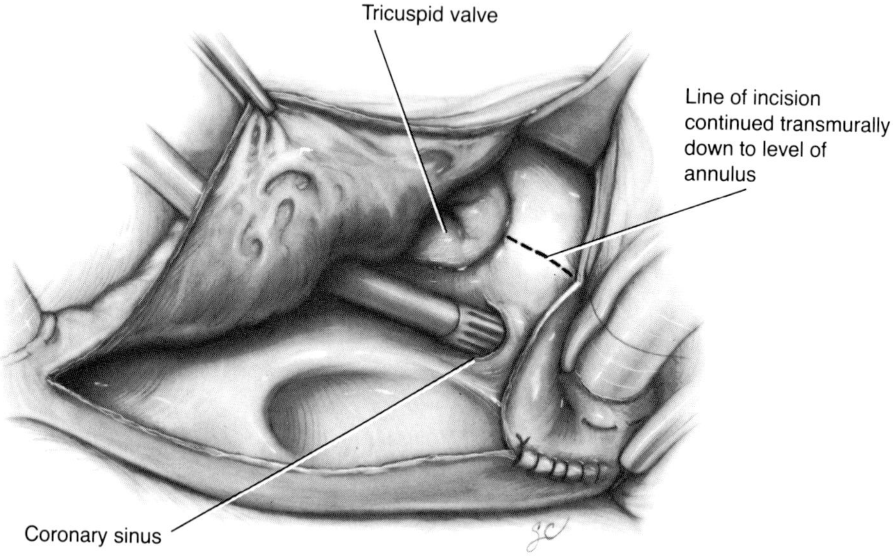

FIGURE 78–4. The right atrial free wall is retracted anteriorly and superiorly. The dashed line shows the planned extension of the T incision to the tricuspid annulus. This continues to be a transmural atriotomy, but underlying this portion of the incision is the fat pad of the right atrioventricular groove that harbors the right coronary artery. Therefore, this portion of the incision must be made with care. Once the atrial wall has been divided transmurally, the fat in the atrioventricular groove is visible.

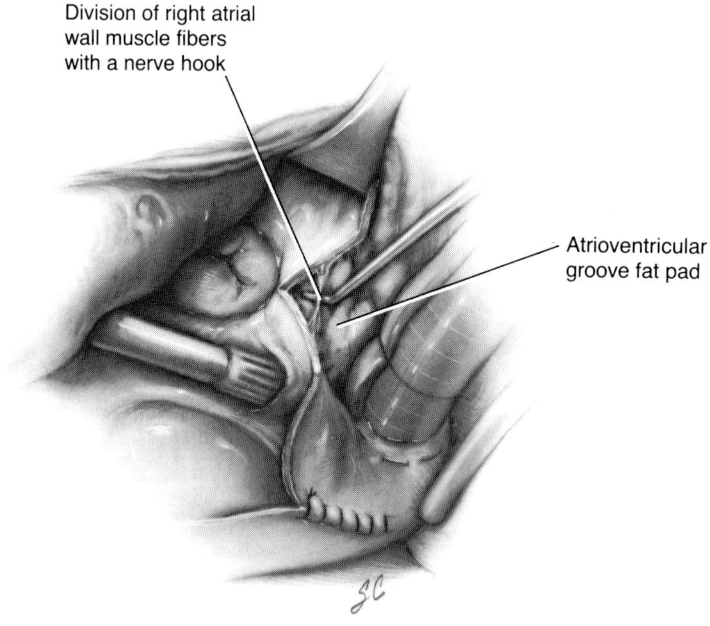

FIGURE 78–5. It is essential to divide all atrial myocardial fibers traversing this portion of the T incision using either a knife or a nerve hook.

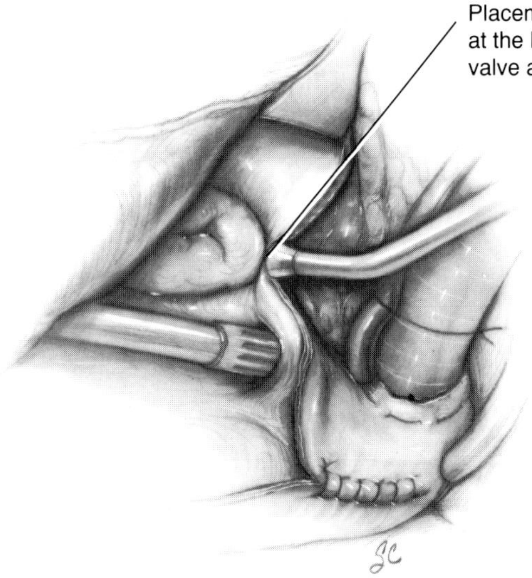

FIGURE 78–6. A cryolesion is placed at the tricuspid end of the T incision to be certain that no remaining fibers traverse the incision at the level of the tricuspid valve annulus. A 3-mm cryoprobe is applied for 2 minutes at −60°C.

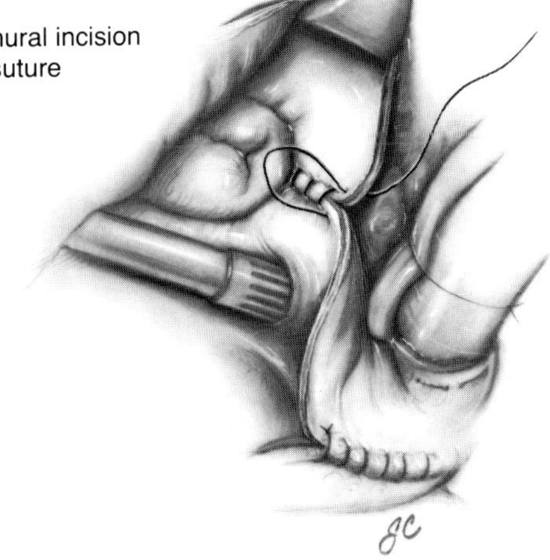

FIGURE 78–7. The tricuspid end of the T incision is closed to the level of the top of the atrioventricular groove. The remainder of the incision is left unclosed in order to attain better surgical exposure during the remainder of the procedure.

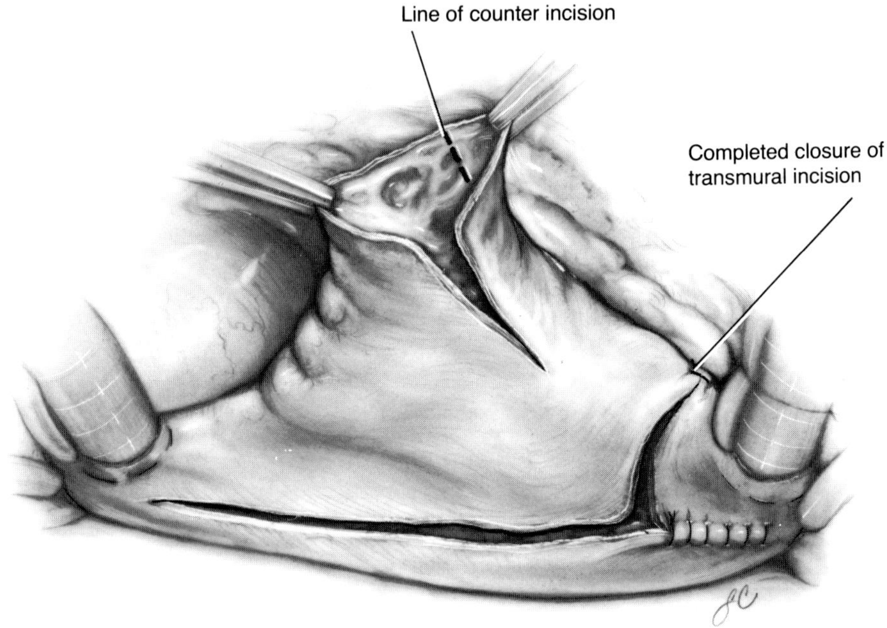

FIGURE 78–8. Once the lower ends of the posterior longitudinal incision and the T incision have been closed, the anterior right atrial counter incision is performed beginning at the anteromedial border of the excised right atrial appendage *(dashed line).* This incision extends to the anteromedial tricuspid valve annulus, and once begun it is easier to complete from within the right atrium.

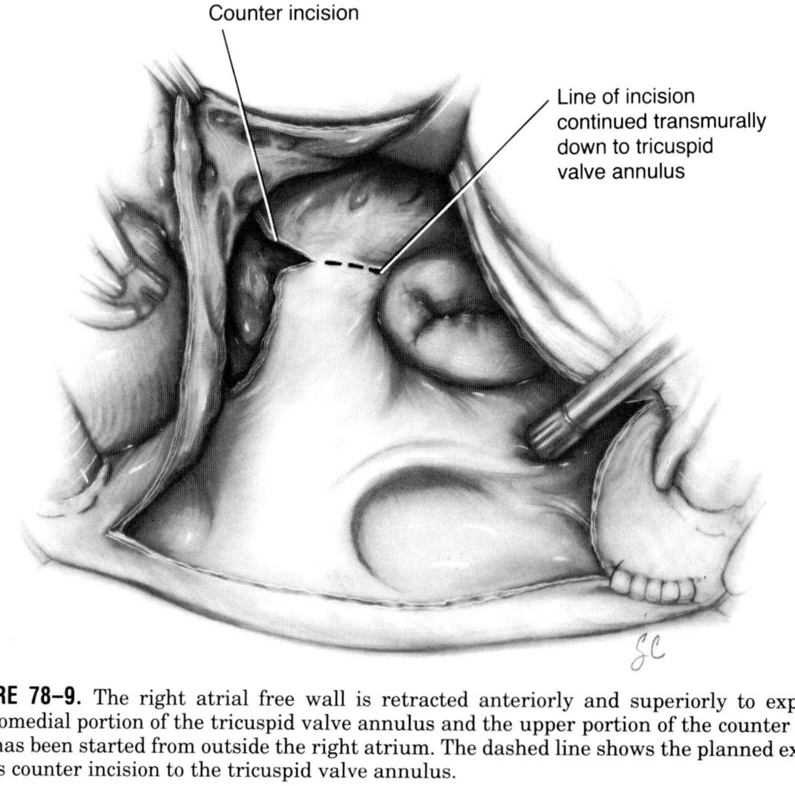

FIGURE 78–9. The right atrial free wall is retracted anteriorly and superiorly to expose the anteromedial portion of the tricuspid valve annulus and the upper portion of the counter incision that has been started from outside the right atrium. The dashed line shows the planned extension of this counter incision to the tricuspid valve annulus.

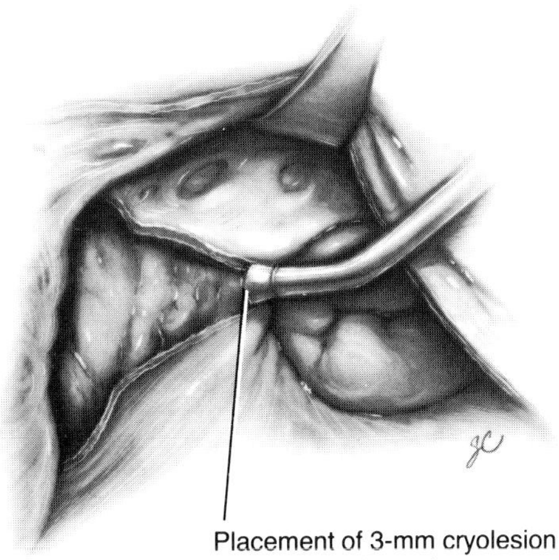

FIGURE 78–10. The counter incision is transmural, but care must be taken in dividing the final myocardial fibers because the right atrioventricular groove fat pad lies immediately beneath the incision. This portion of the right atrioventricular groove corresponds to the anterior septal space. In this case, the incision is approximately 2 to 3 cm anterior to the atrioventricular (AV) node–His bundle complex. The right coronary artery usually has not joined the right atrioventricular groove at this point, although anatomic variations exist. A 3-mm cryolesion is also placed at the tricuspid end of this incision to ensure its completion. This is the final right atrial incision.

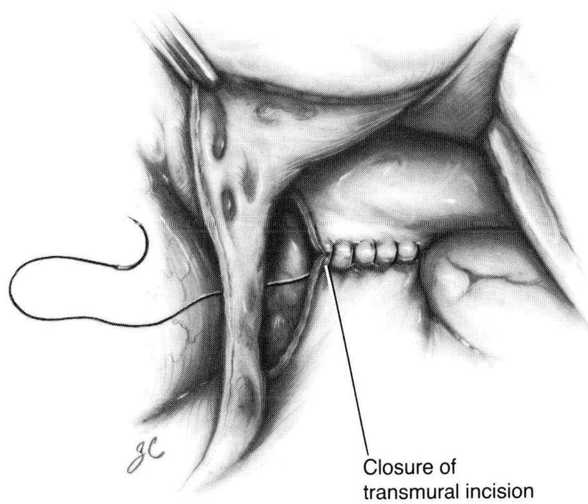

FIGURE 78–11. The entire counter incision is closed to the base of the excised atrial appendage.

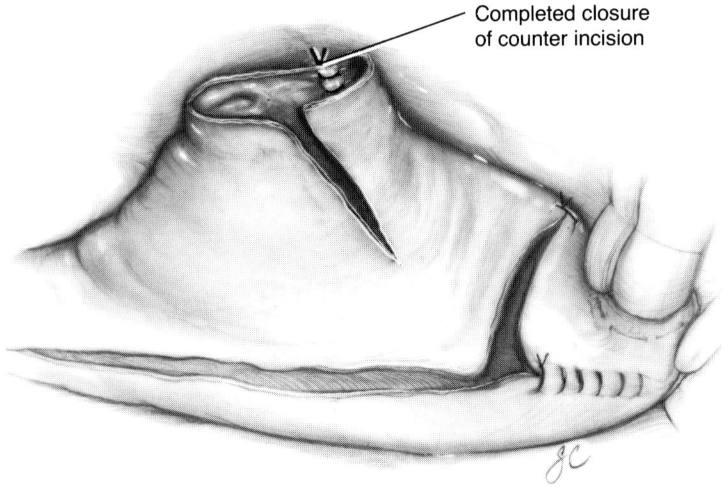

FIGURE 78–12. Once the anteromedial counter incision has been closed, the remaining right atrial incisions are left unclosed until the left atrial procedure has been completed.

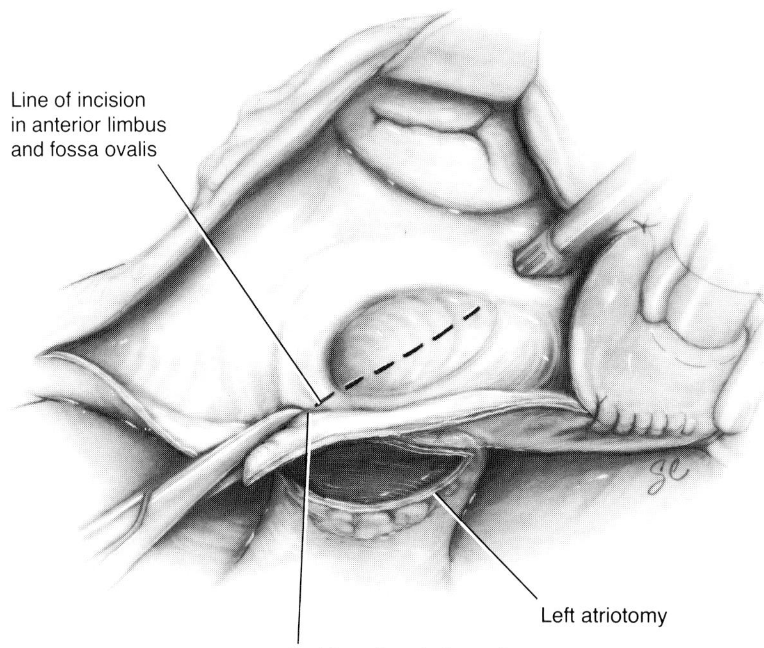

FIGURE 78–13. A standard left atriotomy is performed in the interatrial groove, its lower end being extended around the lower lip of the orifice of the right inferior pulmonary vein. The atrial septum is then divided beginning 2 to 3 cm below the orifice of the superior vena cava, traversing the anterior limbus of the fossa ovalis, and then traversing the fossa ovalis itself *(dashed line)*. This septal incision should be slanted in the general direction of the opening of the coronary sinus, but it is absolutely essential to terminate it at the bottom of the thin portion of the fossa ovalis.

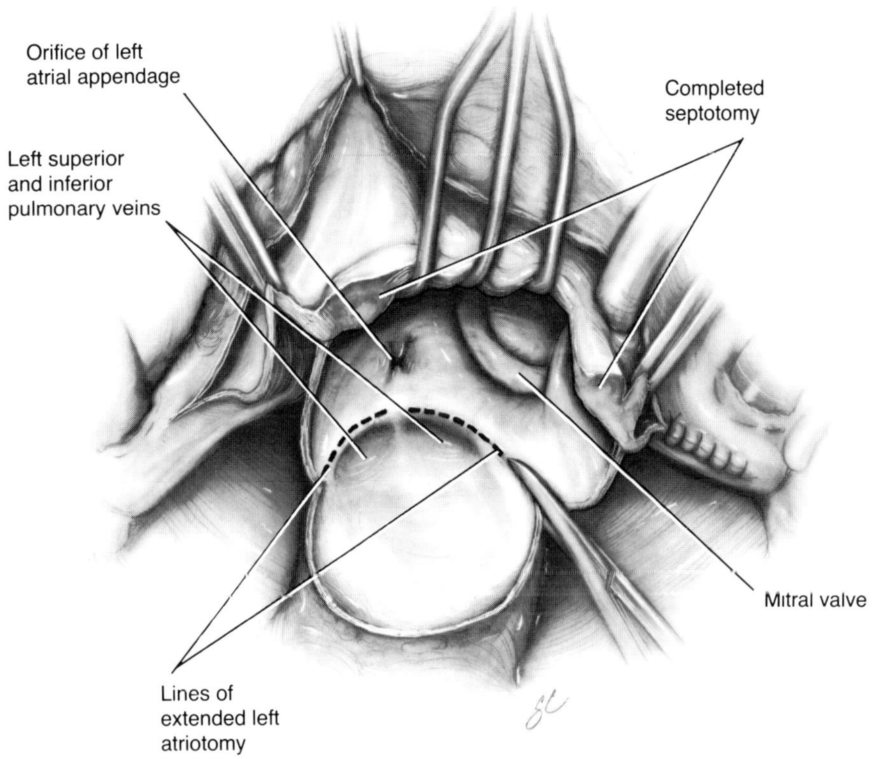

FIGURE 78–14. The atrial septum is retracted for optimal exposure of the left atrium, mitral valve, left pulmonary veins, and orifice of the left atrial appendage. The standard left atriotomy is extended *inferiorly* across the posterior left atrial free wall between the mitral valve and the orifices of the inferior pulmonary veins. Likewise, the *superior* portion of the standard left atriotomy is extended around the lip of the left superior pulmonary vein orifice. Before the two ends of this pulmonary vein isolation incision are joined, the left atrial appendage is excised.

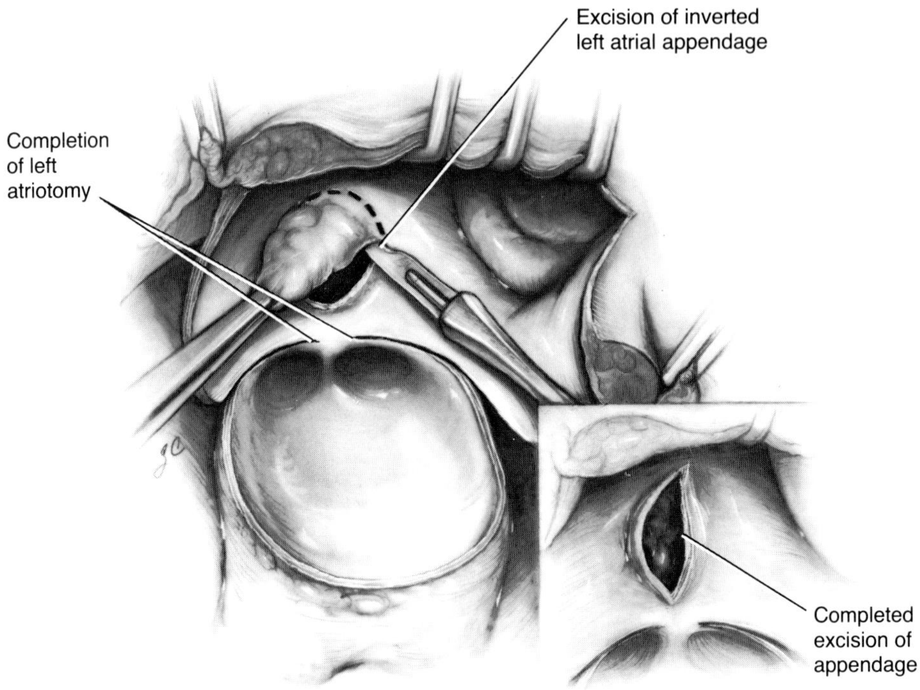

FIGURE 78–15. The left atrial appendage is inverted and amputated at its base. The base of the appendage to the right, as viewed by the surgeon in this orientation, must be approached with special care because the circumflex coronary artery may course very near to this portion of the incision. Once the appendage is excised, a small bridge of tissue remains between the appendage amputation site and the two ends of the pulmonary vein encircling incision (*inset*). This bridge of tissue can be divided and closed with sutures, or it can be left intact and cryoablated.

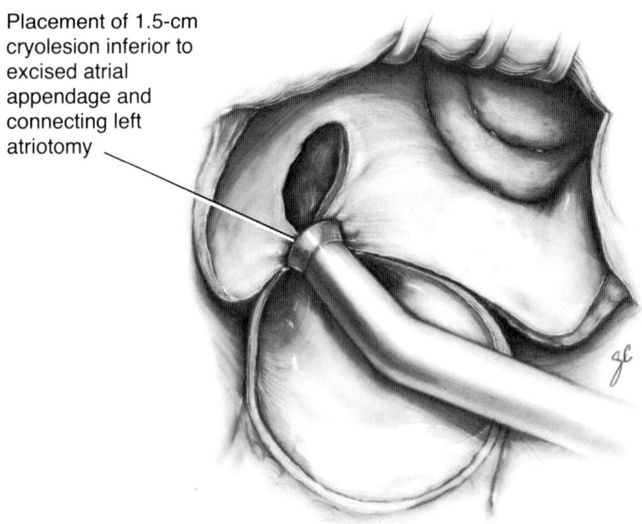

FIGURE 78–16. A 1.5-cm cryoprobe is applied to the bridge of tissue for 2 minutes at –60°C. The isolation incision of the pulmonary vein is much easier to close if this tissue bridge is left intact rather than surgically divided.

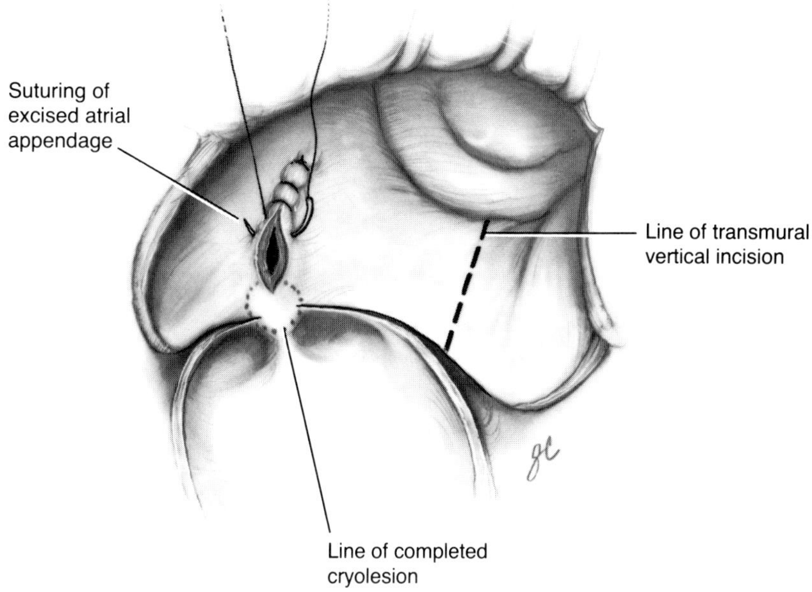

FIGURE 78–17. After the cryolesion is completed *(dotted circle)*, the site of the appendage amputation is closed. The dashed line represents the site of the final incision, a posterior vertical left atriotomy that extends from the pulmonary vein isolation incision to the mitral valve annulus.

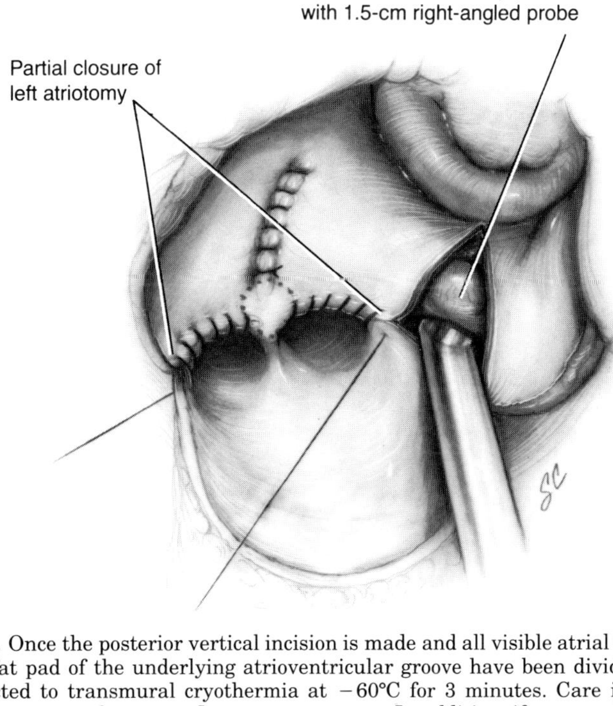

FIGURE 78–18. Once the posterior vertical incision is made and all visible atrial myocardial fibers spanning the fat pad of the underlying atrioventricular groove have been divided, the coronary sinus is subjected to transmural cryothermia at −60°C for 3 minutes. Care is taken to avoid applying cryosurgery to the circumflex coronary artery. In addition, if retrograde cardioplegia is used, the cannula should be removed during this portion of the procedure.

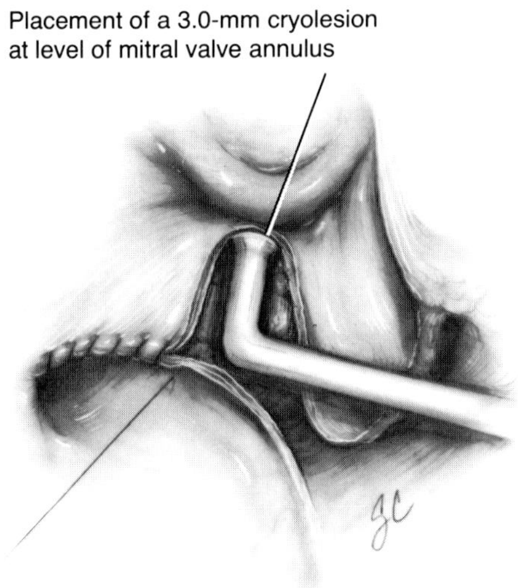

FIGURE 78–19. A 3-mm cryolesion is placed at the lower end of the incision adjacent to the mitral valve annulus.

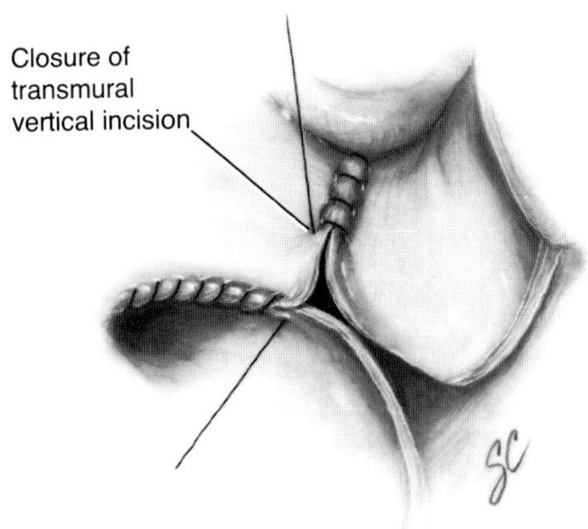

FIGURE 78–20. The posterior vertical left atriotomy is closed.

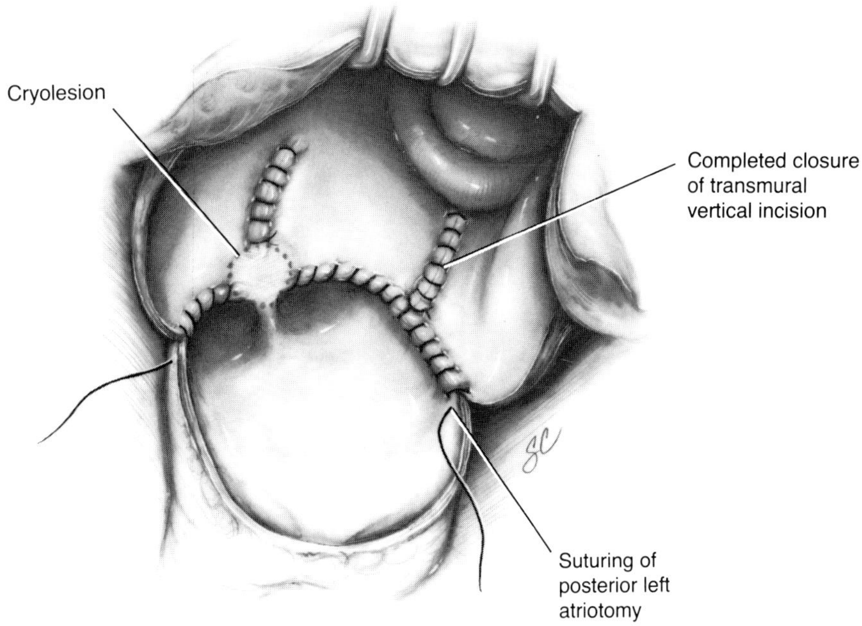

FIGURE 78–21. The lower portion of the pulmonary vein isolation incision is closed across the posteroinferior free wall of the left atrium.

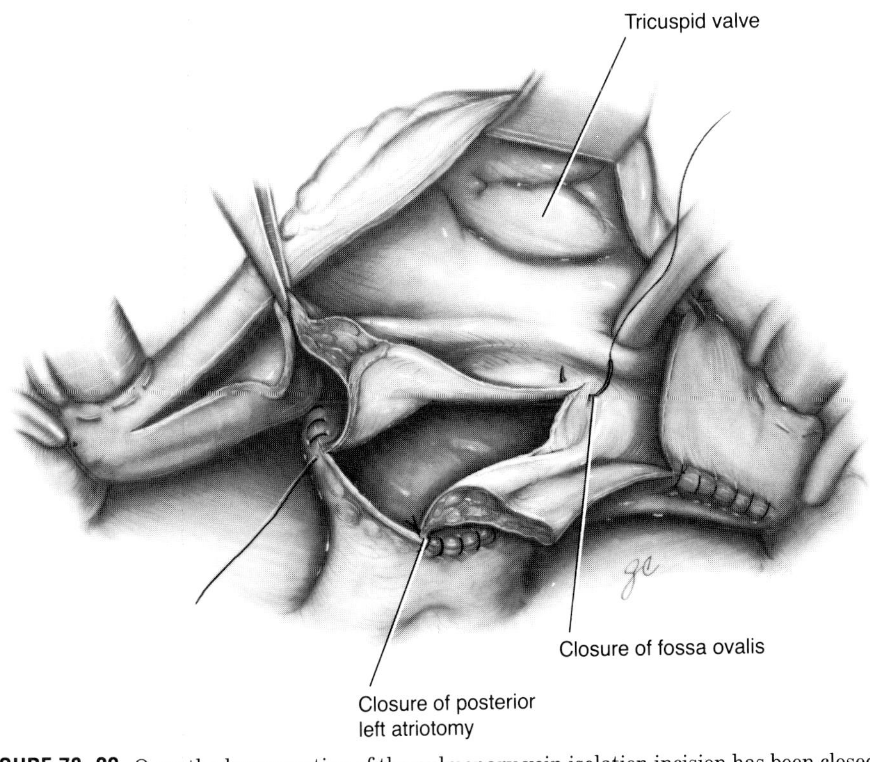

FIGURE 78–22. Once the lower portion of the pulmonary vein isolation incision has been closed to the level of the atrial septum, the incision again resembles a standard atriotomy in the interatrial groove. At this point, the septal incision is closed beginning at its lower end. A retrograde cardioplegia cannula is shown in the os of the coronary sinus.

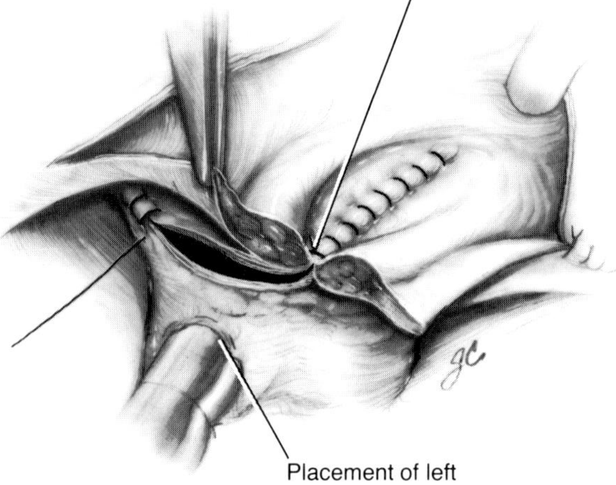

FIGURE 78–23. The thin portion of the fossa ovalis is closed up to the inferior margin of the anterior limbus.

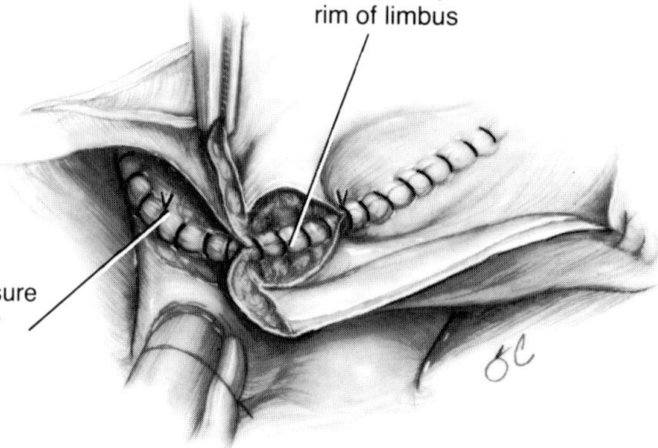

FIGURE 78–24. The left atrial side of the limbus of the fossa ovalis is closed in continuity with the remainder of the superior left atriotomy.

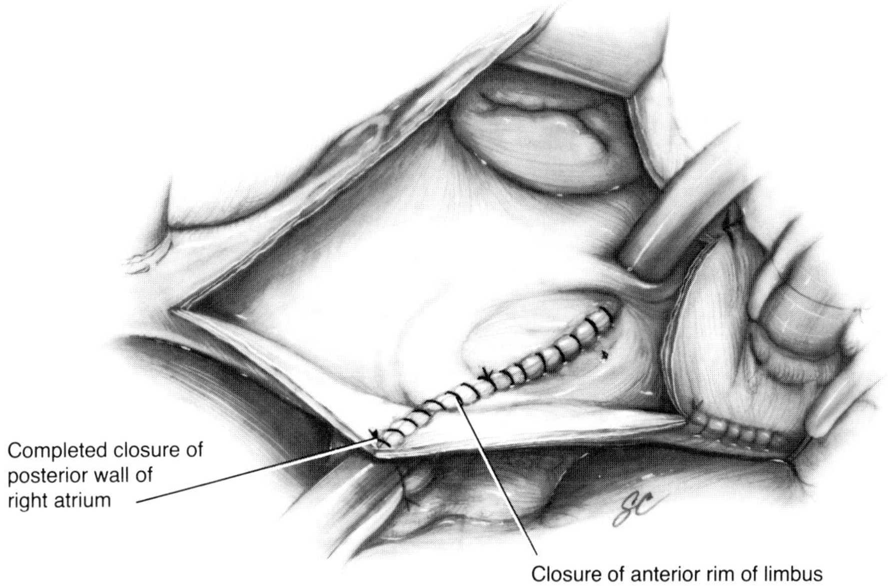

FIGURE 78–25. The right side of the limbus of the fossa ovalis is closed in continuity with the portion of the posterior right atrial free wall that is medial to the posterior longitudinal right atriotomy.

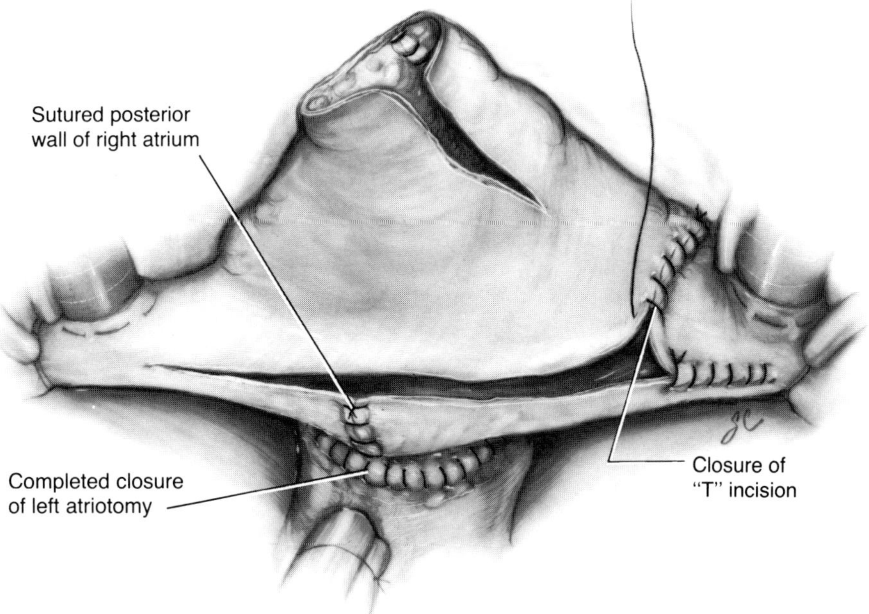

FIGURE 78–26. The remainder of the right atrial T incision is closed.

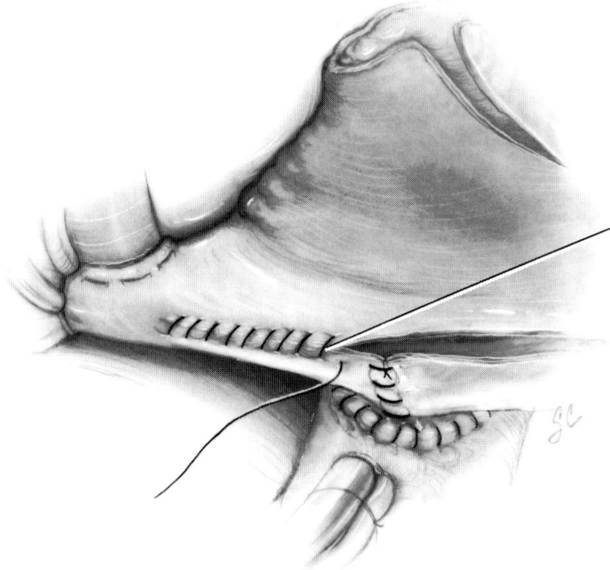

FIGURE 78–27. The remainder of the posterior longitudinal right atriotomy is closed.

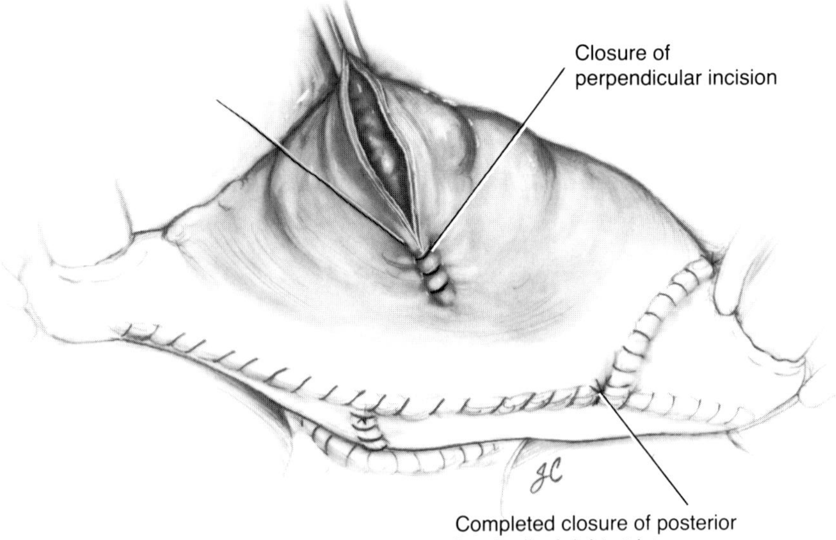

FIGURE 78–28. The lateral right atriotomy and the site of the amputated right atrial appendage are closed in continuity from a lateral to a medial direction.

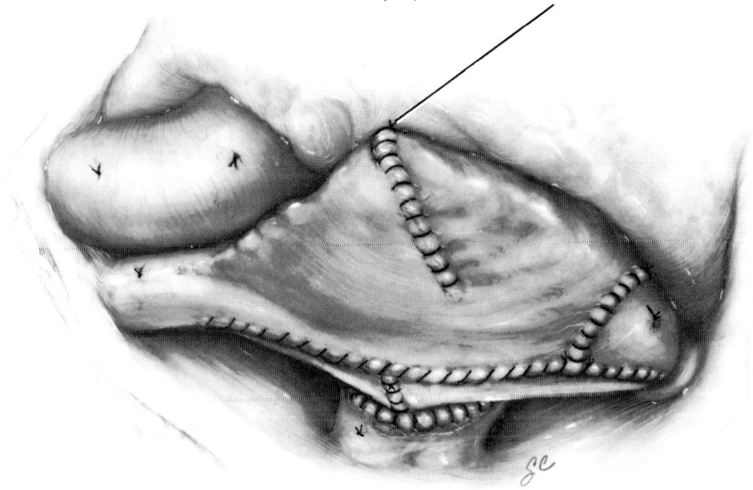

FIGURE 78–29. Appearance of the completed Maze III procedure.

SECTION XV

Myocardial Revascularization

ROBERT H. JONES, M.D.

79

Coronary Artery Bypass Grafts

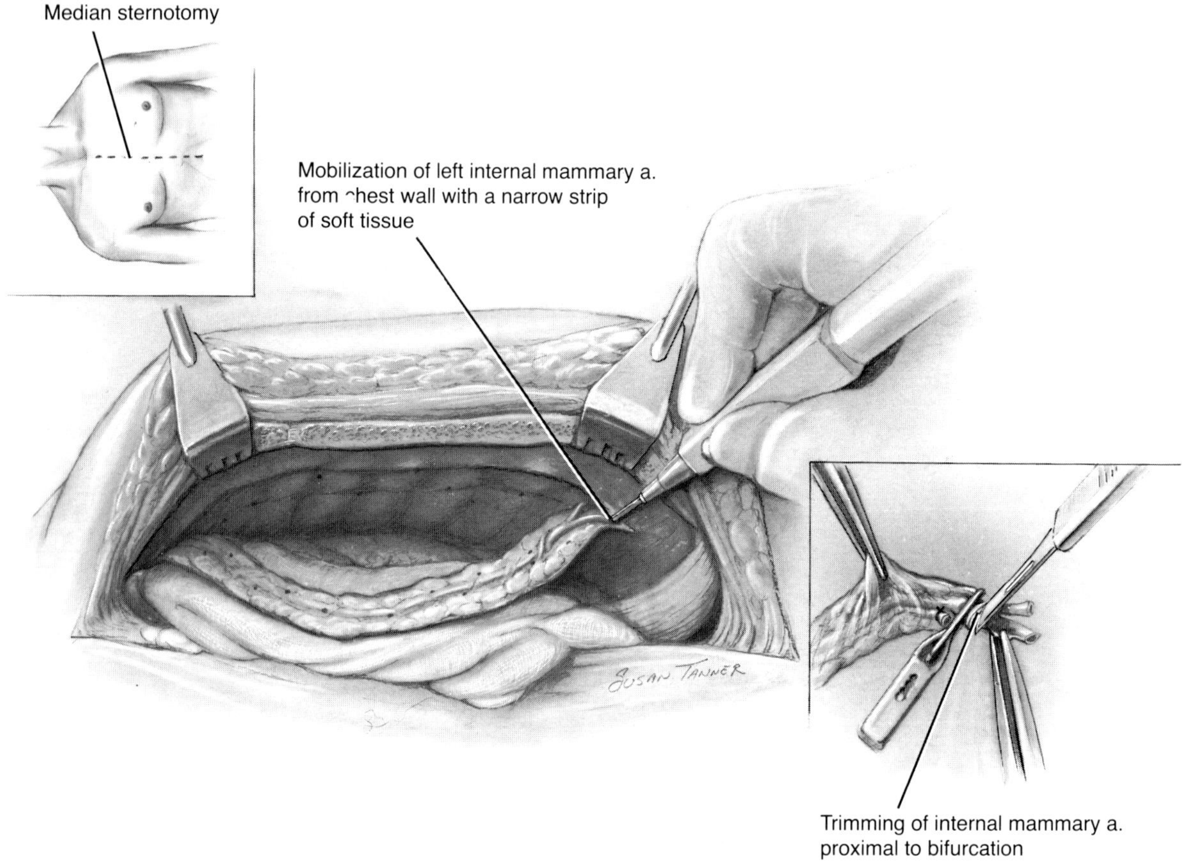

FIGURE 79–1 *See legend on opposite page*

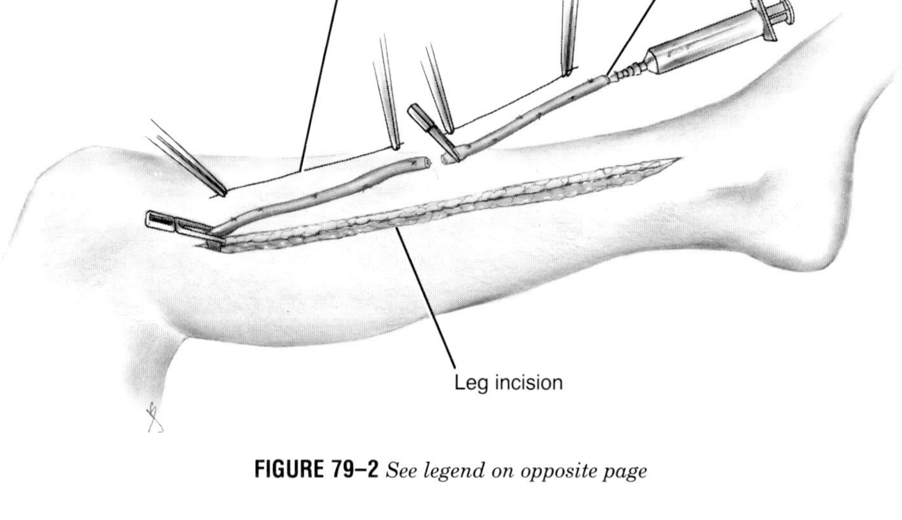

FIGURE 79–2 *See legend on opposite page*

FIGURE 79–1. Coronary bypass procedures are performed through a median sternotomy (*inset*). Simultaneously, harvest of the saphenous vein is undertaken if this conduit is to be used for grafting. Because of favorable long-term patency rates, at least one internal mammary artery is used in almost all bypass procedures. Emergency coronary bypass operations may require institution of cardiopulmonary bypass as a first step of the operation if the patient is hemodynamically unstable. In these situations, the internal mammary artery may be dissected while the patient is fully heparinized and on cardiopulmonary bypass support. However, in most situations, all material for grafting is harvested before heparinization.

The divided sternum is lifted by controlled retraction sufficient to provide exposure but not so excessive as to fracture the sternum or ribs. The pleura can be left intact and dissected from the medial chest wall before mammary harvest. Alternatively, the pleura can be widely opened near the point where it joins the chest wall and left as one surface of the mammary pedicle. The medial mammary vein is used to guide the incision forming the medial border of the pedicle, and dissection usually begins on the chest wall at the point the medial mammary vein is most visible. An electrocautery set at the lowest intensity that is adequate to divide tissue is used for both blunt and sharp dissection. Continuing dissection in the appropriate plane without injury to the intercostal muscle greatly decreases the amount of bleeding in the chest wall. Injury to the lung is prevented by decreasing tidal volume and by covering the lung with a gauze pad.

As dissection proceeds in both directions, arterial and venous branches connecting the internal mammary and intercostal vessels are identified, clipped, and divided by cautery on the chest wall side. Downward tension from gentle traction or the weight of the pedicle enhances exposure. Dissection progresses in both directions until an adequate length of the pedicle is developed to fully expose a 2-cm length of the lateral internal mammary artery vein. An incision through the soft tissue lateral to this vein completes formation of the second border of the pedicle. Dissection continues cephalad until the pedicle loses its upward course along the chest wall and lies flat against the upper mediastinal structures. Dissection continues caudad until adequate length is obtained for the intended graft or the arterial diameter appears too small for use in grafting. The most common point to end dissection inferiorly is at the bifurcation of the internal mammary artery. Heparin must be administered systematically before the internal mammary artery is occluded. Delaying division of the artery until completion of the entire dissection enhances hemostasis of the chest wall.

Occasionally, both branches of the internal mammary artery can be used for grafting separate coronary arteries, but more commonly the internal mammary artery is sharply divided at a site proximal to the bifurcation (*inset*). To prepare the internal mammary artery for grafting, the artery is dissected from the pedicle tissues for 1 cm, and the pedicle is first transected. Thereafter, the artery is sharply divided 1 cm longer than the pedicle and opened longitudinally for a length greater than the intended coronary arteriotomy.

FIGURE 79–2. The greater saphenous vein in the lower leg is most commonly used for coronary artery bypass grafting. The greater saphenous vein from the thigh or lesser saphenous vein from the posterior calf also provides a suitable conduit. The extent of incision of the leg should not exceed the anticipated length of vein needed. An early conservative estimate of length needed may be made after cardiopulmonary bypass is instituted and the final sites of graft insertion are identified. An accurate estimate of the length of each graft is obtained by placing an epicardial suture at each coronary site and leading these sutures through the anticipated course of the vein graft to the aortic site selected for the proximal anastomosis. The vein is gently distended with fluid to ensure that all tributaries are individually ligated. Preparing segments of vein to correspond accurately to the length of each suture permits harvest of the vein needed with only a slight excess to permit trimming to avoid branches or sites of valves within the vein.

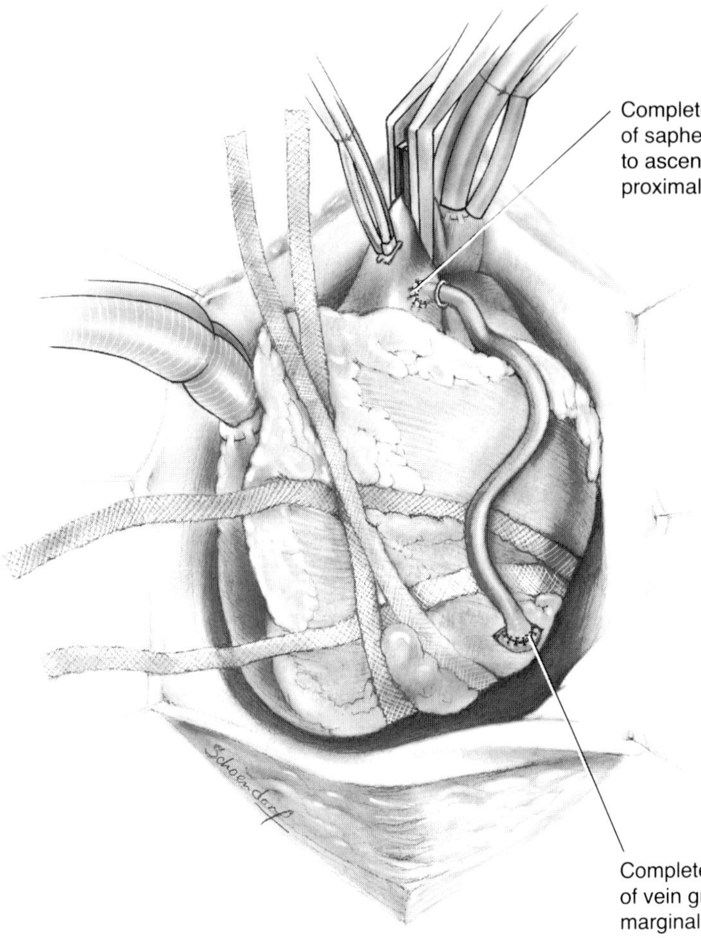

FIGURE 79–3. The sequence of anastomosis of vein grafts between the aorta and coronary arteries can be ordered to construct first all the proximal or all the distal anastomoses. Use of partial aortic occlusion permits coronary blood flow during completion of the proximal anastomoses, and total aortic occlusion with hypothermic cardioplegic arrest facilitates completion of the distal anastomoses. Advantages of completing the proximal anastomoses first are that the aortic root infusion of cardioplegia facilitates removal of air from grafts before the distal anastomoses are completed and that each completed vein graft becomes an additional conduit for cardioplegia to myocardium fed by stenotic or occluded coronary arteries. The advantage of completing the distal anastomoses first is that the vein itself can be positioned to assess graft length, thereby avoiding the step of using a suture for this purpose.

Two doubled strips of gauze passed through the transverse sinus and around the inferior vena cava aid exposure for the distal coronary anastomoses. The optimal exposure is first obtained manually, and the free ends of the strips are used to maintain the gentle traction that supports the heart in the desired position optimal for individual coronary arteries. The typical exposure necessary to construct an anastomosis to a marginal branch of the circumflex coronary artery is best obtained by weaving the four strips into a V configuration adjacent to the planned site for anastomosis.

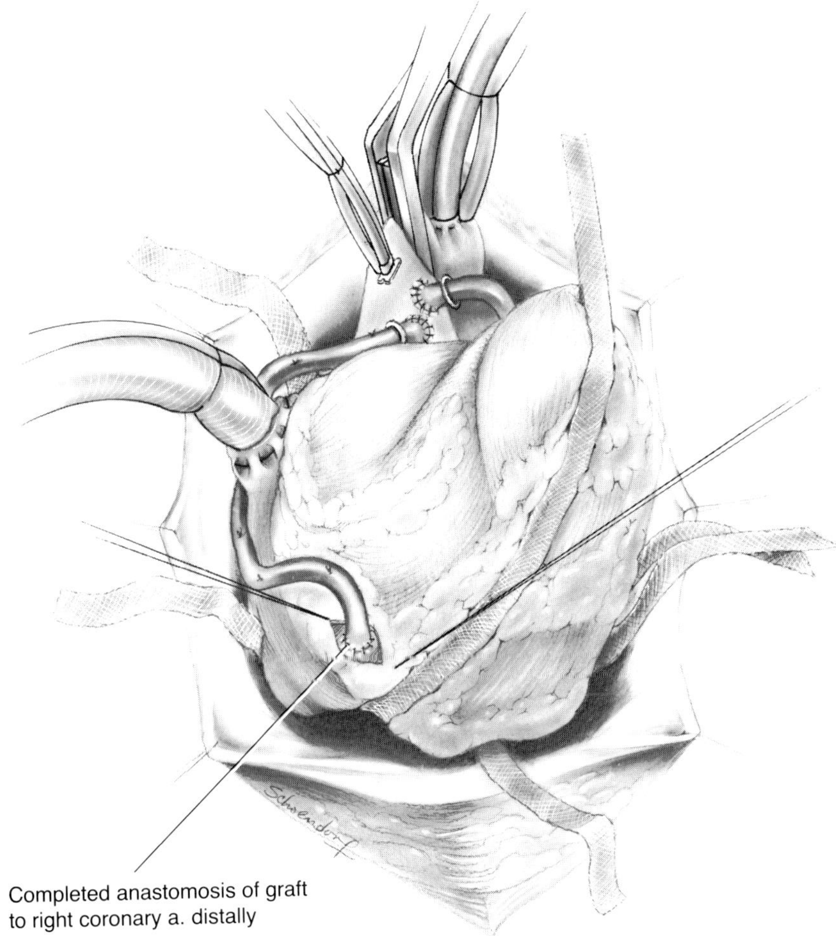

FIGURE 79–4. One or two strips oriented in the direction of the posterior septum may aid exposure for construction of the distal anastomosis to the right coronary artery. Several epicardial sutures are usually needed to optimize exposure of the site selected for graft insertion.

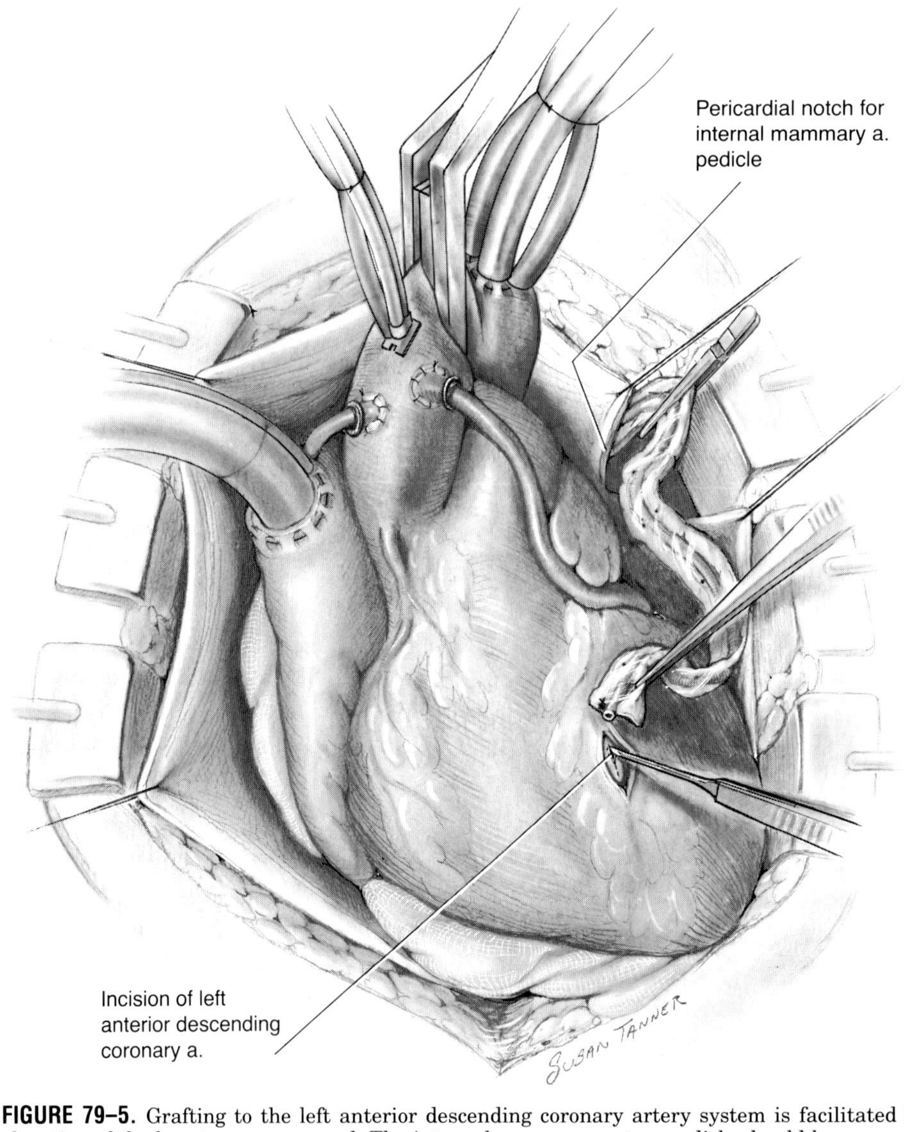

FIGURE 79–5. Grafting to the left anterior descending coronary artery system is facilitated by elevation of the heart on a gauze pad. The internal mammary artery pedicle should be prepared with adequate length to avoid tension from lung inflation when cardiopulmonary bypass is concluded.

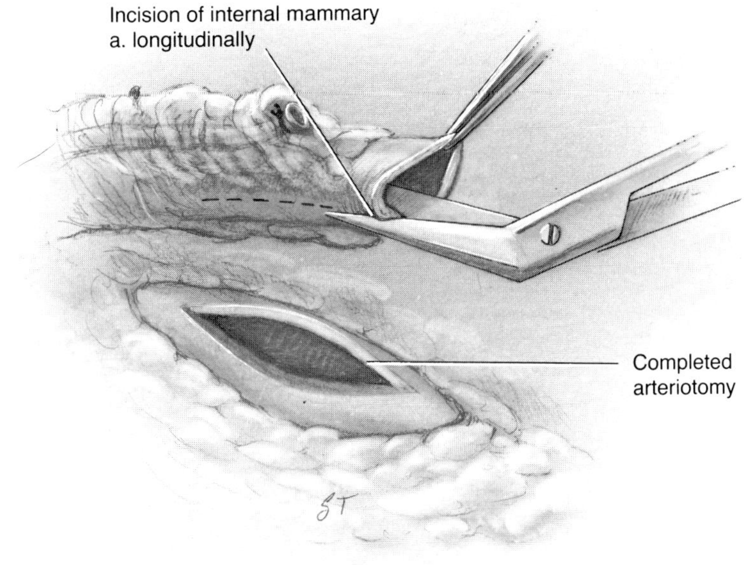

FIGURE 79–6. The technique of anastomosis between the left internal mammary artery and left anterior descending coronary artery illustrates the general principles used to construct all proximal and distal anastomoses. The graft is opened longitudinally to match or exceed the length of the coronary arteriotomy. This opening prevents kinking at the site of the anastomoses of the internal mammary artery and aorta to the saphenous vein. This opening is not necessary at the distal vein anastomotic site, but a slight bevel cut of the distal vein helps prevent kinking of the saphenous vein to the coronary artery anastomoses.

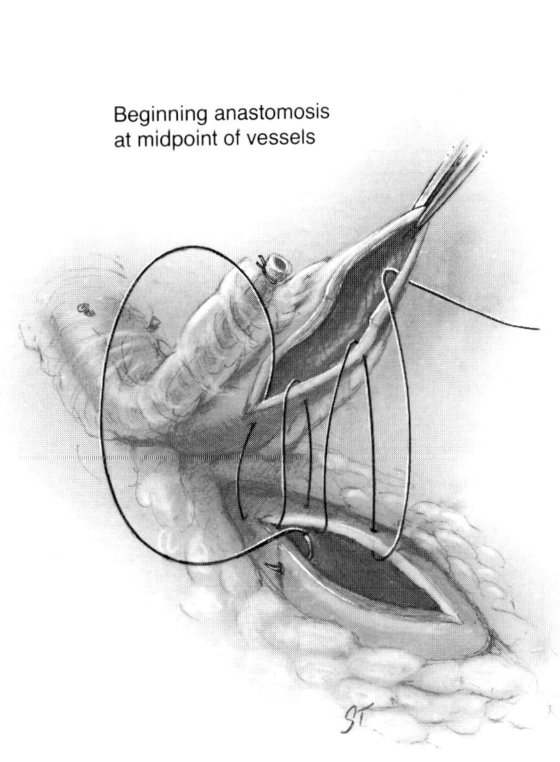

FIGURE 79–7. The anastomosis begins midway along the side of the graft so that the final knot will not be at the most distal or proximal portion of the anastomosis, thereby decreasing the chances of technical error that would impede graft flow. The polypropylene suture permits a portion of the anastomosis to be completed before the two vessels are joined.

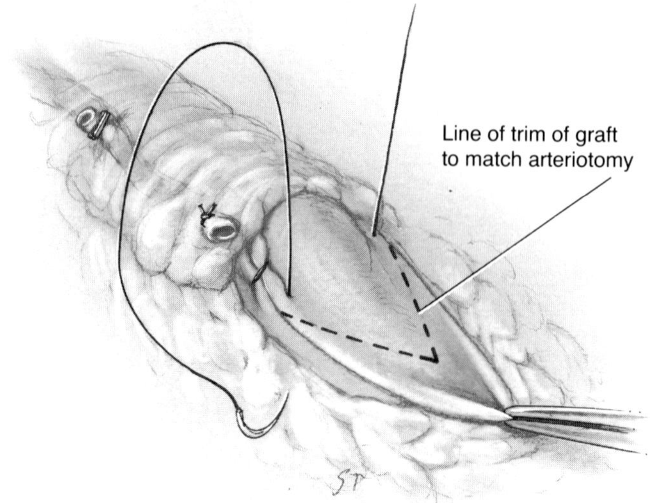

FIGURE 79–8. After gentle tension on both ends of the suture approximates one half of the vessel, the remaining vessel can be accurately cut to the appropriate size if the original longitudinal opening has been excessive.

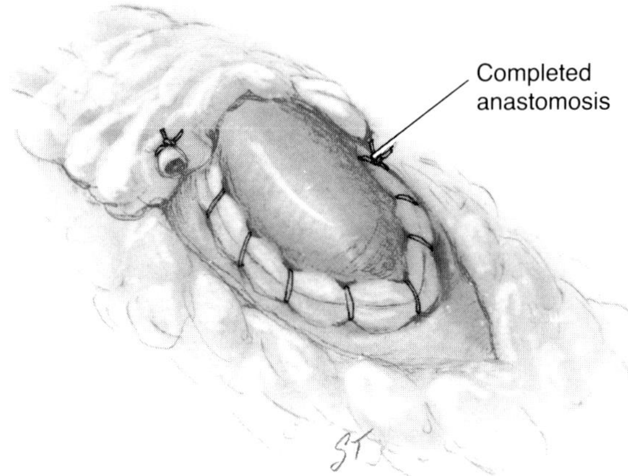

FIGURE 79–9. The integrity of the completed anastomosis can be confirmed by release of internal mammary artery occlusion or aortic instillation of cardioplegic solution for saphenous vein grafts.

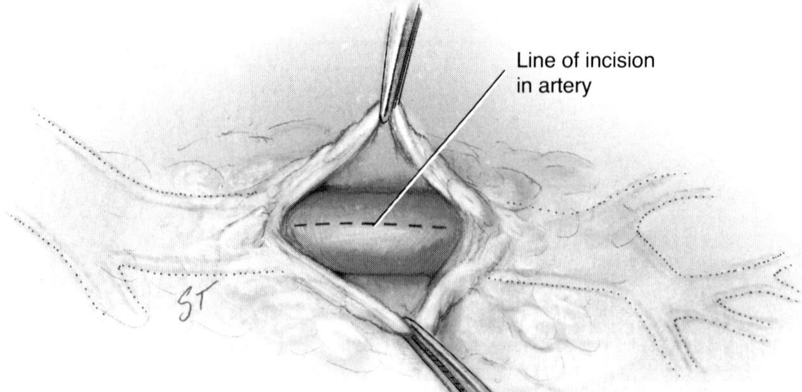

FIGURE 79–10. Coronary endarterectomy may be required before graft insertion in some circumstances. The site of incision in the artery should be proximal to any major bifurcation requiring distal perfusion.

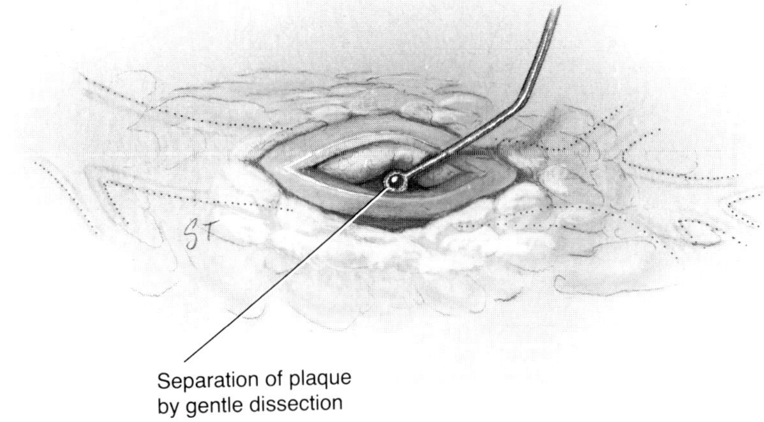

FIGURE 79–11. After the initial arteriotomy, the plaque is separated from the edges of the arteriotomy and is encircled circumferentially.

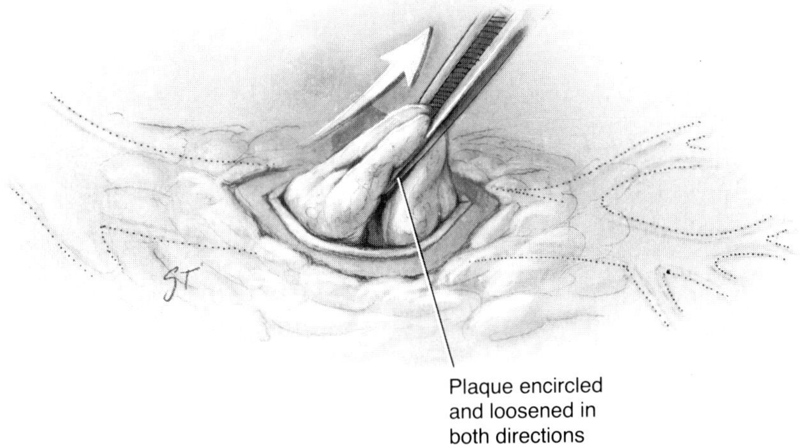

FIGURE 79–12. Intraluminal dissection to gently loosen the plaque in both directions without perforation of the vessel wall is aided by a flexible probe with a bulb tip and wire loops. The proximal plaque is extracted first and may be sharply transected if the plaque involves proximal branches.

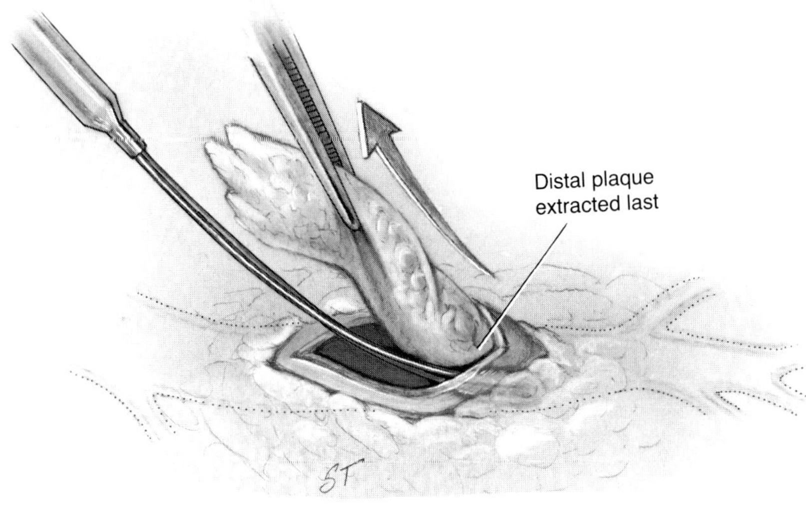

FIGURE 79–13. The distal plaque is extracted by gentle manual traction on the plaque balanced against the sweeping movements of an intraluminal endarterectomy instrument.

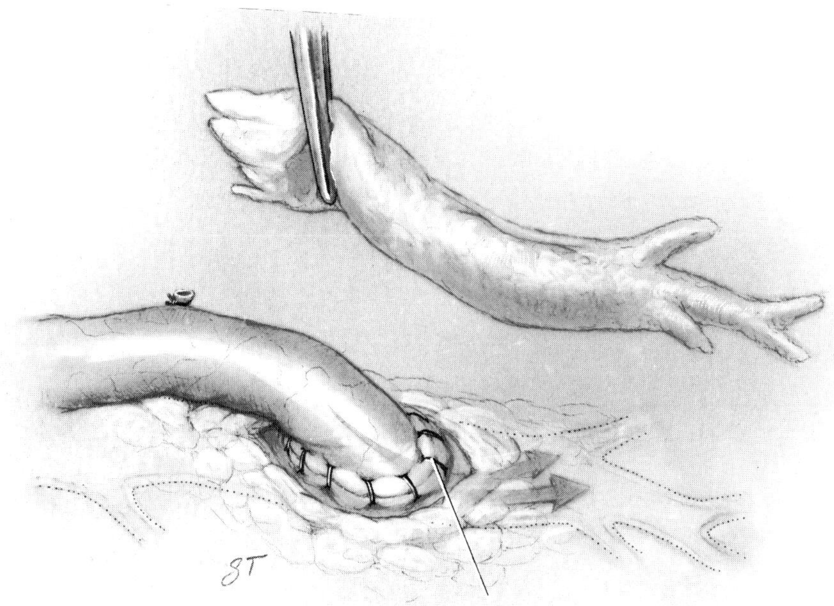

FIGURE 79-14. As vessel bifurcations are encountered, the plaque should be extracted sequentially from each branch to avoid fracturing the plaque. Aortic instillation of cardioplegic solution after the endarterectomy is completed helps cleanse the coronary artery of any fragments of debris left from the endarterectomy.

PETER K. SMITH, M.D.

80

Reoperation for Coronary Artery Bypass Grafting

Reoperation for coronary artery disease exposes the patient to several risks not present during initial revascularization. The primary additional risks are

1. accidental injury to substernal structures (innominate vein, aorta, right ventricle)
2. accidental injury to patent bypass grafts, particularly *in situ* internal mammary artery grafts
3. embolization of atheromatous material from diseased grafts during cardiac dissection
4. less than optimal myocardial preservation
5. incomplete revascularization

Some of these risks can be modified by altering the conduct of the operation, although the wide variety of techniques employed in performing reoperative coronary procedures emphasizes the inability to eliminate these risks completely.

The patient is evaluated for reoperative coronary surgery in the standard manner, with particular attention to the details of the prior operation(s), the status of available conduit for revascularization, and study of the posteroanterior and lateral chest films to assess the degree of obliteration of the retrosternal space. Patients with patent retrosternal bypass grafts, particularly internal mammary grafts, and those with pulmonary hypertension are at increased risk for cardiac injury during median sternotomy. For these patients, consideration may be given to alternative approaches via either right or left thoracotomy or to exposure and even cannulation of the femoral vessels before the repeat sternotomy.

The patient is prepared for operation in the usual manner, invasively monitored, and anesthetized. A defibrillating electrode patch is positioned on the posterior chest to the left of the midline and connected to a cardioverter/defibrillator. Because defibrillation may be required with varying levels of cardiac exposure, the other defibrillator electrode is attached sequentially to a sterile external paddle and a sterile internal paddle, followed by two internal paddles as the operation proceeds.

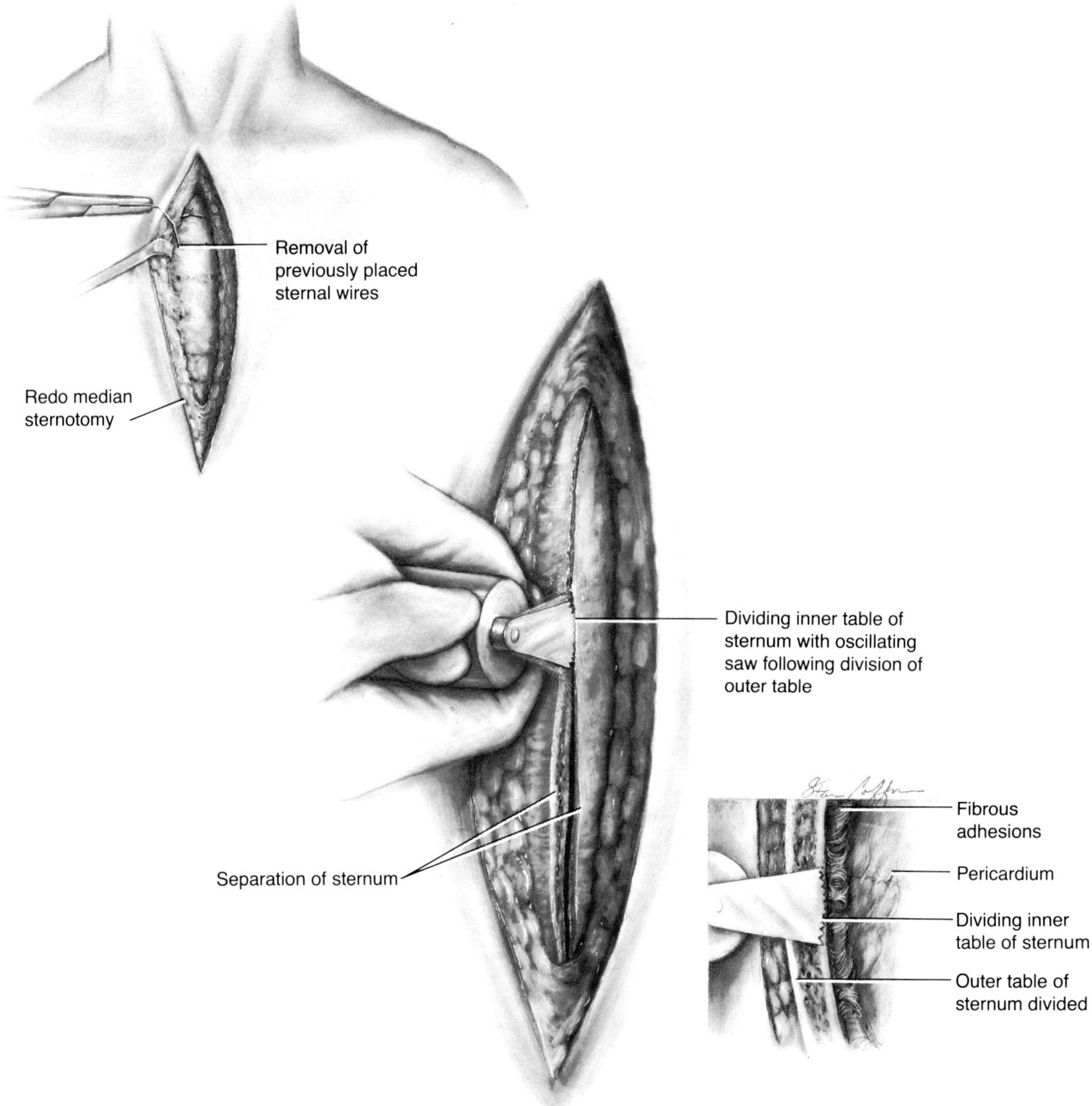

FIGURE 80–1. After removal of the sternal wires, the sternal midline is scored with electrocautery. The patient should be fully heparinized to facilitate emergency cannulation. Shed blood is either returned to the cardiotomy reservoir or salvaged, washed, and reinfused. An oscillating saw is then used to divide the outer table of the sternum, followed by division of the inner table. Areas of potential entry into vascular structures or the heart are dissected last. The saw is used both to divide the sternum and to detect the presence of undivided areas with the saw stopped. Heavy scissors are used to divide fibrous adhesions, particularly in the suprasternal area.

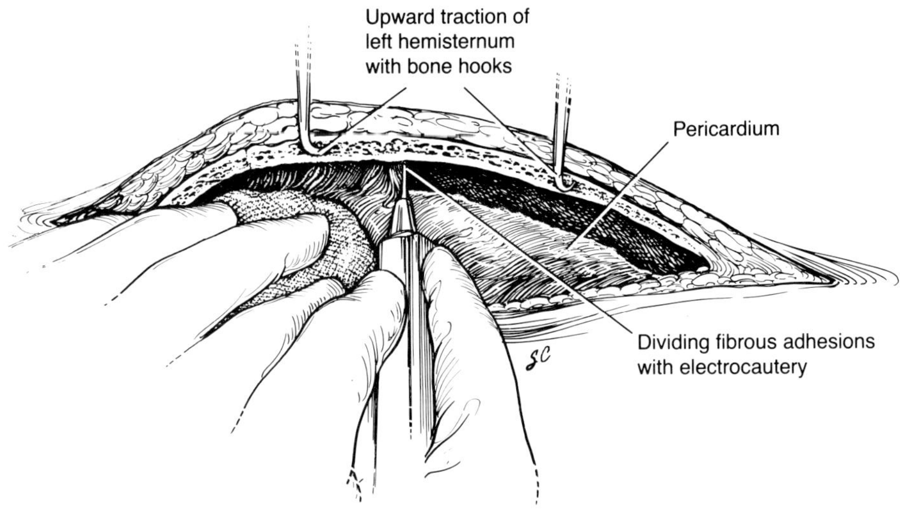

FIGURE 80–2. A bone hook or sharp rake is placed in the body of each hemisternum, and gentle upward traction is applied. The operating table is rotated to the left, and the left hemisternum is dissected sharply from underlying structures. Dissection is accomplished using electrocautery, scissors, or scalpel, according to individual preference, the character of the adhesions, and the relative danger of the dissection. The avoidance of undue traction and blunt dissection is critical to this dissection, as is the concept of dissecting the sternum from the underlying structures. Dissection usually is begun inferiorly on the left side and continued throughout the length of the hemisternum. The dissection is performed laterally, and usually an area free of adhesions rapidly appears. The right hemisternum is then dissected completely in the same manner. This usually is much less difficult than the left-sided dissection.

The sternal retractor is then inserted and opened to permit intrapericardial dissection. Intramediastinal structures should be palpated during sternal retraction, because injury to tethered structures can occur, and unrecognized nontransmural injuries can become transmural as tension is applied.

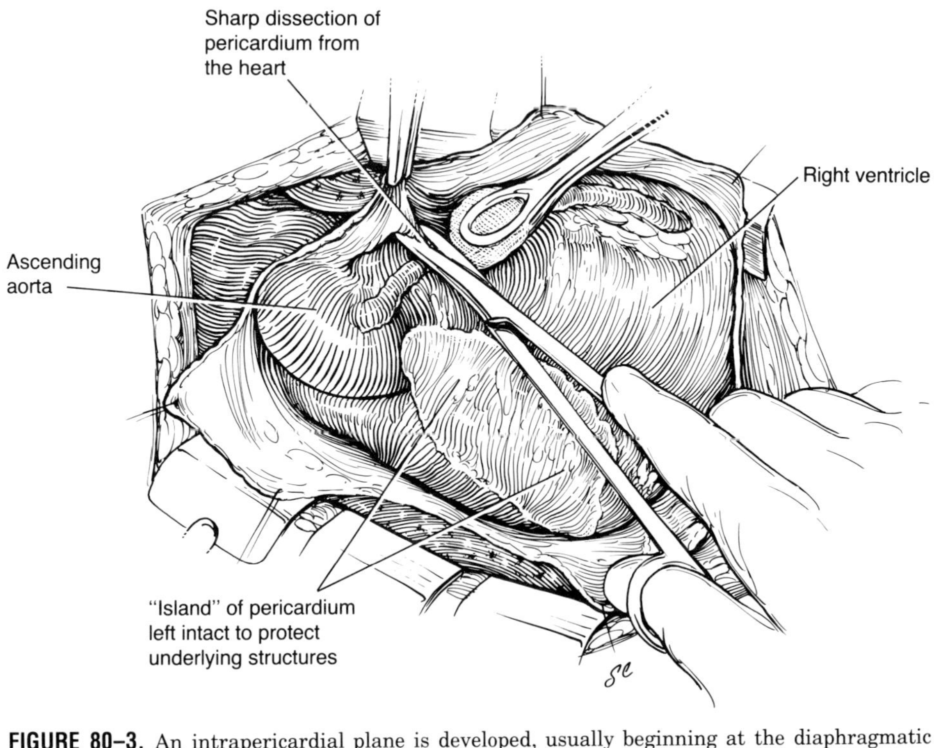

FIGURE 80–3. An intrapericardial plane is developed, usually beginning at the diaphragmatic pericardium. Sharp dissection is again important, as is the concept of dissecting the pericardium from the heart. Attention is focused on exposing the right atrium and aorta to permit early cannulation. Dense adhesions in the area of the right atrium caused by prior cannulation or the presence of a patent right graft usually are bypassed by entering the pleural space and reentering the pericardium to create "islands" that are not directly dissected.

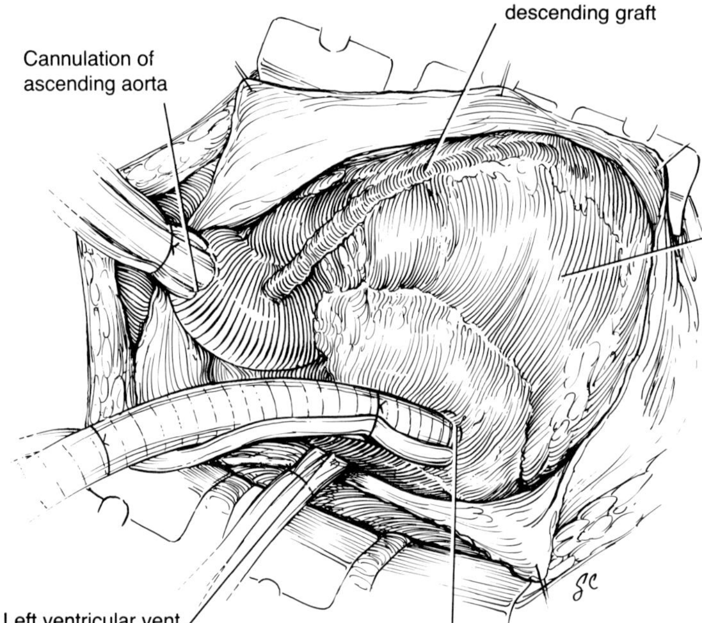

FIGURE 80–4. Once satisfactory exposure has been obtained, usually cannulation is achieved and the patient is placed on cardiopulmonary bypass to facilitate the remainder of the dissection. A single double-stage venous return cannula usually is employed, as is ascending aortic cannulation. If aortic dissection is particularly difficult, or difficulties are anticipated in aortic crossclamping or in placing the grafts, femoral arterial cannulation is performed. The remainder of the dissection is then performed on cardiopulmonary bypass and is facilitated by left ventricular decompression.

After adequate exposure has been established, the remainder of the operation is done with similar techniques and with the goals of primary revascularization. Particular attention must be given to myocardial preservation, which may require profound systemic hypothermia, early ligation of atherosclerotic grafts to prevent embolization, the employment of *retrograde* as well as *antegrade* cardioplegia, and control of a functioning mammary artery graft. Old grafts with significant obstructions and grafts with significant potential for distal embolization despite the lack of physiologic obstruction usually are replaced. New proximal aortic anastomoses may be accomplished more easily under a single cardioplegic arrest, rather than attempting partial aortic occlusion in the presence of multiple prior grafts.

Upon completion of cardiac reoperation, temporary atrial and ventricular pacing wires are routinely positioned. Frequently, atrial pacing wires may have poor thresholds owing to prior adhesions and epicardial scarring. Similarly, ventricular pacing wires must be placed deep within the myocardium to ensure functionality. Hemostasis often is a problem in reoperative coronary operations, and every attempt must be made to achieve excellent surgical hemostasis before closure. Coagulopathy usually is treated with blood component therapy, and local hemostasis may be improved with the use of topical fibrin glue. Sternal closure usually is accomplished with interrupted sternal wires, although a parasternal weave may be employed here more commonly than in primary revascularization.

DAVID C. SABISTON, JR., M.D.

81

Correction of Anomalous Left Coronary Artery Arising from the Pulmonary Artery

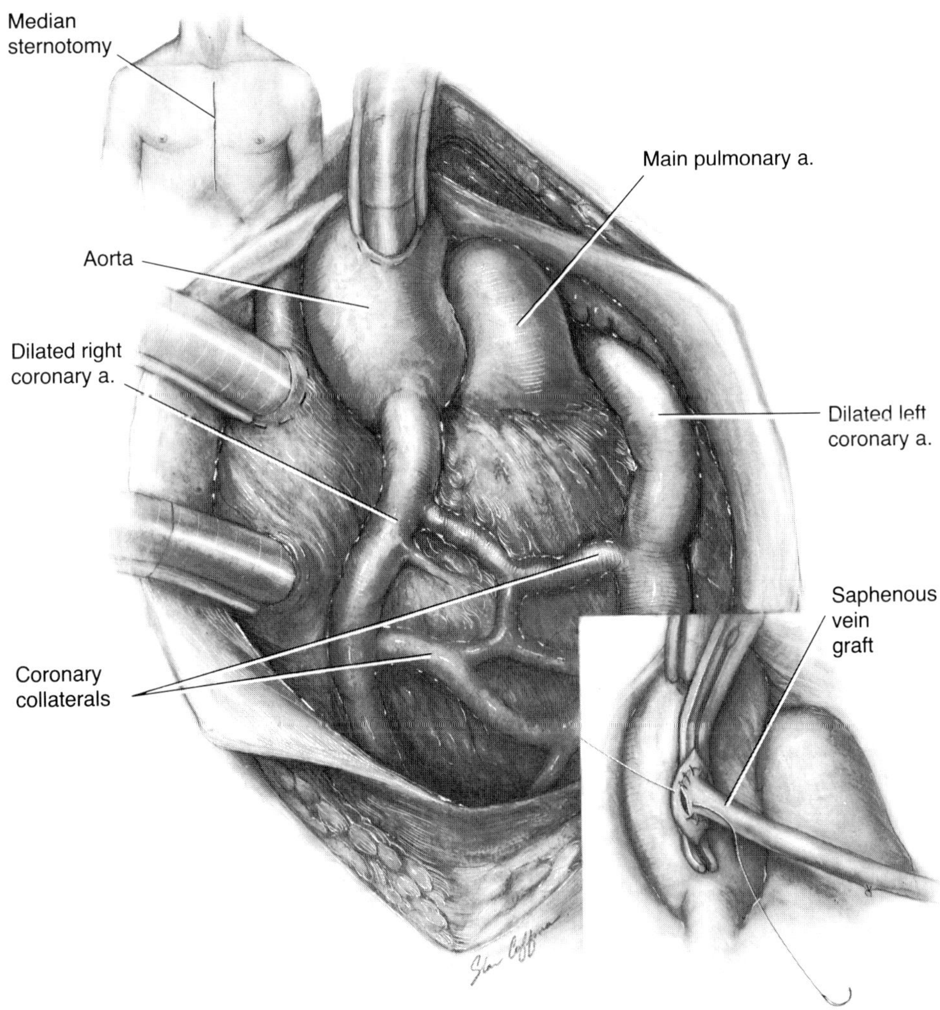

FIGURE 81–1. A median sternotomy is made, and the pericardium is entered. Cardiopulmonary bypass is initiated using separate cannulae in the right atrium, the superior vena cava, and the inferior vena cava, with cannulation of the aorta for arterial inflow. *Inset,* A saphenous vein graft is anastomosed end-to-side to the ascending aorta. The body temperature is lowered, and the ascending aorta is occluded with induction of potassium cardioplegia and topical hypothermia.

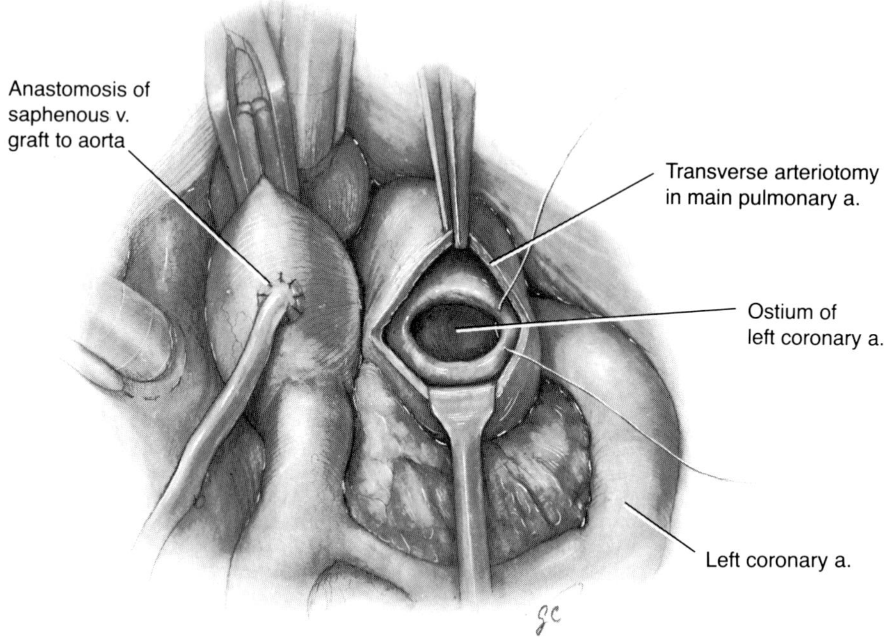

FIGURE 81–2. The main pulmonary artery is opened, with identification of the orifice of the left coronary artery, which usually arises in the posterior cusp of the pulmonary valve.

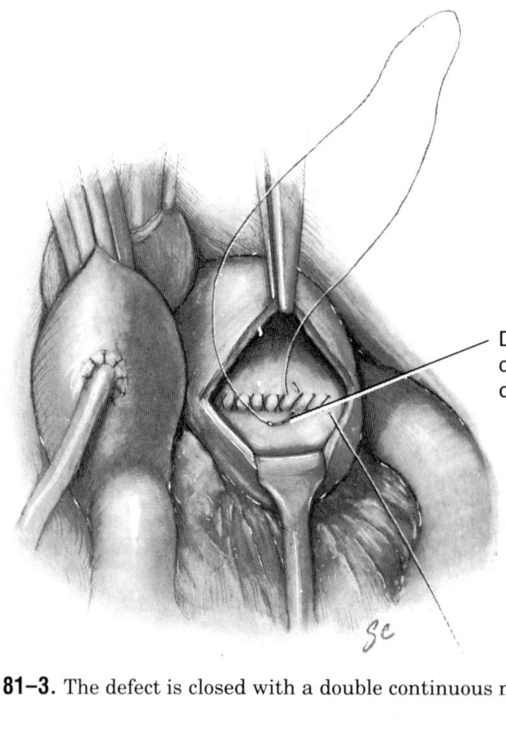

FIGURE 81–3. The defect is closed with a double continuous monofilament suture.

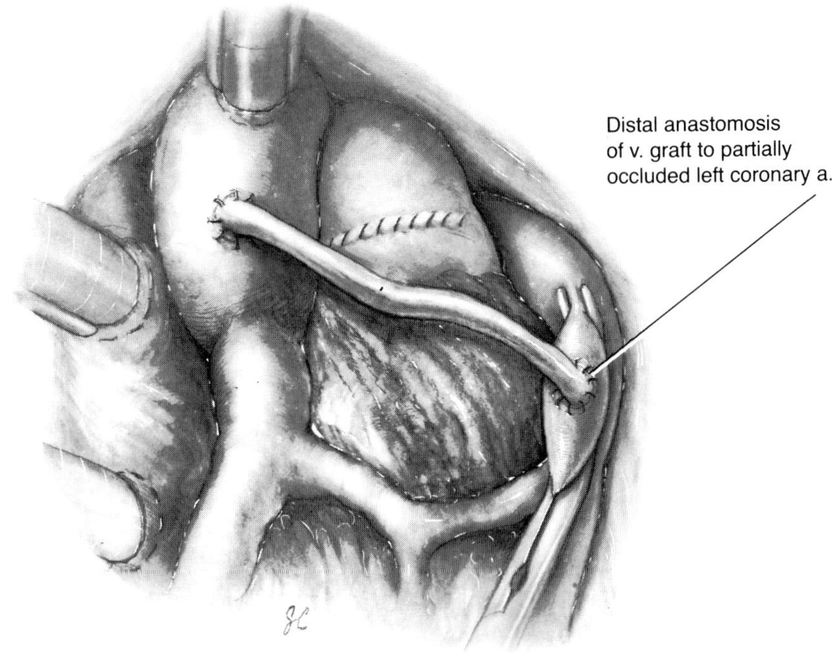

FIGURE 81–4. The pulmonary arteriotomy is closed with a continuous monofilament suture. The distal end of the graft is then sutured either to the left main coronary artery or to the anterior descending coronary artery, end-to-side. In the case shown, the left anterior descending coronary artery measured 23 mm in diameter, and it was possible to use a partial occlusion clamp. The body temperature is raised, and the patient is separated from cardiopulmonary bypass. The incision is then closed.

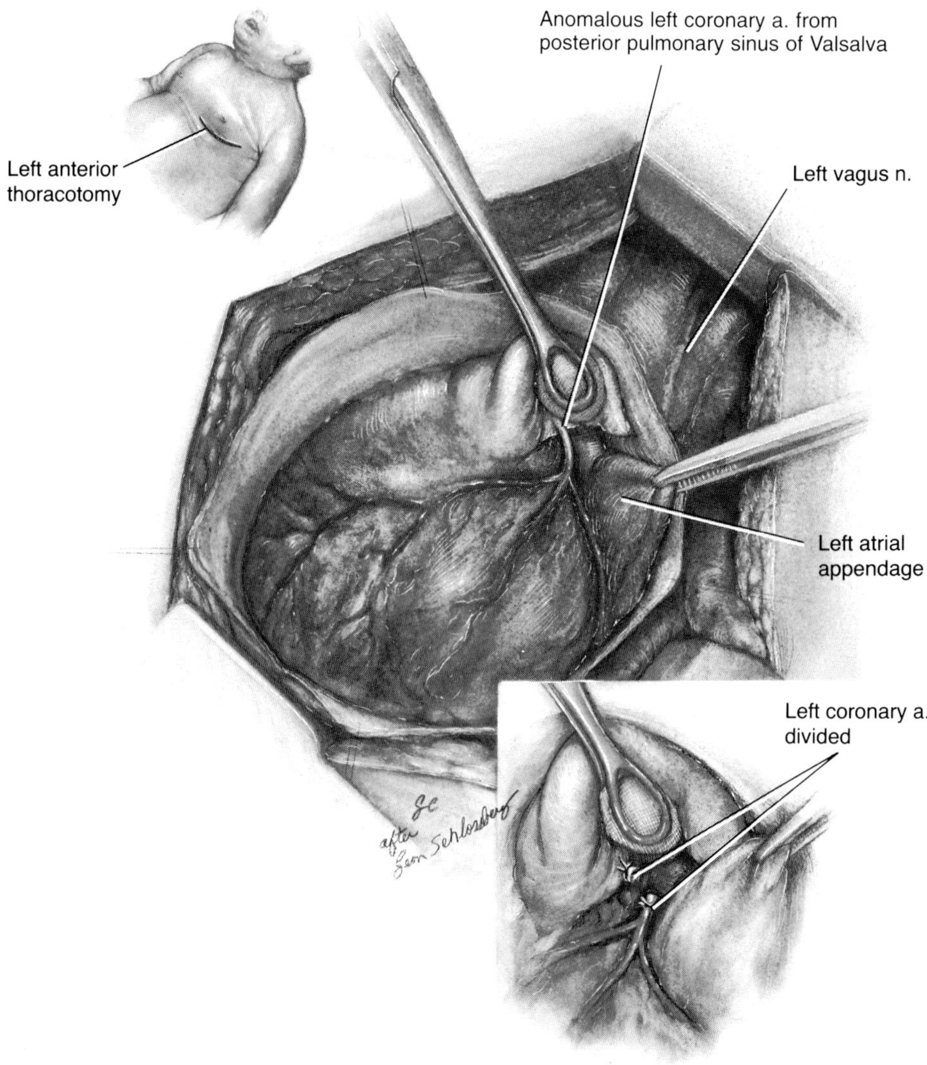

FIGURE 81–5. In infancy (usually within the first several weeks of life), the left coronary artery may be too small for performance of a direct procedure, and ligation of the vessel may be appropriate. A left anterior thoracotomy is performed in the third intercostal space, and the left coronary artery is identified and dissected. It is doubly ligated and divided. The incision is then closed. (Redrawn from Sabiston DC Jr: Surgical management of congenital lesions of the coronary circulation. Ann Surg 157:908–924, 1963.)

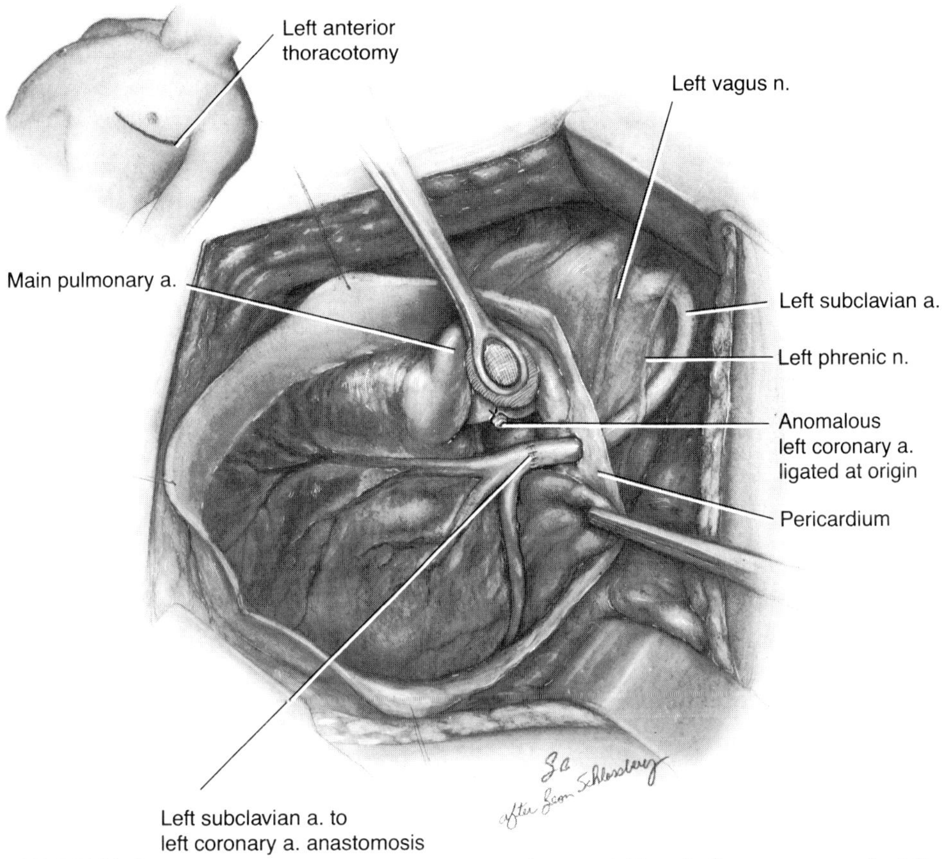

FIGURE 81–6. An alternative operation in infants and young children is direct anastomosis of the subclavian artery to the distal left coronary artery. A left anterior thoracotomy is made, and the chest is entered through the third intercostal space. The subclavian artery is exposed in the upper mediastinum and dissected. The branches are ligated and divided as far distally as possible, and the artery is then drawn inferiorly and brought through a pericardial defect. The left coronary artery is ligated and divided at its origin, and a direct anastomosis is made between the end of the left subclavian artery and the distal end of the left coronary artery. (Redrawn from Lowe JE, Sabiston DC Jr: Congenital coronary malformations. *In* Conn L [ed]: Modern Technics in Surgery, Cardiac-Thoracic Surgery. Mt. Kisco, NY, Futura Publishing, 1981.)

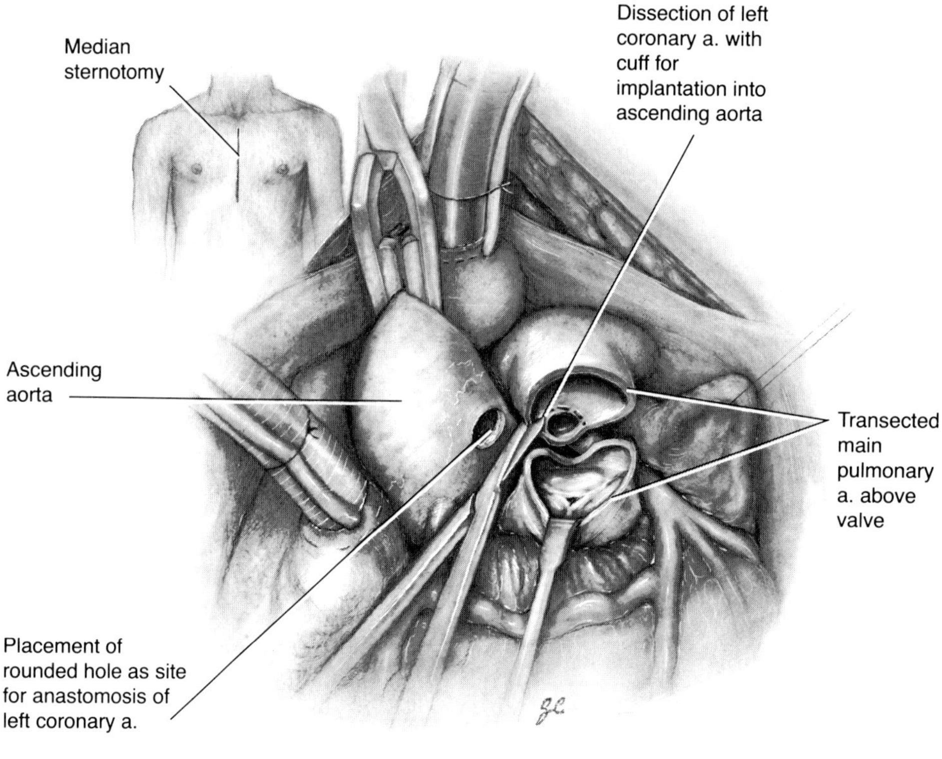

FIGURE 81–7. Using cardiopulmonary bypass with venous cannulation of the right atrium and arterial cannulation of the ascending aorta, the body temperature is lowered. The ascending aorta is occluded, and potassium cardioplegia is introduced. The pulmonary artery is divided, and the orifice of the left coronary artery arising anomalously in the posterior cusp is identified. A ring of pulmonary wall around the origin of the left coronary artery is excised.

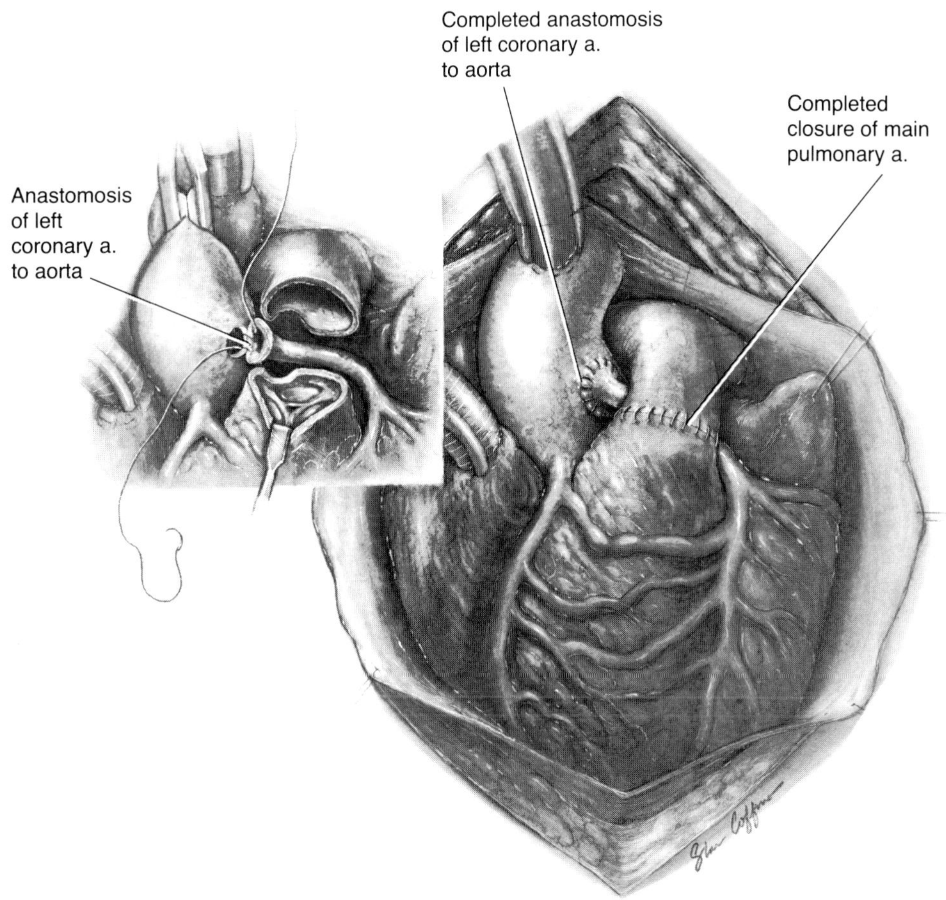

FIGURE 81–8. An incision is made in the ascending aorta, and the left coronary artery is joined to the aorta with a continuous monofilament suture. The pulmonary artery is then rejoined end-to-end with a continuous monofilament suture. The patient's body temperature is rewarmed, with separation from cardiopulmonary bypass.

SECTION XVI

Cardiac Neoplasms

DAVID C. SABISTON, JR., M.D.

82
Excision of Left Atrial Myxoma

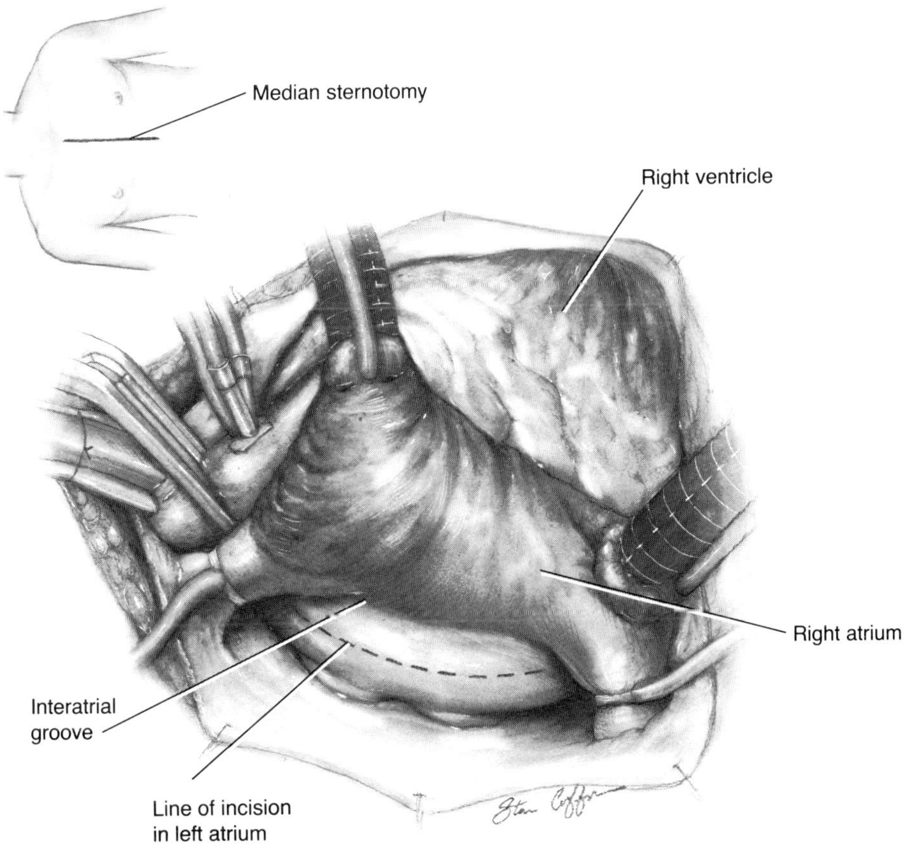

FIGURE 82–1. A median sternotomy provides excellent exposure for excision of left atrial myxomas. Alternatively, a right anterior thoracotomy also provides appropriate exposure and has been used frequently. Cardiac cannulae are inserted into the *right* atrium for venous return, and the ascending aorta is used for the arterial inflow. The body temperature is lowered, and potassium cardioplegia is employed after crossclamping the ascending aorta. A longitudinal incision is made in the left atrium just posterior to the atrial groove and anterior to the right superior and inferior pulmonary veins.

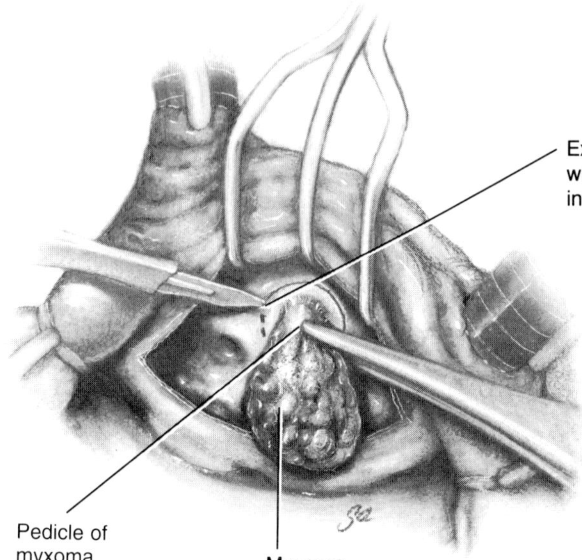

FIGURE 82–2. Retractors are inserted, providing exposure of the left atrium. The myxoma is identified and is usually attached by a stalk to the atrial septum. Because myxoma may invade the base of the stalk and the septum, a margin of atrial septum is taken with the specimen.

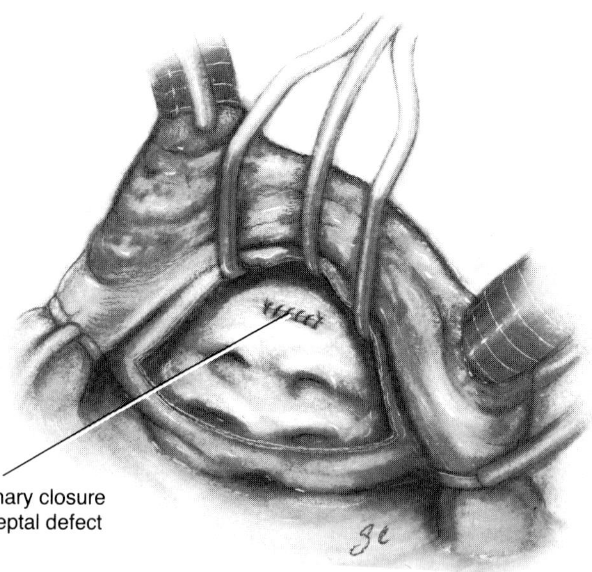

FIGURE 82–3. The subsequent defect is closed with a continuous nonabsorbable suture or a patch of pericardium or plastic prosthesis. The atriotomy incision is closed with a continuous nonabsorbable suture, and air is evacuated prior to tying the final suture in place. The patient is then separated from cardiopulmonary bypass.

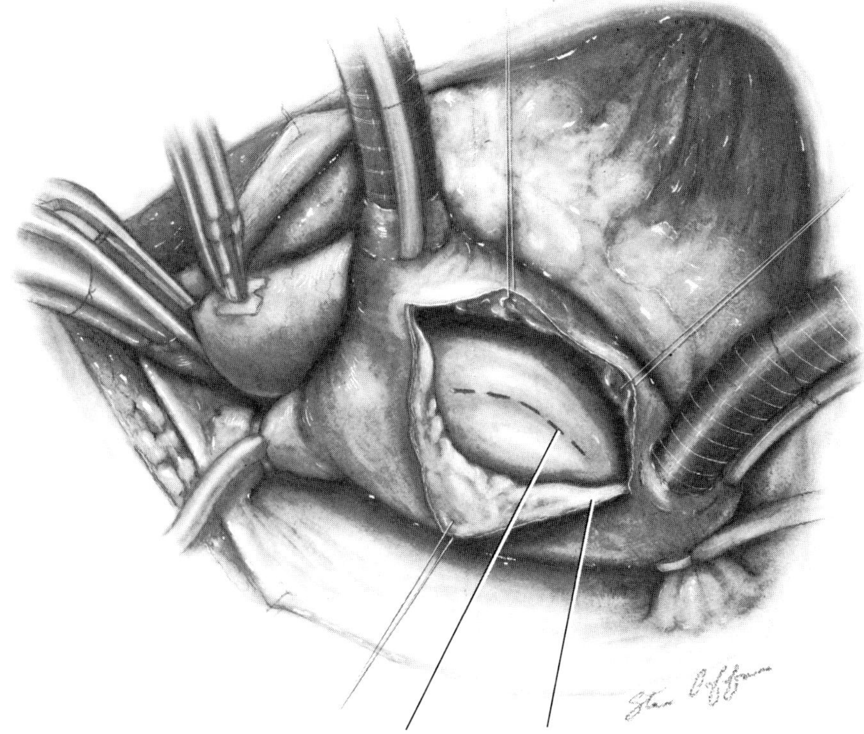

FIGURE 82–4. Occasionally, it is preferable to use the *trans-septal* approach, with entry into the right atrium followed by an incision in the interatrial septum. This incision is made in a longitudinal direction.

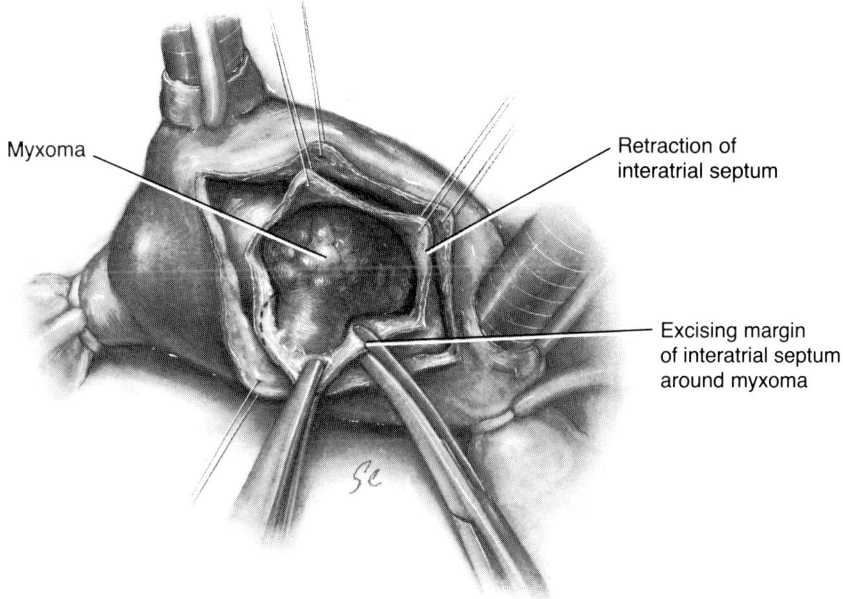

FIGURE 82–5. The myxoma is excised, and a margin of interatrial septum may be included around the stalk of the tumor.

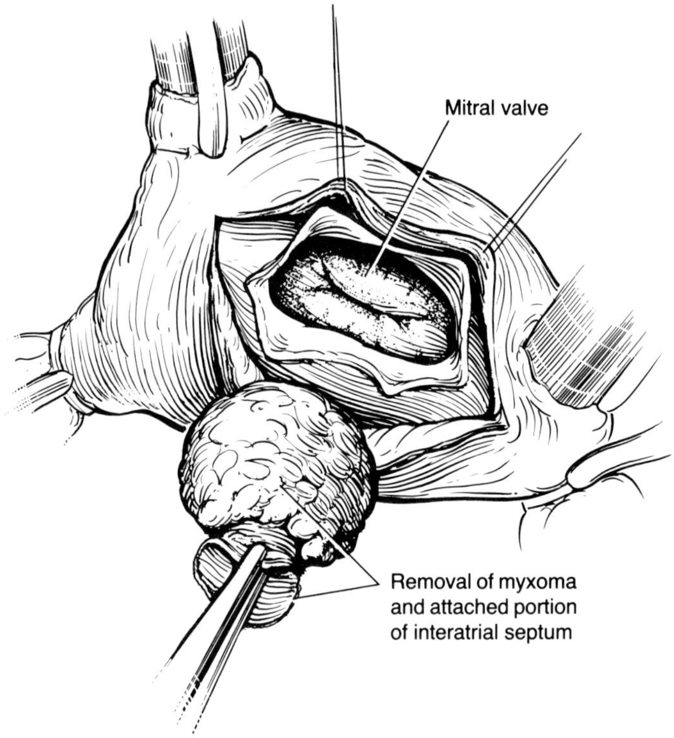

FIGURE 82–6. The atrial myxoma is shown with the attached circumferential border of atrial septum. After removal of the myxoma, the mitral valve is easily apparent.

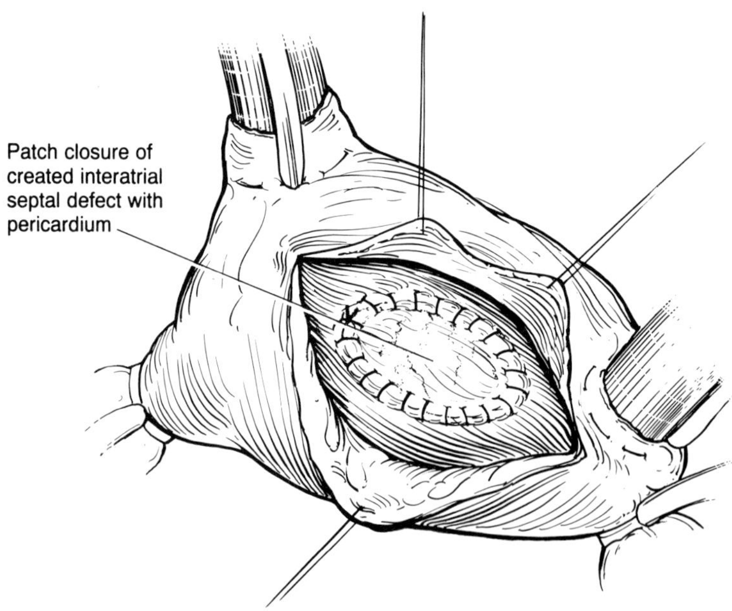

FIGURE 82–7. The defect in the atrial wall can be closed either primarily or usually with a septal patch of pericardium or plastic material. The right atriotomy is closed with a continuous nonabsorbable suture. The patient is separated from cardiopulmonary bypass, and the incision is closed.

SECTION XVII

Transplantation

PETER VAN TRIGT, III, M.D.

83

Cardiac Transplantation

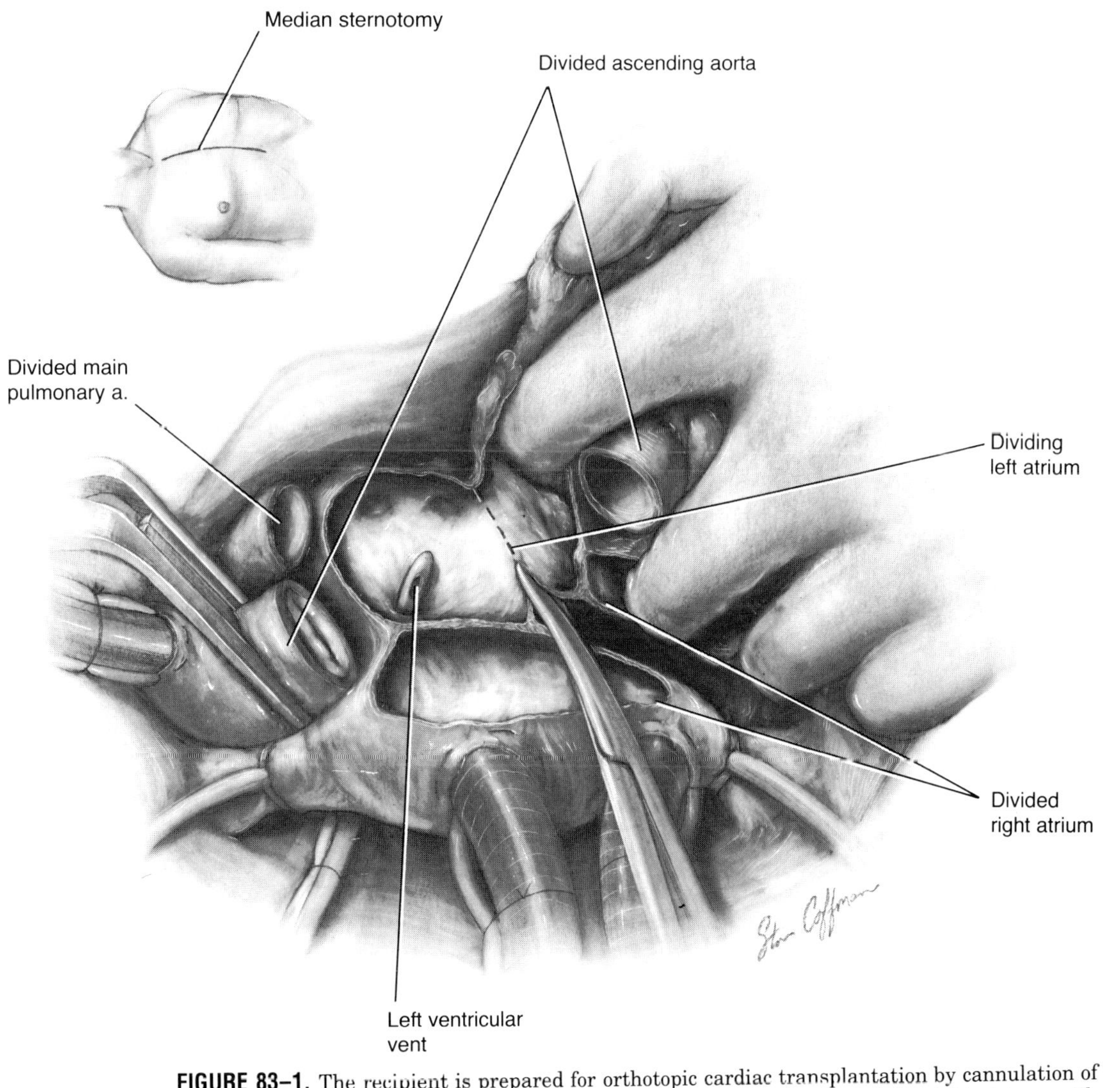

FIGURE 83–1. The recipient is prepared for orthotopic cardiac transplantation by cannulation of the ascending aorta and bicaval cannulation through the lateral aspect of the right atrium, with snares placed around each caval cannula. A left ventricular vent is passed through the right superior pulmonary vein, and the aortic crossclamp is applied. The recipient's heart is excised at the level of the atrioventricular groove and across the great vessels just above the two valves.

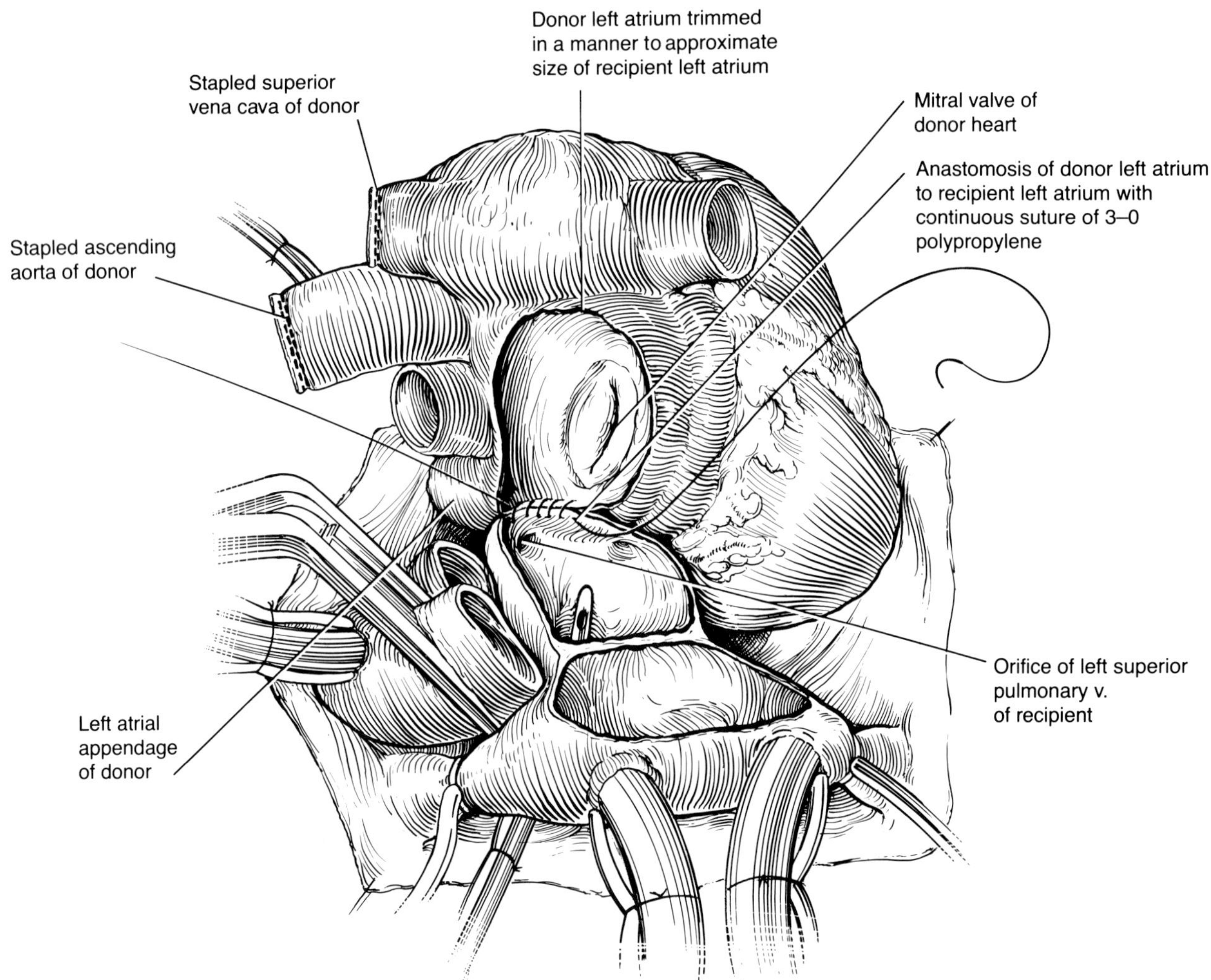

FIGURE 83–2. The donor heart is placed into the pericardial space to expose the left atrium, which has been opened through the pulmonary veins, and trimmed to match the recipient's left atrial cuff. The left atrial anastomosis is done with a continuous 3–0 monofilament polypropylene suture, starting at the area of the left atrial appendage and progressing down the lateral free wall. This anastomosis is completed by extending the other end of the suture to the septum inferiorly. Cardioplegia is delivered to the donor heart after this anastomosis is completed.

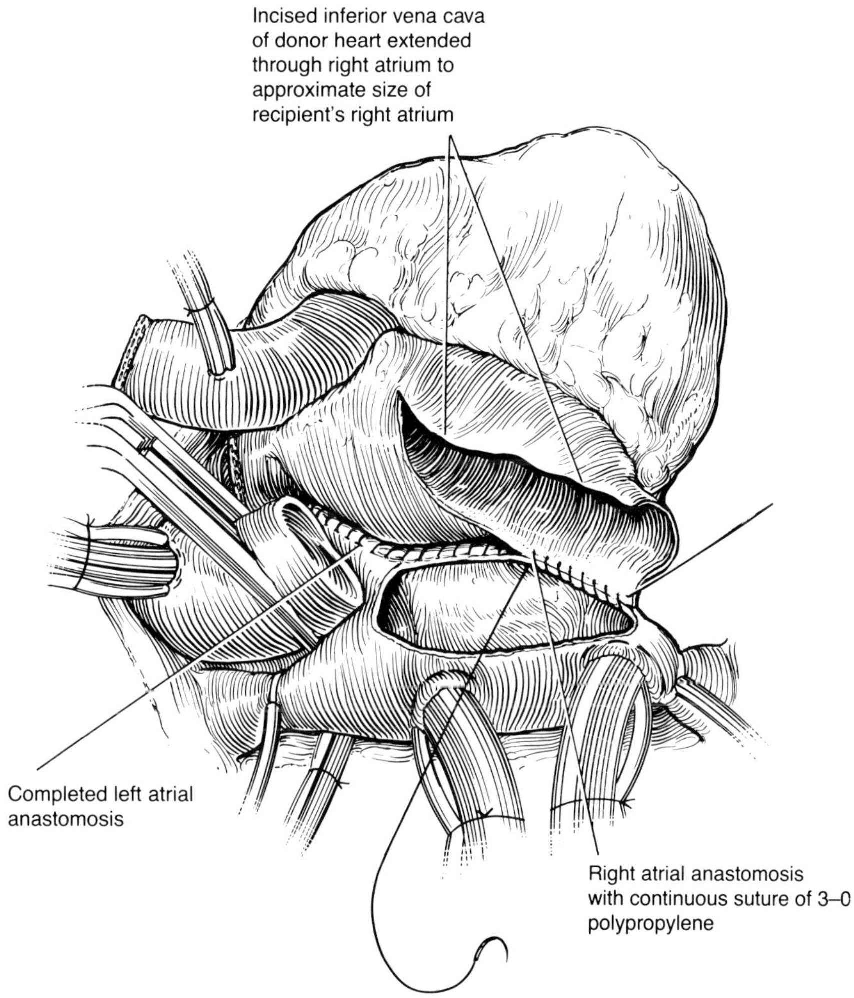

FIGURE 83–3. The donor right atrium is opened with a curvilinear incision from the inferior vena cava to the right atrial appendage, avoiding the area of the sinoatrial node. The right atrial anastomosis is completed with a continuous 3–0 monofilament polypropylene suture, starting close to the inferior vena cava and continuing superiorly along the interatrial septum. After this anastomosis is completed, cardioplegia is again administered through the cannula in the donor ascending aorta.

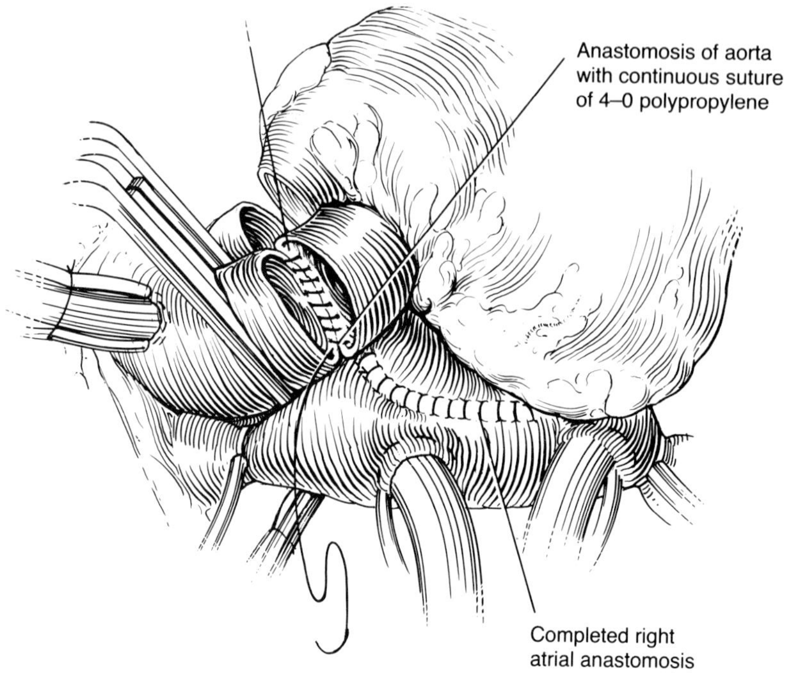

FIGURE 83–4. The ascending aorta of the donor is divided to leave an appropriate match for the end-to-end anastomosis, which is completed using a continuous 4–0 monofilament polypropylene suture. The posterior wall is anastomosed initially, and the sutures are extended anteriorly and tied after air is removed from the donor heart. The aortic crossclamp is released after the donor heart is allowed to fill with blood and all left-sided air is purged through the aortic suture line.

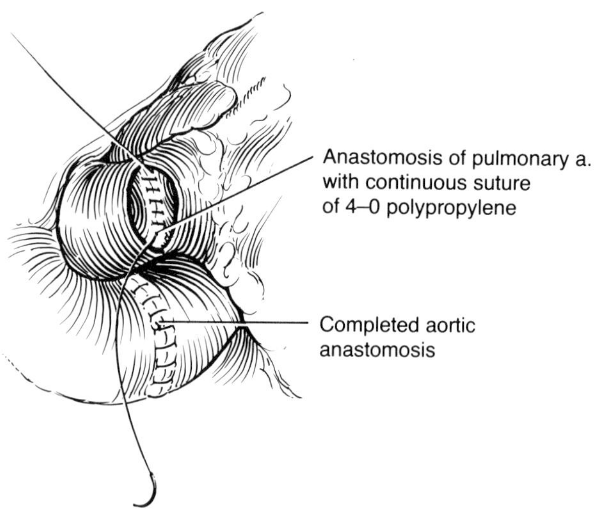

FIGURE 83–5. The pulmonary artery of the donor is trimmed to the appropriate length, and a continuous 4–0 monofilament polypropylene suture is placed while the heart remains fibrillating as the patient is rewarmed on cardiopulmonary bypass.

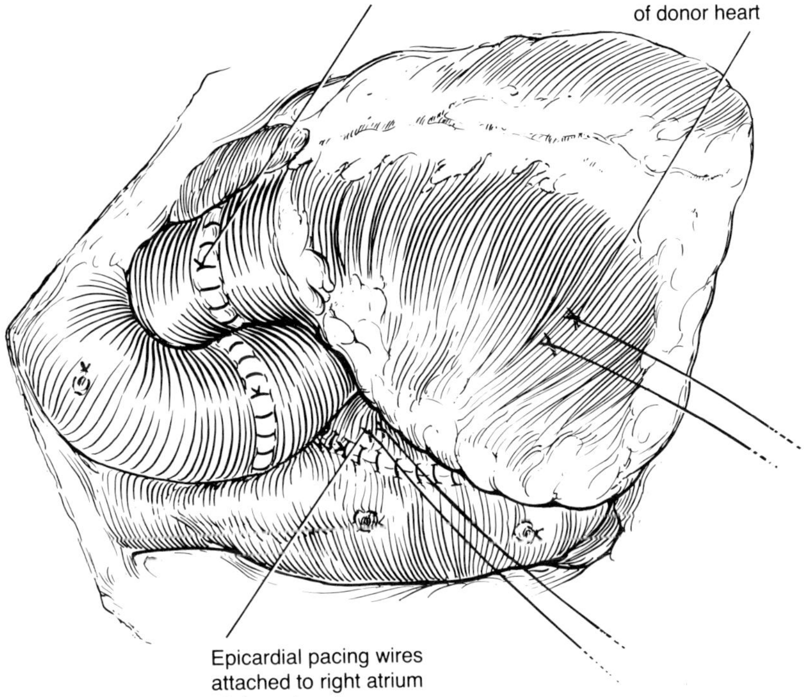

FIGURE 83–6. The heart is cardioverted, and temporary epicardial atrial and ventricular pace wires are attached to the donor heart. After the donor heart has been reperfused and the patient rewarmed, the cannulae are removed after separation from cardiopulmonary bypass.

PETER VAN TRIGT, III, M.D.

84

Right Lung Transplantation

FIGURE 84–1. The patient is intubated with a double-lumen endotracheal tube and placed in a full right lateral position. A posterolateral thoracotomy is performed, and the pleural cavity is entered through the fifth intercostal space. The recipient pneumonectomy is performed in the routine manner, with ligation and division of the pulmonary artery followed by the superior and inferior pulmonary veins. Electrocautery is used to achieve meticulous hemostasis, and enlarged lymph nodes are removed only when they encroach upon the operative field. The right main bronchus is dissected carefully without denuding the surrounding vascular adventitia. Airway division is performed with a scalpel, one ring proximal to the upper lobe orifice. After the airway is divided, the recipient right lung is removed, and the operative field is again examined for hemostasis.

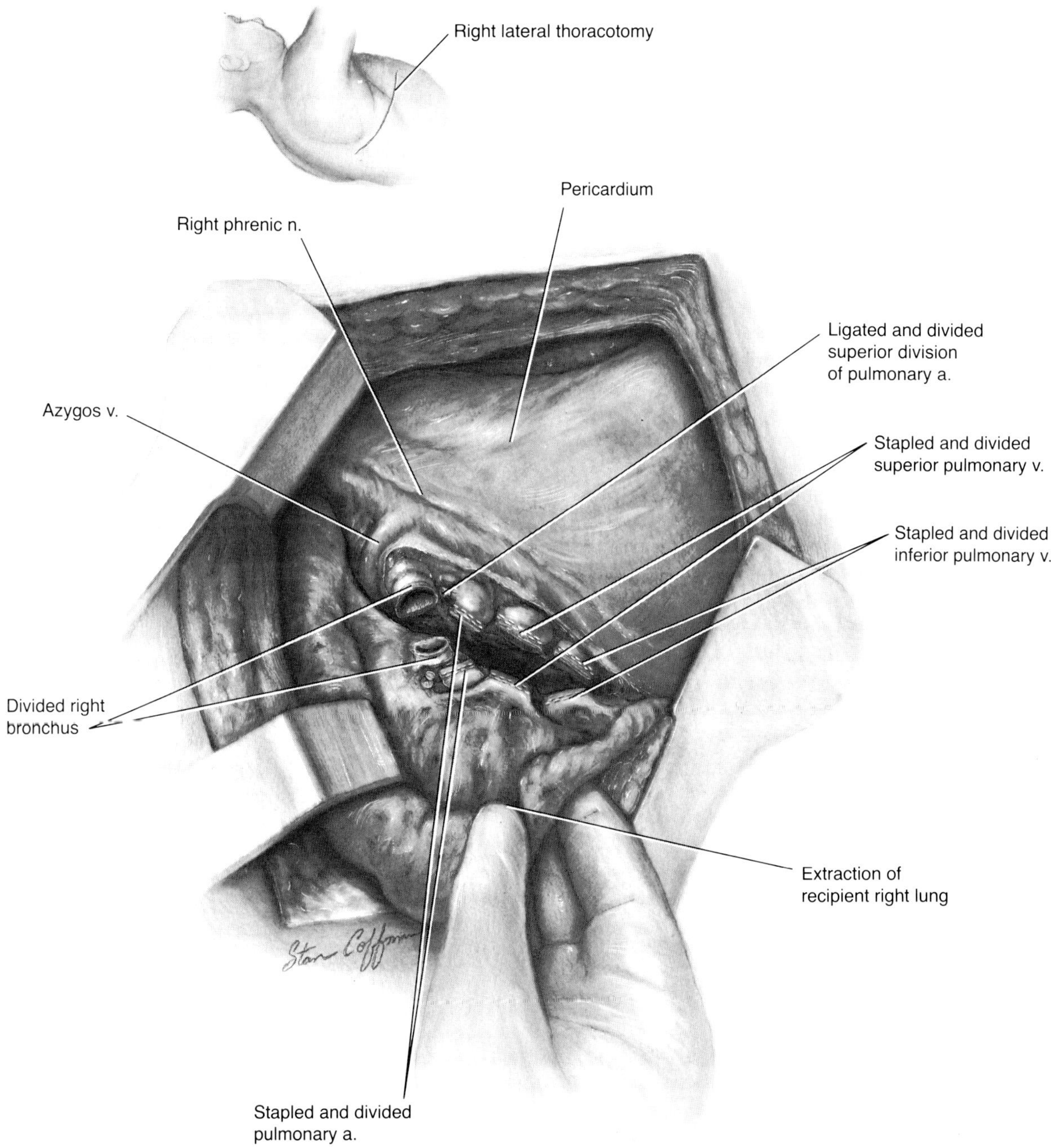

FIGURE 84–1 *See legend on opposite page*

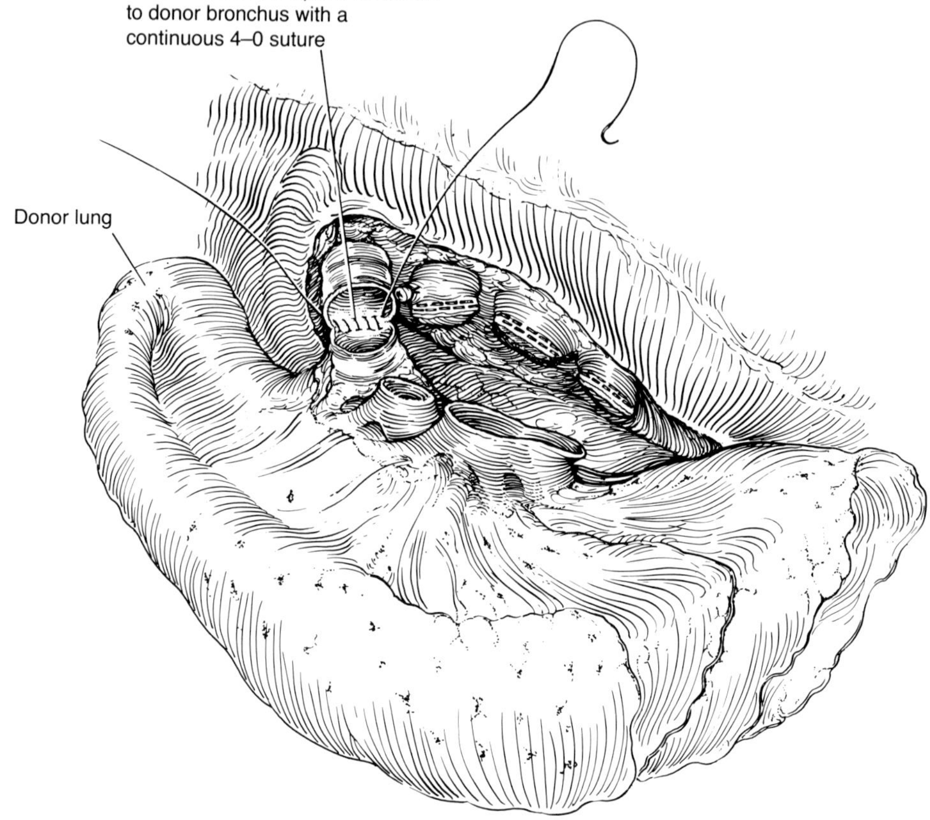

FIGURE 84–2. The right lung is placed in the right pleural cavity, and the bronchial anastomosis is begun along the posterior membranous wall with a continuous 4–0 monofilament (PDS) suture. The ends of this suture are left as stay sutures.

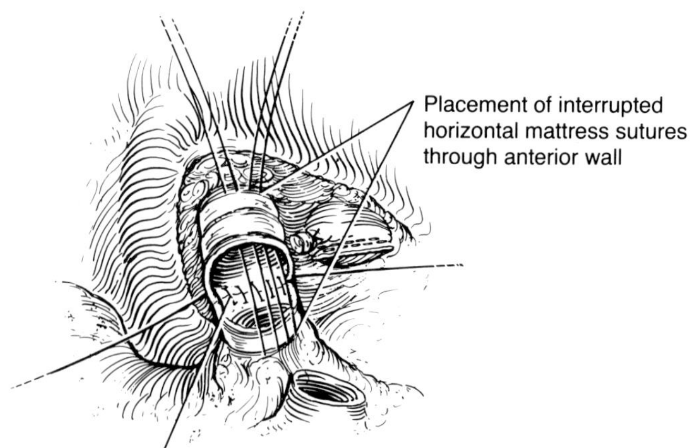

FIGURE 84–3. To achieve telescoping of the donor main bronchus into the recipient requires placement of five or six interrupted horizontal mattress sutures of 4–0 PDS inserted as shown. These mattress sutures are brought out two cartilaginous rings above the end of the recipient's bronchus.

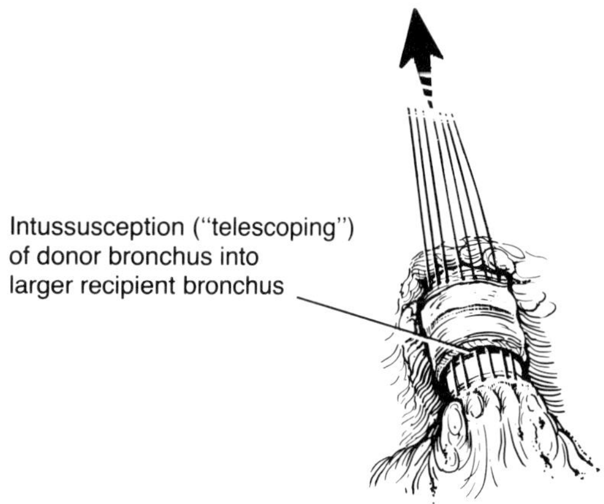

FIGURE 84–4. As the interrupted mattress sutures are drawn tight and tied, the donor bronchus is telescoped into the recipient bronchial stump.

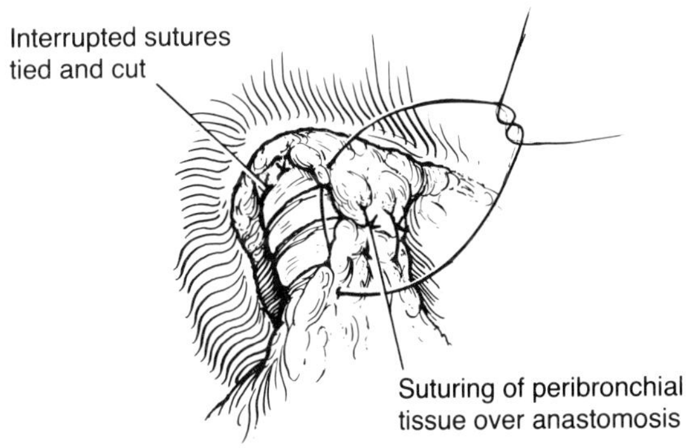

FIGURE 84–5. Peribronchial tissue is approximated over the bronchial anastomosis.

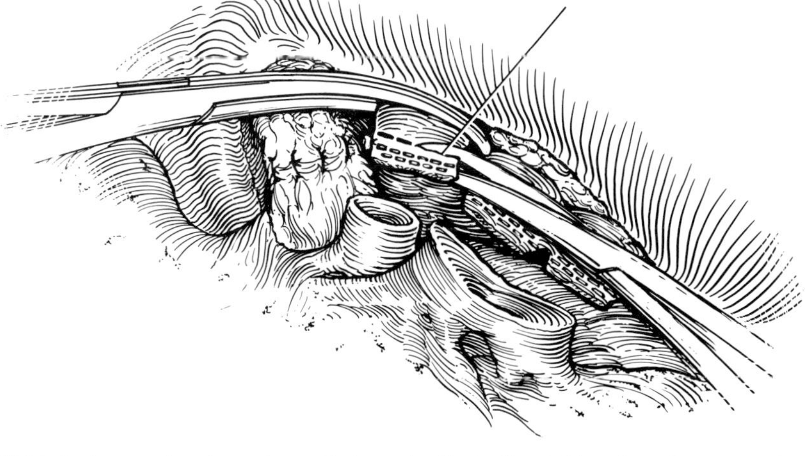

FIGURE 84–6. A vascular clamp is applied proximally to the right main pulmonary artery, and the stapled end trimmed.

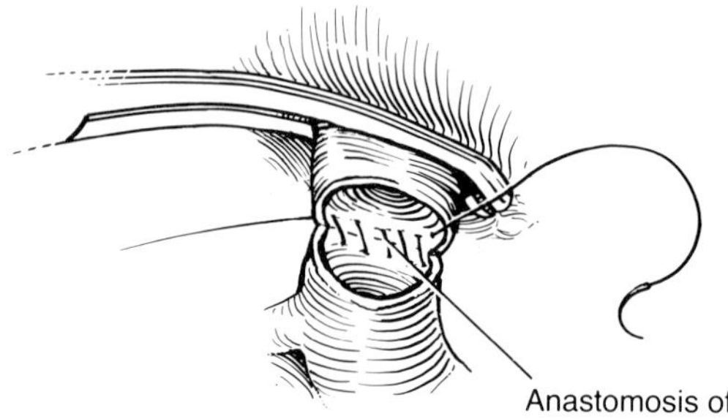

FIGURE 84–7. An end-to-end anastomosis between donor and recipient main pulmonary artery is performed using a continuous 5–0 monofilament suture. Care is taken to assess the length of the donor recipient vessels, because excessive length may be associated with kinking and secondary vascular compromise.

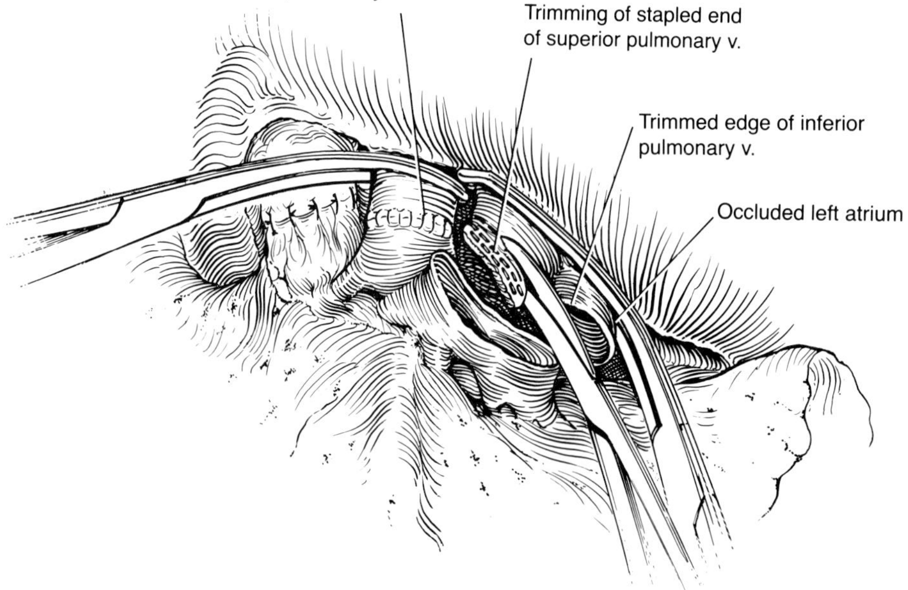

FIGURE 84–8. The anastomosis of the pulmonary artery is tested briefly by release of the proximal vascular clamp, which is then reapplied. The two pulmonary veins are then retracted away from the pericardium, and a Satinsky clamp is placed across the left atrium at the base of the pulmonary veins.

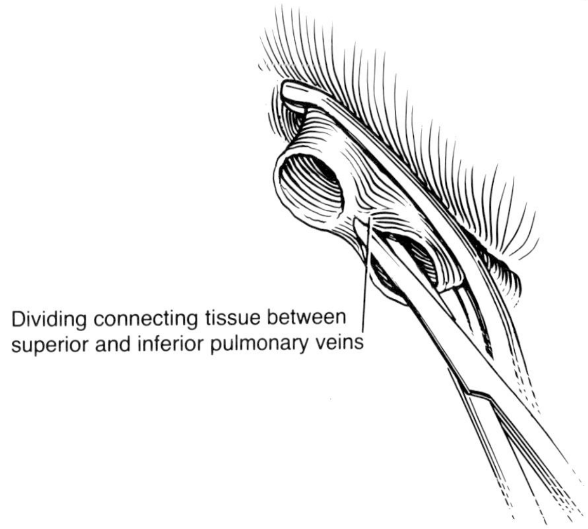

FIGURE 84–9. The recipient's pulmonary veins are trimmed and opened into a single vascular cuff.

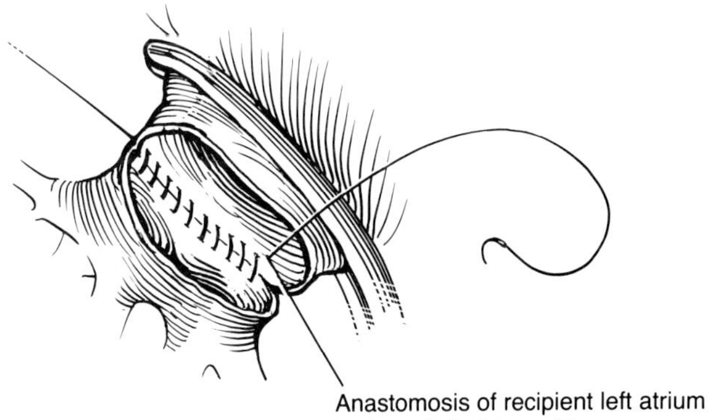

FIGURE 84–10. The left atrial anastomosis is performed using a continuous 4–0 monofilament suture starting posteriorly and finishing anteriorly.

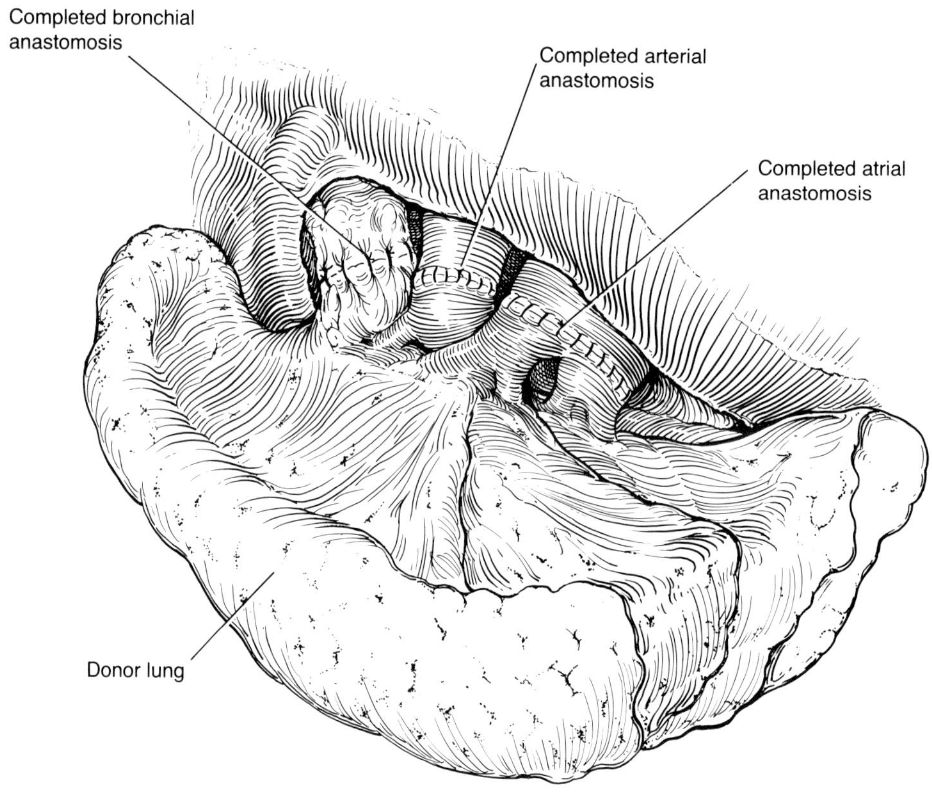

FIGURE 84–11. Air is removed from the pulmonary allograft by slow release of the pulmonary artery clamp. This allows air to be purged through the untied left atrial suture line, which is then tied as the Satinsky clamp is removed. This procedure is performed with the patient in the Trendelenburg position as the lung is gently inflated. The anastomoses are checked carefully after the lung is re-expanded and reperfused.

PETER VAN TRIGT, III, M.D.

85

Cardiopulmonary Transplantation

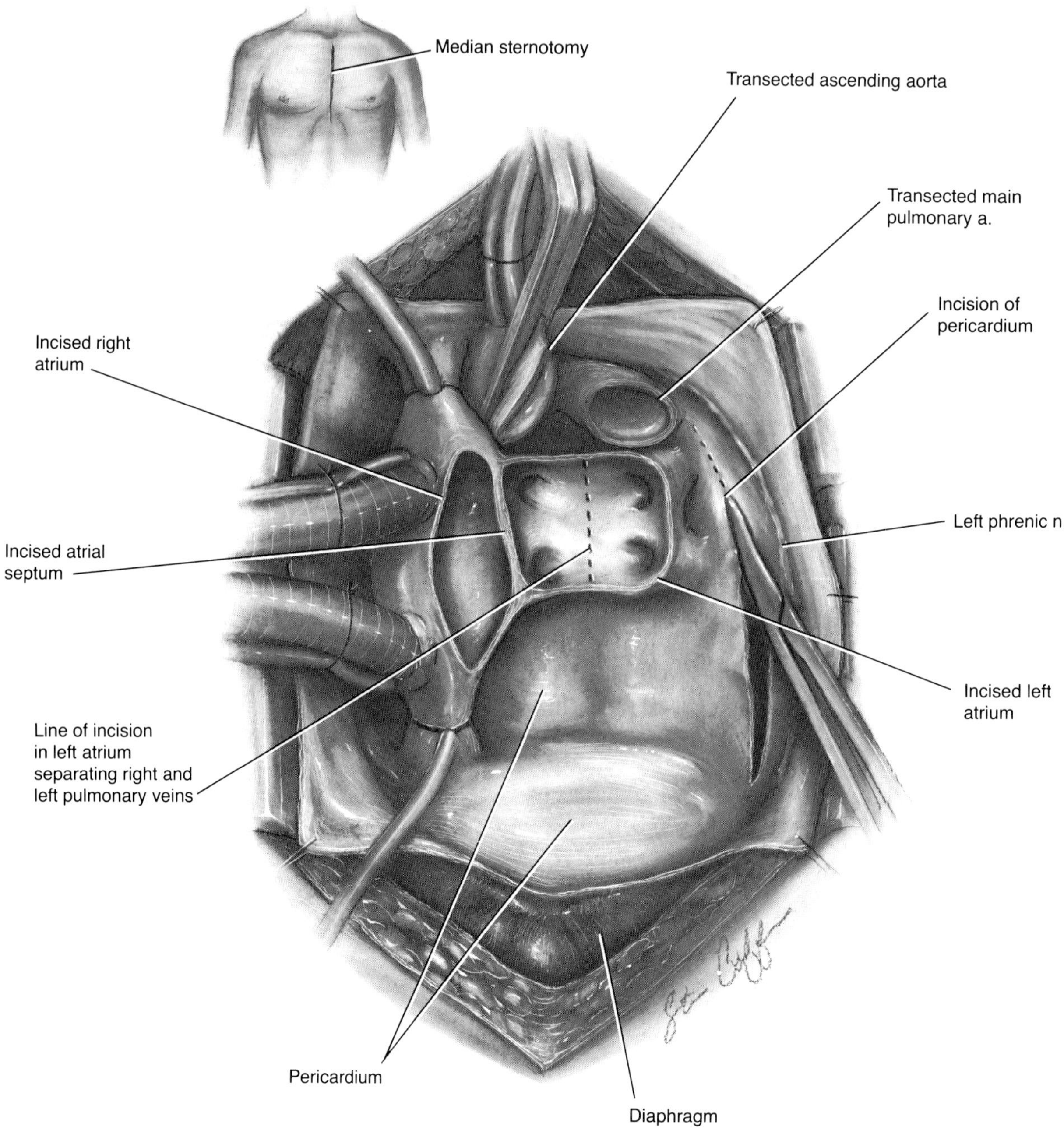

FIGURE 85–1. A median sternotomy is made, and the pleura is incised on both sides. Each pleural space is examined for adhesions, and these are removed with electrocautery as completely as possible before cardiopulmonary bypass and systemic heparinization are initiated. The heart is cannulated as for cardiac transplantation; and after initiation of bypass, the superior and inferior venae cavae are snared. The aorta is crossclamped, and the heart is excised first. The incision follows the atrioventricular groove with removal of the atrial appendages. The ascending aorta and main pulmonary artery are transected, and the heart is removed from the chest. The pericardial edge on the left side is retracted anteriorly, and an incision is made in the pericardium just anterior to the pulmonary veins. The incision is continued inferiorly to the diaphragm, with care taken to stay well behind the course of the left phrenic nerve. A vertical incision divides the left atrium, which effectively separates the right and left pulmonary veins. The left lung is then removed by separating the pulmonary veins from the posterior attachments and dividing the pulmonary artery and inferior pulmonary ligament. The left main bronchus is dissected with careful control of the bronchial arteries. The bronchus is stapled with a TA-30 stapler, and the lung is removed. A similar technique is used to excise the right lung. Because the phrenic nerve lies much closer to the hilum on the right side, care must be taken to prevent injury to the nerve as the pleura is incised posteriorly.

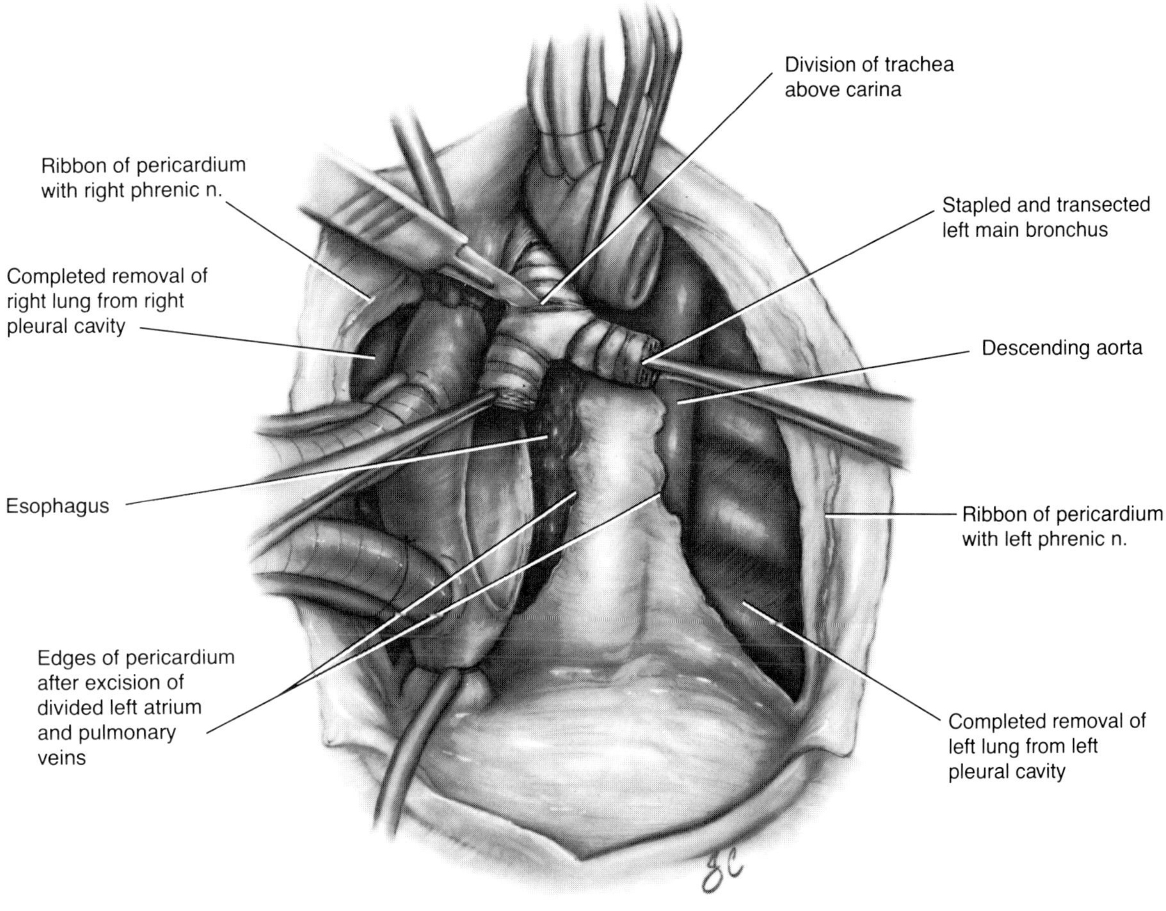

FIGURE 85-2. The aorta is retracted to the left, and the trachea is exposed. The trachea is then divided with a scalpel, and the two freed main bronchi are removed from the field with meticulous hemostasis being obtained.

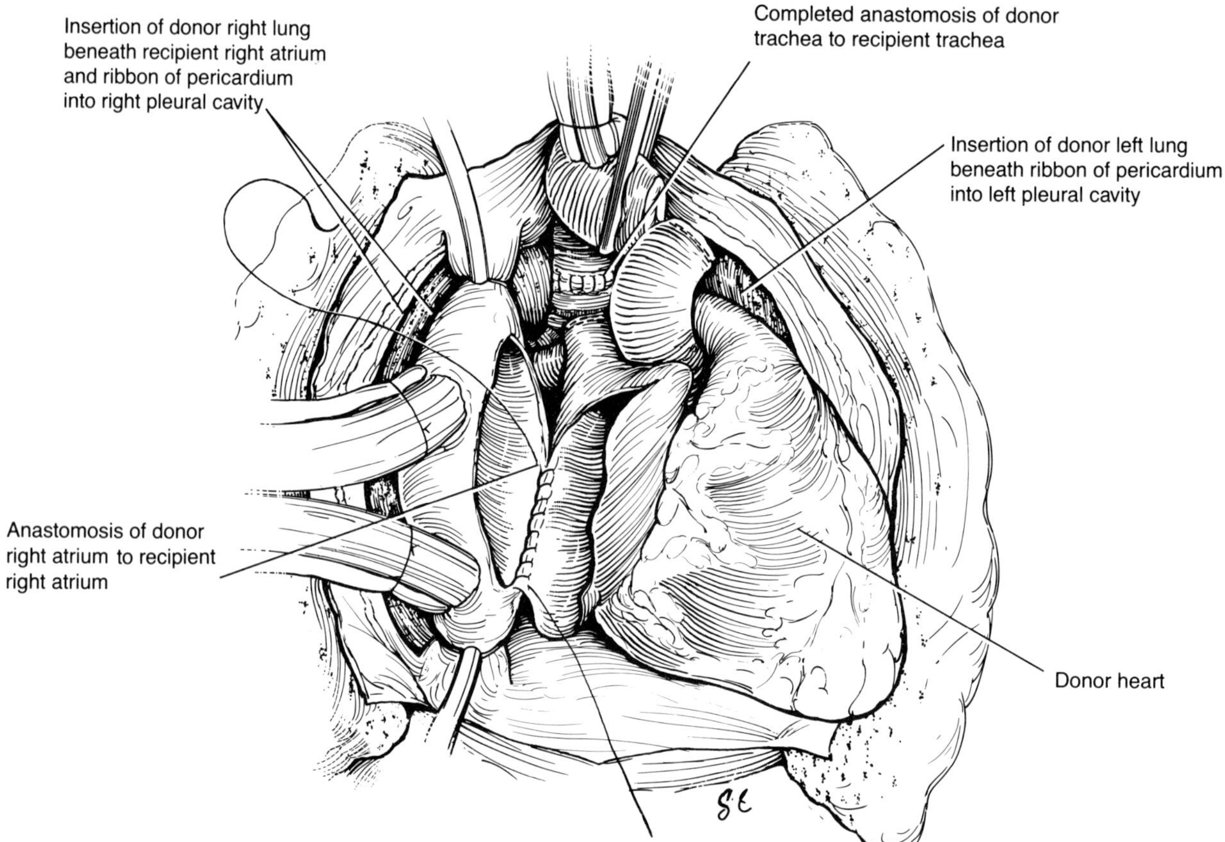

FIGURE 85–3. The donor right lung is passed beneath the right atrium and both venae cavae, and the left lung is passed beneath the left phrenic nerve and its pericardial pedicle. The tracheal anastomosis is performed with a continuous 3–0 polypropylene suture, with incorporation of surrounding tissue to preserve the blood supply of the recipient trachea. The right atrial anastomosis is then performed. The donor right atrium is opened in a curvilinear manner as for cardiac transplantation, avoiding injury to the sinus node. This anastomosis is completed with a continuous 3–0 polypropylene suture.

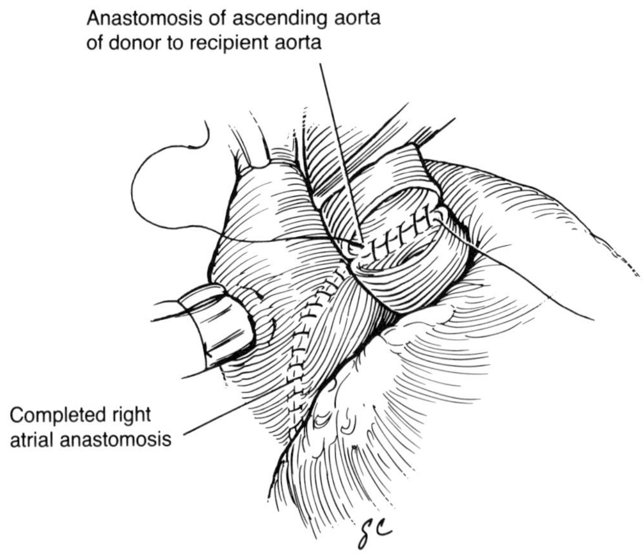

FIGURE 85–4. An end-to-end anastomosis is performed using a continuous 4–0 polypropylene suture, and air is removed from the heart as the aortic crossclamp is removed. The lungs are inflated gently, and the patient is separated from cardiopulmonary bypass.

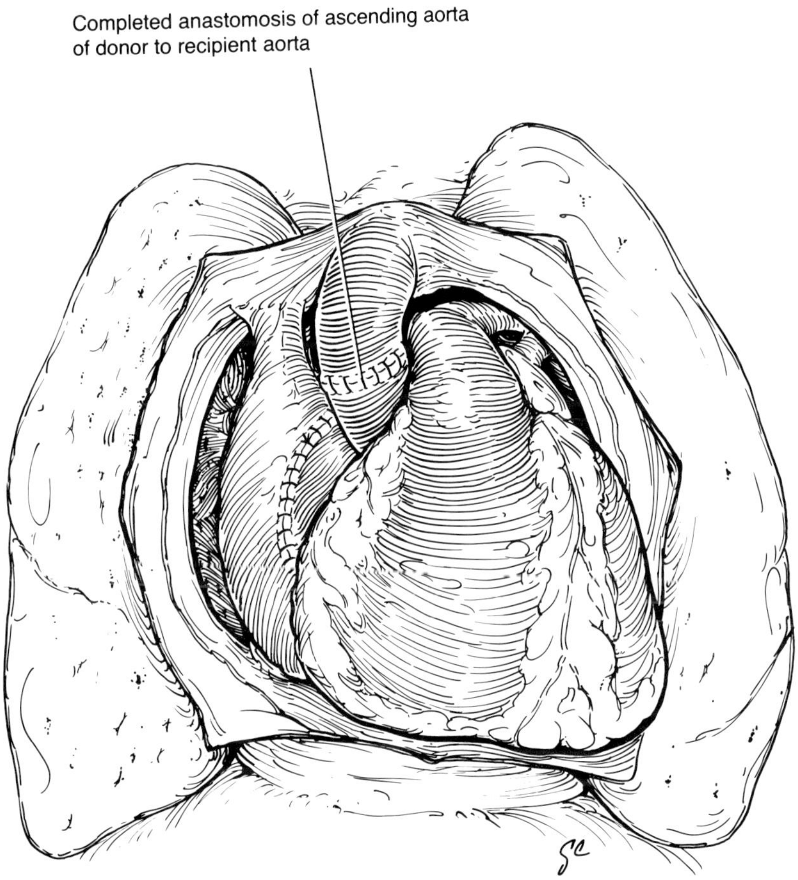

FIGURE 85–5. Cardiopulmonary transplantation is completed.

SECTION XVIII

Ventricular Aneurysms

JAMES E. LOWE, M.D.

86

Resection and Repair of Left Ventricular Aneurysm

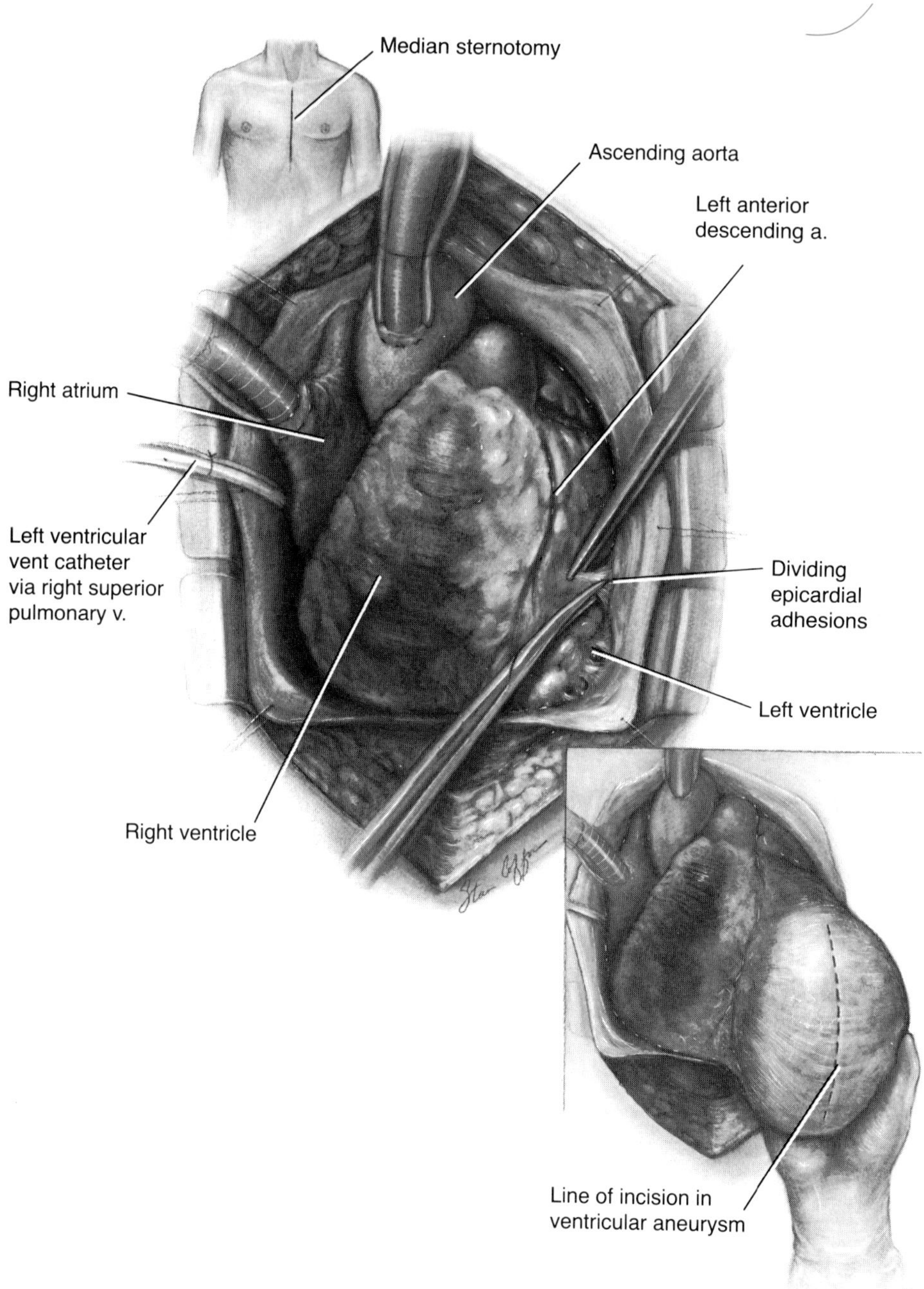

FIGURE 86–1. Left ventricular aneurysms are approached through a standard median sternotomy incision. The pericardium is opened, and any adhesions between the anterior portions of the left and right ventricles are sharply divided in order to create a pericardial cradle. Because many aneurysms contain fresh and old thrombus, care is taken to avoid any manipulation of the heart before institution of cardiopulmonary bypass and left ventricular decompression. The ascending aorta is cannulated for arterial inflow, and venous return is accomplished by placing a two-staged cannula into the right atrium and inferior vena cava through a pursestring suture placed over the right atrial appendage. Cardiopulmonary bypass is then begun, and, with the heart in the empty-beating state, any residual adhesions between the pericardium and epicardial surfaces of the heart are sharply divided. The left ventricle is decompressed by placing a vent catheter into the left ventricle through a pursestring suture placed over the right superior pulmonary vein.

Inset, With the heart completely empty and decompressed through the left ventricular vent, the aneurysm is elevated into the operative field. The aneurysm edges are gently palpated, and the center of the aneurysm is identified. At this point, there are two options: The heart can be arrested by using cold antegrade cardioplegia, or the entire resection and repair can be accomplished while the heart is in the empty-beating state. If concomitant coronary artery bypass grafts are to be placed, cardioplegic arrest is preferred.

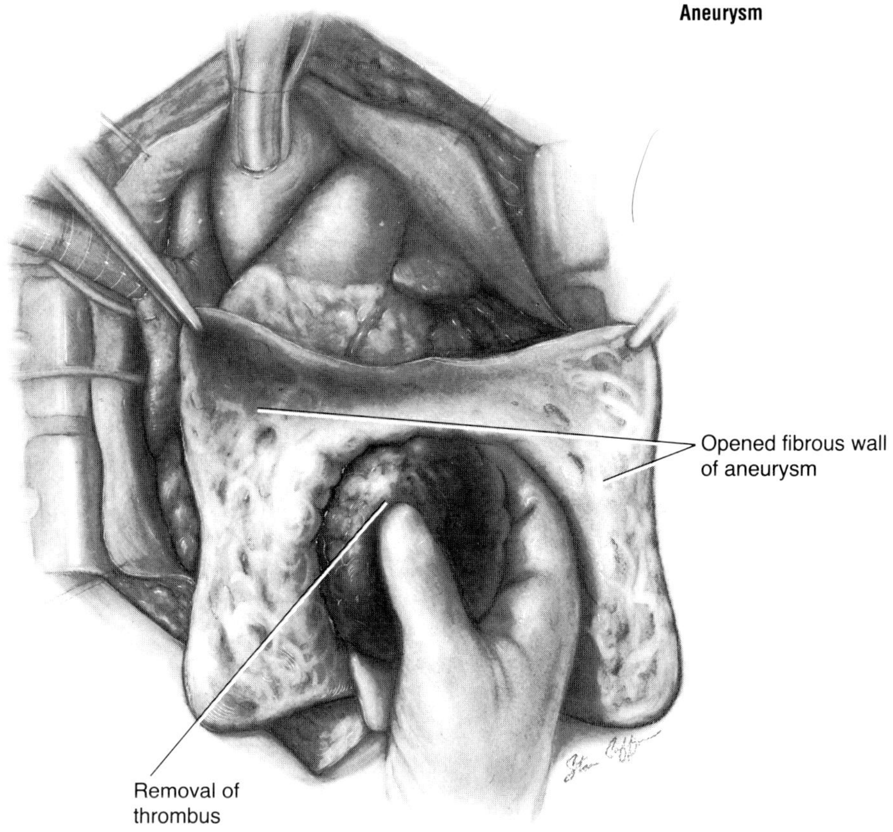

FIGURE 86–2. The aneurysm is opened in its midportion.

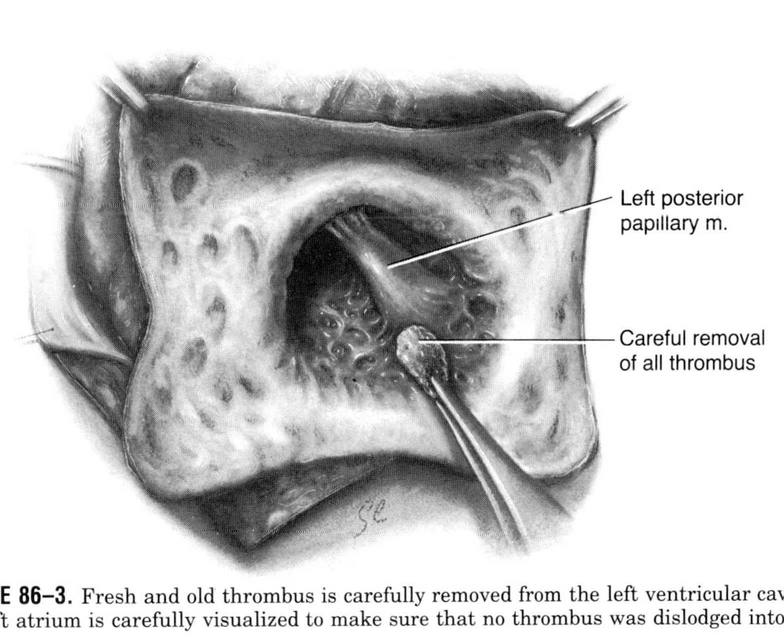

FIGURE 86–3. Fresh and old thrombus is carefully removed from the left ventricular cavity, and the left atrium is carefully visualized to make sure that no thrombus was dislodged into the left atrium.

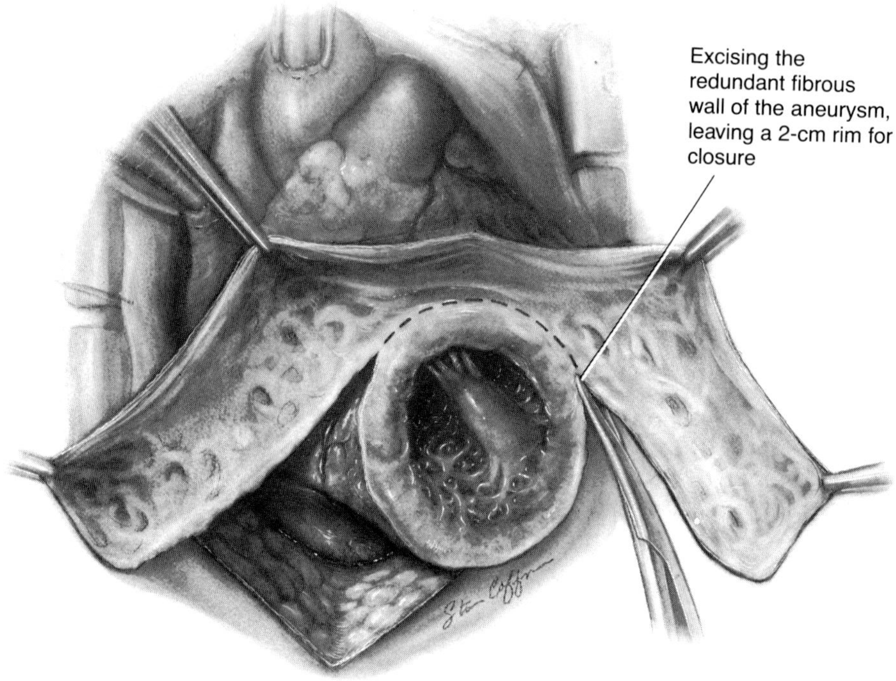

FIGURE 86–4. After complete removal of all thrombus material, the left ventricular cavity is irrigated with saline. The redundant fibrous wall of the aneurysm is then removed, leaving at least a 2-cm rim for closure. In large aneurysms, the redundant fibrous wall is removed before repair is begun. However, in small aneurysms, the geometry of the left ventricle should be set using Teflon felt strips and horizontal mattress sutures before excision of any fibrous rim.

A common mistake in resecting left ventricular aneurysms is to remove too much residual aneurysm neck. Primary repair then produces a small left ventricular cavity, and left ventricular failure may persist postoperatively. Therefore, it is critical that an adequate rim of fibrous tissue be left in place to allow closure without compromising left ventricular end-diastolic volume.

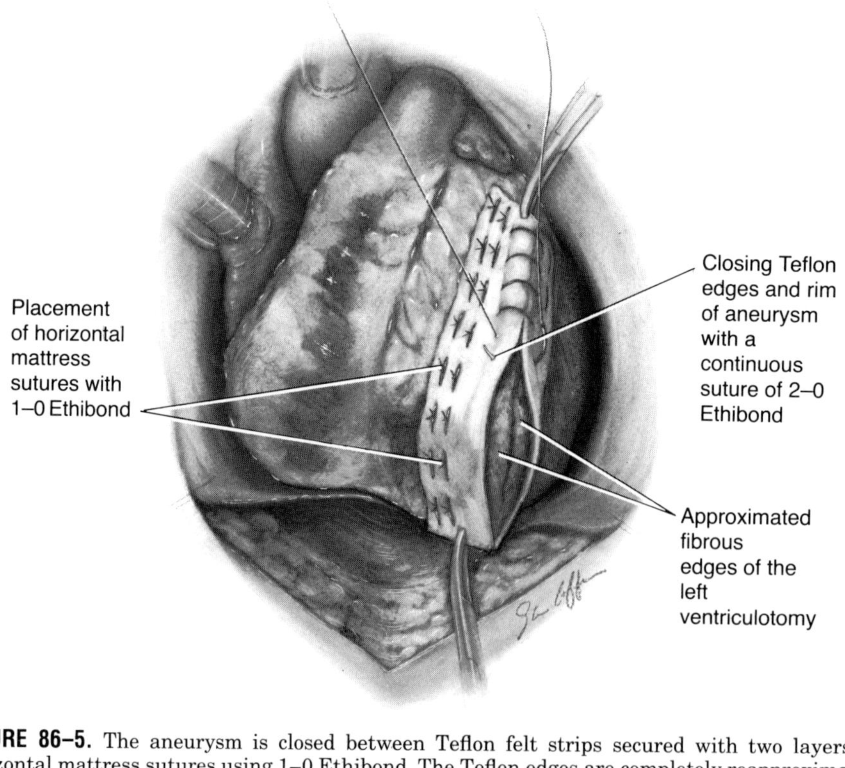

FIGURE 86–5. The aneurysm is closed between Teflon felt strips secured with two layers of horizontal mattress sutures using 1–0 Ethibond. The Teflon edges are completely reapproximated over the apex of the ventricle using two layers of continuous running suture of 2–0 Ethibond.

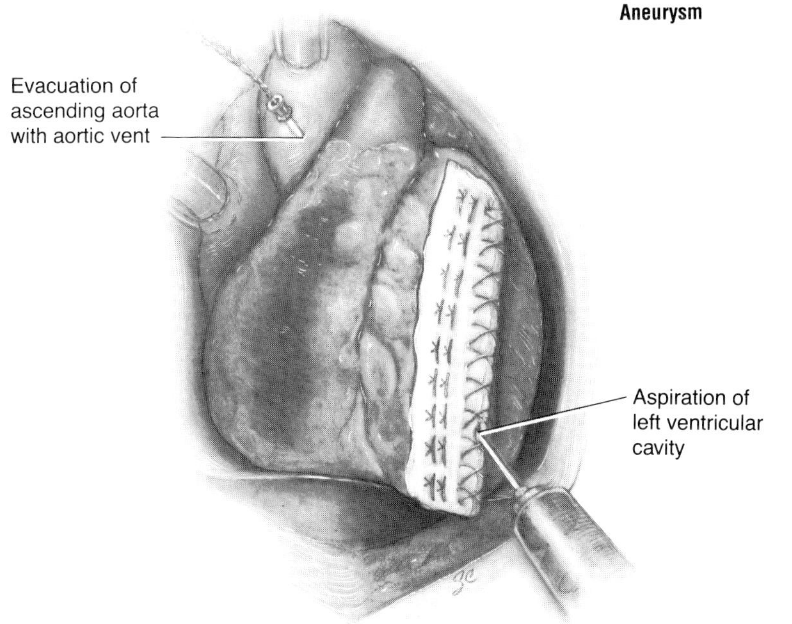

FIGURE 86–6. Transesophageal echo is used to confirm that all intercardiac air has been evacuated. This is accomplished by aspirating the left ventricular cavity through the apical portion of the repair as well as by placing a needle vent over the ascending aorta as the heart is allowed to fill and eject.

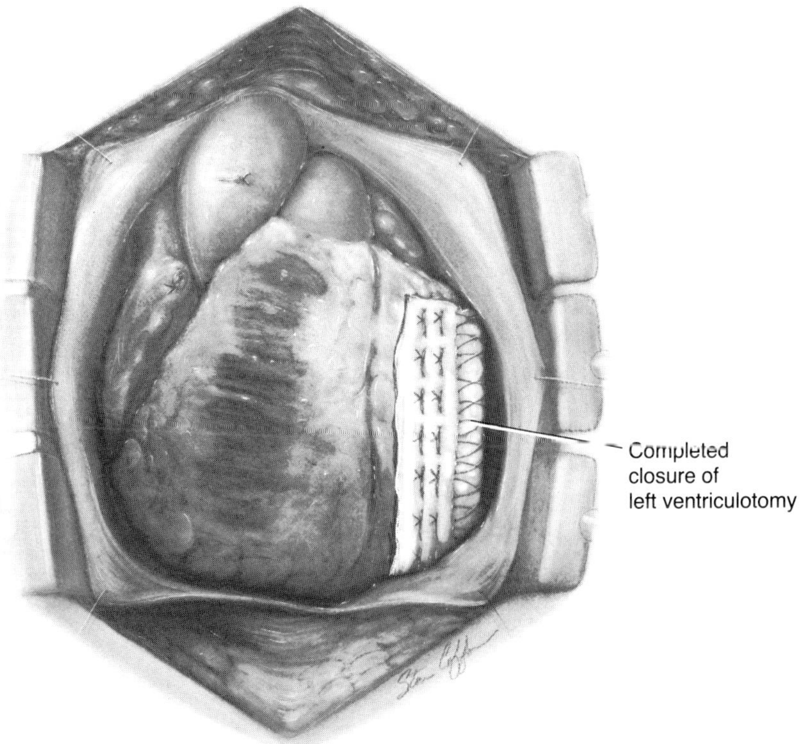

FIGURE 86–7. In this particular approach to the resection and repair of left ventricular aneurysms, a hemostatic closure is used to ensure that an adequate ventricular cavity is created so that left ventricular end-diastolic volume is not compromised. Leaving an adequate rim of fibrous aneurysm for repair ensures that complicated endoaneurysmorrhaphy procedures requiring patches will be unnecessary in most patients.

SECTION XIX

Extracorporeal Membrane Oxygenation

ROSS M. UNGERLEIDER, M.D.

87 Cannulation

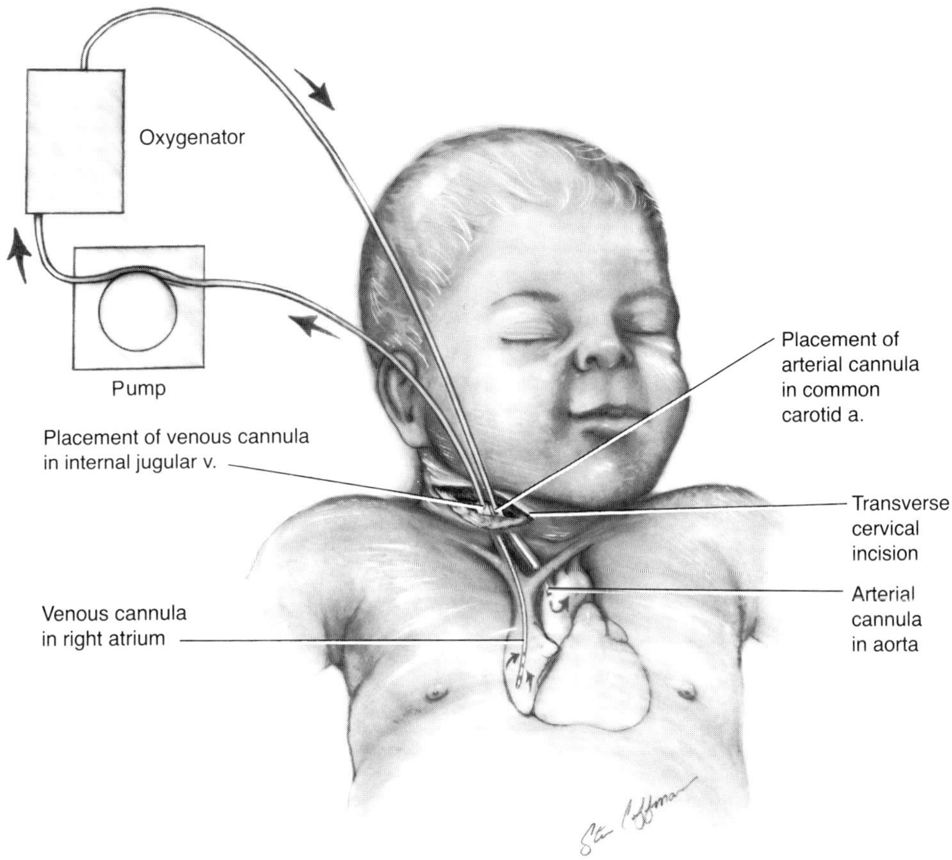

FIGURE 87–1. Venoarterial cannulation is accomplished through a transverse neck incision, which is usually performed in a skin fold halfway between the clavicle and angle of the mandible. This incision needs to be only 1.5 cm in the typical neonate who is placed on extracorporeal membrane oxygenation (ECMO). The platysma is divided to allow identification of the medial border of the sternocleidomastoid muscle. This muscle is retracted laterally to identify the jugular vein and the more posterior and medial carotid artery. Each of these vessels is dissected completely and encircled with ligatures. The patient is then heparinized, and the distal artery and vein are ligated.

Before the distal portion of the jugular vein is ligated, it is helpful to occlude the proximal portion with a vascular clamp. This creates venous distention that does not decompress with distal ligation—thus making subsequent venotomy for cannula insertion easier. Appropriate-size arterial and venous cannulae are selected. The arterial cannula is placed into the carotid artery and advanced so that its tip lies at the juncture of the innominate artery with the ascending aorta (approximately 3 cm) and is then securely tied in place with ligatures placed over the proximal carotid artery. It is helpful to tie these ligatures over a small rubber "vessel loop" so that when the cannula is later removed the ties can be cut over this material to avoid injury to the underlying carotid artery. The jugular venous cannula is placed in a similar manner, except that it is advanced proximally into the right atrium before it is secured. These cannulae are then attached to the appropriate pump lines, with care taken not to leave any air bubbles in the lines.

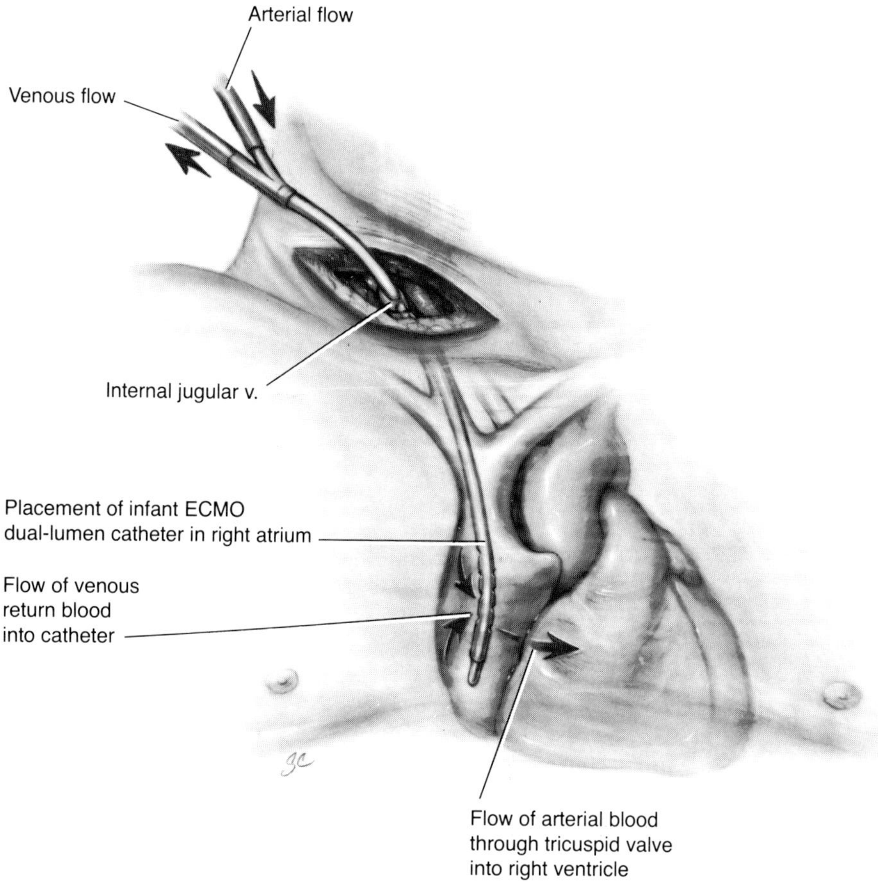

FIGURE 87–2. In patients who are appropriate candidates for venovenous ECMO, the jugular vein and carotid artery should be identified and dissected free of surrounding tissue, as described in Figure 87–1. It is important to dissect the carotid artery so that if the patient needs to be converted to venoarterial ECMO, the artery will be readily available. A dual-lumen venovenous cannula is then inserted into the jugular vein, advanced, and oriented in the appropriate manner. The cannula is secured to the vein over a vessel loop, as described in Figure 87–1. Pump lines are attached to the appropriate ports of the cannula. It is important to understand that venovenous ECMO will provide adequate gas exchange but no hemodynamic support, and must therefore be used only in properly selected patients.

SECTION XX

Thoracoscopic Procedures

IVO HANKE, M.D.
JAMES M. DOUGLAS, JR., M.D.

88

General Approach to Video-Assisted Thoracoscopic Surgery

The introduction and subsequent refinement of video technology have initiated an intense interest in video-assisted laparoscopic and, subsequently, thoracoscopic procedures. Improvements in optical equipment and surgical instrumentation continue to advance rapidly. Nonetheless, adherence to certain basic principles remains quite important for the safe and facile performance of video-assisted endosurgical procedures. Although video-assisted laparoscopic techniques share certain considerations with video-assisted thoracoscopic procedures, the constraints imposed by a rigid thoracic cavity and the physiologic consequences of intrathoracic operations using single-lung ventilation present special potential problems. This section presents the considerations of importance to all thoracic surgeons performing video-assisted thoracoscopic techniques. Because of the widely varying available instrumentation and ongoing technologic advancements, it is impractical to focus on specific instrumentation. Instead, areas that are operator-dependent and more consistently important are discussed.

EQUIPMENT

Video-assisted thoracoscopic procedures basically require a fiberoptic light source with associated video camera system, monitors, and an assortment of endoscopic graspers, clamps, and surgical staplers. Several excellent camera systems are available, with varying degrees of optical excellence. Resolution and color are currently greatest with the three-chip technology. Of greatest importance is that a reliable system with dependable service backup be obtained.

Both rigid and flexible endoscopes may be used for thoracoscopy. The rigid endoscope has been the most useful because of the increased field of view, resolution, and simplicity. The zero-degree rigid endoscope provides a field of vision that is directly in front of the scope. This system is useful in all procedures. However, rigid scopes are also available that have an angled field of vision, usually 30 or 60 degrees away from the in-line angle of incidence. These scopes provide views of areas that are at sharp angles to the normal field of vision. Although they are frequently useful, the viewing angle may be confusing to the untrained observer.

The thoracoscopic surgeon should have a variety of instruments designed for grasping small areas of tissue as well as large portions, such as lung parenchyma. An endoscopic stapling system is indispensable for pulmonary

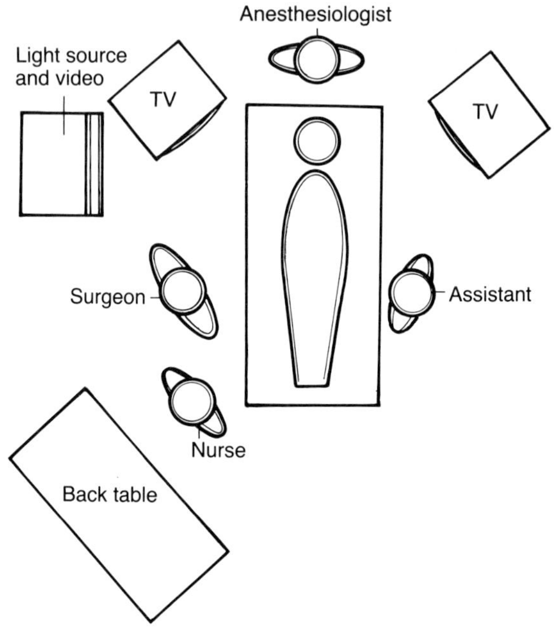

FIGURE 88–1. Typical operating room environment. Two video monitors are suggested so that the operator and assistants can easily visualize the ongoing procedure.

operations. Additionally, a suction-irrigation system should be available for all cases. Endoscopic laser instrumentation may be useful in selected cases; however, laser equipment is rarely a necessary adjunct.

Although most thoracoscopic procedures can be performed without the use of carbon dioxide insufflation, its availability is encouraged. Occasionally, infusion of carbon dioxide at an intrathoracic pressure of less than 10 mm Hg can assist in the collapse of the lung.

ANESTHESIA

General anesthesia with single-lung ventilation is currently the anesthetic technique of choice for all thoracoscopic procedures. There are several possible techniques for lung separation. The simplest approach, now used only for emergencies, is to advance the endotracheal tube into the mainstem bronchus of the unoperated side. Another option is to fiberoptically place a bronchial blocker. This is often necessary in children and small adults, because double-lumen endobronchial tubes are not available for patients who weigh less than 50 kg. Although the bronchial blocker technique has been recently refined, these tubes still tend to back out of the bronchus to the trachea and partially obstruct it. Furthermore, the distal lumen of the blocker is too small to be effective for suctioning. Therefore, the use of a double-lumen tube is preferred.

Both right- and left-sided tubes can be used for separated ventilation on either side. The right-sided tube, when applied for left lung collapse, has a risk of obstructing the upper-lobe bronchus. The left-sided double-lumen tube, because of its ease in handling, has a lower risk of improper placement and has become the instrument of choice for most cases of one-lung anesthesia. It is essential to confirm proper positioning of the tube with a flexible bronchoscope after the patient is turned into the lateral decubitus position.

Continuous monitoring of the patient's oxygenation during the procedure is a basic requirement. The lung should be ventilated with a tidal volume of approximately 10 ml/kg, and the respiratory rate adjusted to maintain the

$PaCO_2$ around 40 mm Hg. If hypoxemia persists, positive end-expiratory pressure (PEEP) or continuous positive airway pressure (CPAP) or a combination of both should be applied. If necessary, the operation should be interrupted to allow temporary reinflation of the collapsed lung.

POSITION

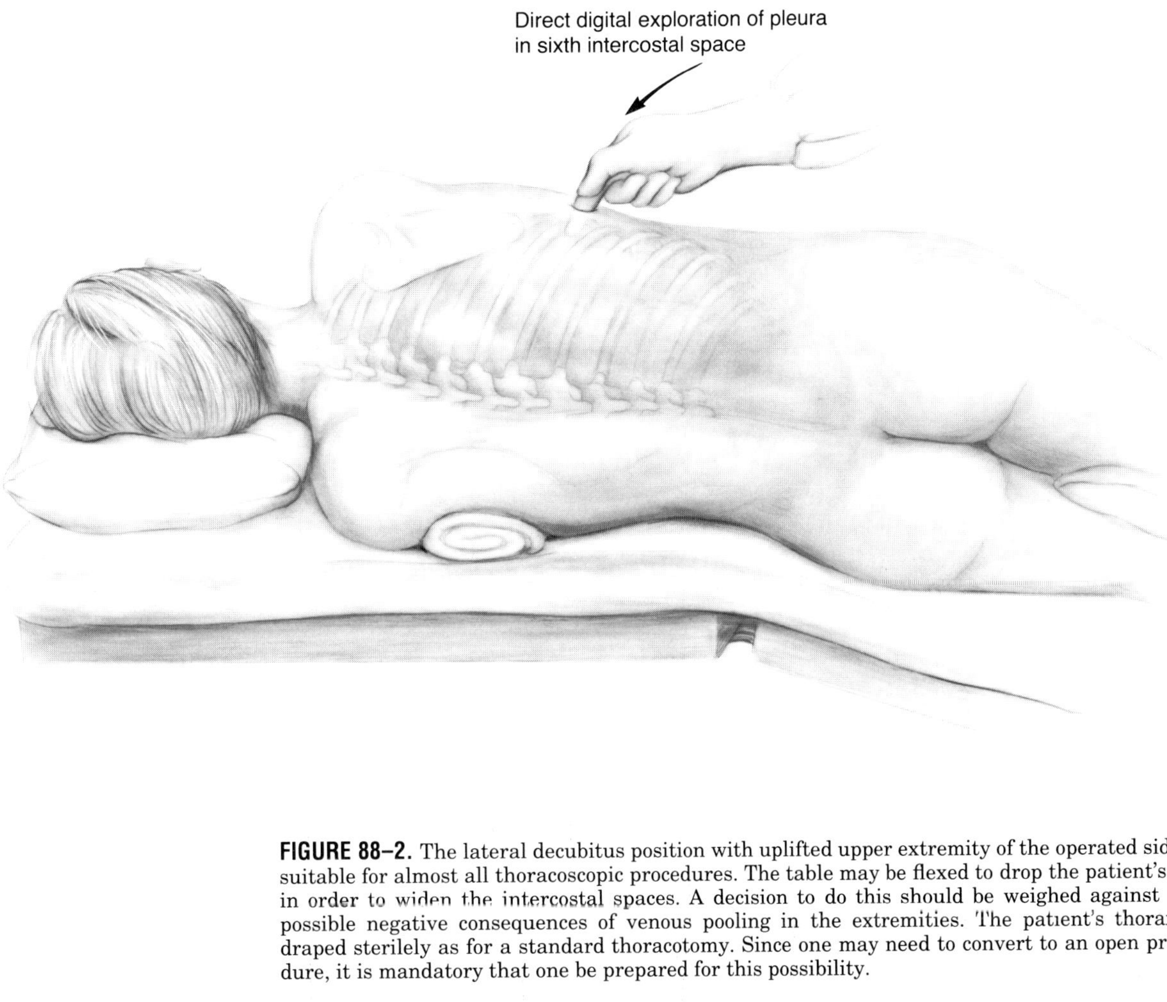

FIGURE 88–2. The lateral decubitus position with uplifted upper extremity of the operated side is suitable for almost all thoracoscopic procedures. The table may be flexed to drop the patient's hip in order to widen the intercostal spaces. A decision to do this should be weighed against any possible negative consequences of venous pooling in the extremities. The patient's thorax is draped sterilely as for a standard thoracotomy. Since one may need to convert to an open procedure, it is mandatory that one be prepared for this possibility.

PROCEDURE

The initial, and probably the most important, part of the thoracoscopic procedure is design of a strategy for placement of ports for the camera and other instruments. Improper placement of the ports during laparoscopy can often be compensated for by the extensive compliance and flexibility of the abdominal wall. However, because the thoracic cavity is rigid, a misplaced thoracic port complicates or may lead to failure of the procedure.

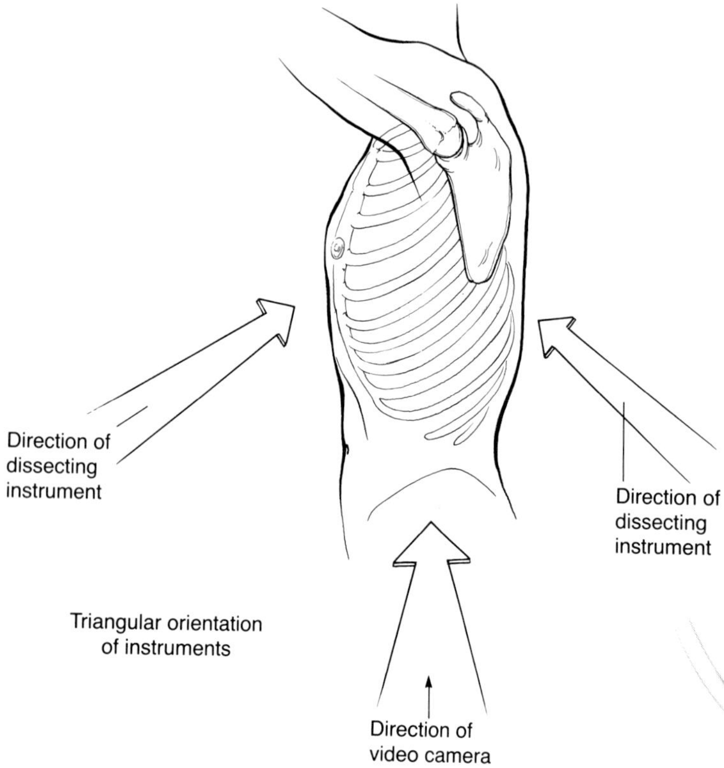

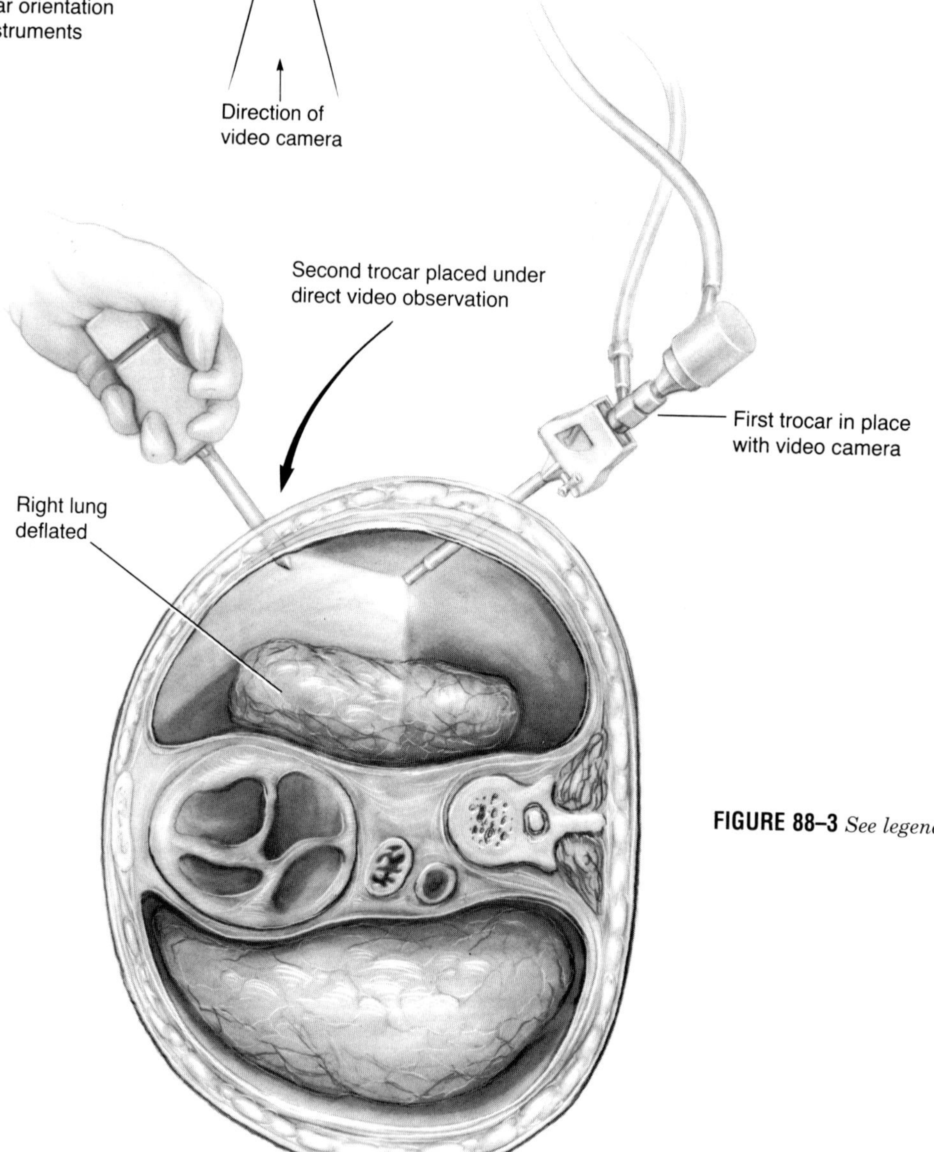

FIGURE 88–3 *See legend on opposite page*

FIGURE 88–3. It is important to orient the endoscopic instruments and camera in the same direction, toward the target of interest. This helps to avoid the mirror-image effect, which can further complicate an already technically demanding procedure. Triangulation of the scope and the accessory instruments prevents the interference of one instrument with the others during the operation. Generally speaking, it is most suitable initially to place the scope within the fifth to seventh intercostal space in the anterior to posterior axillary line. The intercostal spaces are maximally widened in this area, and a panoramic view of the thorax can be obtained. Repositioning may be helpful later, depending on the procedure being performed.

Before the trocars are inserted, the lung should be deflated. Because collapse of the alveoli takes some time, it is useful to request lung deflation as soon as the patient is positioned. Usually two to four trocars are necessary to complete the procedure. Incisions for the placement of trocars are from 1 to 2 cm long, depending on the size of the instruments. When the initial trocar is placed, the subcutaneous tissue and underlying musculature are divided with cautery under direct visual control until the pleural space is entered. By introducing the finger into the thorax, the surgeon can be assured that there are no adhesions and that the lung is collapsed. By this approach the initial trocar and camera can be inserted safely into the pleural cavity, and injury to the lung parenchyma is avoided.

If the lung is not completely collapsed, inflating the pleural cavity with CO_2, keeping the pressure below 10 mm Hg, can be helpful. The remaining trocars are inserted under direct endoscopic visualization. They are inserted above the edge of the lower rib to avoid injury to the intercostal bundle. Some form of thoracoscopic port should always be used for passage of the scope. However, direct passage of instruments through the chest wall is an acceptable technique, particularly when standard thoracic instruments are being used.

After the procedure is completed, hemostasis of the operative site and the trocar sites should be confirmed. Generally a chest tube is introduced through one of the incisions. The tube is fixed to the skin with sutures. After all instruments are removed, the incisions are closed in layers. The lung is re-expanded, and the tube is connected to suction. The chest tube is removed when all air leaks are sealed and drainage is less than 100 ml per day.

CHUNG-PING HSU, M.D.
JAMES M. DOUGLAS, JR., M.D.

89

Thoracoscopic Wedge Resection for Indeterminate Pulmonary Nodule

Video-assisted thoracoscopic surgery provides an excellent modality for wedge resection of peripheral pulmonary nodules. It is particularly useful for the diagnosis of metastatic disease or infectious and inflammatory nodules. In patients with poor pulmonary function, it may provide a means of surgical resection of a primary carcinoma that might otherwise go unresected. In general, wedge resection of primary carcinomas of the lung in patients who are candidates for standard lobectomy remains a controversial topic. The availability of a thoracoscopic approach should not be the determining factor in making the decision to proceed with that mode of therapy. Furthermore, if thoracoscopic wedge resection is chosen as a technique for removal of a possible isolated carcinoma, time-honored thoracic surgical principles, including adequate surgical margins, must be adhered to. Because currently employed endoscopic stapling systems do not allow for the degree of margin that is possible with standard open stapling techniques, a thoracoscopically assisted technique for wedge resection is preferred when a narrow margin becomes a concern. In that circumstance, the thoracoscope is employed to identify the nodule, following which a mini-thoracotomy over the area of interest is performed. Open stapling techniques are then used to perform the wedge resection.

The thoracoscopic approach is best suited for pulmonary nodules that lie on or just beneath the surface of the lung. Nodules larger than 2 cm in diameter may be evaluated with incisional biopsy, but are problematic for wedge excision with the current endoscopic stapling device. Although experience with the techniques described here allows superficial nodules to be identified by the surgeon, preoperative needle localization may help identify nodules smaller than 1 cm in diameter and those more than 1 cm beneath the surface of the lung.

Several factors limit the utility of thoracoscopic wedge resection: small nodule (<1 cm), subpleural lesion, lesions in the interlobar fissure or diaphragmatic surface, diffuse parenchymal disease or emphysema, and inexperience. With improvements in instrumentation, and especially the surgeon's experience, most indeterminate peripheral pulmonary nodules can be thoracoscopically resected safely.

PATIENT PREPARATION

Consent for possible open thoracotomy should be obtained before operation. The patient should have no oral intake for at least 8 hours. No specific medication is needed except overnight oral sedative, if necessary. The axillary hair should be shaved. One problem specific to this category of patient is the method of localization for subpleural pulmonary nodule before the thoracoscopic procedure. The current available methods for preoperative localization of the pulmonary nodule include computed tomography (CT) scan examination, needle localization (CT or sono-guided), and methylene blue stain. Even with these techniques, small nodules (<1 cm) still present with some difficulties for localization. Under such circumstances, instrumental palpation, digital palpation, or even intraoperative ultrasound detection will be imperative.

ANESTHESIA

General anesthesia with a double-lumen endobronchial tube is used. The lateral decubitus position is standard. If the patient has a localization needle in the chest, the lung should not be collapsed hastily before the thoracoscope is introduced. Dislodgement of the needle may compel the surgeon to make a limited thoracotomy for identification and resection of the nodule.

PROCEDURE

The skin is sterilized and draped as in standard thoracotomy.

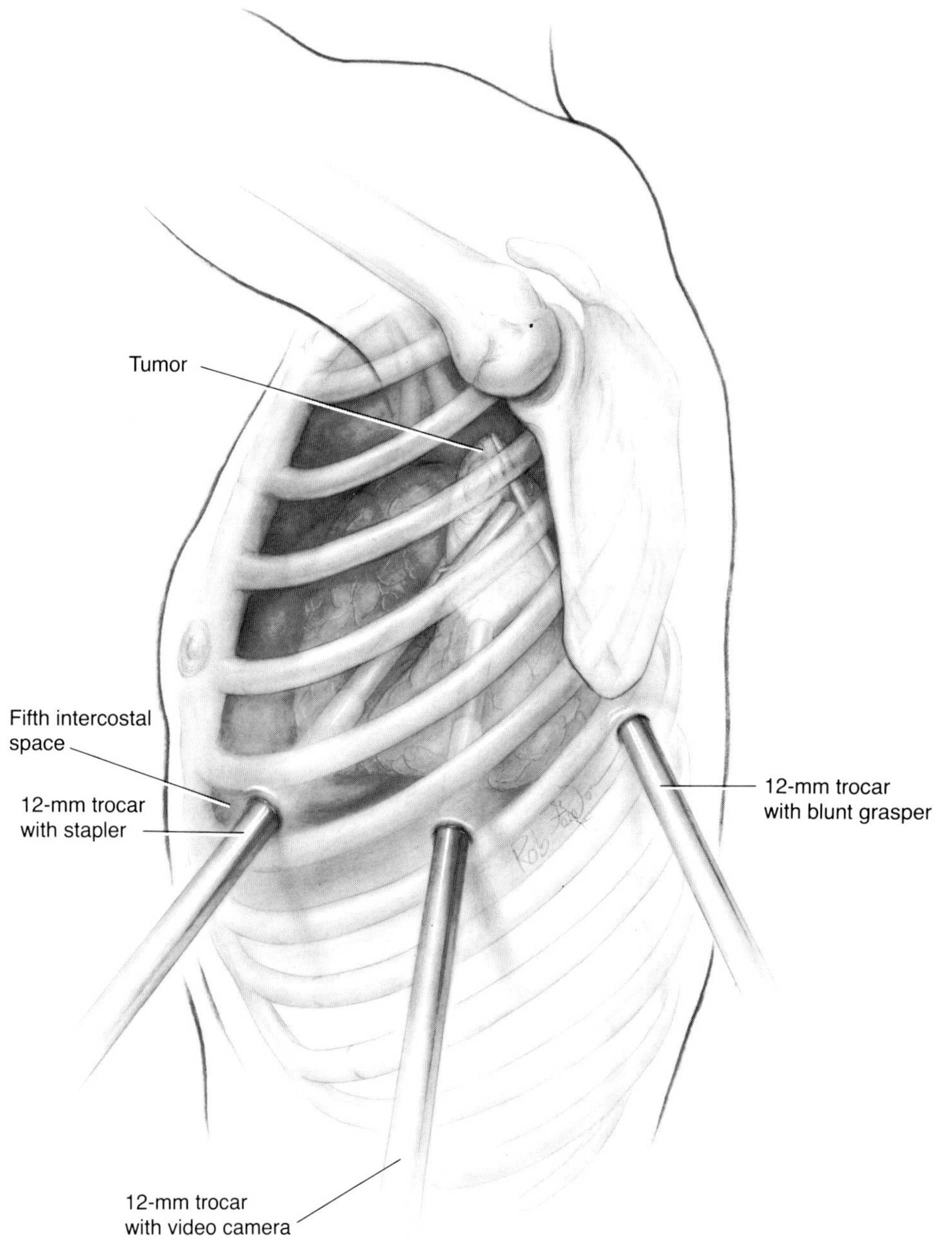

FIGURE 89–1 *See legend on opposite page*

FIGURE 89–1. The initial incision is made at the fifth to seventh intercostal space (ICS) in the middle or posterior axillary lines (according to the site of the lesion) for introduction of the thoracoscope. The nodule is lifted, and the stapler is applied at a 2-cm distance on the healthy lung tissue. Other incisions for accessory ICS access sites should be made under direct visual control by the thoracoscope. Usually two more ICS access sites are required to complete the pulmonary wedge resection. These access sites should aim at the pathologic site of interest and form the so-called "triangulation" for easy instrumental manipulation and prevention of mirror image. Sites should be placed at least 10 cm apart in order to prevent "dueling" of the instruments.

It is essential to perform a digital exploration before insertion of the initial trocar. Loose intrapleural adhesions can be easily taken down. However, diffuse and dense intrapleural adhesions prohibit further attempts at thoracoscopy. Conversion to a mini-thoracotomy shortens the operative time and decreases the operative risk.

With the operated lung collapsed by one-lung anesthesia, the thoracoscope is introduced through the initial port site. After a thorough exploratory thoracoscopy, the accessory ICS access sites for lung resection are selected, aimed at the areas of interest under direct visual control. The first step is to identify the pulmonary nodule. If the nodule has been marked preoperatively, there will be little problem in recognizing the lesion. If not, the nodule can be identified by endoscopic inspection, by instrumental palpation, by digital examination, or even by ultrasound. Some nodules show hypervascularity or scarring of the overlying visceral pleura, and others show effacement of the pulmonary parenchyma surrounding the nodule. All of these are clues for recognizing the lesions. If the nodule cannot be found by inspection, then instrumental palpation should be performed. Our experiences show that a soft-tipped stick dissector is particularly useful for instrumental palpation. Alternatively, under partial inflation of the lung, one can use the finger to identify the nodule. Intraoperative ultrasonic detection is under investigation; however, few people have this experience. Most of the lesions can be localized by the methods described here. Only rarely is an open thoracotomy necessary because of inability to identify the nodule. Fortunately, accumulation of experience will lower the incidence of open thoracotomy.

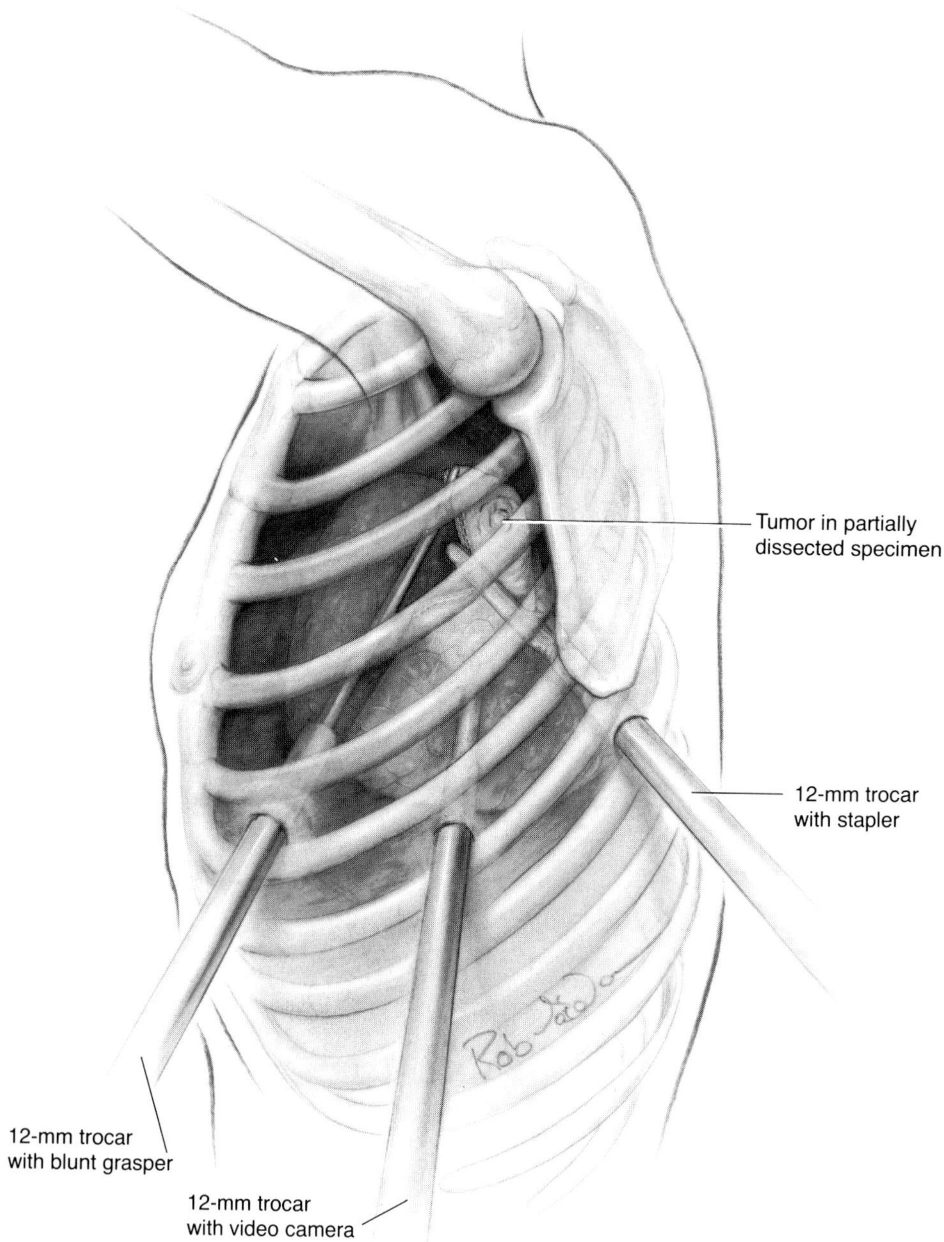

FIGURE 89–2. The nodule is grasped and resected with stapling techniques. The port sites of the stapler and the grasper are switched to complete the wedge resection.

A nodule lying on the interlobar fissure or diaphragmatic surface is not easily resected with an endoscopic stapling device. Persistent attempts in such circumstances may lead to parenchymal laceration of the staple line with air leak and bleeding. Core excision with laser techniques has been successful in some surgeons' experience. Usually, the whole procedure can be completed with two or three staplings. The resected specimen can be extracted from one of the access sites. Before removal, the specimen can be placed in a specially designed bag or finger of a sterile surgical glove. The specimen is sent for frozen section pathologic study. If the result is inconclusive, thoracotomy may be required. After hemostasis is ensured, a chest tube is inserted into the pleural cavity through the lowest access site and connected to an underwater sealed drain. The other incisions are closed in layers.

CHUNG-PING HSU, M.D.
JAMES M. DOUGLAS, JR., M.D.

90

Thoracoscopic Pulmonary Biopsy for Diffuse Lung Disease

Open-lung biopsy has long been the standard approach for the diagnosis of diffuse lung disease. But since the introduction of the endoscopic stapler in the early 1990s, this standard has changed because the thoracoscopic approach is effective and less invasive. However, patients who require mechanical ventilation are not good candidates for a thoracoscopic procedure. For critically ill patients, open thoracotomy can be done without the need for endotracheal tube manipulation for one-lung ventilation and its attendant risks.

PATIENT PREPARATION

The patient should have no oral intake for at least 8 hours. No specific premedication is necessary except an overnight oral sedative, if desired. Preoperative preparation should be the same as that for routine thoracotomies.

ANESTHESIA

General anesthesia for all patients is preferred. In most circumstances, a left-sided double-lumen endobronchial tube is used. We routinely use a pulse oximeter for detection of the peripheral O_2 saturation during the operation.

PROCEDURE

The patient is placed in the lateral decubitus position. A rolling pad is put under the dependent axilla to protect the neurovascular bundles.

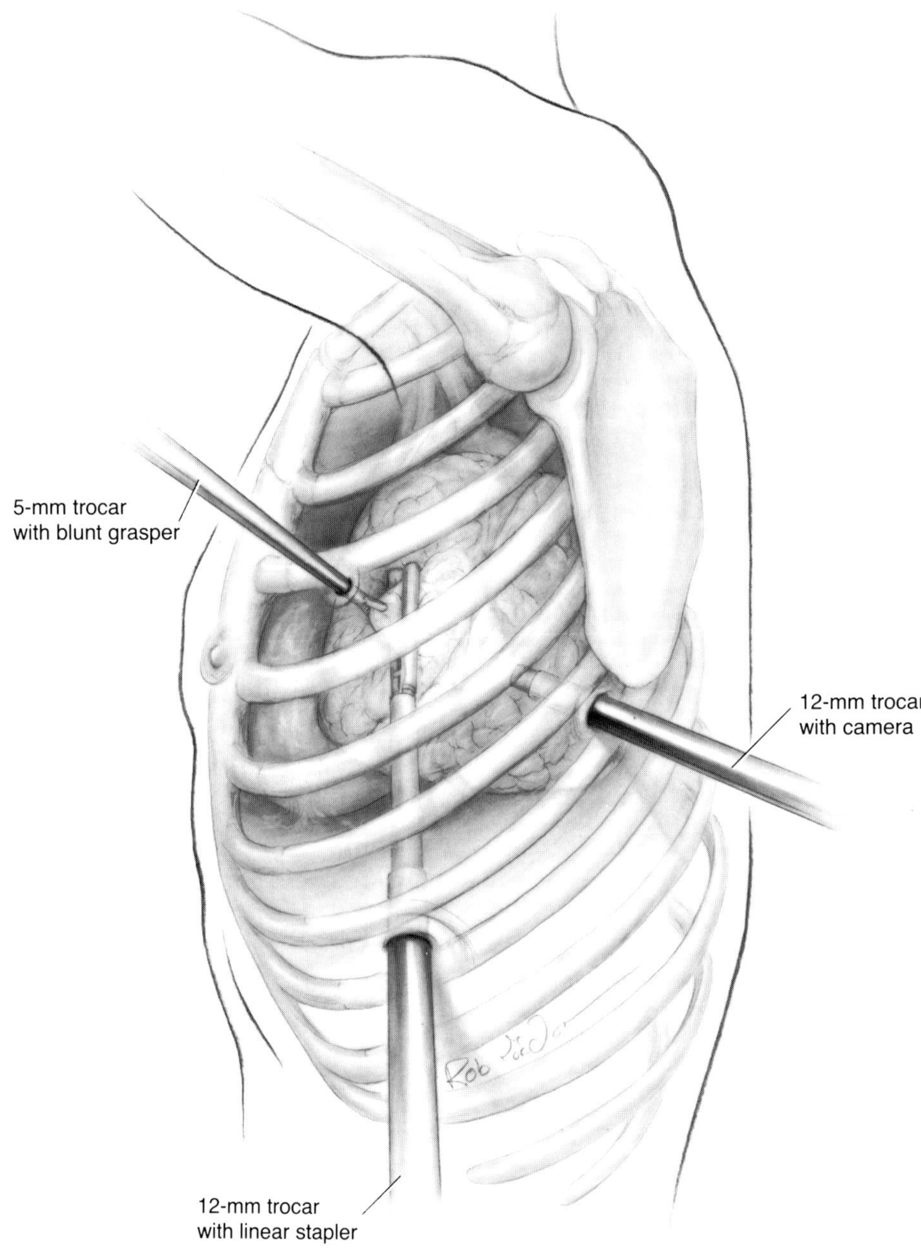

FIGURE 90–1. With the operated lung collapsed by one-lung ventilation, the thoracoscope is introduced through an initial port site placed in the fifth to seventh intercostal spaces in the mid- to posterior axillary line. After a thorough exploratory thoracoscopy, the accessory access sites for lung biopsy are selected, aimed at the areas of interest under direct visual control. Two additional access sites are typically required. They should be placed at least 10 cm apart in the anterior axillary line and the posterior axillary to midscapular line. The lung is grasped in the area of interest for application of stapler. Specially designed endoscopic lung clamps may be used. Alternatively, one can introduce the traditional thoracotomy instruments (ring forceps, lung forceps, or Kelly forceps) through the access site without using the thoracoscopic port. The endoscopic stapler is introduced through another access site for pulmonary biopsy. Usually, the procedure can be completed with two or three staplings. Multiple biopsies from different lobes can be obtained. The resected specimen can be pulled out from one of the access sites and is sent for pathologic and microbiologic studies. Air leakage can be checked by instillation of saline on the suture line. Adequate homeostasis is essential. A chest tube is inserted into the pleural cavity through the lowest access site for underwater sealed drainage. The incisions are closed in layers.

IVO HANKE, M.D.
JAMES M. DOUGLAS, JR., M.D.

91

Thoracoscopic Resection of Blebs and Pleurodesis

The thoracoscopic approach to the resection of pulmonary blebs and pleurodesis is ideally suited for patients with recurrent spontaneous pneumothorax. This approach provides visualization of the entire thoracic cavity, and the instrumentation is sophisticated enough to allow treatment identical to that afforded by the open operation. Recovery from thoracoscopic bleb resection and pleurodesis is quicker than for any of the open approaches, and the results appear to be comparable.

PROCEDURE

The patient is placed in the lateral decubitus position with a double-lumen endotracheal tube in place and is prepared as for standard thoracotomy. No specific considerations for the thoracoscopic approach are necessary. If the patient has undergone previous chest tube placement in a standard lateral fifth or sixth intercostal space, this entry site will be used for insertion of the thoracoscope. The skin incision is re-excised after extensive sterile skin preparation. Ideally, the initial insertion site for the scope is within the fifth to sixth intercostal space in the anterior axillary line. The accessory ports are then inserted at a distance of more than 10 cm laterally in the fourth intercostal space and posteriorly in the fourth or fifth intercostal space under direct thoracoscopic visualization. The underlying disease process and the consequences of chest tube insertion are regularly associated with the formation of adhesions. The filmy adhesions can be taken down easily with blunt dissection. When more firm and solid adhesions are formed, the use of electrocautery and scissors is necessary.

Commonly the blebs are large enough to be easily recognized. If not, the air leak in the bleb can be visualized by partial inflation of the lung. Most commonly they are located in the apex of the upper lobe and the superior segment of the lower lobe.

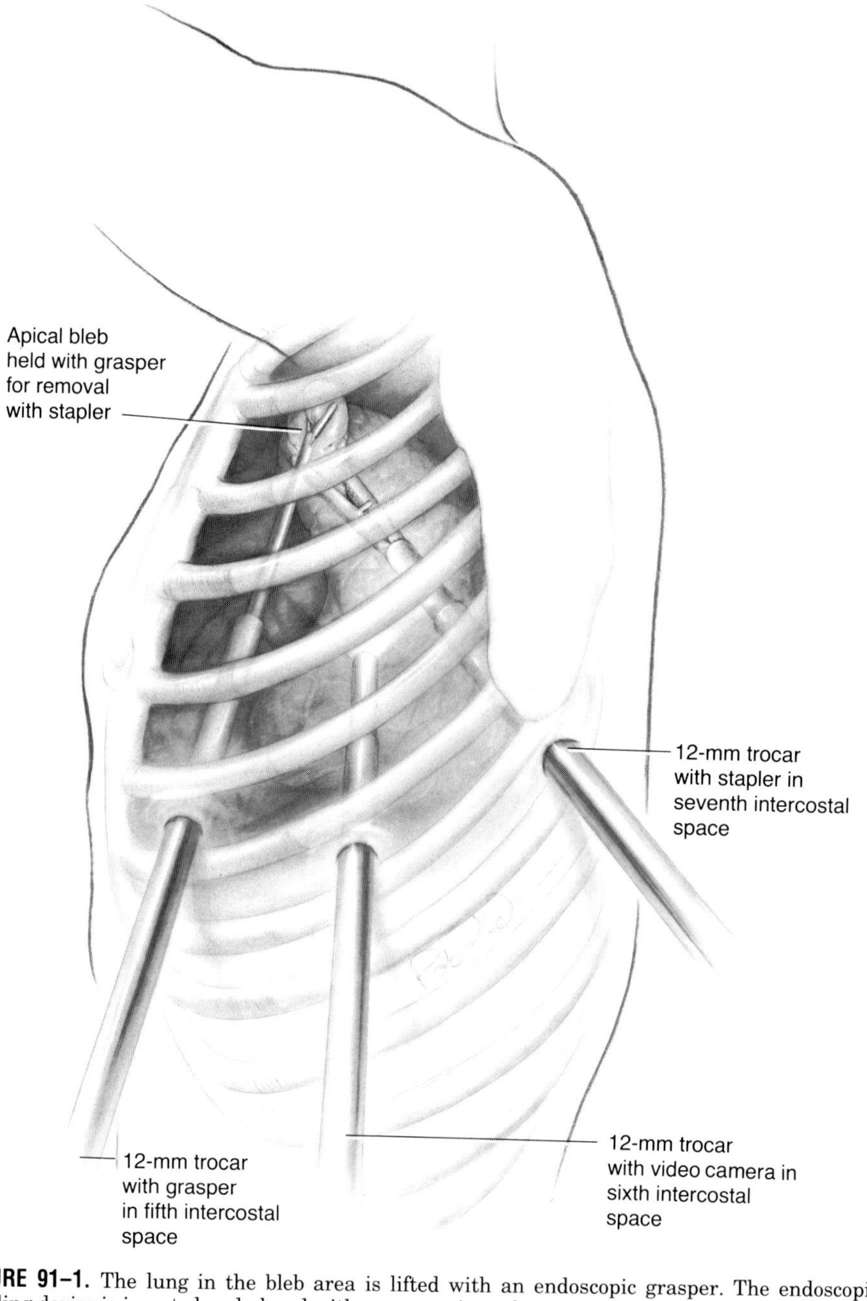

FIGURE 91–1. The lung in the bleb area is lifted with an endoscopic grasper. The endoscopic stapling device is inserted and placed with an approximately 1-cm safe margin from the bleb onto the healthy lung tissue. The stapler is then fired and the bleb resected. Usually the bleb resection can be completed with two or three reload staplings. It is advisable to approach the target from different directions, by switching the position of the grasper and the stapler.

After the specimen is extracted from the thorax, the pleural cavity is irrigated with saline solution. Then the patient is moved into the Trendelenburg position so that the suture line is under the water level. The lung is inflated, and any air leak can be easily found. Subsequently all irrigation fluid is removed with suction.

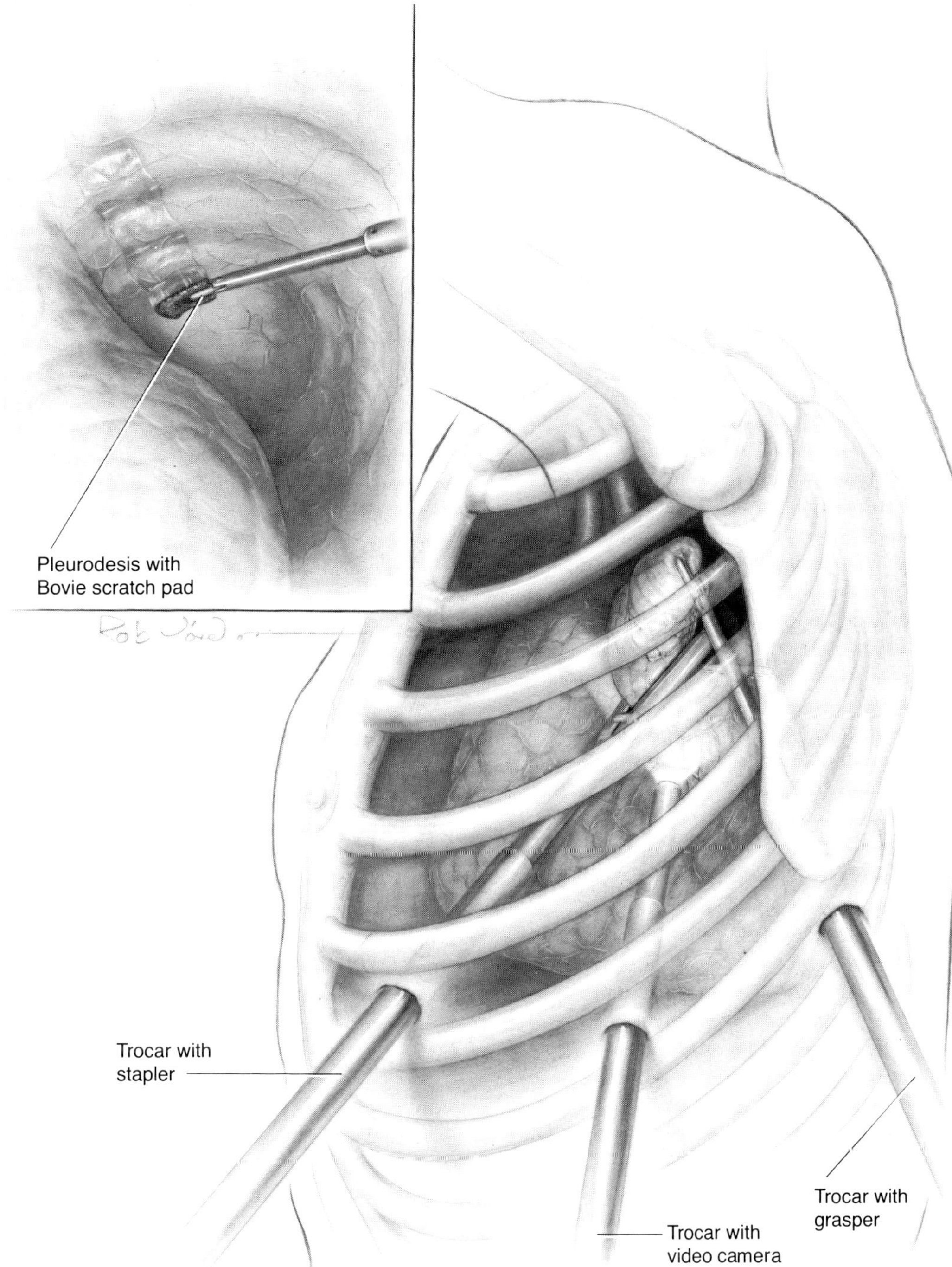

FIGURE 91–2. In order to decrease the probability of recurrent pneumothorax, pleurodesis should also be performed. Several techniques can be applied. The simplest, time-honored method is mechanical abrasion. This can be accomplished thoracoscopically using either a Bovie scratch pad on a long Kelly clamp or a sponge on a long ring forceps. Under direct vision the apical part of the thoracic cavity and then the rest of parietal pleura are abraded.

When the procedure is completed, a chest tube is inserted through a lower trocar site and placed to underwater suction. An extra hole cut out of the tube near the chest wall entry site allows better fluid drainage. Care should be taken to be certain that the extra hole remains within the pleural space and that the size is comparable to the manufacturer's holes.

CHUNG-PING HSU, M.D.
JAMES M. DOUGLAS, JR., M.D.

92

Thoracoscopic Approach to the Aorticopulmonary Window

The classic mediastinoscopy for lung cancer staging gives limited access to the aorticopulmonary window and subcarinal regions. The Chamberlain incision for anterior mediastinoscopy was the standard approach to the aorticopulmonary window before the introduction of video-assisted thoracoscopy. The merits of video-assisted thoracoscopic exploration of the thoracic cavity and biopsy are still under investigation. However, the advantages include the following: The entire thoracic cavity can be examined at the same time; tumor staging under direct visualization is possible; and the subcarinal and anterior mediastinal lymph nodes can be accessed easily.

PATIENT PREPARATION

Consent for possible open thoracotomy should be obtained before the procedure. The patient should have no oral intake for at least 8 hours. No specific medication is needed except an overnight oral sedative, if desired. The axillary hair should be shaved.

ANESTHESIA

General anesthesia with selected lung ventilation by way of a double-lumen endobronchial tube is required for all patients. The intraoperative monitoring is the same as for other video-assisted thoracoscopic (VATS) procedures.

PROCEDURE

The patient lies in the left lateral decubitus position as for standard thoracotomy. A rolling pad is placed under the right axilla for protection of the neurovascular bundles. The skin is sterilized and draped as for standard thoracotomy. A 1-cm incision is made at the sixth or seventh intercostal space in the midaxillary line for introduction of the thoracoscope. Another incision can be made in the posterior axillary line, one intercostal space below the thoracoscopic port, for introduction of a lung retractor if needed. Usually, two other access sites, one in the fourth intercostal space in the anterior axillary line and the other in the fifth intercostal space posterior to the medial border of the scapula, are made. The vagus nerve and phrenic nerve should be identified before any dissection of the aorticopulmonary window.

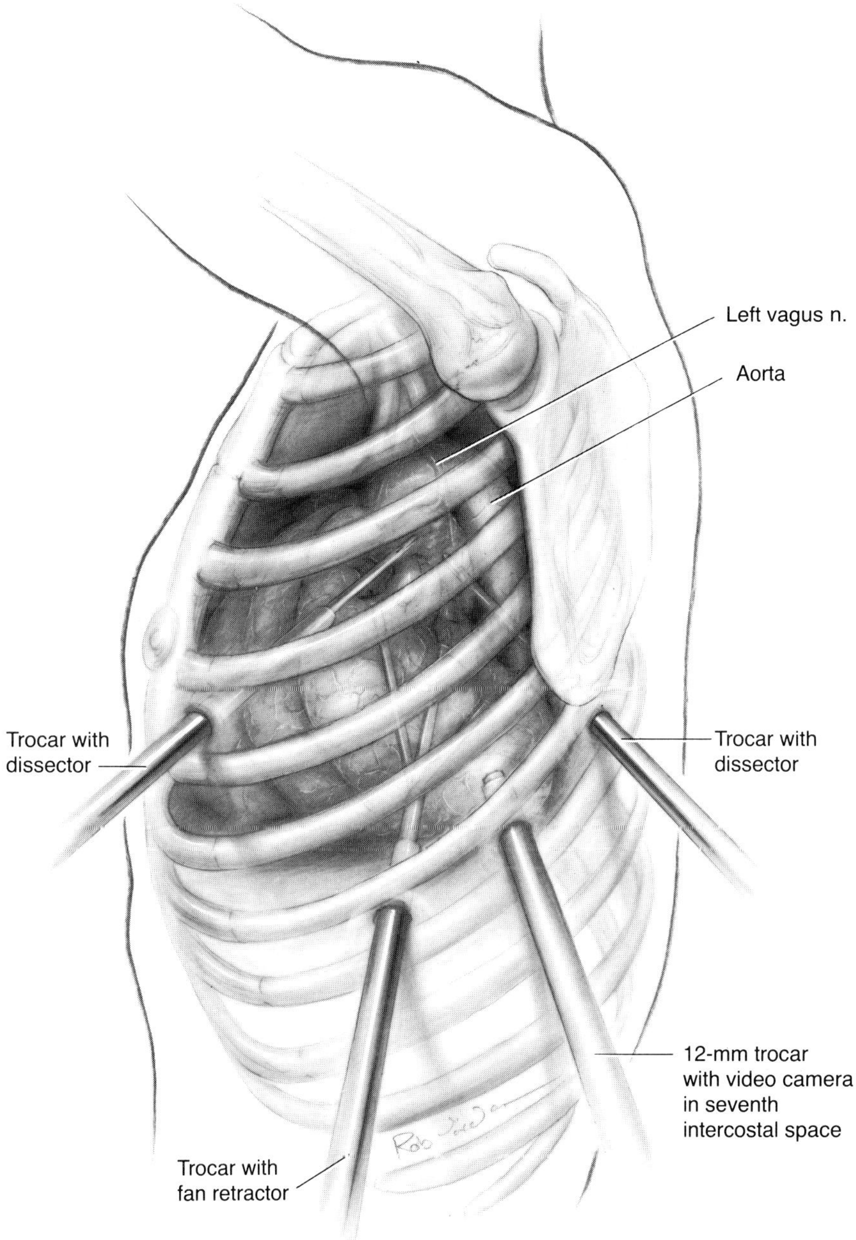

FIGURE 92–1. The pleural covering over the lymph node is opened and the lymph node dissected carefully without interfering with the recurrent laryngeal nerve. The vascular pedicle can be secured with endoscopic clips. Meticulous dissection to avoid injury to the aorta and main pulmonary artery is essential. After adequate hemostasis, a chest tube is inserted into the pleural cavity through the lowest access site for underwater sealed drainage. The other incisions are closed with absorbable sutures.

CHUNG-PING HSU, M.D.
JAMES M. DOUGLAS, JR., M.D.

93

Video-Assisted Thoracoscopic Surgery for Posterior Mediastinal Tumors

Most posterior mediastinal tumors are benign neurogenic tumors. They are frequently detected by incidental chest film before they become symptomatic. These tumors are usually small, lie in the costovertebral recess, and are readily accessible for video-assisted thoracoscopic surgery (VATS) resection. However, a preoperative computed tomography (CT) scan is essential to exclude the possibility of spinal cord invasion (dumbbell tumor) or direct mediastinal organ invasion. With these findings, a thoracoscopic approach is not suitable. Tumors larger than 5 cm in diameter are probably better approached through a limited posterolateral thoracotomy for resection en bloc. Once the tumor size exceeds 5 cm, the malignant potential increases. We suggest open thoracotomy rather than VATS for radical and curative resection of malignant neoplasms.

PATIENT PREPARATION

The patient should have no oral intake for at least 8 hours. No specific medication is needed except overnight oral sedative, if desired. The axillary hair should be shaved. The possibility of open thoracotomy for tumor resection should be discussed before operation.

ANESTHESIA

General anesthesia with single-lung ventilation capability is required for all patients. Pulse oximeter for monitor of peripheral O_2 saturation is routinely used during the period of selected lung ventilation. The collapsed lung should be ventilated every 30 minutes or whenever the O_2 saturation falls below 90%.

POSITION

The patient lies in the lateral decubitus position, as for standard thoracotomy. A rolling pad is put under the dependent axilla to protect the neurovascular bundles. The exposure can be improved by putting the patient in a "jackknife" position, which spreads the intercostal spaces and facilitates manipulation of the instruments.

PROCEDURE

The skin is sterilized and draped as in standard thoracotomy.

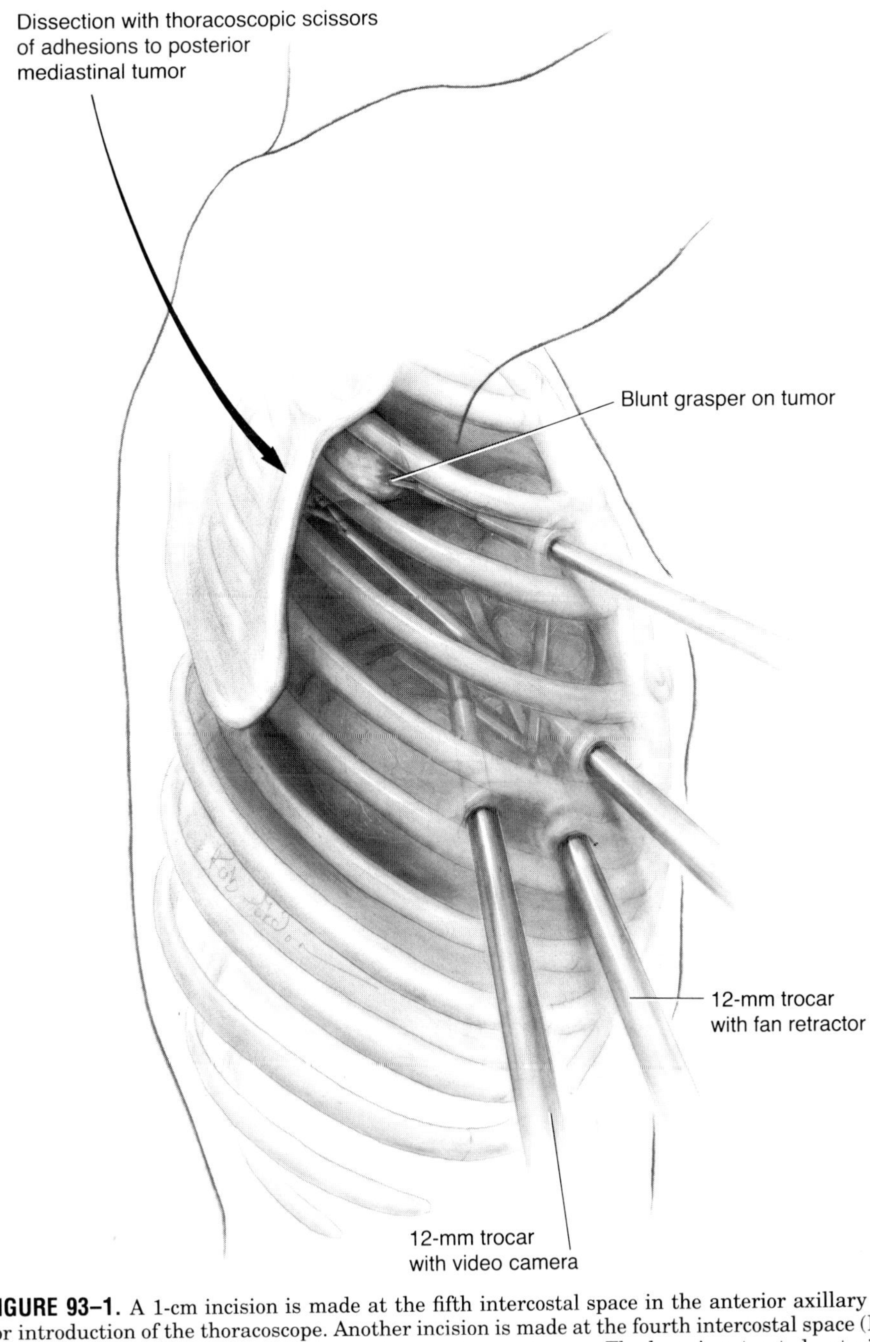

FIGURE 93–1. A 1-cm incision is made at the fifth intercostal space in the anterior axillary line for introduction of the thoracoscope. Another incision is made at the fourth intercostal space (ICS) in the anterior axillary line for introduction of a lung retractor. The lung is retracted anteriorly with a fan retractor. For upper and middle posterior mediastinal tumors, the accessory ICS access sites should be made at anterior to middle axillary lines between the second to fourth intercostal spaces. For lower posterior mediastinal tumors, the accessory ICS access sites should be made at the midaxillary line between the fifth and seventh intercostal spaces. A slight tilting of the operative table to the ventral side of the patient allows the lung to shift anteriorly and improves the endoscopic visual fields.

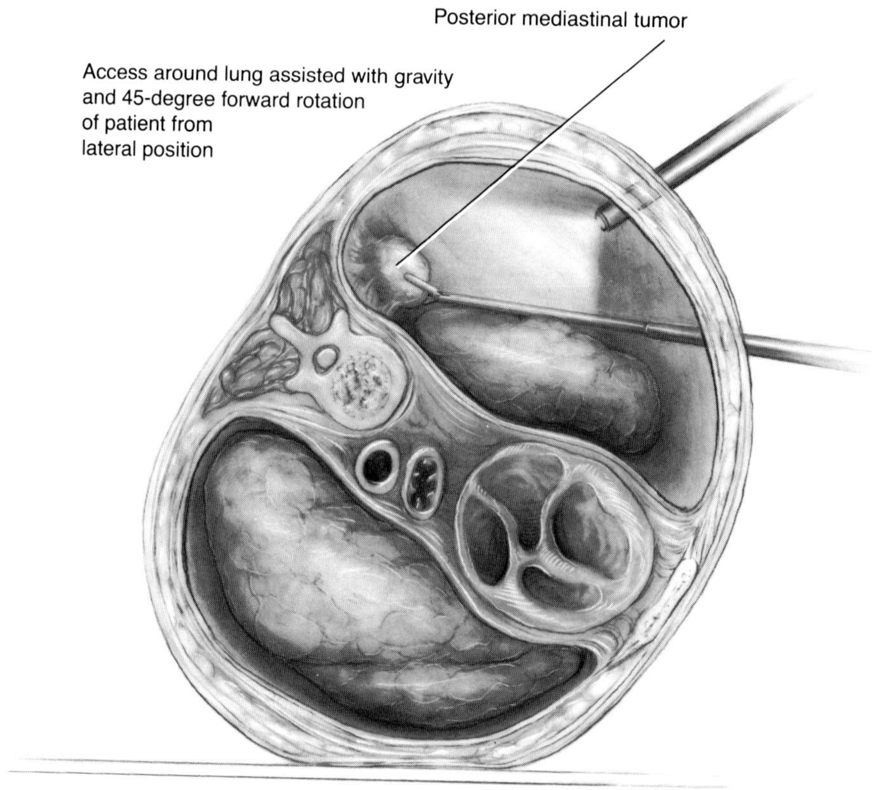

FIGURE 93–2. The endoscopic dissector, scissors, and grasper can be introduced into the pleural cavity through the accessory ICS access sites to complete the tumor resection. The resected tumor can be put into a plastic bag and withdrawn through one of the access sites. The access site may have to be extended to allow tumor removal. Adequate hemostasis is essential. A chest tube (French 28) is inserted into the pleural cavity through the lowest access site for underwater sealed drainage. The other incisions are closed with sutures.

IVO HANKE, M.D.
JAMES M. DOUGLAS, JR., M.D.

94

Pericardial Window

Thoracoscopic pericardial window may be performed from either the left or the right side. Extensive pericardial effusion obliterating the greater part of the left hemithorax is more conveniently approached from the right side. Moderate to small effusions may be approached from either side, but, because of most surgeons' experience, the left side is preferred. The thoracoscopic approach should especially be considered in patients who would otherwise be subjected to thoracotomy. A standard subxiphoidal pericardial window remains an excellent technique for treatment of patients with poor prognoses.

POSITION AND ANESTHESIA

The patient is placed in the lateral decubitus position under general anesthesia with a double-lumen endotracheal tube in place. Standard monitoring is employed. The patient's thorax is draped to create a sterile field, as in thoracotomy. An external defibrillator with sterile paddles should be available.

PROCEDURE

After the lung is collapsed, the initial trocar for the camera is placed within the eighth intercostal space in the posterior axillary line. The pleural space is inspected with the scope. When full anatomic orientation has been achieved, the other instruments should be inserted through the fifth intercostal space in the posterior axillary line and the seventh intercostal space in the anterior axillary line. The pericardial resection can be performed anteriorly or posteriorly to the phrenic nerve.

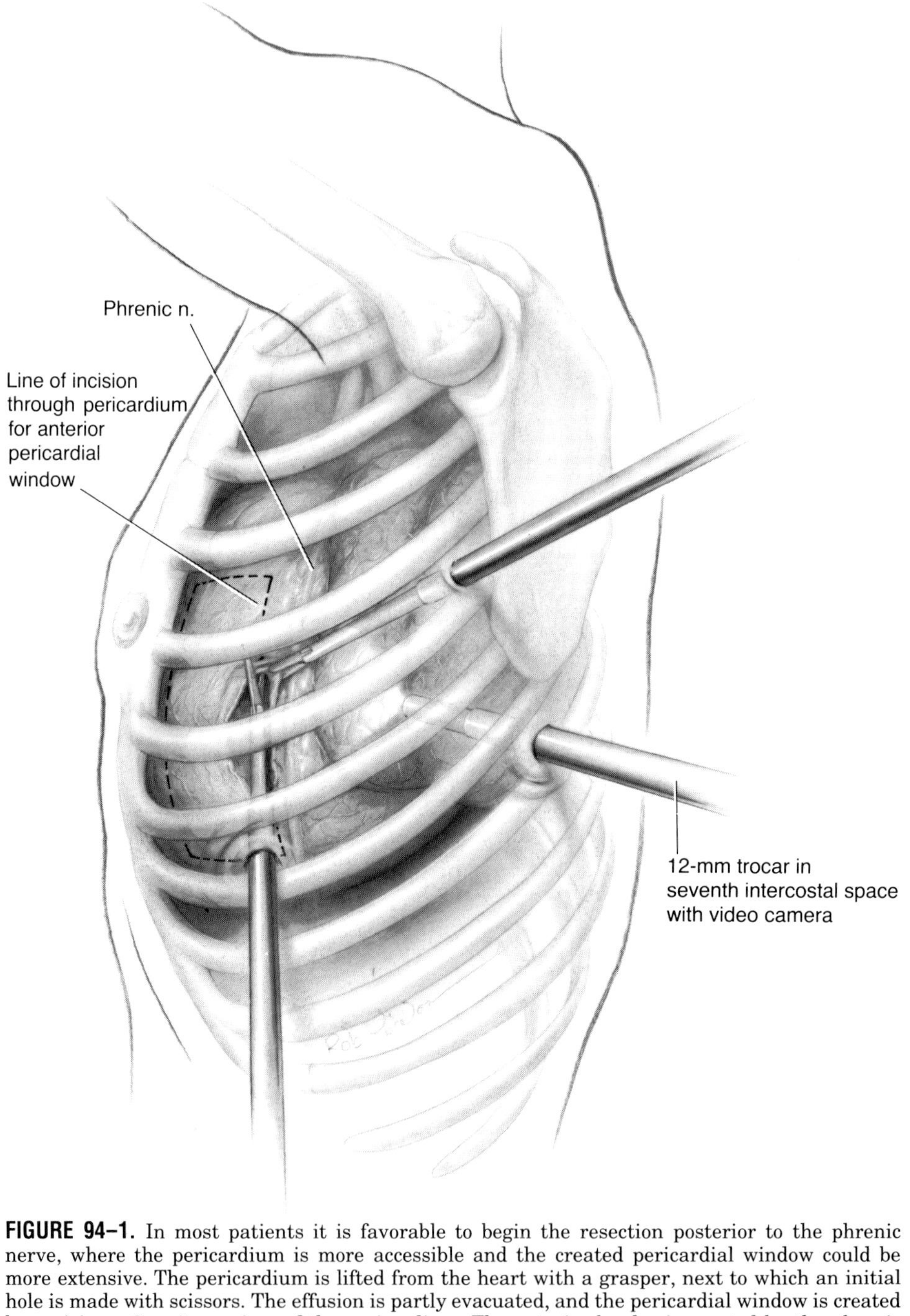

FIGURE 94–1. In most patients it is favorable to begin the resection posterior to the phrenic nerve, where the pericardium is more accessible and the created pericardial window could be more extensive. The pericardium is lifted from the heart with a grasper, next to which an initial hole is made with scissors. The effusion is partly evacuated, and the pericardial window is created by excising a 3 × 5 cm piece of the pericardium. The anterior border is created by the phrenic nerve. When the pericardium is particularly vascular and the fat thick, they may be divided using an endoscopic stapler.

Filmy intrapericardial adhesions can be dissected easily with a soft-tipped stick dissector. All sources of bleeding are meticulously controlled, and the chest tube is placed through one of the trocar's sites. Consequently, all instruments are extracted one after the other. The possibility of bleeding from the chest wall is ruled out by visualization of the port sites with the scope. The incisions are closed in layers.

IVO HANKE, M.D.
JAMES M. DOUGLAS, JR., M.D.

95

Video-Assisted Thoracoscopic Surgical Approach to the Anterior Mediastinum

The diagnosis and treatment of anterior mediastinal disorders traditionally have been challenging. The thoracoscopic approach to this area is useful for both diagnosis and treatment, and is gaining popularity and importance. As with traditional surgical approaches, the most frequent procedures in the anterior mediastinum are biopsies of masses and lymph nodes suggestive of hematopoietic neoplasms and diseases. Less frequently performed procedures include thymectomy for myasthenia gravis and resection of thymic, bronchial, or pericardial cysts. Other procedures still remain in the stage of clinical trials and are not currently recommended for routine practice.

POSITION AND ANESTHESIA

Although the lateral decubitus position with uplifted upper extremity of the operated side is suitable for the operation, it is convenient to rotate the patient slightly posteriorly. This position allows the mediastinum and lung to rest more posteriorly, and thereby facilitates the dissection. The patient is routinely anesthetized with a double-lumen tube and separated lung ventilation. Standard monitoring is required.

PROCEDURE

The anterior mediastinum is bounded by the innominate vein superiorly and the left ventricular prominence inferiorly. The lateral borders are formed by the left and right phrenic nerves. The superior surface is the posterior sternum, and the floor is the pericardium. When possible, the anterior mediastinum should be approached from the left side using the heart and pericardium as landmarks.

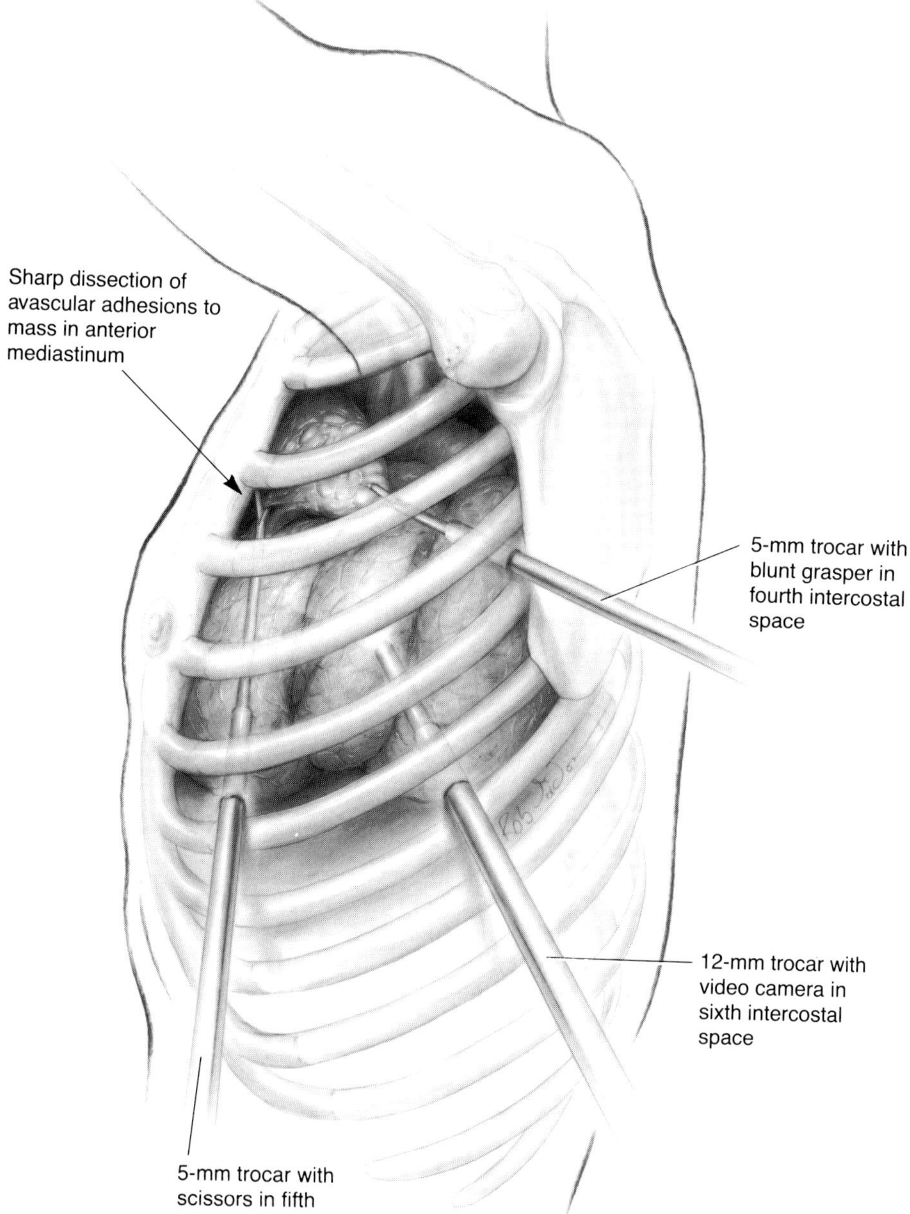

FIGURE 95–1. The initial trocar for the camera is placed within the mid- to posterior axillary line in the fifth intercostal space. The other ports for instruments are placed in the fifth intercostal space in the anterior axillary line and in the third intercostal space in the posterior axillary line. This properly triangulates the instrumentation and enables one to add more ports if necessary. The initial recognition of the innominate vein, its branches, and the phrenic nerve is essential for safe conduct of the operation. The anterior mediastinal tumor is drawn posteriorly with a grasper and dissected with endoscopic scissors. The dissection of the pathology is begun inferiorly and laterally and extended medially, with meticulous clipping and coagulation of all bleeders, especially branches of the innominate vein.

When the procedure is completed and the surgeon is assured that there is no bleeding from the port sites, a chest tube is inserted through one of the port sites and connected to the underwater suction.

JAMES M. DOUGLAS, JR., M.D.

96

Modified Heller Esophagomyotomy for Achalasia

Although balloon dilatation has become extremely popular for the treatment of achalasia, the accepted standard for efficacy and long-term success remains the modified Heller esophagomyotomy performed through a left posterolateral thoracotomy. Recently, experience has been gained with a thoracoscopic approach to this operation. This procedure ideally should yield results comparable to those of the open technique with less patient morbidity. Although the long-term effects of the thoracoscopic approach have yet to be elucidated, this technique is promising and is worthy of description.

PATIENT PREPARATION

The patient is prepared for operation as for a standard Heller esophagomyotomy. Nothing by mouth is given for at least 8 hours before operation. Patients who have the potential to retain food particles in a megaesophagus must have these contents evacuated with special precautions to avoid aspiration. Anesthesia using single-lung ventilation facilitates the procedure. The patient is placed in the right lateral decubitus position as for a standard left posterolateral thoracotomy. Intraoperative monitoring is the same as previously discussed.

EQUIPMENT

Standard thoracoscopic video equipment and instrumentation are required. Additionally, the operation should be done with an endoscopist as part of the team. A flexible gastroscope should be passed transorally, with cooperation between the endoscopist and the anesthesiologist. Passage of the scope may be performed before or after the patient is put in the lateral decubitus position. In either case, care must be taken to protect the endotracheal tube, and undue torque of the endoscope must be avoided to prevent esophageal injury. With the patient in the lateral position, the chest is prepared as for a standard thoracotomy.

PROCEDURE

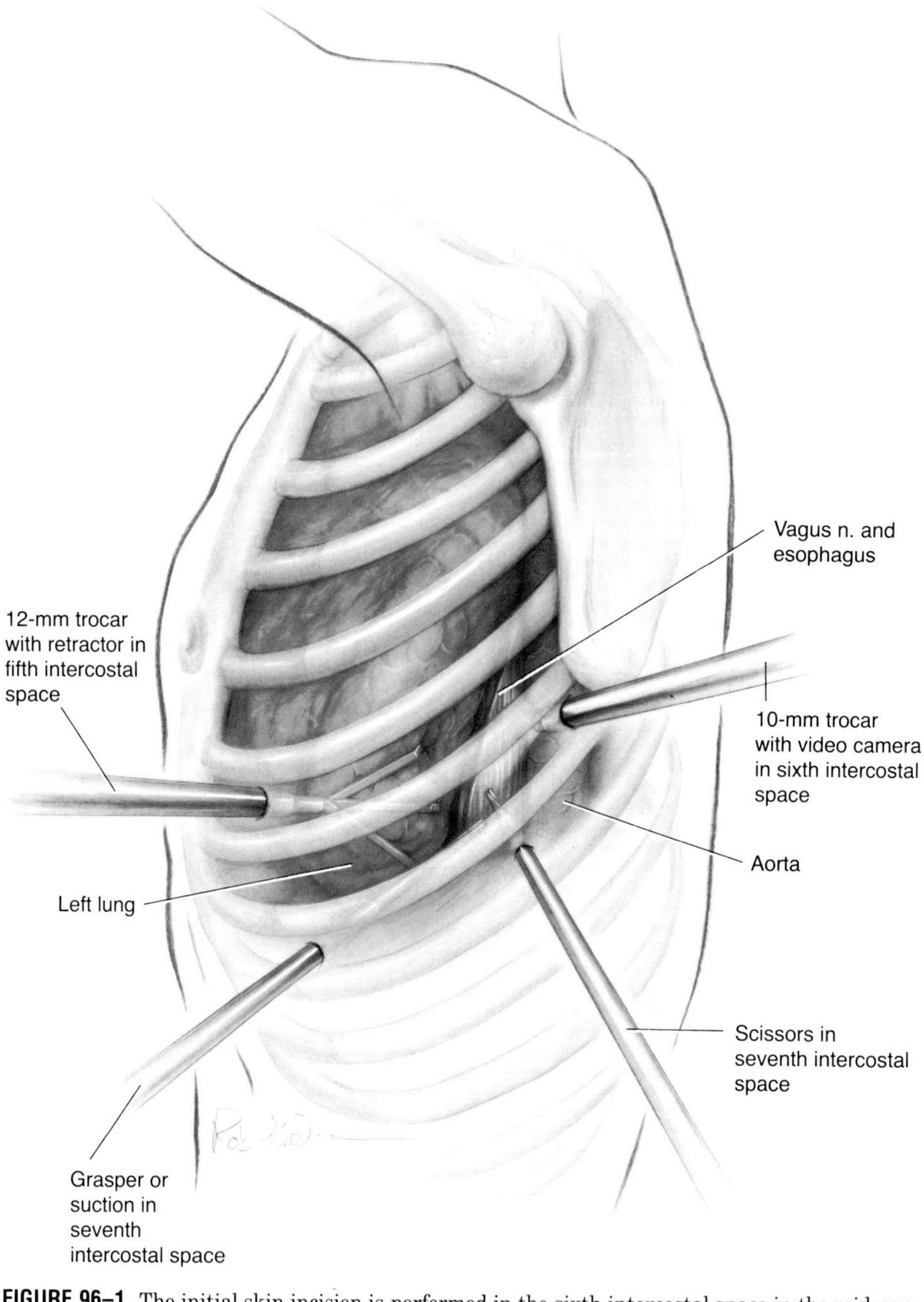

FIGURE 96–1. The initial skin incision is performed in the sixth intercostal space in the midscapular line. Under direct vision, the left hemithorax is entered and a straight, rigid thoracoscope inserted. The hemithorax is visually explored. A 10-mm trocar is then passed through a small incision in the fifth intercostal space in the anterior axillary line. A lung retractor is passed through this trocar, and the left lung is retracted superiorly to reveal the region of the esophageal hiatus. A third trocar is then passed through the seventh intercostal space in the anterior axillary line. This port is used for suction catheters, grasping instruments, and dissectors, as needed. A fourth incision in the seventh intercostal space in the posterior scapular line is used for insertion of scissors and graspers.

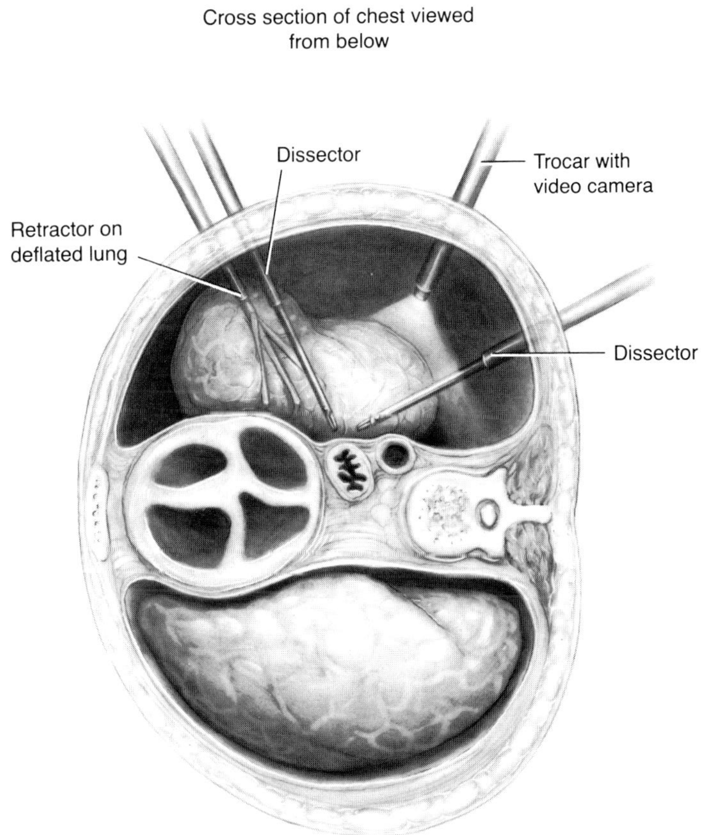

FIGURE 96–2. A cross section of the chest is shown, as viewed from below.

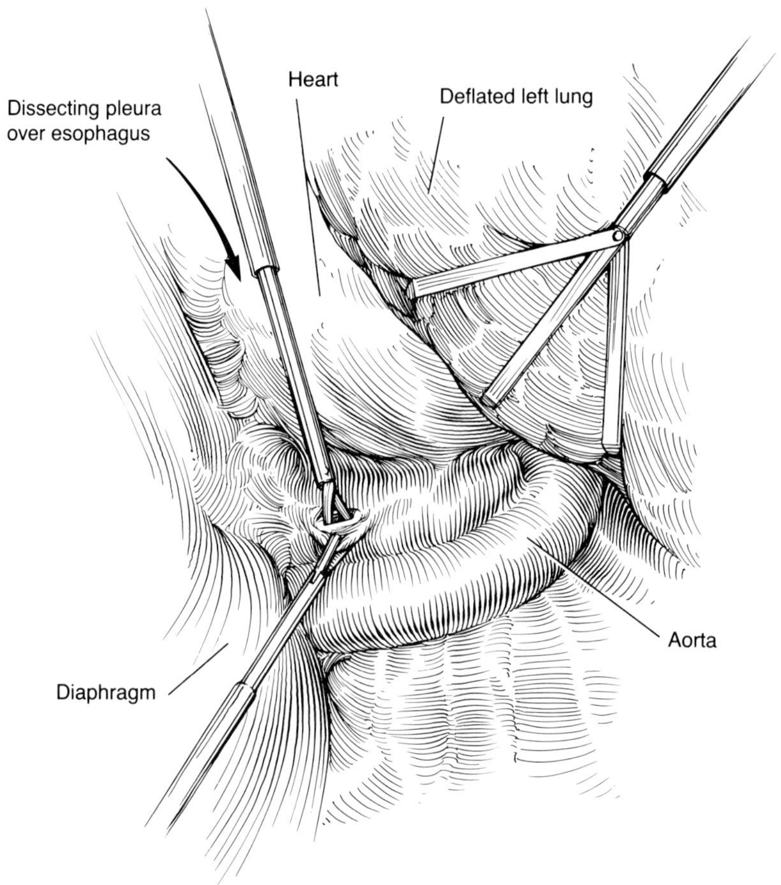

FIGURE 96–3. After the lung is retracted, the mediastinal pleura overlying the lower esophagus is dissected free using blunt and sharp dissection. The gastroscope is passed by the endoscopist with the light on in order to improve visualization of the esophagus. Otherwise, during the course of the dissection, the gastroscope light should be turned on only when necessary. This avoids inadvertent burning of the esophageal mucosa secondary to excessive light source use.

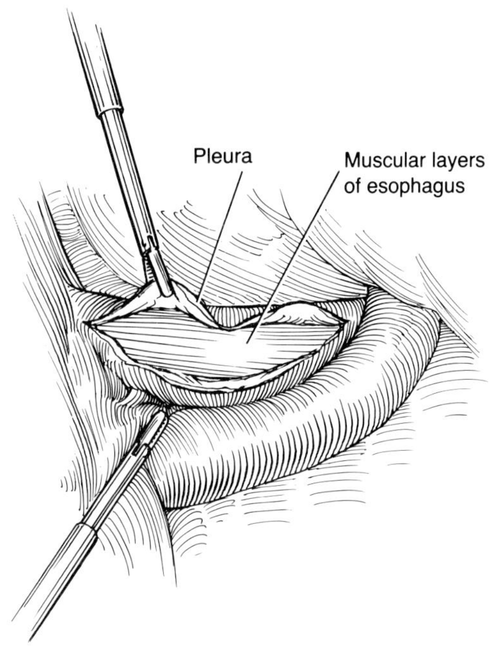

FIGURE 96–4

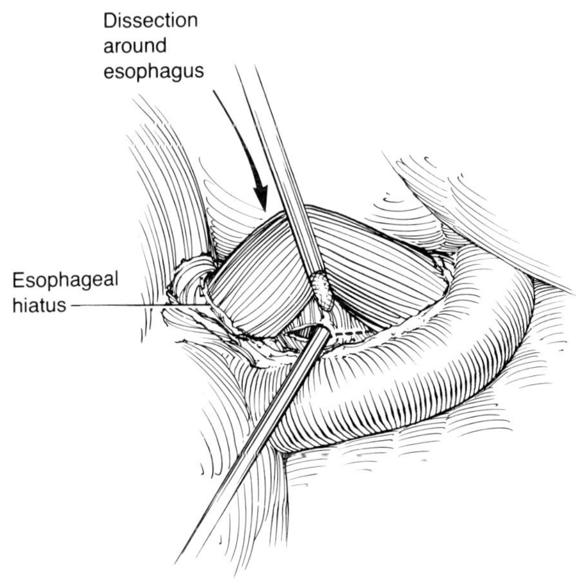

FIGURE 96–5

FIGURES 96–4 and 96–5. The lower esophagus is dissected laterally and medially away from the aorta and pericardium. The gastroscope is left in place just past the esophagogastric junction to serve as a stent and aid for delineation of the esophagus.

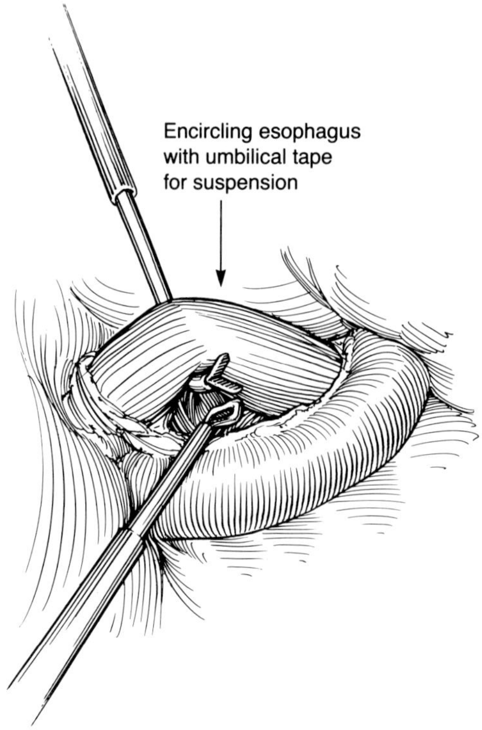

FIGURE 96–6. With a right-angle instrument or reticulating instrument, an umbilical tape is passed around the lower esophagus for retraction.

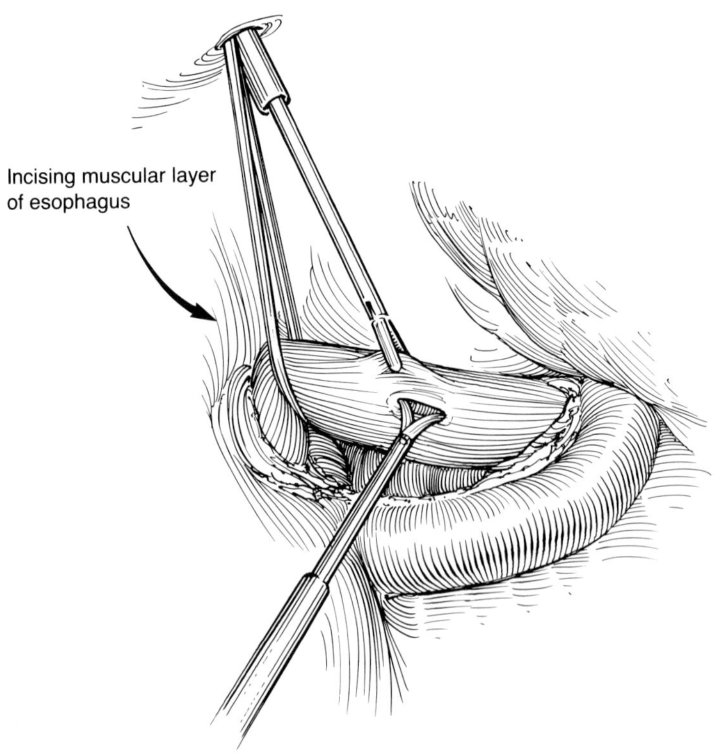

FIGURE 96–7. The initial esophagomyotomy is made with scissor dissection in a longitudinal manner approximately 3 cm above the diaphragmatic hiatus.

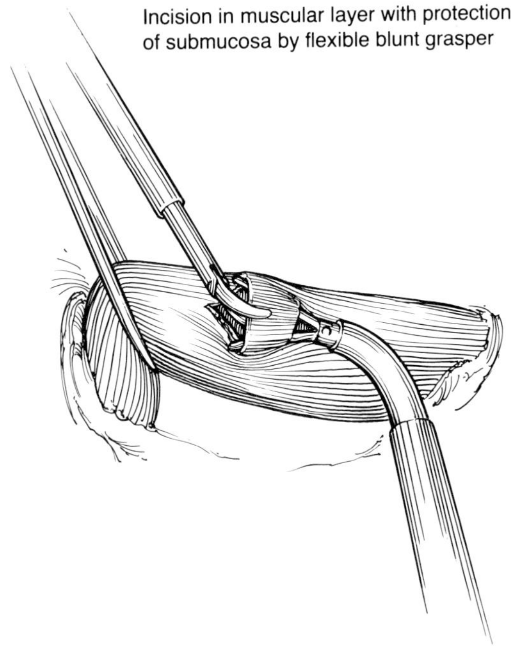

FIGURE 96–8

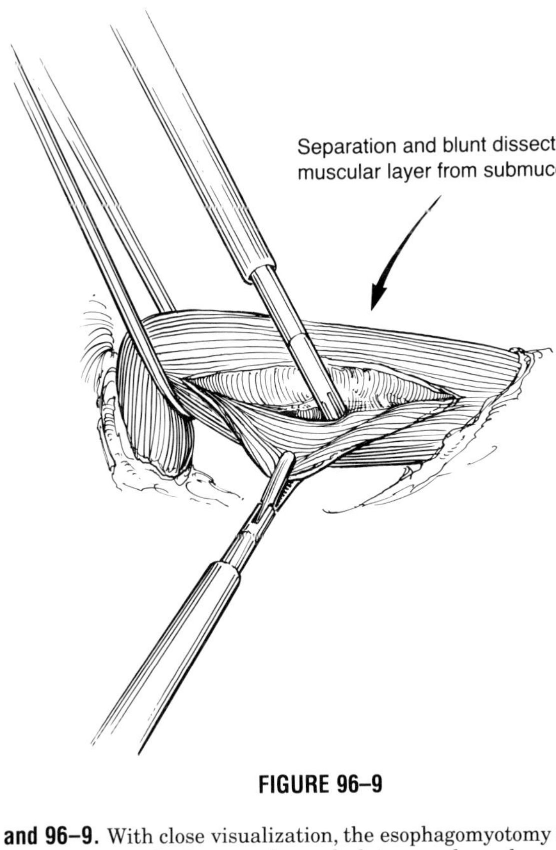

FIGURE 96–9

FIGURES 96–8 and 96–9. With close visualization, the esophagomyotomy is extended through the longitudinal and circular muscle down to the underlying esophageal mucosa. During the course of this dissection, electrocautery is specifically avoided. Although some bleeding is evident, as with a standard open esophagomyotomy, this bleeding is minimal and can be cleared with intermittent irrigation and patience. Because the esophageal mucosa may be damaged in a less than obvious manner with use of the electrocautery, only the most troublesome bleeders should be coagulated, and these should be coagulated extremely precisely.

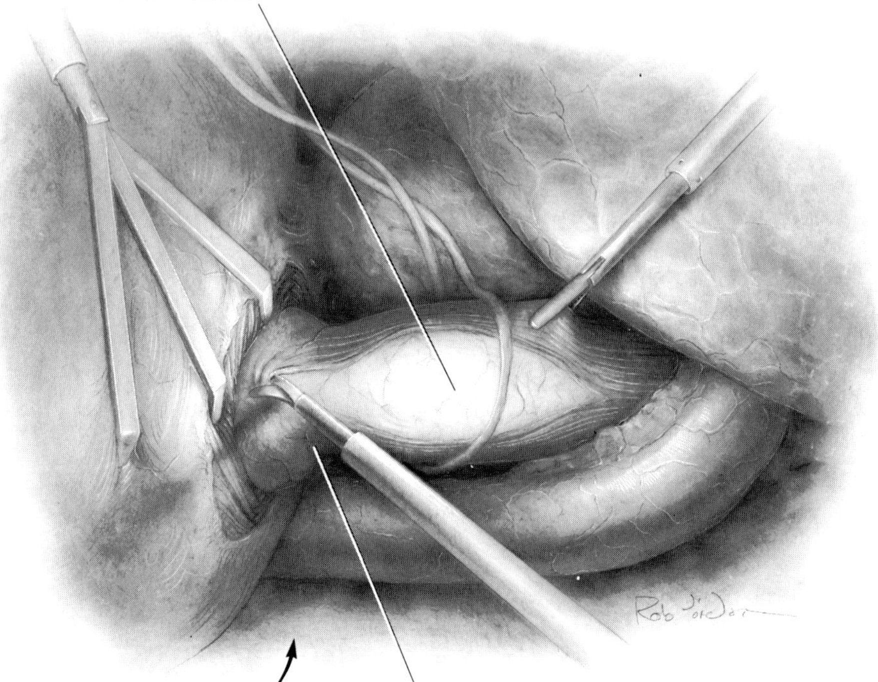

FIGURE 96–10. The esophagomyotomy is continued in a caudal direction while the endoscopist visualizes the gastroesophageal junction. The lung retractor may be switched to a lower port to provide downward retraction on the diaphragm. This allows better visualization of the gastroesophageal junction. The circular muscles and transverse veins that typically identify the lower esophageal sphincter area may be difficult to distinguish. Because of this, the gastroscope is an extremely useful tool. Once the lower esophageal sphincter has been divided, the endoscopist will readily see frank relaxation of the constriction at the lower esophageal sphincter area.

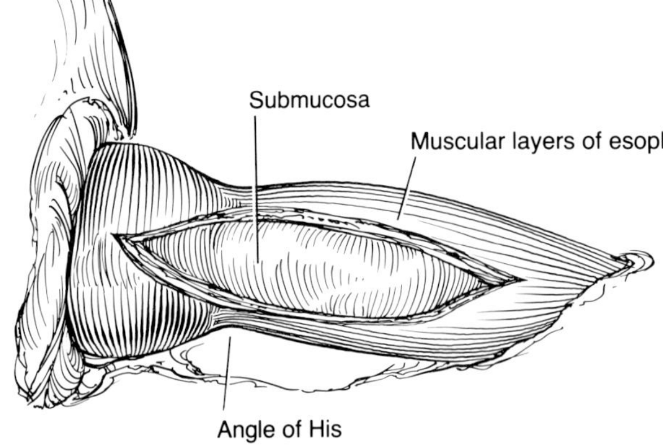

FIGURE 96–11. After the sphincter is divided, the esophagomyotomy is continued in a cephalad direction. Insufflation of the esophagus will allow ballooning of the esophageal mucosa and aid in dissection of the muscular layers away from the underlying mucosal region. The esophagomyotomy is continued superiorly to the level of the inferior pulmonary vein. If the surgeon decides to pass a nasogastric tube, this should be done under direct visualization by the thoracoscope. Because the esophageal mucosa is extremely thin, perforation can occur with blind passage of the nasogastric tube. Once the tube is in place, it should be fixed securely at the patient's nose, and strict instructions should be given to avoid manipulation of this tube. A chest tube is usually inserted through one of the lower thoracoscopic ports and placed on underwater sealed drainage. It is removed when complete lung expansion is ensured and chest drainage is minimal. Oral feedings can be started as early as the first postoperative day if the patient has no ileus or nausea.

CHUNG-PING HSU, M.D.
JAMES M. DOUGLAS, JR., M.D.

97

Thoracoscopic Sympathectomy

Upper thoracic sympathectomy is the treatment of choice for hyperhidrosis palmaris, and the sympathectomy can be confined to the T2 sympathetic ganglion alone. Other indications for upper thoracic sympathectomy include vascular occlusive disease, Raynaud's disease, shoulder-hand syndrome, causalgia, and visceral pain. For these, the extent of sympathectomy should be modified according to the clinical problem.

PATIENT PREPARATION

The procedure can be done either on an outpatient or inpatient basis, with no oral intake for at least 8 hours. No specific medication is needed except an overnight oral sedative, if desired. The axillary hair should be shaved.

ANESTHESIA

Even though the procedure can be accomplished under local anesthesia, we recommend general anesthesia for all patients. In most circumstances, a left-sided double-lumen endobronchial tube is used for anesthesia. Also required are a pulse oximeter for monitoring of peripheral O_2 saturation and a surface temperature recorder to detect peripheral temperature change due to vasodilatation after sympathectomy. However, for an experienced surgeon or in particular situations (e.g., young patient), anesthesia with an ordinary endotracheal tube is acceptable. In these conditions, the lungs can be collapsed simultaneously (with the patient in apneic condition), and the sympathectomy can be accomplished within 3 to 5 minutes. During the period of apnea, special attention should be given to the peripheral O_2 saturation. Once the saturation falls below 90%, the procedure should be suspended and the lung ventilated with 100% oxygen. The procedure can then be continued in the next turn of apnea.

POSITION

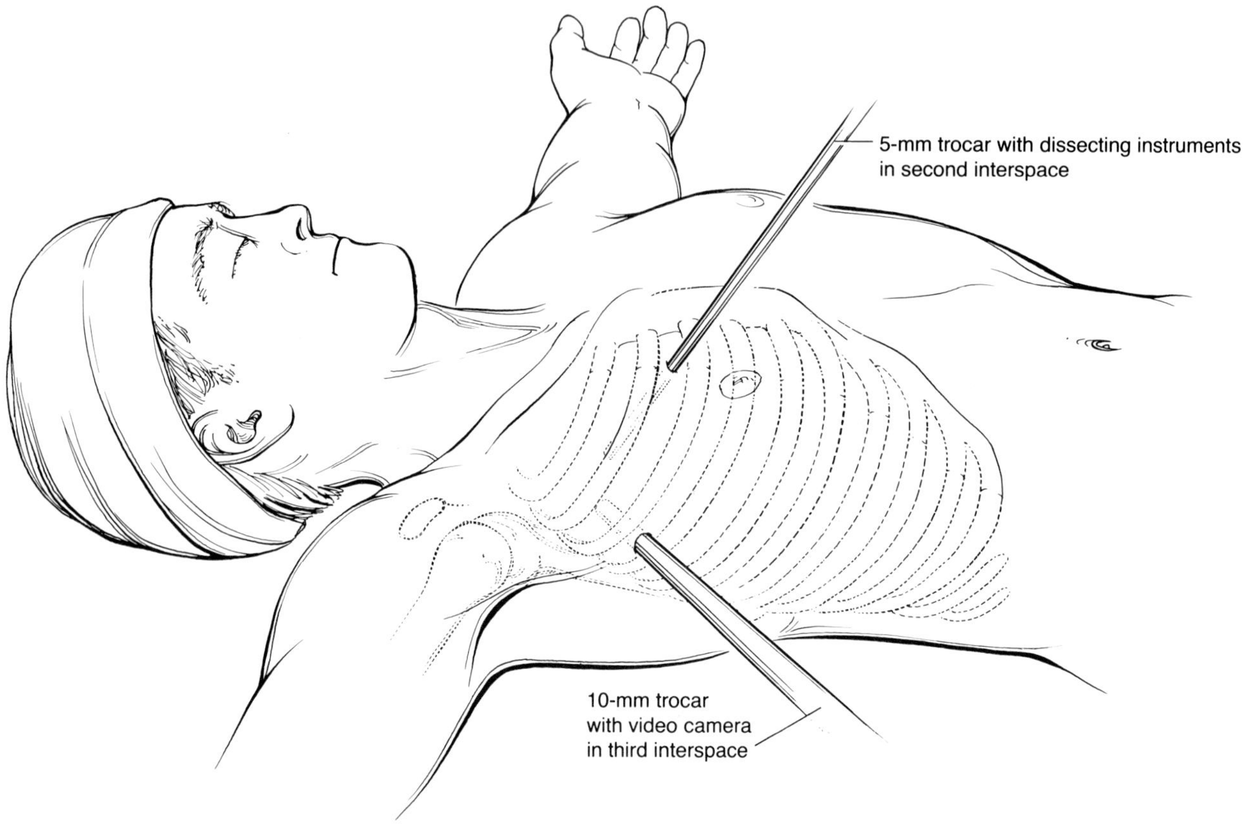

FIGURE 97–1. The patient lies in the supine position. A pad or sandbag is placed in the interscapular region in order to hyperextend the upper thoracic spine. Both of the upper limbs are abducted 90 degrees. The surface temperature recorder is attached to the tip of the middle finger on the operated side.

PROCEDURE

The skin is sterilized and draped to expose both sides of the axillary region. A 1-cm incision is made on the operated side axilla along the skin fold, just lateral to the margin of the pectoralis major muscle. After the incision is made, the anesthesiologist is asked to collapse the lung on the operated side. Routine use of CO_2 insufflation is not necessary. Usually, with the operated side endobronchial tube open to the atmosphere, the lung collapses in minutes. If suction is applied to the endobronchial tube, the lung collapses even more quickly. At this point, a Kelly forceps is used to dissect the intercostal muscles of the third intercostal space, and the pleural cavity is entered. Digital exploration of the pleural cavity through the stab wound is important before the trocar is inserted. After it is certain that there are no major intrapleural adhesions around the stab site, a 10-mm trocar is introduced into the pleural cavity for insertion of the thoracoscope. A 10-mm rigid thoracoscope with a 5-mm operating channel is preferred. An initial panoramic view of the upper pleural cavity and mediastinal structures is required for anatomic orientation. The sympathetic chain lies just lateral to the articulation between the ribs and the transverse processes of the thoracic vertebrae. The primary strategy of the whole procedure is to precisely localize the second rib. We have found that the most reliable method for identification of the second rib is to visualize the internal intercostal muscles from the first rib above and terminating at the upper margin of the second rib.

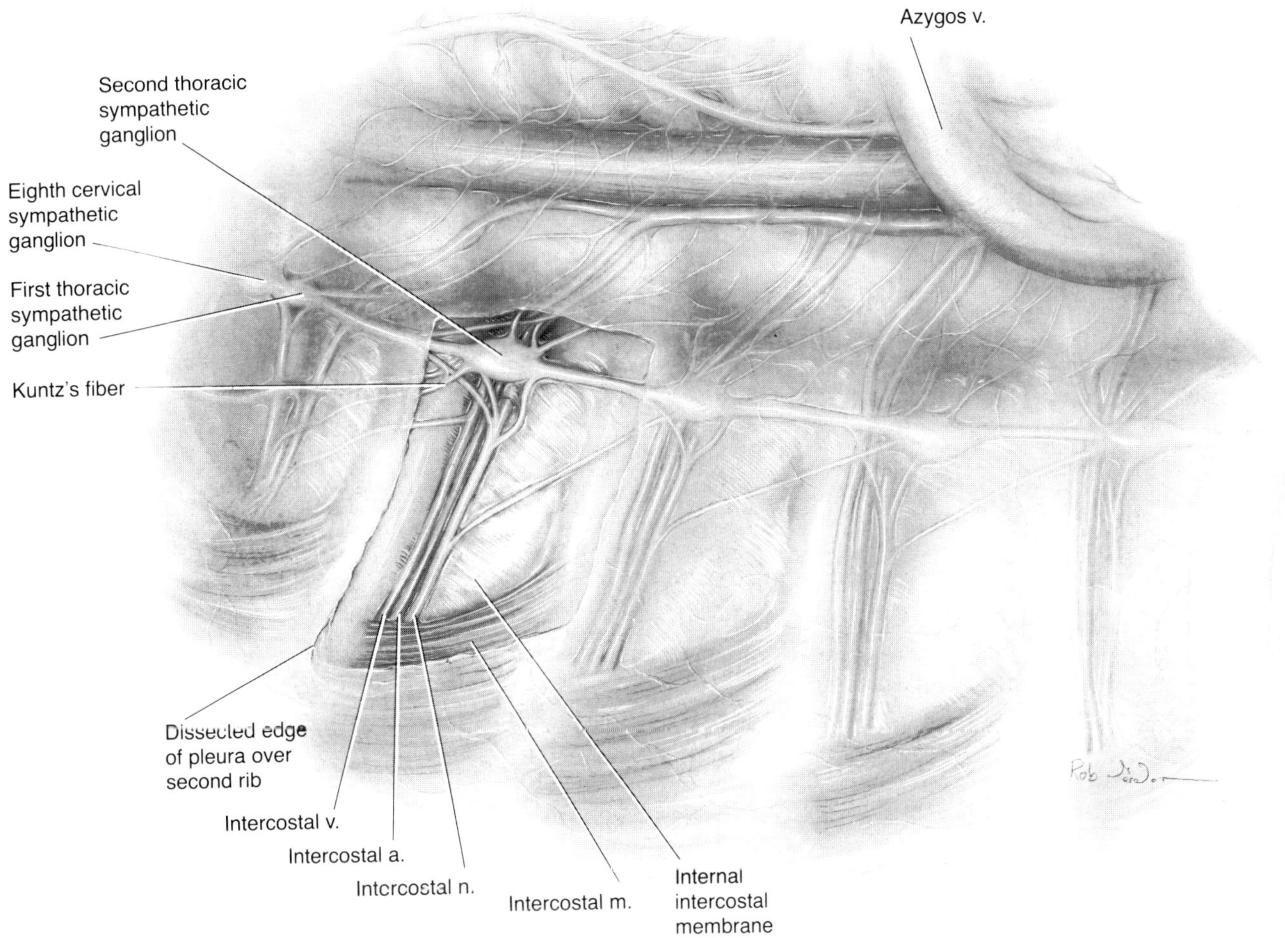

FIGURE 97–2. The pleura overlying the sympathetic chain is opened with the electrocautery, and a segment of sympathetic chain between the second and third ribs (including the second thoracic sympathetic ganglion) is dissected and freed. This segment of sympathetic chain is then totally destroyed with the electrocautery. It is usually unnecessary to remove the specimen for pathologic confirmation if one can observe the effect of sympathectomy on the surface temperature recorder. Usually, the temperature rises to a plateau within 5 minutes. However, if a pathologic confirmation is necessary, a 5-mm incision can be made at the midclavicular line of the second intercostal space, and endoscopic scissors introduced to resect the sympathetic chain. Finally, a segment of pleura (5 cm in length) of the pleura overlying the second (and third) rib is unroofed for transection of possible existing Kuntz's fiber.

These procedures make an inverted L- or U-shaped brand of cauterization on the pleura. A 20 Fr (or smaller) thoracic catheter is inserted into the pleura through the stab wound previously made for passage of the scope. The anesthesiologist starts to inflate the lung, and the operator moves to the opposite side of table for sympathectomy of the other side. The procedure for a left-sided sympathectomy is similar to that of the right side, except that the dome of the left pleural cavity is somewhat lower, and the pleural fat is somewhat more prominent. If there is definitely no injury to the lung during the operation, both chest tubes can be removed after re-expansion of the lungs by positive inflation and closure of the incisions. A postoperative chest film is essential for every patient. The patient may be discharged after negative chest film findings, either the same day of operation or the day after the operation.

JAMES M. DOUGLAS, JR., M.D.

98

Thoracoscopic Splanchnicectomy

The treatment of chronic visceral pain has long been a difficult problem. Division of the splanchnic nerves formerly was performed often, particularly for the treatment of chronic pain secondary to pancreatitis or pancreatic cancer. However, because of unpredictable results and the associated morbidity from open operations, enthusiasm for the procedure waned. The advent of thoracoscopic techniques has led to a resurgence of interest in ablative surgery of the autonomic nervous system. The minimally invasive nature of this approach makes thoracoscopic division of these nerves a feasible option. Experience continues to show that the effectiveness of the procedure is unpredictable. Although perhaps as many as 50% of patients with chronic pancreatic pain may experience relief following division of the splanchnic nerves, long-term relief of pain is less likely. It remains unclear to what degree other associated nerves, including the sympathetic trunk and vagus nerves, should be ablated in order to improve results. The necessity of bilateral versus unilateral neurectomy is also debatable. Because of these vagaries, it is currently recommended that consideration of thoracoscopic splanchnicectomy be given only for patients with terminal pancreatic cancer who have pain refractory to other treatment. As more experience is gained, it is possible that results will improve and that the required extent of neuroablation will be better defined.

PATIENT PREPARATION

The routine preoperative management as indicated for standard thoracotomy is required. General anesthesia with single-lung ventilation is preferable.

PROCEDURE

In general, a left thoracic splanchnicectomy including division of the greater, lesser, and least splanchnic nerves is planned. In refractory patients, a similar procedure may be performed in a staged manner on the right side.

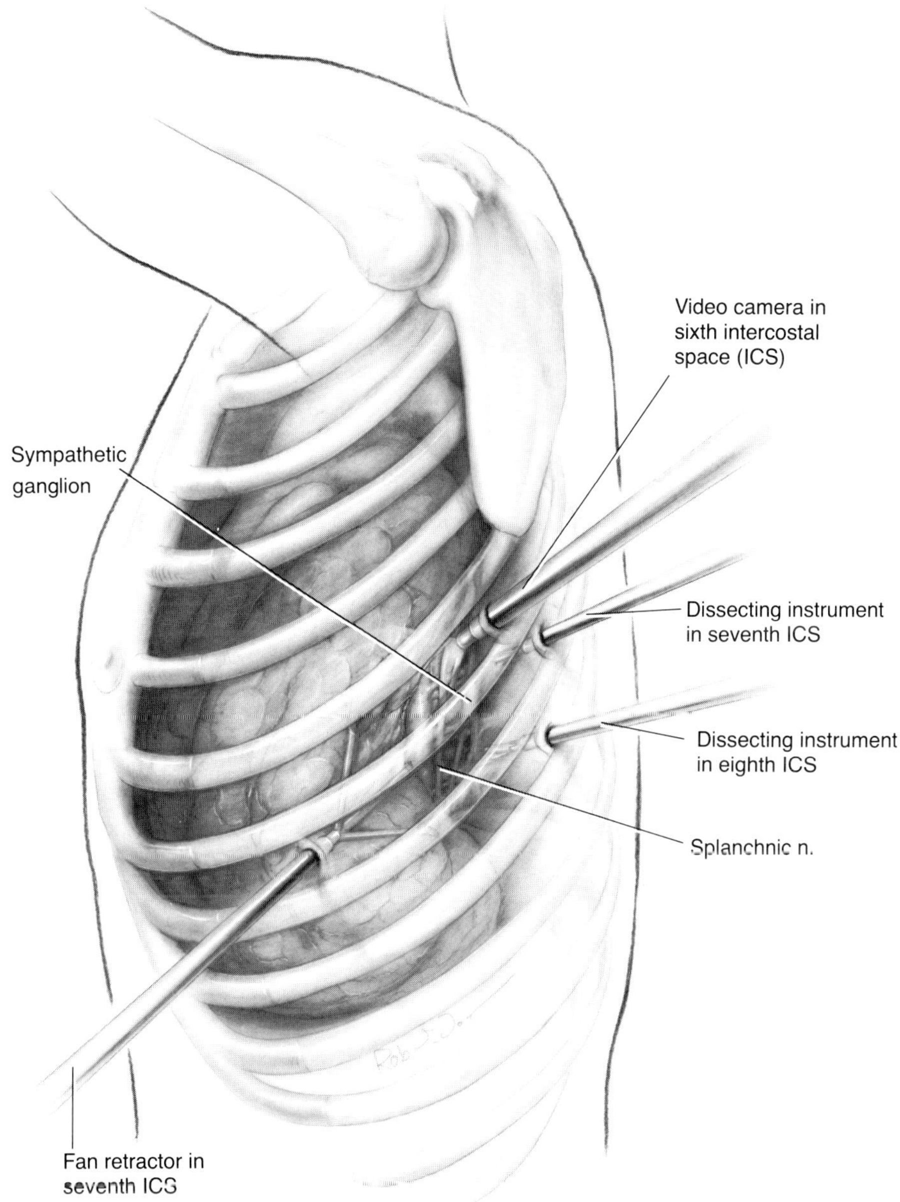

FIGURE 98–1. The patient is usually placed in the right lateral decubitus position, and standard sterile skin preparation and draping for thoracotomy is performed. The initial skin incision is made in the sixth intercostal space in the posterior axillary line. Following collapse of the left lung, dissection is extended through the chest wall under direct vision. The chest is entered and digital palpation used to confirm a free pleural space, and a 10-mm trocar is passed through this entry site. The laparoscope is then inserted and the hemithorax explored routinely. A second trocar is passed under vision through a small incision located in the anterior axillary line through the seventh intercostal space. A fan retractor is passed directly through this incision or through a 10-mm port. Graspers and scissors are then passed through two additional ports located in the seventh and eighth intercostal spaces in the posterior scapular line.

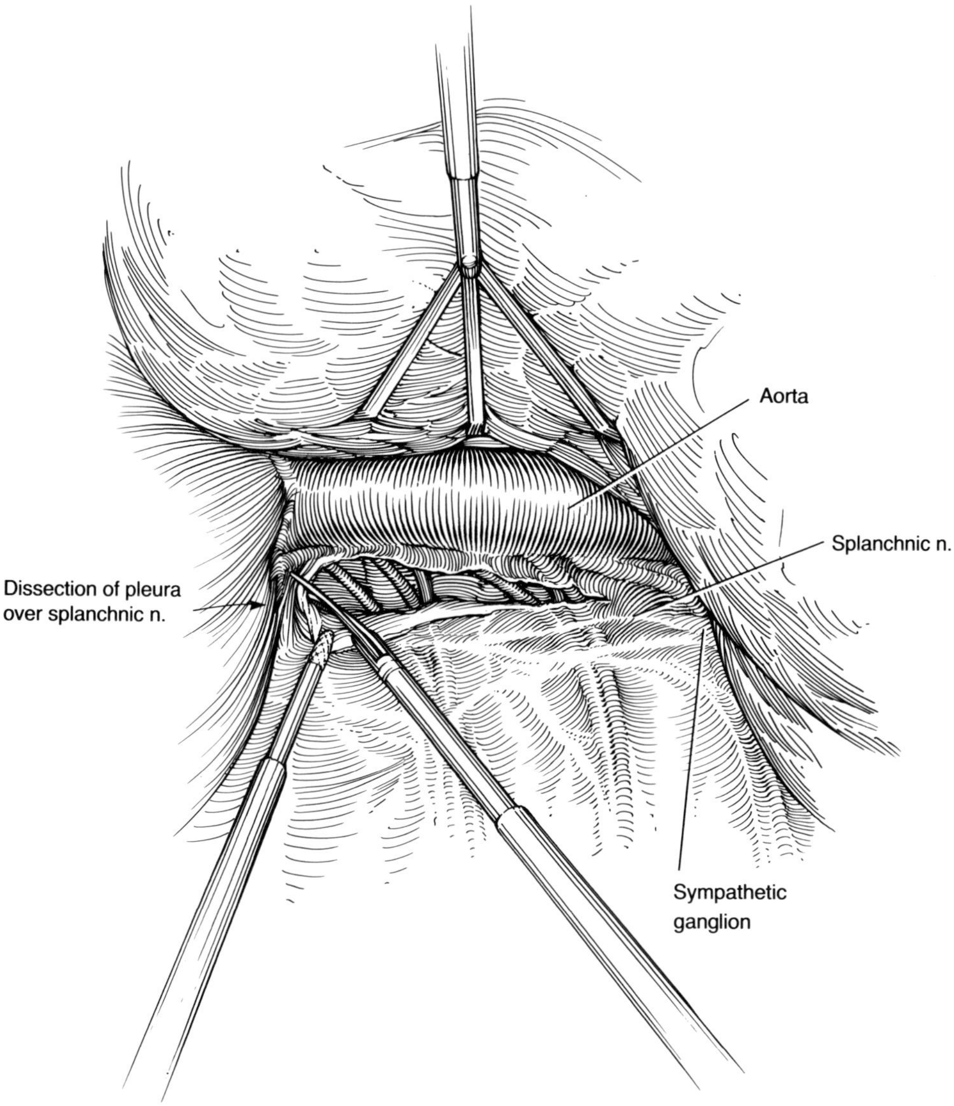

FIGURE 98–2. The parietal pleura lateral to the aorta is carefully divided, and hemostasis is meticulously maintained. The sympathetic chain is identified in its position in the costovertebral angle. The greater splanchnic nerve is seen to course medially and caudally between the aorta and the sympathetic chain.

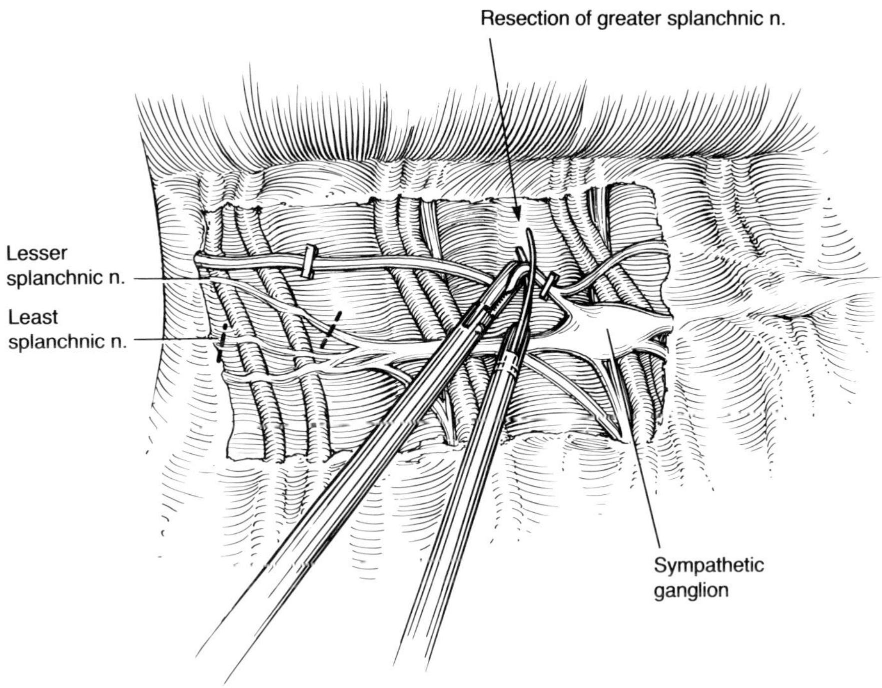

FIGURE 98–3. In most patients, the greater and lesser splanchnic nerves are easily identified. These nerves should be clipped and divided quite distally, just above the aortic hiatus. The least splanchnic nerve should also be identified and divided if possible. The nerve sections are sent for pathologic confirmation. The instruments are then withdrawn. A 24 French chest tube is passed through the most anterior trocar site, and the lung is re-expanded. The incisions are closed in layers, and the chest tube is fixed securely at the skin level. The tube may be removed at the end of the procedure if hemostasis is complete and no air leaks are identified.

JAMES M. DOUGLAS, JR., M.D.

99

Thoracoscopic Truncal Vagotomy

Although isolated truncal vagotomy is not a commonly required procedure, in those special circumstances in which vagotomy may be indicated, the thoracoscopic approach avoids an open thoracotomy and currently appears to be a very reasonable procedure.

PATIENT PREPARATION

The patient is allowed nothing by mouth for approximately 8 hours before the procedure. Routine preoperative sedatives are administered, and prophylactic antibiotics are generally given. General anesthesia with a double-lumen endotracheal tube is required.

PROCEDURE

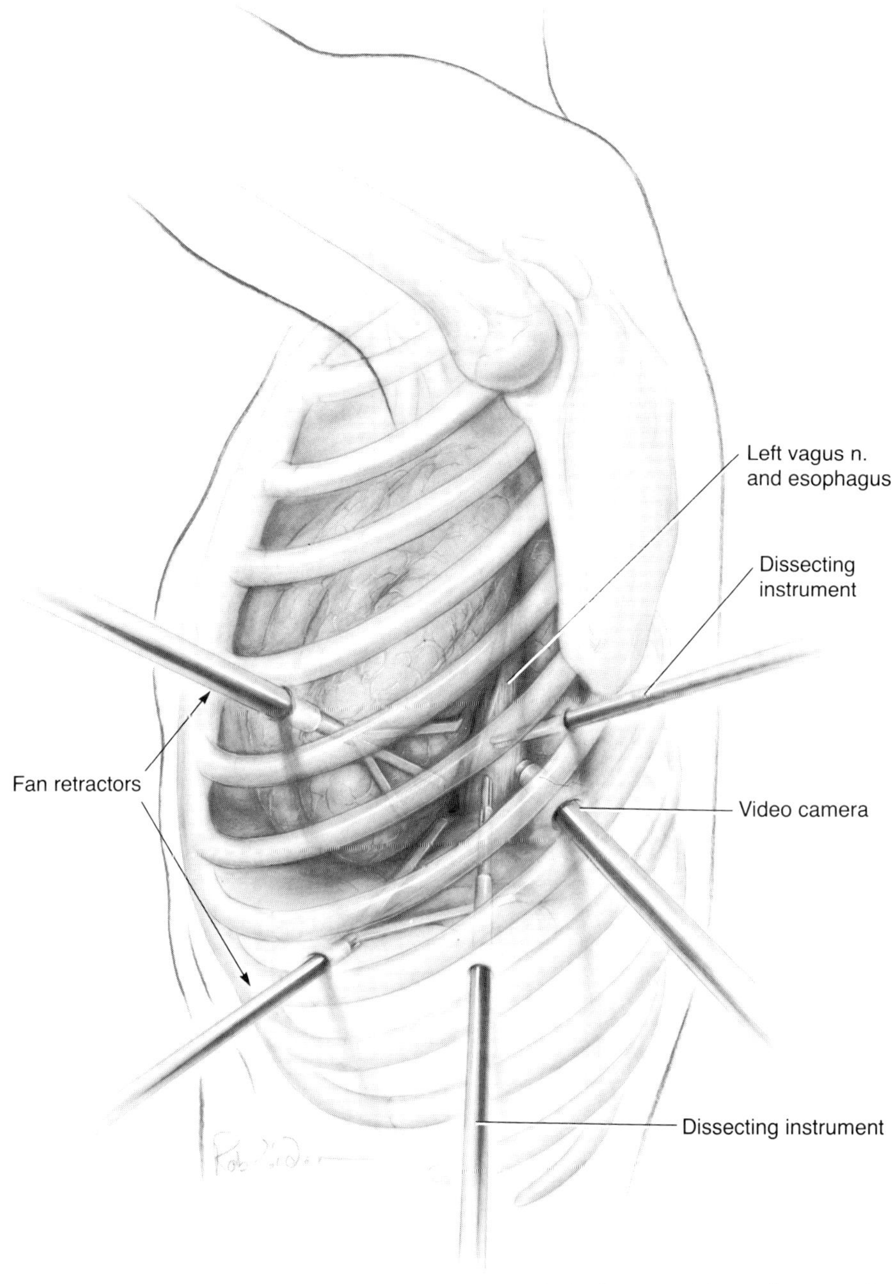

FIGURE 99–1. The patient is placed in the right lateral decubitus position and prepared and draped as for a standard left lateral thoracotomy. Passage of a 36 French esophageal bougie facilitates later dissection of the esophagus from surrounding tissues. An initial incision is placed in the eighth intercostal space in the posterior axillary line for subsequent passage of the laparoscope. As usual, dissection through the chest wall is performed under direct visualization to prevent inadvertent injury to the underlying lung tissue. A 10-mm trocar generally is passed to allow standard scope placement. With the lung collapsed, a brief examination of the left hemithorax is performed. Subsequent trocars are then placed in the fourth and eighth intercostal spaces in the anterior axillary line for passage of retracting instruments. The dissecting instruments are passed through the sixth intercostal space in the midscapular line and the ninth intercostal space in the midaxillary line.

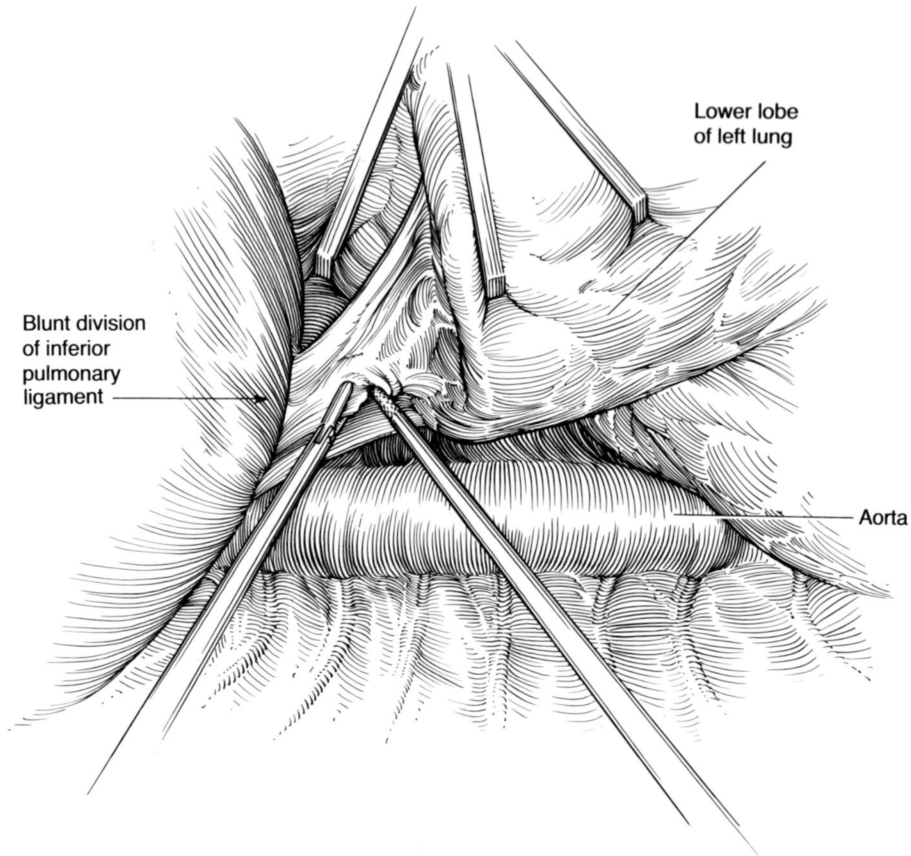

FIGURE 99–2. With the lung retracted medially, the inferior pulmonary ligament is divided with a combination of blunt and sharp dissection.

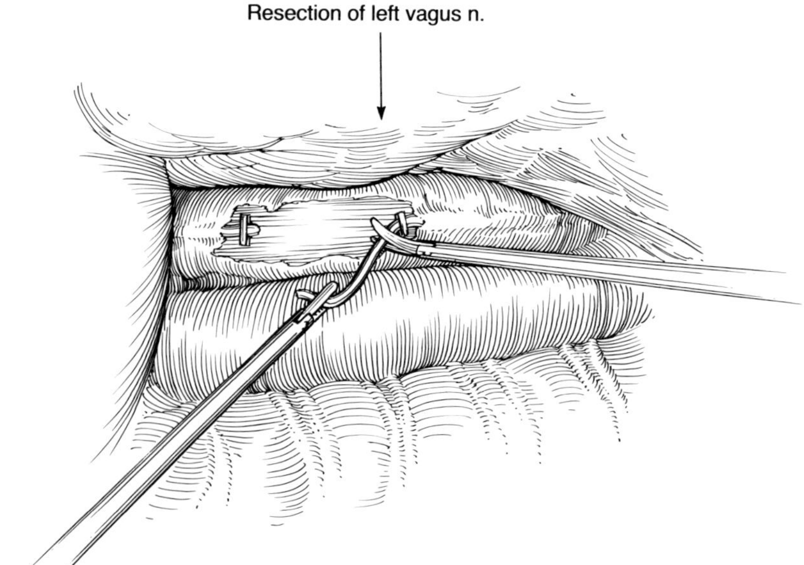

FIGURE 99–3. The anterior vagus nerve is easily identified as it passes along the surface of the esophagus. This nerve is doubly clipped, and a segment is removed for pathologic confirmation.

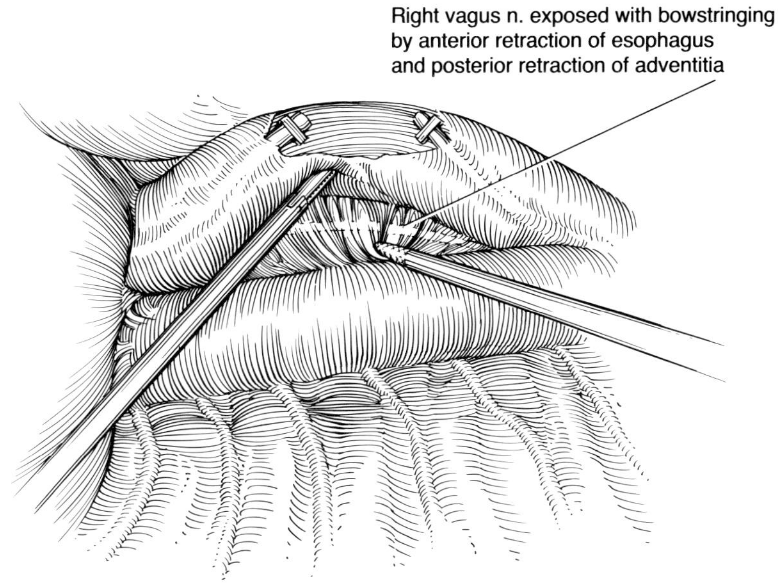

FIGURE 99–4. The esophagus is bluntly dissected from surrounding tissues in order to localize the posterior vagus nerve. The previous placement of a bougie allows easier initial manipulation of the esophagus. However, once the plane of dissection is defined, it may be safer to withdraw the bougie to prevent undue pressure of the esophageal tissue against the internal stent. The posterior vagus will be found to bow-string within the surrounding tissues immediately adjacent to the esophagus. The endoscopic blunt cotton-tipped dissector is an excellent instrument for defining and dissecting these tissues.

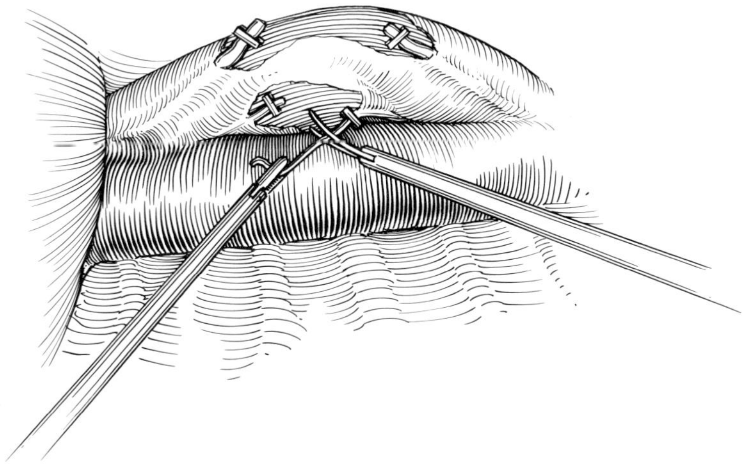

FIGURE 99–5. Once the posterior nerve is identified, it is doubly clipped and a segment excised for pathologic evaluation. Following assurance of hemostasis, a small chest tube is usually passed through one of the more anteroinferior ports. The lung is reinflated under direct visualization. All trocar sites are closed in layers. The chest tube is placed on underwater sealed drainage and removed when insignificant drainage and no air leak are documented.

CHUNG-PING HSU, M.D.
JAMES M. DOUGLAS, JR., M.D.

100

Thoracoscopic Lobectomy for Lung Cancer

It is generally accepted that thoracoscopic surgery can provide excellent visualization, decrease the severity of pain, shorten the hospital stay, and improve the cosmetic appearance. However, loss of tactile sensation makes dissection of the major pulmonary vessels and lobar bronchus more difficult, and this can prolong operative time and dilute the benefits of the thoracoscopic approach. This procedure demands much skill and is certainly not a procedure for the novice. A patient considered for thoracoscopic resection should have a clinically resectable peripheral tumor. Although any anatomic resection may be performed thoracoscopically, a left lower lobectomy is described here.

PATIENT PREPARATION

Consent for possible open thoracotomy should be obtained. The patient should have nothing by mouth for at least 8 hours. The axilla should be shaved, and the instruments necessary for open thoracotomy should be available.

ANESTHESIA

General anesthesia is required for the procedure. A left-sided double-lumen endobronchial tube is preferred. The oxygen saturation and end-tidal carbon dioxide levels should be monitored throughout the procedure. Epidural analgesia or intercostal nerve block with bupivacaine at the end of operation should be considered.

PROCEDURE

The patient is placed in the right lateral decubitus position (jackknifed) as in a standard left thoracotomy. A rolling pad is put under the dependent axilla to protect the patient's neurovascular bundles. The skin is sterilized and draped as for open thoracotomy. The lung on the operative side is kept collapsed with selective lung ventilation. The operator can stand either anterior or posterior to the patient.

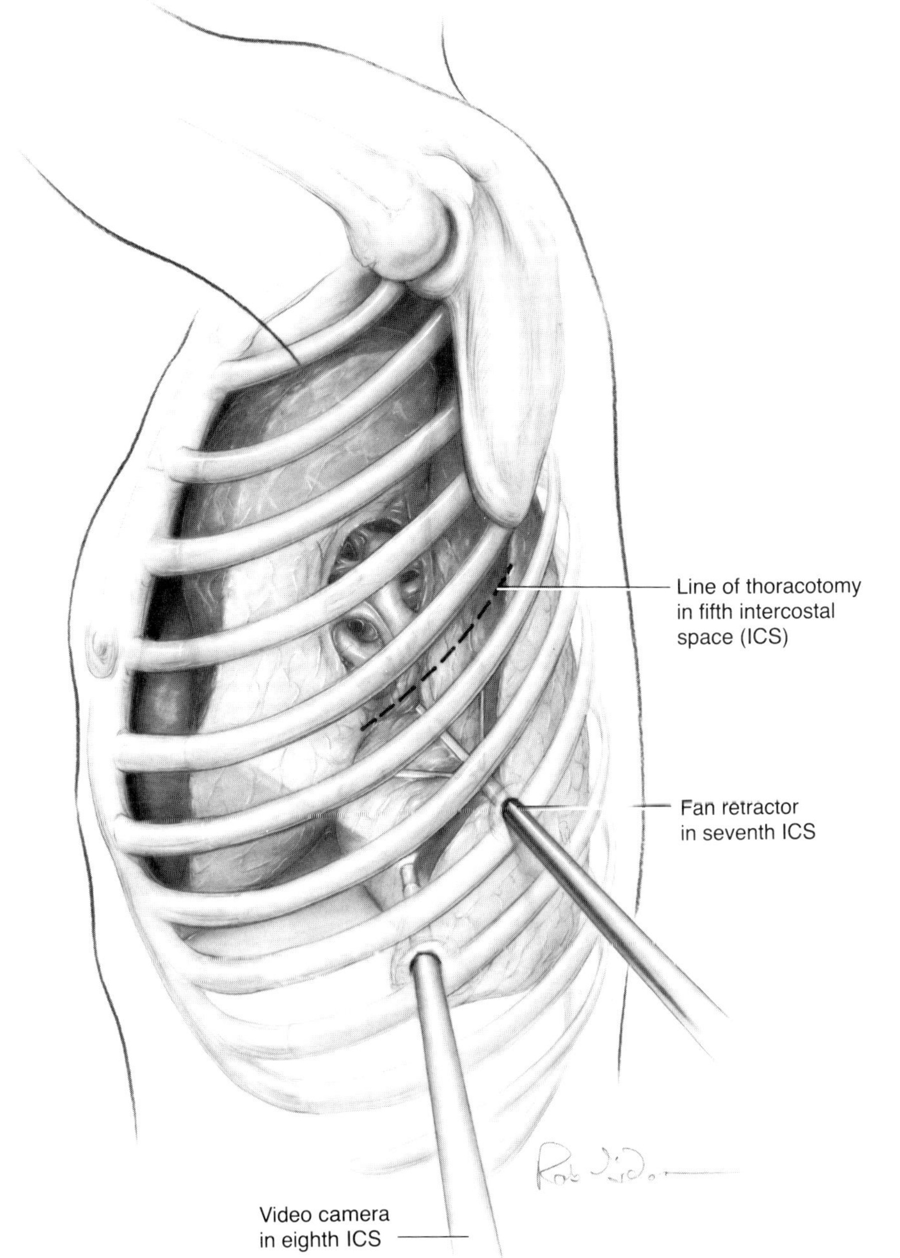

FIGURE 100–1. The thoracoscope is inserted through the eighth intercostal space in the anterior to middle axillary line. Carbon dioxide insufflation to facilitate lung collapse is unnecessary because an access mini-thoracotomy is made later. An initial thoracoscopic exploration of the pleural cavity is performed. If no evidence of intrapleural spreading or N_2 lymph node involvement can be identified, an oblique 8- to 10-cm access mini-thoracotomy just above the major interlobar fissure is performed under direct thoracoscopic guidance. Usually, the incision is made at the fifth intercostal space between the anterior and posterior axillary lines. A second port site is made at the seventh to eighth intercostal space in the posterior axillary line to introduce a fan retractor or other endoscopic instruments. The initial step is to open the interlobar fusion if the fissure is not complete. The dissection should be performed through the access thoracotomy using traditional long thoracic instruments or specifically designed thoracoscopic instruments. Usually the interlobar pulmonary artery and its branches can be identified just posterior to the center of the major fissure. After the interlobar pulmonary artery is found, adequate exposure of the artery should be obtained. If there is no direct tumor invasion of lymph node adhesion, the perivascular space should be easily accessed. The superior segmental artery above the lingular artery is divided with double endoscopic clips.

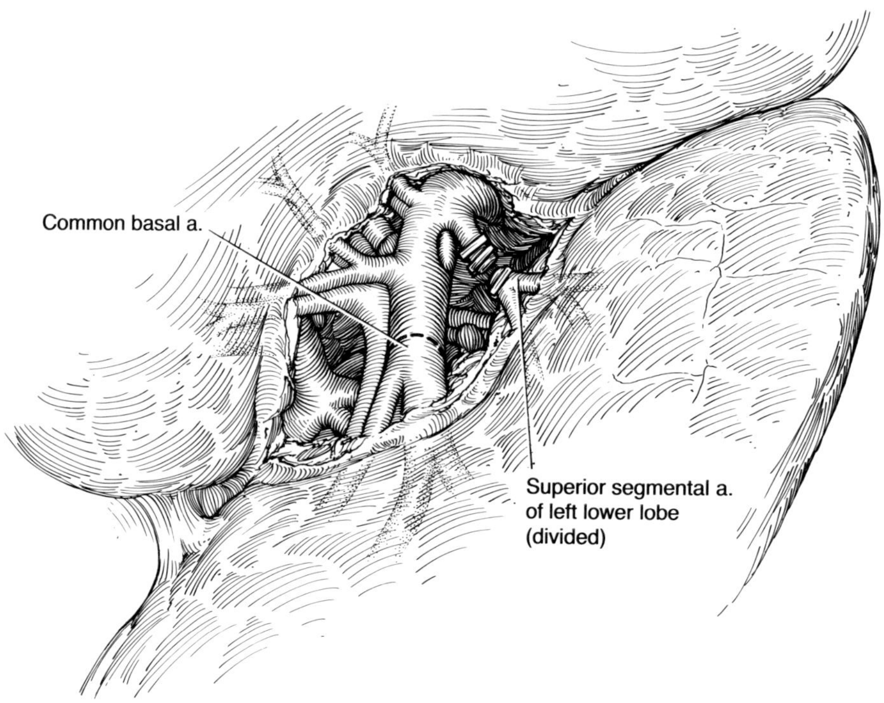

FIGURE 100–2. The common basal artery is divided by an endoscopic vascular stapler just below the origin of the lingular artery. The patient is placed in Trendelenburg position and rotated toward the ventral side. With upward traction of the left lower lobe, the inferior pulmonary ligament is divided with endoscopic scissors through the second access port site. The inferior pulmonary vein is completely freed for an adequate length and stapled with an endoscopic vascular stapler just outside the pericardium. After all the appropriate pulmonary vessels have been divided, the residual incomplete interlobar fissures can be separated with an endoscopic stapler. The mediastinal pleura overlying the lobar bronchus is opened with anterior traction on the lung.

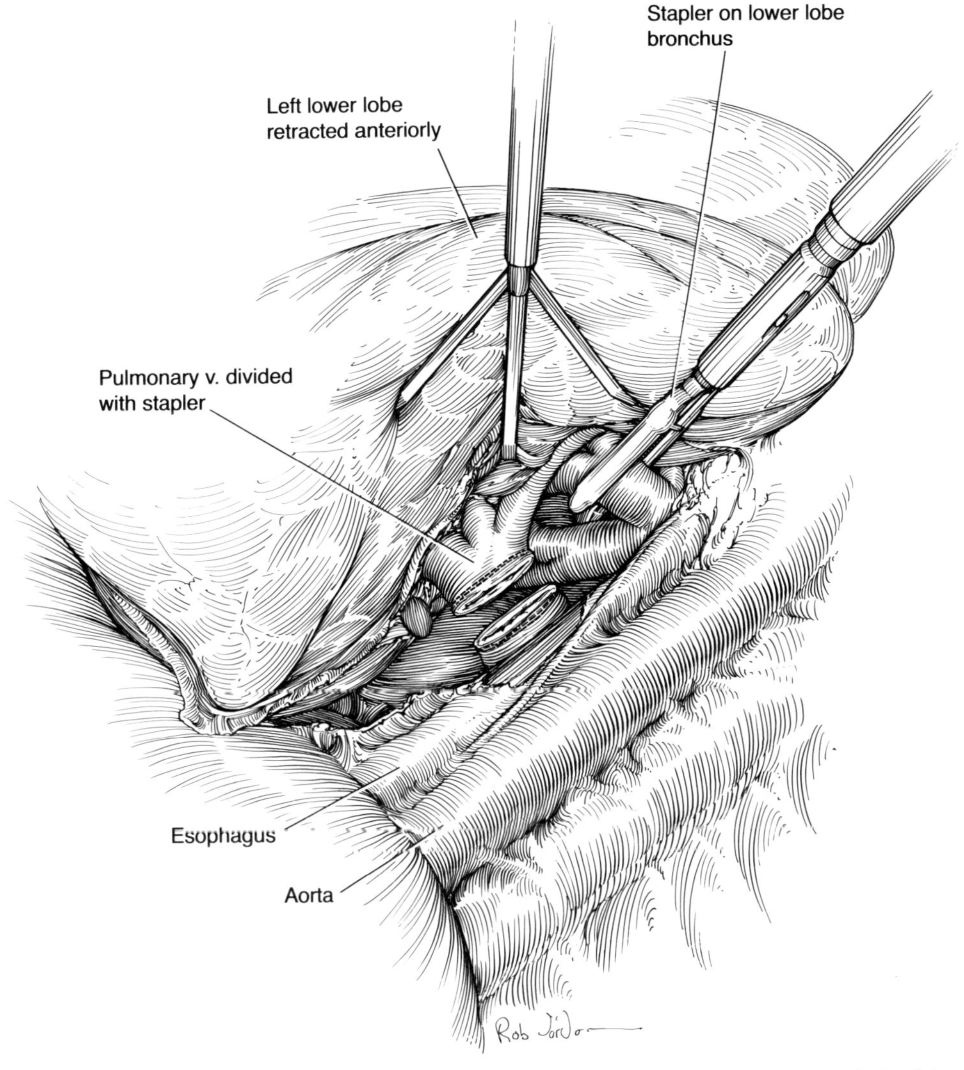

FIGURE 100–3. The lung is retracted anteriorly to expose the main bronchus and the lobar bronchi. An endoscopic stapler is introduced through the access thoracotomy and applied to the common basal bronchus proximal to the orifice of the superior segmental bronchus in preparation for transection of the left lower lobe bronchus. The lower lobe bronchus should be carefully trimmed of the peribronchial tissues and lymph nodes and then secured with an endoscopic or traditional stapler. If the superior segmental bronchus is quite close to the upper lobe bronchus, it should be transected separately to prevent compromise of the lumen of the left upper lobe bronchus. Sometimes it may be necessary to use a rib spreader to deliver the resected lobe through the access thoracotomy. The mediastinal lymph nodes are dissected through the mini-thoracotomy for complete tumor staging. The bronchial stump is immersed under saline to be certain that it is airtight. Good homeostasis is essential. A French 32 or 36 thoracic drainage tube is inserted through one of the access ports and connected to underwater sealed drain. The other incisions are closed in layers.

INDEX

Note: Page numbers in *italics* refer to illustrations.

A

Abdomen, scaphoid, *224*
viscera of, in diaphragmatic hernia, *226*
Achalasia, correction of, *218–219*
modified Heller esophagomyotomy for, 565, *566–572*
Adhesions, in coronary bypass reoperation, *490–491*
thoracoscopic resection of, *554, 562*
in wedge resection of pulmonary nodule, 545, 549
Air, removal of, from aorta, *340*
from left atrium, *280–281, 284, 289, 304, 504*
from right atrium, *383*
in aortic valve replacement, *416*
in cardiac transplantation, *512*
in extracorporeal membrane oxygenation, *537*
in mitral valve replacement, 396–397
in pulmonary transplantation, *520*
in ventricular aneurysm repair, *533*
Air embolism, prevention of, 424
Air insufflation, in flexible esophagoscopy, *21,* 22
Air leak, in lung, 553, 554
Anastomosis(es), end-to-end, in coarctation of aorta, *271–272*
in coronary artery bypass grafting, *482–483, 485–486, 488*
in tracheoesophageal fistula repair, *179–181*
of aortic graft, *429–433, 436–437, 441–442*
of left atrium, to pulmonary venous confluence, *290–294*
of stomach and esophagus, in esophagogastrectomy, Ivor Lewis, *205–206*
Sweet procedure, *196–197*
transhiatal, *216–217*
Anesthesia, in esophagoscopy, 21
in fiberoptic bronchoscopy, 11, 12
in thoracoscopic surgery, 542–543
for lobectomy, 584
for mediastinal tumor resection, 558
for pericardial window approach, 561
for procedures on anterior mediastinum, 563
for procedures on aorticopulmonary window, 556
for pulmonary biopsy, 551
for sympathectomy, 573
for wedge resection of pulmonary nodule, 547
local, for thoracostomy, *67*
Aneurysms, aortic arch, *434–437*
ascending aorta, *426–433*
Aneurysms *(Continued)*
dissecting, *431–433*
descending aorta, *438–442*
of sinus of Valsalva, *276–278*
ventricular, *527–533*
scar tissue of, re-entrant tachycardia and, *458*
Angioplasty catheter, balloon, *328*
Angle of His, in modified Heller esophagomyotomy, *572*
Annuloplasty ring, for aortic valve, *415, 419–420*
for mitral valve repair, *409–412*
for tricuspid valve repair, 384, *385–388*
Annulus. See also names of specific valves.
between mitral and tricuspid valves, atrial septal defect and, *287–288*
pulmonary, in repair of tetralogy of Fallot, *313–316*
Anomalous pulmonary venous return, repair of, *290–296*
subdiaphragmatic, *293–294*
to coronary sinus, *295–296*
Aorta, anastomoses of, *271–272, 334, 342–343, 512*
anomalous left coronary artery attached to, *498–499*
ascending, air removal from, *340*
aneurysms of, *426–433*
in extracorporeal membrane oxygenation, *537*
wounds of, repair of, *421*
coarctation of, by end-to-end anastomosis, *271–272*
by patch aortoplasty, *266–267*
by subclavian flap aortoplasty, *268–270*
via sternotomy with patient on cardiopulmonary bypass, *273–275*
descending, aneurysms of, *438–442*
visualization of, *49*
wounds of, repair of, *425*
dextrorotated, in tetralogy of Fallot, *311*
repair of, in transposition of great arteries, *346*
in truncus arteriosus, *321, 324*
separation from pulmonary artery, *260–265*
Aortic arch, incision of, in coarctation of aorta, *273*
in hypoplastic left heart syndrome, *357–359*
interruption of, *341–345*
transverse, aneurysms of, aortic valve replacement and, *437*
repair of, *434–437*
in patent ductus arteriosus, *256*
visualization of, *49*
wounds of, repair of, *424–425*
Aortic stenosis. See also *Aortic valve.*
congenital, repair of, *325–340*
division of fused commissures in, *327–328*
physiology of, *325*
subaortic, *329–330*
subvalvar left ventricular outflow tract narrowing and, *335–337*
supravalvular, *339–340*
valve replacement in, *331–334, 336, 413–416*
Aortic valve, commissures of, *327–328*
competence of, aortic aneurysm repair and, *431–433*
mitral valve examination and, 401
incompetence of, aortic aneurysm repair and, *426–431*
valve replacement for, *417–420*
muscle wedge removed from, *329–330*
prosthetic, placement of, *415–416*
sizing of, *419, 428*
replacement of, *336*
for aortic aneurysm repair, *428*
for aortic arch aneurysm repair, *437*
for aortic insufficiency, *417–420*
for aortic stenosis, *331–334, 336, 413–416*
procedure for, *415–416*
sizing of, *419, 428*
Aorticopulmonary window, thoracoscopic approach to, 556, *557*
Aortoplasty, patch, *266–267*
for coarctation of aorta, *266–267*
subclavian flap, *268–270*
Aortopulmonary shunt, in infants, *362*
in pulmonary atresia, *355*
in tetralogy of Fallot, *319*
in tricuspid atresia, *362*
Fontan procedure and, *366–368*
Aortopulmonary window, repair of, *260–265*
Aortoventriculoplasty, in aortic stenosis repair, *337–339*
Argon beam coagulation, of re-entrant tachycardic focus, in interventricular septum, *459*
Arrhythmias, cardiac, 443–475. See also names of specific conditions (i.e., *Tachycardia*).
surgical procedures for, 448–459
for automatic atrial tachycardias, *453–457*
for concealed atrioventricular connections, *448–452*
for re-entrant ventricular tachycardia, *458–459*
for Wolff-Parkinson-White syndrome, *448–452*
Artery(ies), basal, *586*
basilar trunk of, *148, 153, 157*
brachiocephalic, in aortic aneurysm repair, *434–436*

Artery(ies) *(Continued)*
bronchial, *165*
carotid, *50, 52*
in aortic aneurysm repair, *434–436*
in extracorporeal membrane oxygenation, *537–538*
circumflex coronary, in coronary artery bypass grafting, *482*
in Maze III procedure, *468–469*
in transposition of great vessels, *348*
coronary, bypass grafts of, 479, *480–488*
reoperation for, 489, *490–492*
in aortic aneurysm repair, *429*
in aortic stenosis, *335, 337, 339–340*
in aortic valve replacement, *417*
in transposition of great arteries, *346–348, 351*
left anterior descending, anomalous, arising from pulmonary artery, *493–499*
in tetralogy of Fallot, *311, 316, 319*
in coronary artery bypass grafting, *484–486*
wounds of, closure of, *380*
epigastric, *126*
gastric epiploic, *128–129*
great, transposition of, *346–351*
innominate, 42
in coarctation of aorta, *271*
in extracorporeal membrane oxygenation, *537*
in hypoplastic left heart syndrome, *361*
in palliation of tetralogy of Fallot, *319*
in tricuspid atresia, *362*
wounds of, repair of, *423*
intercostal, in aortic aneurysm repair, *440*
internal mammary, 26, *46–47*
harvest of, *480–481*
in coronary artery bypass grafting, *121, 484–486,* 492
lingular, *148, 585–586*
middle lobe, *137, 140*
plaque extraction from, *487–488*
pulmonary, anastomosis of, in cardiac transplantation, *512*
in right lung transplantation, *517–518*
anomalous, in tetralogy of Fallot, *311*
anomalous left coronary artery arising from, *493–499*
as neo-aorta in repair of transposed great vessels, *347–349*
bifurcation of, homograft repair of, *361*
in Lecompte maneuver, *259, 349*
in transposed great vessel repair, *351*
branches of, in coarctation of aorta, *273*
in embolectomy, *170–171, 173*
catheter in, 292
dissection of, *162–163, 165, 169*
enlarged, *172*
excision of, in truncus arteriosus, *320–324*
homograft of, in tetralogy of Fallot, *316–318*
in truncus arteriosus, *322–324*
hypoplastic, in tetralogy of Fallot, *317–318*

Artery(ies) *(Continued)*
in tricuspid atresia, *364–365*
in embolectomy, *166–168, 170–173*
in hypoplastic left heart syndrome, *356–357*
in interrupted aortic arch, *341, 345*
in left lower lobectomy, *152*
in pulmonary atresia, *352–353*
in tetralogy of Fallot, *311, 313–318*
in tracheal resection, *83*
in transposition of great arteries, *346–349*
in tricuspid atresia, *362–369*
interlobar, *585*
main, cannulation of, in hypoplastic left heart syndrome, *356*
hypoplasia of, in tricuspid atresia, *364–365*
in aortic arch reconstruction, *359–361*
in tetralogy of Fallot, *313, 315–317*
in truncus arteriosus, *320–324*
right, anastomosis to main pulmonary artery, *264–265*
"hemi-truncus" defect of, *262–265*
right ventricular communication with, reconstruction of, *316–318, 334, 352–355*
separation of aorta from, *260–265*
reimplantation of, in congenital aortic stenosis, *331–334*
segmental, *143, 148*
superior, *585*
segmental posterior, in right upper lobectomy, *138*
subclavian, anastomosed to left coronary artery, *497*
in aortic aneurysm repair, *435, 438–440*
in patent ductus arteriosus repair, *256*
in thoracic outlet syndrome correction, *104*
left, in coarctation of aorta, *268–269, 271*
surgical approaches to, *46–50*
right, *51–52*
thoracoacromial, *123*
thyrocervical trunk, *46*
vertebral, *46*
in coarctation of aorta, *268–269*
Aryepiglottic folds, in flexible esophagoscopy, 22
Arytenoid cartilage, in esophagoscopy, *16, 21,* 22
Atrial appendages, in cardiopulmonary transplantation, *522*
left, in Maze III procedure, *467–468*
mitral valve and, in anomalous pulmonary venous return to coronary sinus, 295–296
right, excision of, *454–455, 460, 474*
Atrial fibrillation, Maze III procedure for, 460–475
Atrial septal defect, anomalous pulmonary venous return and, *292, 294–296*
in Fontan procedure, *366–368*
primum, Ebstein's anomaly and, *373*
repair of, *287–289*
secundum, Ebstein's anomaly and, *373*
repair of, *279–282*
sinus venosus repair in, *283–286*
Atrioventricular connections, accessory, *448*

Atrioventricular connections *(Continued)*
division of, *450–452*
operative approach to, left-sided, *451–452*
right-sided, *449–450*
Atrioventricular groove, fat pad of, in Maze III procedure, *461–462, 465, 469*
in surgery for Wolff-Parkinson-White syndrome, *452*
in cardiac transplantation, *509*
in cardiopulmonary transplantation, *522*
Atrioventricular node, in Maze III procedure, *465*
Atrioventricular septal defect, complete, Rastelli type A, *297–301*
Rastelli type C, *302–304*
repair of, *297–304*
partial, repair of, *287–289*
Atrioventricular valve, distention of, *298*
left, in complete atrioventricular septal defect, *300, 303*
Atrium. See also under *Atrial.*
in sinus venosus repair, *283–285*
injuries of, *377–378*
left, anastomosis of, in right lung transplantation, *519*
to pulmonary venous confluence, *290–294*
"de-airing" of, *280–281, 284, 289, 304, 504*
in cardiac transplantation, *510*
in cardiopulmonary transplantation, 522
in Maze III procedure, *466–470*
in ventricular aneurysm repair, *531*
myxoma of, excision of, *503–506*
right, anastomosis of, in cardiopulmonary transplantation, *524*
"de-airing" of, *383*
in cardiac transplantation, *511*
in Ebstein's anomaly, *372–373*
in extracorporeal membrane oxygenation, *537*
in Maze III procedure, *461–465*
incision of, *385*
repair of, in transposed great vessels, *350*
wall of, excision of, *456–457*
septum of, in hypoplastic left heart syndrome, *360*
Axillary hair line, *37*
Azygos vein, *29, 39, 178, 202, 205*

B

Belsey procedure, for correction of hiatal hernia, *185–190*
Bio-Medicus pump, in aortic aneurysm repair, *438–439*
Biopsy, pulmonary, thoracoscopic, 551, *552*
Blebs, thoracoscopic resection of, 553, *554–555*
Blood, circulation of, in extracorporeal membrane oxygenation, *225*
Blood supply, lateral segmental, in tracheal resection, 81
Bovie scratch pad, *555*
Brachiocephalic vessels, in hypoplastic left heart syndrome, *356–357*
Bronchial blockers, in thoracoscopic surgery, 542

Bronchoscope, flexible fiberoptic, 11, 12, *13*
rigid, insertion of, *4–6*
Bronchoscopy, flexible, 11–12, *13*
rigid, 3–11, *4–10*
bronchial examination in, *8–10*
diagnostic and therapeutic uses of, 3
technique of, 3, *4–10*
termination of, 11
Bronchus, left main, dissection of, *165*
in cardiopulmonary transplantation, 522
in flexible fiberoptic bronchoscopy, *13*
in rigid bronchoscopy, *8–10*
lower lobe, *587*
stapling and division of, *145, 156–157*
middle lobe, stapling of, *141*
right main, in right lung transplantation, *514–517*
in right pneumonectomy, *160*
in rigid bronchoscopy, *8–9*
stapling of, *160*
superior segmental, *587*
stapling and division of, *145*
upper lobe, *587*
division of, *150–151*
stapling of, *138*
Bulla, emphysematous, *135*

C

Calcium, annular, in aortic valve, *414*
Cameras, in thoracoscopic surgery, 541, 543, *544,* 545
Cancer, pancreatic, splanchnicectomy for, 576
Cannulation, for anomalous left coronary artery correction, *493*
for anomalous pulmonary venous return, *290, 293, 295*
for aortic aneurysms, *426, 438–439*
for aortic stenosis, *326*
for aortic valve replacement, *413, 417–418*
for aortic wounds, *422*
for aortopulmonary window repair, *260*
for atrial septal defect repair, *287*
for cardiac transplantation, *509*
for cardiopulmonary transplantation, *522*
for complete atrioventricular septal defect, *297*
for coronary bypass reoperation, *492*
for dissecting aortic aneurysms, 432, *432*
for Ebstein's anomaly, *372*
for extracorporeal membrane oxygenation, *537–538*
for hypoplastic left heart syndrome, *356*
for interrupted aortic arch, *341*
for left atrial myxoma excision, *503*
for Maze III procedure, *460–461*
for mitral valve repair, 399
for mitral valve replacement, *390*
for pulmonary atresia with intact right ventricle, *352–353*
for sinus venosus repair, *283–286*
for tetralogy of Fallot, *311*
for transposition of great arteries, *346*
for tricuspid atresia, *363, 365–366, 368*
for tricuspid valve replacement, *381*
Cannulation *(Continued)*
for truncus arteriosus, *320*
for ventricular aneurysm, *529*
for ventricular septal defect, *305*
for Wolff-Parkinson-White syndrome, *449*
Carbon dioxide, in thoracoscopic surgery, 542, 545, 585
Cardiac arrest, for coarctation of aorta repair, *273*
for examination of mitral valve, 401, 402
for ventricular septal defect repair, *305*
with cardioplegic solution. See *Cardioplegia.*
Cardiac arrhythmias, 443–475. See also names of specific conditions (e.g., *Tachycardia*).
implantable defibrillation device for, *445–447*
pacemaker insertion for, *229–231,* 492, *513*
surgical procedures for, 448–459
for automatic atrial tachycardias, *453–457*
for concealed atrioventricular connections, *448–452*
for re-entrant ventricular tachycardia, *458–459*
for Wolff-Parkinson-White syndrome, *448–452*
Cardiac defibrillation, for coronary bypass reoperation, 489
implantable device for, placement of, *445–447*
Cardiac tamponade, 238
Cardiac transplantation, *509–513*
Cardiac valvular disease, acquired, 375–442
Cardioplegia, 260, 263
coronary sinus route for delivery of, 390
for aneurysm of sinus of Valsalva, *276*
for anomalous pulmonary venous return, *290, 293, 295*
for aortic aneurysms, *426*
for aortic stenosis, *329*
for aortic valve replacement, *413, 417–418*
for aortic wounds, *422*
for atrial septal defect repair, *287*
for automatic atrial tachycardia, 453
for cardiac transplantation, *510–511*
for complete atrioventricular septal defect, *297*
for coronary artery bypass grafting, order of, 482, 486, 488
for dissecting aortic aneurysms, 432
for Ebstein's anomaly, *372*
for Maze III procedure, *460*
for mitral valve replacement, *390*
for tetralogy of Fallot, *311*
for transposition of great arteries, *347*
for tricuspid atresia, *364, 366, 368*
for truncus arteriosus, *320*
for ventricular aneurysm repair, *529*
for ventricular septal defect, *305*
in Fontan procedure, for tricuspid atresia, *366*
potassium and, for anomalous left coronary artery correction, *493, 498*
for left atrial myxoma excision, *503*
retrograde and antegrade, in coronary bypass reoperation, *492*
Cardiopulmonary bypass, for aneurysm of sinus of Valsalva, *276*
Cardiopulmonary bypass *(Continued)*
for anomalous left coronary artery, *493, 498*
for anomalous pulmonary venous return, *290, 293, 295*
for aortic aneurysms, *426*
for aortic arch aneurysms, *434*
for aortic stenosis, *326*
for aortic valve stenosis, 331
for aortic wounds, *422*
for atrial septal defect, *287*
for coarctation of aorta, *273–275*
for complete atrioventricular septal defect, *297*
for coronary artery bypass grafting, *480–481*
for coronary bypass reoperation, *492*
for Ebstein's anomaly, *372*
for embolectomy, 166, 168, *169, 173*
for hypoplastic left heart syndrome, *356–357, 361*
for interrupted aortic arch, *341, 344–345*
for Maze III procedure, 460
for mitral valve repair, 399
for mitral valve replacement, *390,* 396–397
for pulmonary atresia with intact right ventricle, *352–353*
for sinus venosus, *283*
for tetralogy of Fallot, *311*
for transposition of great arteries, *346*
for tricuspid atresia, *362, 368*
for tricuspid valve repair, 384
for tricuspid valve replacement, *381*
for truncus arteriosus, *320*
for ventricular aneurysms, *529*
for ventricular septal defect, *305*
standby, for closure of penetrating wounds of heart, *377*
Cardiotomy sucker, for aortic stenosis, *328*
for Maze III procedure, *461*
for tetralogy of Fallot, *312*
for tricuspid atresia, *363*
for truncus arteriosus, *322*
for ventricular septal defect, *309*
Cardioversion, in cardiac transplantation, *513*
Cardioverter-defibrillator, for coronary bypass reoperation, 489
Carpentier retractor, 391
Carpentier tricuspid annuloplasty ring, 384
sizing and orientation of, *386*
suturing of, *387–388*
Carpentier-Edwards prosthetic valves, aortic, *420*
tricuspid, *382–383*
Cartilage, arytenoid, *21,* 22
costal, *57, 63–64*
dissection of, *87–89, 97*
exposure of, *87*
cricoid, identification of, *73*
infected, removal of, *120*
posterior laryngeal, in rigid bronchoscopy, *6*
Catheter, angioplasty balloon, for repair of aortic stenosis, *328*
Fogarty, in embolectomy, *167, 171, 173*
in tracheoesophageal fistula repair, *180*
pulmonary arterial, 292
Cauterization, silver nitrate, 77
Cervicothoracic incisions, 45, *46–52*

Cetacaine, in flexible fiberoptic bronchoscopy, 12
Chamberlain incision, vs. thoracoscopic techniques, 556
Chest, cross-section of, *567*
Chest film, for confirmation of chest tube placement, 70
  in right pneumonectomy, 161
  postoperative, in thoracoscopic sympathectomy, *575*
Chest tube(s), for achalasia, *219*
  for aortic aneurysm repair, *442*
  for esophagogastrectomy, Ivor Lewis, *206*
    Sweet procedure, *198*
  for lobectomy, *138,* 141, 146
  for pericardiectomy, *239, 241*
  for pneumothorax, 65, *66–70*
  for thoracic outlet syndrome correction, *106*
  for thoracoabdominal incision closure, *62–63*
  for thoracostomy, *67, 69, 70*
  in pericardial window, *237*
  in pleural space, *34*
  in thoracoscopic surgery, 545
    for approach to aorticopulmonary window, *557*
    for pulmonary biopsy, 552
    for resection of mediastinal tumors, *560*
    for resection of pericardial effusion, *562*
    for splanchnicectomy, *579*
  indications for, 65
  placement of, *62*
Chest wall, anterior, tumors of, *249–251*
  posterior, tumors of, 245, *246–248*
Children, anomalous left coronary artery in, alternative procedure for, *497*
Clagett operation, for thoracic outlet syndrome correction, *104*
Coarctation of aorta, by end-to-end anastomosis, *271–272*
  by patch aortoplasty, *266–267*
  by subclavian flap aortoplasty, *268–270*
  via sternotomy with patient on cardiopulmonary bypass, *273–275*
Conduction tissue, protection of, *288*
    in complete atrioventricular septal defect repair, *298*
    in Ebstein's anomaly repair, *373*
    in subaortic stenosis repair, *330*
    in tetralogy of Fallot repair, *313*
    in tricuspid annuloplasty, *386*
    in tricuspid valve replacement, *381–382*
    in ventricular septal defect repair, *306, 310*
Congenital anomalies, aortic stenosis, *325–340*
  diaphragmatic hernia, 223, *224–228*
  esophageal atresia, 177
  of sternum, 85–99
    pectus carinatum, *94–96*
    pectus excavatum, *87–93*
    sternal cleft, *97–99*
Congenital heart disease, 253–373
  specific types of, aneurysm of sinus of Valsalva, *276–278*
    anomalous pulmonary venous return, *290–296*
    aortic stenosis, *325–340*
    aortopulmonary window, *260–265*
    atrial septal defect, *279–289*
Congenital heart disease *(Continued)*
    atrioventricular septal defect, *297–304*
    coarctation of aorta, *266–275*
    Ebstein's anomaly, *372–373*
    hypoplastic left heart syndrome, *356–361*
    interrupted aortic arch, *341–345*
    patent ductus arteriosus, *255–259*
    pulmonary atresia, *352–355*
    tetralogy of Fallot, *311–319*
    transposition of great arteries, *346–351*
    tricuspid atresia, *362–371*
    truncus arteriosus, *320–324*
    ventricular septal defect, *305–310*
Continuous positive airway pressure, in thoracoscopic surgery, 543
Coronary artery(ies), anomalous left, arising from pulmonary artery, *493–499*
    attached to aorta, *498–499*
    ligation of, *496*
  bypass grafts of, 479, *480–488*
    reoperation for, 489, *490–492*
      preparation for, 489
      risks of, 489
  reimplantation of, in congenital aortic stenosis, *331–334*
  translocation of, in transposition of great arteries, *346–348, 351*
Coronary ostium, in aneurysm of sinus of Valsalva, *276*
Coronary sinus, anomalous pulmonary venous return to, *295–296*
  atrial septal defect and, *287–288*
  in complete atrioventricular septal defect, *301*
  in Maze III procedure, *469*
Cosgrove retractor, 391
Costal cartilage, *57, 63–64*
  dissection of, *87–89, 97*
  exposure of, *87*
Costovertebral angle, *578*
Cricoid cartilage, identification of, *73*
Cricopharyngeus muscle, *15*
  for Zenker's diverticulum resection, *184*
  in esophagoscopy, *15, 17–18,* 22
Cricothyrotomy, tracheostomy and, 74
Cryotherapy, in ectopic atrial tachycardia, *457*
  in Maze III procedure for atrial fibrillation, *463, 465, 468–470*

D

Defibrillation, for coronary bypass reoperation, 489
  implantable device for, placement of, *445–447*
Diaphragm, 221–231
  closure of, *62, 192, 198*
  division of, *59–60*
  hernia of, congenital, 223, *224–228*
  in esophagogastrectomy (Sweet procedure), *192, 198*
  retroperitoneal dissection of, *60–61*
Digital pressure, for closure of heart wounds, *378–380*
Diverticulum, atrial, excision of, *454–455*
Doyen periosteal elevator, *56*
Drains, for muscle flaps for mediastinitis, *125, 127*
Drains *(Continued)*
  in Belsey procedure for hiatal hernia, *190*
  in esophagogastrectomy, *198, 206, 217*
  in Zenker's diverticulum resection, *184*
  pleural, *248*
  suction (Jackson-Pratt), for pectus carinatum, *96*
    for pectus excavatum, *93*
Ductus arteriosus, in coarctation of aorta, *266, 268, 271, 273*
  in tetralogy of Fallot, *311*
  patent, in congenital aortic stenosis, *325–326, 329*
    in hypoplastic left heart syndrome, *356–357*
    in interrupted aortic arch, *341–342*
    in pulmonary atresia with intact right ventricle, *352–353*
    in transposition of great arteries, *346*
  repair of, *255–259*
    during intracardiac repair, *259*

E

Ebstein's anomaly, *372–373*
Echocardiography, transesophageal, for ventricular aneurysm repair, *533*
    for Wolff-Parkinson-White syndrome, 449
ECMO. See *Extracorporeal membrane oxygenation.*
Electrocautery, for cardiopulmonary transplantation, *522*
  for chest wall tumor removal, *246*
  for coronary bypass reoperation, *490*
  for harvesting of vessels for coronary artery bypass grafting, *480–481*
  for median sternotomy, *40–42*
  for modified Heller esophagomyotomy, *571*
  for pectus excavatum repair, *88–89*
  for rib excision, *55*
  for right lung transplantation, *514*
  for thoracoscopic sympathectomy, 575
Electrode (pacemaker), diaphragmatic, placement of, *229–231*
Embolectomy, for acute pulmonary embolism, *166–168*
  for chronic pulmonary embolism, *169–173*
Embolism, prevention of, *424*
    in coronary bypass reoperation, *492*
Emphysematous bulla, excision of, *135*
Endobronchial tubes, in thoracoscopic surgery, 542, 547
    for resection of pulmonary nodule, 547
    for sympathectomy, 573, 574
Endoscopes, in thoracoscopic surgery, 541
Endoscopic lung clamps, in thoracoscopic surgery, *552*
Endoscopic staplers, in thoracoscopic surgery, 541–542, 546, *550, 552, 554–555, 587*
Endoscopy, 2–22. See also *Bronchoscopy; Esophagoscopy; Thoracoscopic surgery.*
Endotracheal granulations, 77
Endotracheal tube, bronchoscope insertion and, *4*
  double lumen, *147, 158, 514*

Endotracheal tube *(Continued)*
for thoracoscopic sympathectomy, 573
in esophagoscopy, 6–7, 20, 22
in left upper lobectomy, *147*
in modified Heller esophagomyotomy, 565
in tracheal resection, *82–83*
in tracheal stenosis correction, *79–80*
in tracheostomy, *76–77*
Epicardium, in pericardiectomy, *239, 241*
Epiglottis, in bronchoscopy, *5–6,* 11
Epimysium, in muscle flaps for mediastinitis, *121, 125*
Esophagogastrectomy, Ivor Lewis, *199–206*
left transthoracic approach for, (Sweet procedure), *191–198*
transhiatal (Orringer), *207–217*
Esophagogastric junction, in achalasia correction, *219*
in Belsey procedure for hiatal hernia, *188, 190*
Esophagomyotomy, Heller (modified), for achalasia, 565, *566–572*
Esophagoscopy, 14–22
diagnostic and therapeutic uses of, 14
flexible, technique of, *21–22*
rigid, contraindications to, 14
technique of, *16–20, 22*
Esophagus, anatomy of, *15*
atresia of, with distal tracheoesophageal fistula, 177, *178–181*
benign lesions of, 177, *178–190*
cervical, in transhiatal esophagogastrectomy, *210*
dissection of, *583*
hiatus of, *208*
in esophagogastrectomy, Ivor Lewis type, *200, 202, 204–206*
Sweet procedure, *191–198*
transhiatal, *212*
in modified Heller esophagomyotomy, *566, 568–572*
lumen of, identification of, *17–18*
perforation of, 22
malignant lesions of, *191–219*
mobilization of, in Belsey procedure for hiatal hernia, *185*
in tracheoesophageal fistula repair, *179*
in transhiatal esophagogastrectomy, *211*
"short," in Belsey procedure for hiatal hernia, *185*
sphincter of, in modified Heller esophagomyotomy, *572*
Zenker's diverticulum resection and, *182–184*
External oblique muscle, closure of, *63*
division of, *54, 58*
Extracorporeal membrane oxygenation, 535–538
cannulation for, *537–538*
in correction of congenital diaphragmatic hernia, 223, *225*

F

Fat pad, of atrioventricular groove, in Maze III procedure, *461–462, 465, 469*
in surgery for Wolff-Parkinson-White syndrome, *452*
over gastroesophageal junction, in Belsey procedure for hiatal hernia, *187*
Fiberoptic light source, in thoracoscopic surgery, 541
Fibrin glue, topical, in coronary bypass reoperation, 492
Fistula, H-type, 177
tracheoesophageal, esophageal atresia and, 177, *178–181*
Fluoroscopy, in placement of implantable cardiac defibrillator, 445
Fogarty catheter, in embolectomy, *167, 171, 173*
in tracheoesophageal fistula repair, *180*
Fontan procedure, after previous bidirectional Glenn operation, *368–369*
for Ebstein's anomaly repair, *373*
for tricuspid atresia repair, *366–368*
hypoplastic left heart syndrome and, *369–371*
lateral tunnel, *369–371*
Forceps, in embolectomy, *167, 169*
thoracotomy, 552
Fossa ovalis, atrial septal defect secundum and, 283
in Maze III procedure, *466, 472, 473*
Frozen section, in thoracoscopic surgery, 550
of lymph nodes, *136, 158*

G

Gastroesophageal junction, *15, 19*
in Belsey procedure for hiatal hernia, *187, 190*
in esophagogastrectomy, *193, 203, 214*
tumor in, *193, 203*
Gastroesophageal reflux, diaphragmatic hernia and, *227*
tracheoesophageal fistula repair and, 177, *179*
Gastroscope, in thoracoscopic esophagomyotomy, 565, *568–569, 572*
Gastrostomy, tracheoesophageal fistula repair and, 177
GIA staplers, in left lower lobectomy, *153, 156*
in pulmonary wedge resection, *134*
Glenn shunt, in repair of tricuspid atresia, *364–366*
Gore-Tex patch, for aneurysm of sinus of Valsalva, *277–278*
for atrial septal defect, *279–282, 288–289, 296*
for coarctation of aorta, *267, 274*
for complete atrioventricular septal defect, *298–304*
for diaphragmatic hernia, *228*
for sinus of Valsalva aneurysm repair, *277–278*
for sinus venosus repair, *283*
for tetralogy of Fallot, *312–314*
supra-annular, *315*
transannular, 311, *314*
with monocusp, *317–318*
for tricuspid atresia repair, *365, 370–371*
for truncus arteriosus, *321*
Gore-Tex shunt, for hypoplastic left heart syndrome, *361*
for tricuspid atresia, *362*
Gore-Tex suture, for ruptured mitral valve chords, *408*
Graft. See also *Patch.*
Graft *(Continued)*
saphenous vein, for anomalous left coronary artery correction, *493*
wedge, for pectus excavatum repair, *91–92*
Great vessels, access to, incisions for, *48*

H

Heart, access to, incisions for, *48*
and lung, transplantation of, *521–525*
revascularization of, 477–499
in anomalous left coronary artery repair, *493–499*
in coronary artery bypass grafts, 479, *480–488*
reoperation for, *489–492*
superior view of, *448*
transplantation of, *509–513*
wounds of, closure of, *377–380*
Heart disease, congenital, 253–373
Heart valves, acquired disease of, 375–442
aneurysms of ascending aorta, *426–433*
aneurysms of descending aorta, *438–442*
aneurysms of transverse aortic arch, *434–437*
aortic valve repair, *417–420*
aortic valve replacement, *413–416*
aortic wounds, *421–425*
heart wounds, *377–380*
mitral valve repair, *398–412*
mitral valve replacement, *390–397*
tricuspid valve repair, *384–388*
tricuspid valve replacement, *381–383*
Heller esophagomyotomy, modified, for achalasia, 565, *566–572*
Hemisternum, dissection of, *491*
Hemithorax, in modified Heller esophagomyotomy, *566*
pressure in, 161
Hemi-truncus defect, of right pulmonary artery, *262–265*
Hemoclips, for obliteration of patent ductus arteriosus, *258*
in coarctation of aorta, *266–271*
Hemostasis, in coronary bypass reoperation, 492
in penetrating heart wounds, *378–380*
in thoracoscopic splanchnicectomy, *578–579*
in thoracoscopic surgery, 545
in ventricular aneurysm repair, *533*
Heparin, 481
in cardiopulmonary transplantation, *522*
in coronary bypass reoperation, 490
in extracorporeal membrane oxygenation, *537*
Hernia, congenital diaphragmatic, 223, *224–228*
hiatal, Belsey procedure for, *185–190*
His bundle, in Maze III procedure, *465*
in surgery for Wolff-Parkinson-White syndrome, *449*
Hypopharynx, in bronchoscopy, 11
in esophagoscopy, 22
Hypoplastic left heart syndrome, *356–361*
Fontan procedure and, *369–371*
Hypothermia. See also *Cardioplegia.*
for anomalous left coronary artery correction, *493, 498*

Hypothermia *(Continued)*
for aortic aneurysm repair, *426*
for aortic valve replacement, *417–418*
for coarctation of aorta, *273–275*
for coronary artery bypass grafting, 482
for coronary bypass reoperation, *492*
for dissecting aortic aneurysms, 432
for mitral valve examination, 401
for transposition of great vessels, *350*

I

Implantable cardiac defibrillator, placement of, *445–447*
Incisions, Chamberlain, vs. thoracoscopic techniques, 556
collar, 81
for access to great vessels, *48*
for esophagogastrectomy, transhiatal, *207*
for first rib resection, *104, 107*
for pectus carinatum, *94*
for pectus excavatum, *87*
for placement of implantable cardiac defibrillator, *445–446*
for sternal cleft correction, *97*
for thoracostomy, skin, *66–67*
for thymectomy, *112*
for tracheostomy, *76*
for Zenker's diverticulum resection, *182–183*
infraclavicular, *445–446*
neck, in transhiatal esophagogastrectomy, *207, 210*
of parietal pleura, *58*
specific techniques of, cervicothoracic, 45, *46–52*
for diaphragmatic division, *59–60*
inframammary, *26*
median sternotomy, *40–44*
of latissmus dorsi, *27, 31–32, 35, 63*
of pectoralis major, *26*
of serratus anterior, *31–32*
posterolateral, *49*
supraclavicular, *46, 48*
thoracoabdominal, 53, *54–64*
abdominal wall layer division in, *58*
closure of, *62–64*
patient position for, *54*
rib excision for, *55–57*
uses of, *54*
thoracosupraclavicular, *51*
thoracotomy, anterior, 25, *26–29*
posterolateral, *30–36*
transaxillary, *37–39*
trans-sternal bilateral, *48*
trap-door, *48*
subcostal, *226, 445–446*
submammary, *87, 112*
subxiphoid, for pericardial window, *235*
thoracic, 23–70
Infants, anomalous left coronary artery in, alternative procedure for, *497*
ligation of, *496*
aortic valve replacement in, *331–334*
congenital diaphragmatic hernia in, 223
Ebstein's anomaly in, 372
extracorporeal membrane oxygenation in, 535–538
premature, obliteration of patent ductus arteriosus in, *258*
Infants *(Continued)*
total correction of pulmonary atresia with VSD in, *317–318*
ventricular septal defect in, *305*
Infectious nodules, pulmonary, thoracoscopic surgery and, 546–550
Infundibular muscle, in tetralogy of Fallot repair, *315*
Intercostal bundles, in correction of pectus excavatum, *89*
Intercostal muscles, closure of, *64*
division of, *32*
in chest wall tumor removal, *246*
in localization of second rib, 574
incision of, *27*
Intercostal perforators, in creation of pectoralis muscle flaps, *123*
Intercostal space, eighth, *585*
fifth, 27, 32, 49, 158, 438, 553, *559*
for entry into pleural cavity, *172*
fourth, *27, 32, 48, 49,* 81, *82, 238,* 438, *559*
in thoracostomy, *66–67*
seventh, *185, 191, 218*
sixth, *27, 32, 191,* 553, 577
sutures in, in median sternotomy, *44*
third, *38,* 574
thoracoscope insertion into, *549*
Internal oblique muscle, division of, *58*
Interventricular septum, incision into, *335, 337*
re-entrant ventricular tachycardia and, argon beam coagulation of, *459*
Ivor Lewis esophagogastrectomy, *199–206*

J

Jackson-Pratt drain, *93, 96, 99*
Joseph elevator, *88*

K

Kelly clamp, *68–69,* 555
Kelly forceps, 574
Koch, triangle of, *386*
Kocher clamp, in thoracic outlet syndrome correction, *105*
Kuntz's fiber, in thoracoscopic sympathectomy, 575, *575*

L

Laryngoscope, for lifting epiglottis, *6*
Larynx, exposure of, *6*
Laser techniques, in thoracoscopic surgery, 542, 550
Lateral tunnel Fontan procedure, *371*
Latissimus dorsi, closure of, *35, 63*
division of, *54*
incision of, *27, 31*
mobilization of, *38*
Lecompte maneuver, *259, 349*
Lidocaine, in thoracostomy, *67*
Ligament(s), pulmonary, inferior, *82, 150–151, 154–155, 158, 159, 164, 582, 586*
suprasternal, in median sternotomy, *42–43*
Ligatures, in patent ductus arteriosus, *256–257, 259*
Line, inframammary, *30*
Line *(Continued)*
of Douglas, *126*
Linea alba, closure of, 44
in creation of pericardial window, *235, 237*
Lobectomy, fissure lines in, *586*
development and division of, *137, 140–141, 143, 148, 152–153*
lower, *142–146, 152–157*
middle, *139–141*
thoracoscopic, for lung cancer, 584, *585–587*
upper, *136–138, 147–151*
Lung. See also under *Bronchus; Lobectomy; Pulmonary.*
and heart, transplantation of, *521–525*
blebs of, thoracoscopic resection of, 553, *554–555*
cancer in, thoracoscopic lobectomy for, 584, *585–587*
collapse of, in thoracoscopic sympathectomy, 574
deflation of, in thoracoscopic surgery, 545, *549,* 574
diffuse disease in, thoracoscopic pulmonary biopsy for, 551, *552*
exposure of, in anterior thoracotomy, *28–29*
hypoplastic, in congenital diaphragmatic hernia, *224*
injury to, left posterolateral thoracotomy and, *49*
transplantation of, *514–520*
Lung cancer, thoracoscopic lobectomy for, 584, *585–587*
Lymph nodes, dissection of, *158, 557*
frozen section of, *136, 158, 557*

M

Manubrium, in median sternotomy, *42, 44*
Mapping, intraoperative, 453, *456,* 458
Marlex mesh and methyl methacrylate prosthetic patch, in chest wall tumor removal, *251*
Maze III procedure for atrial fibrillation, 460–475
atrial septal incision in, *466, 471*
completed appearance of, *475*
cryolesions in, *463, 465, 468–470*
fossa ovalis incision in, *466, 472, 473*
lateral incision in, *461*
posterior longitudinal incision in, *461, 464, 474*
posterior vertical incision in, *469–470*
pulmonary vein isolation incision in, *467–468, 471*
right atrial counterincision in, *464–465*
T incision in, *461–463, 473*
Mediastinitis, 119
Mediastinum, 109–129
anterior, thoracoscopic approach to, 563, *564*
tumors of, 563, *564*
exposure of, *28–29, 33, 39*
infection of, muscle and omental flaps for, *119–129*
posterior, thoracoscopic approach to, 558, *559–560*
tumors of, 558, *559–560*
thymectomy and, 111–114
tumors of, excision of, *115–118,* 558, *559–560,* 563, *564*

Mitral valve, atrial appendages and, in anomalous pulmonary venous return to coronary sinus, 295–296
chordal attachments of, 399, *400*
elongation of, *404–405*
excision of, *392*
preservation of, *391–392*
rupture of, *406–408*
commissures of, identification of, *399*
examination of, 401
exposure of, 389, *399, 402*
in atrial septal defect repair, *287–288*
in surgery for Wolff-Parkinson-White syndrome, *450–452*
insufficiency of, chordal elongation and, *404–405*
chordal rupture and, *406–408*
commissural prolapse and, 409
leaflet deformities and, 411
leaflet perforation and, 411
prolapse and, analysis of, 401, *401–402*
treatment of, *402–403*
repair of, 401–412
ring annuloplasty and, *409–412*
placement of, *410, 412*
sizing of, *409,* 411, *411–412*
systolic anterior motion of, causing LV outflow obstruction, 411
leaflets of, *399–400*
excision of, *391–392*
in aortoventriculoplasty, *337–339*
in sizing of annuloplasty ring, *409, 411–412*
preservation of, *391–393*
prolapse of, *401–403, 411–412*
papillary muscle sliding plasty of, *404*
prosthetic, orientation of, *395–396*
St. Jude, *396*
sizing of, *393*
strutted, hazards of, 396
suturing of, *394*
repair of, 398–412
vs. valve replacement, 398, 400
replacement of, 389, *390–397*
air removal from, 396–397
atrial closure in, 396–397
rewarming of patient with, 396
separation from cardiopulmonary bypass in, 396
stenosis of, repair of, 398–400
Mouth guard, *13, 21*
Mucosa, esophageal, *18, 20*
in modified Heller esophagomyotomy, *571–572*
gastric, *20*
Muscle flaps. See also names of specific muscles (e.g., *Pectoralis major*).
for mediastinitis, *119–129*
Myasthenia gravis, thymectomy for, 114
Myotomy, for achalasia, *219*
for Zenker's diverticulum resection, *184*
Myxoma, left atrial, *503–506*

N

Nasogastric tube, in modified Heller esophagomyotomy, *572*
Nasopharynx, in flexible bronchoscopy, 11
Neck, anatomy of, *73*
Neonates. See also *Infants.*
extracorporeal membrane oxygenation in, *537*
Neonates *(Continued)*
repair of aortic stenosis in, *326*
Nerve(s), intercostobrachial, *37*
phrenic, 556, *564*
excision of, *161*
identification of, *46*
in pericardiectomy, *240*
left, *33, 49–50*
preservation of, *59, 424,* 522
in thymectomy, *112–114, 116*
right, *29, 51*
in placement of diaphragmatic pacemaker, *229–231*
recurrent laryngeal, *50, 52,* 557
in patent ductus arteriosus, *256*
in transhiatal esophagogastrectomy, *210*
preservation of, *78, 424*
spinal accessory, in thoracic outlet syndrome correction, *104*
splanchnic, thoracoscopic division of, 576, *577–579*
sympathetic trunk, *39*
thoracoscopic division of, 575, *575*
vagus, *33, 47, 49, 50,* 556
anterior, *582*
posterior, *583*
Neurovascular bundles, *63,* 556, 584
Nodules, pulmonary, thoracoscopic surgery and, 546–550

O

Omentum, patch of, in esophagogastrectomy, *198*
transposition flaps of, for treatment of mediastinitis, *128–129*
Orringer esophagogastrectomy, *207–217*
Oscillating saw, in coronary bypass reoperation, *490*
Osteomyelitis, treatment of, 119
Osteotomy, in sternomanubrial joint, *90–93*
Oxygen saturation, in thoracoscopic surgery, 542–543, 573, 584

P

Pacemaker, diaphragmatic, *229–231*
in cardiac transplantation, *513*
in coronary bypass reoperation, 492
Pain, chronic, splanchnicectomy for, 576
Pancreatic cancer, splanchnicectomy for, 576
Paraspinous muscle, in posterolateral thoracotomy, *32*
Parietal band, in tetralogy of Fallot, *311*
Patch, for aortic stenosis repair, *340*
for aortopulmonary window repair, *261–262*
for complete atrioventricular septal defect, *298–304*
for diaphragmatic hernia, *228*
for sinus venosus repair, *283–286*
for truncus arteriosus repair, *321, 323–324*
for ventricular septal defect repair, *305–310*
Gore-Tex. See *Gore-Tex patch.*
in chest wall tumor removal, *249–251*
Marlex mesh and methyl methacrylate, in chest wall tumor removal, *251*
pericardial. See *Pericardial patch.*
Patch *(Continued)*
PTFE. See *Gore-Tex patch.*
Patent ductus arteriosus. See *Ductus arteriosus, patent.*
Pectoralis major, dissection of, *249*
flaps of, for mediastinitis, *121–125*
in sternal cleft correction, *99*
incision of, *26*
for thoracostomy, *66*
insertion of, *40–41*
mobilization of, *38*
reflection of, *87, 94*
sutures of, *93, 96*
Pectoralis minor, flaps of, for mediastinitis, *122–123*
Pectus carinatum, correction of, *94–96*
Pectus excavatum, correction of, *87–93*
Pericardial cradle, for ventricular aneurysm repair, *529*
Pericardial effusion, pericardiectomy for, *238–239*
thoracoscopic resection of, 561, *562*
Pericardial patch, for atrial septal defect, *288–289, 296*
closure of, *279–282*
for coarctation of aorta, *274*
for complete atrioventricular septal defect, *298–304*
for left atrial myxoma excision, *504, 506*
for pulmonary atresia with intact right ventricle, *354*
for sinus venosus repair, *283–284, 286*
for tetralogy of Fallot, *312–314*
supra-annular, *315*
transannular, 311, *314*
with monocusp, *317–318*
in embolectomy, *171, 173*
Pericardial window, thoracoscopic approach to, 561, *562*
Pericardiectomy, for chronic constrictive pericarditis, *240–241*
for pericardial effusion, *238–239*
Pericarditis, pericardiectomy for, *240–241*
Pericardium, 233–241
approach to, *161*
creation of window into, *235–237*
dissection of, in coronary bypass reoperation, *491*
excision of, *238–239*
exposure of, *28–29*
in thymectomy, *112*
Perichondrium, dissection of, in correction of sternal cleft, *97–98*
in pectus carinatum, *94–95*
in pectus excavatum, *88–89*
Periosteal elevator, in rib excision, *55–56*
Periosteum, closure of, *63–64*
in rib excision, *55–56*
Peritoneal cavity, in Belsey procedure for hiatal hernia, *185*
Peritoneal sac, in diaphragmatic hernia, *224*
Peritoneum, blunt mobilization of, *60*
incision of, in diaphragmatic hernia, *227*
Pharynx, perforation of, in flexible esophagoscopy, 22
Pleura, in left pneumonectomy, *162*
in left upper lobectomy, *147*
in thoracic outlet syndrome, *106*
in thoracoscopic sympathectomy, *575*
in thymoma dissection, *116*
mediastinal, in diaphragmatic pacemaker placement, *229–231*

Pleura *(Continued)*
in patent ductus arteriosus, *255–256*
over splanchnic nerve, *578*
parietal, *58, 178*
Pleural flap, in left pneumonectomy, *165*
Pleural space, in Belsey procedure for hiatal hernia, *185*
in posterolateral thoracotomy, *33–34*
in thoracostomy, *68–69*
Pleurodesis, thoracoscopic procedure for, 553, *555*
Pneumonectomy, left, *162–165*
recipient, for right lung transplantation, *514*
right, *158–161*
Pneumothorax, chest tube placement for, 65, *66–70*
needle aspiration for, 65
recurrent, 555
tension, 65
Position of patient, for first rib resection, *107*
for tracheostomy, *74*
in thoracoscopic surgery, 542–543, *543*
for approach to anterior mediastinum, 563
for pericardial window approach, 561
for resection of mediastinal tumors, 558
in transhiatal esophagogastrectomy, *207*
jacknife, 558
reverse Trendelenburg, *74*
right lateral, for right lung transplantation, *514*
semi-Fowler, 74
Trendelenburg, 520
Positive end-expiratory pressure, in thoracoscopic surgery, 543
Prostaglandin E_1, in congenital aortic stenosis, 325, 329
in Ebstein's anomaly, 372
in patent ductus arteriosus, *355*
Prosthetic patch. See *Gore-Tex patch; Patch; Pericardial patch.*
PTFE patch. See *Gore-Tex patch.*
Pulmonary artery. See *Artery(ies), pulmonary.*
Pulmonary atresia, with intact ventricular septum, *352–355*
with ventricular septal defect, total correction of, *317–318*
Pulmonary homograft, in reconstruction of aortic arch, *35–39*
Pulmonary hypertension, coronary bypass reoperation and, 489
in congenital aortic stenosis, 325
postoperative, 292
Pulmonary hypoplasia, in congenital diaphragmatic hernia, 223
Pulmonary nodule, intraoperative localization of, 549
preoperative localization of, 547
wedge resection of, thoracoscopic surgery for, 546-550
Pulmonary procedures, 131–173
embolectomy, for acute pulmonary embolism, *166–168*
for chronic pulmonary embolism, *169–173*
excision of pulmonary bullae, *135*
lobectomy, left lower, *152–157*
left upper, *147–151*
right lower, *142–146*
right middle, *139–141*
Pulmonary procedures *(Continued)*
right upper, *136–138*
pneumonectomy, left, *162–165*
right, *158–161*
pulmonary wedge excision, 133, *134*
Pulmonary valve, autograft of, in aortic valve replacement, *331–334*
in pulmonary atresia with intact right ventricle, *352–353*
preservation of, in tetralogy of Fallot, *315, 316*
Pulmonary vascular bed, protection of, *341*
Pulmonary venous return, anomalous, repair of, *290–296*
Pulmonary wedge resection, thoracoscopic, 546–550
Pulse oximeter, in thoracoscopic surgery, 542, 573
Pursestringing, prevention of, *364*
Pyloromyotomy, in esophagogastrectomy, *193, 201, 209*
Pylorus, visualization of, *21*
Pyriform sinus, *6, 17*

R

Radiographs. See also *Chest film.*
contrast swallow, in Zenker's diverticulum resection, *184*
Rectus abdominis, flap of, *126*
in pectus carinatum correction, *94, 96*
pocket in, *446*
Rheumatic heart disease, 398
Rhomboid muscle, in chest wall tumor removal, *246–248*
in thoracic outlet syndrome correction, *104*
Ribs, division of, *32, 158, 246, 250*
fifth, *32, 158*
first, in thoracic outlet syndrome correction, *104–108*
fourth, *178*
in chest wall tumor removal, *246, 250*
reapproximation of, *34*
in esophagogastrectomy, *198*
removal of, *55–57, 104–108*
periosteal closure with, *63–64*
second, localization of in thoracoscopic sympathectomy, 574
Rumel tourniquets, for mitral valve replacement, *390–391*

S

St. Jude prosthetic valve, aortic, *415*
mitral, *396*
Saphenous vein, graft of, for anomalous left coronary artery correction, *493*
Satinsky clamp, in right lung transplantation, *518, 520*
Scalene muscle, anterior, tendon of, in thoracic outlet syndrome correction, *105*
Scaphoid abdomen, in congenital diaphragmatic hernia, *224*
Scapula, in chest wall tumor removal, *246–248*
mobilization of, in thoracic outlet syndrome correction, *104*
Serratus anterior, closure of, *35*
division of, *38*
incision of, *31*
Silver nitrate cauterization, for tracheostomy healing, 77
Sinoatrial node, protection of, 285, 449
Sinus, transverse, in truncus arteriosus, *320*
Sinus of Valsalva, aneurysm of, *276–278*
Sinus venosus, repair of, *283–286*
Skin stapler, in posterolateral thoracotomy, *36*
Skin wheal, for thoracostomy, *67*
Splanchnicectomy, thoracoscopic, 576, *577–579*
Spleen, preservation of, *193, 226*
Staplers, EEA, in esophagogastrectomy, *197, 206*
endoscopic, *552,* 554–555
in thoracoscopic surgery, 541–542, 546, *550, 587*
GIA, in lobectomy, left lower, *153, 156*
in pulmonary wedge resection, *134*
in emphysematous bulla excision, *135*
in lobectomy, left lower, *153, 155–156*
left upper, *148–150*
right lower, *144–146*
right upper, *137–138*
TA–30, in lobectomy, *149–150, 155–156*
in pneumonectomy, *165*
vascular, in pneumonectomy, left, *163–165*
right, *158–160*
Steinmann pin, *92*
Sternal notch, *40–41*
Sternal saw, in median sternotomy, *43*
Sternocleidomastoid muscle, clavicular head of, *46*
in extracorporeal membrane oxygenation, *537*
in left cervicothoracic incision, *50*
Zenker's diverticulum resection and, *182–183*
Sternohyoid muscle, in tracheostomy, *75*
Sternomanubrial joint, osteotomy in, *90–93*
Sternotomy, median, *40–44, 115*
cervicothoracic incision and, *50*
for aneurysm of sinus of Valsalva, *276*
for anomalous pulmonary venous return, *290, 293, 295*
for aortic aneurysms, *426*
for aortic arch aneurysms, *434*
for aortic stenosis, *326*
for aortopulmonary window, *260*
for atrial myxoma excision, *503*
for atrial septal defect, *279, 287*
for cardiac transplantation, *509*
for closure of penetrating cardiac wounds, *377*
for coarctation of aorta, *273–275*
for complete atrioventricular septal defect, *297*
for coronary artery bypass grafting, *480–481*
for Ebstein's anomaly, *372–373*
for embolectomy, *166*
for hypoplastic left heart syndrome, *356*
for interrupted aortic arch, *341*
for mitral valve repair, *389, 399*
for pericardiectomy, *240*
for sinus venosus, *283*
for tetralogy of Fallot, *311*
for thymectomy, 112
for tricuspid atresia, *362*
for truncus arteriosus, *320*

Sternotomy *(Continued)*
for ventricular aneurysm, *529*
for ventricular septal defect, *305*
reopening of incision for, *120*
repeat, for coronary bypass reoperation, *490*
thoracosupraclavicular incision and, *51*
Sternum, 26
cleft of, *97–99*
congenital deformities of, 85–99
divided, closure of, *44*
division of, for chest wall tumor removal, *250*
for coronary bypass reoperation, *490*
for pectus excavatum, *89–93*
Stomach, in Belsey procedure for hiatal hernia, *185*
in esophagogastrectomy, Ivor Lewis procedure, *200, 203*
Sweet procedure, *194–198*
transhiatal procedure, *215, 216*
visualization of, in esophagoscopy, *20–21,* 22
Strap muscles, in tracheostomy, *75*
Subclavian steal syndrome, in repair of coarctation of aorta, *269*
Subcutaneous tissue, closure of, *35*
Submucosa, in correction of achalasia, *219*
Suction equipment, in thoracoscopic surgery, 542
Suprasternal ligament, in median sternotomy, *42–43*
Sutures, Ethibond, in ventricular aneurysm repair, *532*
for thoracoabdominal incision, *62–64*
for tracheal stenosis, *79–80*
Gore-Tex, for ruptured mitral valve chords, *408*
in mitral valve replacement, *394*
in posterolateral thoracotomy, *35*
in tracheal resection, *83–84*
pericostal, *34*
pledgeted mattress, for aortic wound repair, *421*
for closure of heart wounds, *379–380*
in prosthetic aortic valve placement, *415, 419–420*
pursestringing, distortion from, 269, 272
reefing, in pectus carinatum correction, *95*
tracheal, traction, *79*
wire, in median sternotomy, *44*
Sweet procedure, for esophagogastrectomy, *191–198*
Sympathectomy, thoracoscopic, 573–574, *574–575*
upper thoracic, indications for, 573

T

Tachycardia, automatic atrial, *453–457*
paroxysmal supraventricular, accessory atrioventricular pathways producing, *448*
supraventricular, *453–457*
intraoperative mapping for, 453, *456*
ventricular, re-entrant, *458–459*
Tamponade, atrial injuries and, 377
Teeth, maxillary incisor, in measurement of esophageal lesions, 18
Telescopes, angled-view, in rigid bronchoscopy, *9–10*
Tension pneumothorax, chest tube placement and, 65
Tet atresia, in infants, *317–318*
Tetracaine, in flexible bronchoscopy, 11, 12
Tetralogy of Fallot, repair of, *311–319*
Thoracic incisions, 23–70
Thoracic outlet syndrome, correction of, *101–108*
posterior approach for, *103–106*
transaxillary approach for, *107–108*
Thoracoscopic surgery, 540–587
equipment needed for, 541–542, 565, *566*
general approach to, 541–545
operating room arrangement for, *542*
patient position for, 542–543, *543*
specific procedures in, approach to anterior mediastinum, 563, *564*
approach to aorticopulmonary window, 556, *557*
lobectomy for lung cancer, 584, *585–587*
mediastinal tumor resection, 558, *559–560*
modified Heller esophagomyotomy, 565, *566–572*
pericardial window approach, 561, *562*
pulmonary biopsy for diffuse disease, 551, *552*
resection of blebs and pleurodesis, 553, *554–555*
splanchnicectomy, 576, *577–579*
sympathectomy, 573–574, *574–575*
truncal vagotomy, 580, *581–583*
wedge resection of lung nodule, 546–547, *548–550*
technique of, 543, *544,* 545
Thoracostomy, 65, *66–70*
anesthetic infiltration for, *67*
Thoracostomy tube, in diaphragmatic hernia, *228*
Thoracotomy, anterior, 25, *26–29*
for access to heart and great vessels, *48*
for access to subclavian artery, *46–47*
for embolectomy, *169, 172*
anterolateral, for diaphragmatic pacemaker placement, *229*
for pericardiectomy, *238*
for aortic aneurysms, 438
for emphysematous bulla excision, *135*
lateral, division of ductus arteriosus through, *258*
for achalasia, *218*
for coarctation of aorta, *266, 268*
for left upper lobectomy, *147*
for patent ductus arteriosus, *255*
for right lower lobectomy, *142*
phrenic, anterolateral, for placement of diaphragmatic pacemaker, *229*
posterolateral, for access to left subclavian artery, *49*
for access to subclavian artery, *46*
for chest wall tumor removal, *246*
for repair of aortic wounds, *425*
for right lung transplantation, *514*
for right pneumonectomy, *158*
for right upper lobectomy, *136*
for tracheal resection, 81, *82*
incisions for, *30–36*
transaxillary, *37–39*
Thromboplastic agents, topical, *267*
Thrombus, in ventricular aneurysm repair, *531–532*
Thymoma, malignant, 114
thymectomy for, 114, *115–118*
Thymus, anatomy of, 112
Thyroid gland, isthmus of, in tracheostomy, *75*
Total anomalous pulmonary venous return, repair of, *290–292*
Trachea, anastomosis of, *83, 84*
approximation of, *79*
exposure of, *76*
in bronchoscopy, 11, 12
in cardiopulmonary transplantation, *523–524*
in tracheoesophageal fistula repair, *179*
lumen of, in bronchoscopy, *7–8*
resection of, 81–84
for tumors, 81, *82–84*
stenosis of, correction of, 78–80
surgical procedures on, 71–84
Tracheobronchial tree, anesthesia of, 12
Tracheoesophageal fistula, esophageal atresia and, 177, *178–181*
Tracheostomy, 73–77
closure of, *77*
dissection in, *75–76*
extubation from, 77
healing of, 77
incision for, *74–75*
operating room location and, 73
patient position for, *74*
Transhiatal (Orringer) esophagogastrectomy, *207–217*
Transplantation, 507–525
cardiac, *509–513*
cardiopulmonary, *521–525*
pulmonary, right, *514–520*
Transversalis muscle, division of, *58*
Trap-door incision, *48*
Trapezius, closure of, *35*
in chest wall tumor removal, *246–248*
in thoracic outlet syndrome correction, *104*
Trendelenburg position, 520, *555*
Triangle of Koch, *386*
Tricuspid atresia, *362–371*
Fontan procedure and, *366–368*
Glenn shunt and, *364–366, 368*
hypoplastic pulmonary arteries and, *365–366*
in Ebstein's anomaly, *373*
Tricuspid stenosis, tricuspid valve replacement for, *381–383*
Tricuspid valve, annulus of, in Maze III procedure, *462–464*
Carpentier-Edwards prosthetic, sizing and placement of, *382–383*
chordal attachments of, *306, 308, 382*
in complete atrioventricular septal defect, *301, 304*
in Ebstein's anomaly, *373*
in surgery for Wolff-Parkinson-White syndrome, *449, 451*
in ventricular septal defect, *305–308*
prosthetic, orientation and placement of, *386*
sizing of, *386*
suturing of, *387–388*
repair of (annuloplasty), 384, *385–388*
replacement of, for tricuspid stenosis, *381–383*
Trocars, in thoracoscopic surgery, *544,* 545
Trousseau dilator, 76
Truncal vagotomy, thoracoscopic, 580, *581–583*

Truncus arteriosus, *320–324*
Tuffier retractor, in thoracic outlet syndrome correction, *104*
Tumors, chest wall, 243–251
posterior, 245, *246–248*
dumbbell, 558
malignant, thoracoscopic approach to, 558
mediastinal, *115–118*
anterior, thoracoscopic approach to, 563, *564*
posterior, thoracoscopic approach to, 558, *559–560*
tracheal, 81, *82–84*

V

VACTERL anomalies, esophageal atresia and, 177
Vagotomy, truncal, thoracoscopic, 580, *581–583*
Vallecula, in rigid bronchoscopy, *5*
Vascular clamps, for closure of heart wounds, *378*
in coarctation of aorta repair, *266–267*
Vein(s), azygos, *29, 39*
in Ivor Lewis esophagogastrectomy, *202, 205*
in tracheoesophageal fistula repair, *178*
innominate, *564*
in thymectomy, *114, 116, 117*
jugular, *50, 52*
in extracorporeal membrane oxygenation, *537–538*
middle lobe, *136–138, 141*
pulmonary, in anomalous pulmonary venous return, *290–294*
in right lung transplantation, *518–519*
inferior, *143, 144, 154–155, 157, 586*
division of, *159–160, 164–165*
superior, *136–137*
division of, *163, 165*
in left upper lobectomy, *149, 151*
stapling of, *159*
saphenous, graft of, *493*
subclavian, in placement of implantable cardiac defibrillator, *445*
in thoracic outlet syndrome correction, *104*
Vein(s) *(Continued)*
thoracoacromial, *123*
thymic, *117*
vertical, *290–291, 293*
Vena cava, inferior, cannulation of, for atrial septal defect repair, *283*
in transposition of great arteries, *346*
in tricuspid atresia, *370–371*
superior, cannulation of, for atrial septal defect repair, *283–288*
in sinus venosus repair, *283, 285–286*
in tetralogy of Fallot, *311*
in transposition of great arteries, *346*
in tricuspid atresia, *362–369*
Ventricle(s), left, aneurysms of, *529–533*
outflow tract of, in aortic stenosis, *336, 338*
mitral valve insufficiency and, 411
right, communication with pulmonary artery, in aortic stenosis, *334*
in tetralogy of Fallot, *316–318*
reconstruction of, *337, 339, 352–355*
hypoplastic, *352*
in aneurysm of sinus of Valsalva, *277*
outflow tract of, hypoplastic, pulmonary atresia and, *353–354*
in aortic valve replacement, *331, 334*
in tetralogy of Fallot, *311, 313–319*
pulmonary atresia and, aortopulmonary shunt and, *355*
reconstruction of, in aortic stenosis, *337, 339*
penetrating wounds of, closure of, *379–380*
Ventricular fibrillation, in truncus arteriosus, 320
Ventricular septal defect, closure of, in complete atrioventricular septal defect, *298–299, 303*
in interrupted aortic arch, *344*
in tetralogy of Fallot, *311–313, 315*
in truncus arteriosus, *321–322*
in transposition of great arteries, *346*
inlet, *308*
perimembranous, *308–310*
Ventricular septal defect *(Continued)*
repair of, *305–310*
unrepaired, in tetralogy of Fallot, *318*
Ventricular tachycardia, re-entrant, treatment of, *458–459*
Ventriculotomy, right, in aortic stenosis, *335*
in tetralogy of Fallot, *311, 313–319*
Vertebral artery, *46*
in coarctation of aorta, *268–269*
Vessels, brachiocephalic, in hypoplastic left heart syndrome, *356–357*
gastric, in esophagogastrectomy, *200–201, 208–209*
gastric epiploic, in esophagogastrectomy, *193, 200, 208*
internal mammary, in chest wall tumor removal, *250*
in placement of diaphragmatic pacemaker, *229*
Video-assisted thoracoscopic surgery. See *Thoracoscopic surgery.*
Vocal cords, in flexible bronchoscopy, 11
in rigid bronchoscopy, *6–7*

W

Wires, sternal, *120*
Wolff-Parkinson-White syndrome, accessory atrioventricular pathways producing, *448*
right-sided, *449–451*
Wounds, aortic, repair of, *421–425*
cardiac, closure of, *377–380*

X

Xiphoid process, *40–41*
debridement of, *126*
dissection of, in pectus excavatum, *89*
excision of, for creation of pericardial window, *235*

Z

Zenker's diverticulum, resection of, *182–184*

ISBN 0-7216-3498-2

90038

9 780721 634982